Fundamentals of Pediatric Dentistry

Fundamentals of Pediatric Dentistry

Third Edition

Richard J. Mathewson, DDS, MS, PhD
Professor, Chairman, Department of Pediatric Dentistry
College of Dentistry, University of Oklahoma

Robert E. Primosch, DDS, MS, MEd
Professor, Department of Pediatric Dentistry
College of Dentistry, University of Florida

Illustrations
Jack T. Morrison, DDS

quintessence
books

Quintessence Publishing Co, Inc
Chicago, Berlin, London, Tokyo, São Paulo, Moscow, Prague, and Warsaw

Dedicated to the students,
teachers, and practitioners
of dentistry for children—
those of the past, the present,
and most important,
those of the future

Library of Congress Cataloging-in-Publication Data
Mathewson, Richard J.
  Fundamentals of pediatric dentistry/ Richard J. Mathewson, Robert
E. Primosch ; illustrations, Jack T. Morrison. — 3rd ed.
    p.   cm.
  Includes bibliographical references and index.
  ISBN 0–86715–262–1 (pbk. : alk. paper)
  1. Pedodontics.   I. Primosch, Robert E.   II. Title.
  [DNLM: 1. Pediatric Dentistry.   WU 480 M429f 1995]
  RK55.C5M43   1995
  94–43277—dc20
  DNLM/DLC
  for Library of Congress   94–43277
                                                CIP

Published by Quintessence Publishing Co, Inc
551 North Kimberly Drive
Carol Stream, IL 60188

Composition: Focus Graphics, St Louis, Missouri
Printing: Ovid Bell Press, Fulton, Missouri
Printed in USA

Contents

Preface

As in previous editions, our objectives are to assist students and dentists in the provision of excellent oral health care for children and adolescent patients. Our style has been to present step-by-step guidelines for all phases of pediatric dentistry.

This purpose and form characterize this third edition, into which we have incorporated many recent changes in management styles and clinical methods.

We have revised, rewritten, and reorganized most of the chapters from previous editions. Several chapters have been combined for ease of use, and in some instances, entirely new chapters have been added. These revisions will be of assistance to those who serve the oral health needs of children.

In any undertaking, many people are asked to give of their time and intellectual effort. Our thanks to the following individuals for providing photographs, x-rays, and professional advice: James R. Delaney, T.J. Guthrie, Dean Johnson, Jerome Miller, James Murtaugh, Donald Porter, James Roane, Daniel Shaw, and James Walton.

Special thanks go to Dr Jack Austerman, Department of Orthodontics, College of Dentistry, University of Oklahoma, for manuscript review of chapters 2 and 23; Drs Ram S. Nanda and G. Frans Currier, Department of Orthodontics, for their contributions in the areas of preventive orthodontics, growth, and development of the child and adolescent; to Drs Theresa M. White and Daniel P. Dalzell, Department of Pediatric Dentistry, College of Dentistry, University of Oklahoma, for photographs and professional advice; and to Dr Roger G. Sanger, private practitioner of pediatric dentistry, Salinas, California, for his contributions to the original manuscripts.

Our apologies to those peers from whom we may have inadvertently borrowed or imitated while writing this book.

Last, but not least, our thanks to our wives, Alice and Lori, for their long-standing support and understanding through the years and, most importantly, during completion of this book.

Chapter 1

Behavioral and Physical Assessment

Objectives

After studying this chapter, the student should be able to:
1. Understand the salient features of a health history questionnaire.
2. Discuss the medicolegal basis of appropriate documentation of care.
3. Comprehend the factors influencing child behavior.
4. Describe the behavioral characteristic of normal child behavior during the various stages of child development.
5. Discuss useful methods to describe and classify behavioral characteristics.
6. Describe the anticipated dentist-patient behavioral interactions.
7. Discuss the components of the physical assessment of a child dental patient.
8. Comprehend the chronologic sequence of events contributing to physical development of the child, especially dental development.

Health history

In general, health histories are obtained from self-administered questionnaires completed by the parents of the child. The questionnaire should be designed to provide a preliminary screening of relevant medical, behavioral, familial, and dental conditions. The intention of the questionnaire is not to attempt a comprehensive medical assessment of the child but rather to focus attention to certain factors that might influence precaution or require special care in delivering dental treatment (LeMasney, 1977).

The health questionnaire form should be thorough, orderly, functional, and easy to understand. In addition, the form should be designed to permit easy completion by the parent and quick review by the dentist (Currier, 1982). It would be wrong to assume that parents will provide valid information when given a self-administered questionnaire alone. A recent investigation of health history questionnaires revealed that 32% contained incorrect or missing information (Brady and Martinoff, 1980). This report indicated that the degree of accuracy and thoroughness obtained from self-administered questionnaires depended on several factors; a "no" answer may have meant that (1) the parent did not understand the question or the condition being questioned; (2) the parent failed to perceive the relationship or the relevance of the question to providing

dental care for the child and therefore did not take it seriously; or (3) the emotional state of the parent influenced the reading or interpretation of the question.

If the questionnaire does not stimulate appropriate interest, answers describing potentially significant conditions may be omitted. If parents are not sufficiently stimulated to answer specific questions about their child's health, they may be reluctant or embarrassed to offer this information voluntarily. Therefore, following review of the questionnaire, the dentist must interview and closely interrogate the parent to uncover suspected problems. The completed health questionnaire provides a valuable mechanism to vigorously pursue a follow-up interview of the parents. Health information obtained from personal interviewing is more valid than that obtained from self-administered questionnaires alone (Norheim and Heloe, 1977) but must be gathered in a diplomatic and objectively sympathetic manner.

Because the child is constantly being transformed by his or her physical and emotional environment, an annual updating of the health history form is mandatory. An openly reviewed health history is essential to the establishment of a treatment plan that is harmonious with the child's overall health status.

The following is a listing and explanation of some of the essential components of a health history questionnaire for the child patient:

1. Personal history. The name, age, sex address, telephone number, and place and type of employment of the parents are usually determined first. Many children have nicknames, but not all prefer their use. The child should be asked what name he or she prefers. This simple question shows interest in the child and may help establish trust. The parent's employment information may be helpful in determining financial responsibility and insight into the socioeconomic limitations that may be a factor in establishing a successful preventive program.

2. Medical history. The name and address of the child's physician are important if a medical consultation is required. Likewise, it is prudent to ascertain if the child receives regular medical examinations and if the physician is currently treating the child for any conditions. If medications were dispensed, it is necessary to know what medications, how much, and for how long the child has been taking these medications. The history of present illnesses and medications must be considered for potential adverse reactions and complications before dental treatment is delivered.

The history of past conditions is as important as current conditions when the patient's health questionnaire is reviewed. The investigation must include, but not be limited to, information on the occurrences of any of the following concerns: allergic or unfavorable reactions to any medications; prior hospitalization; rheumatic fever; heart problems; anemia; bleeding problems; birth defects; seizures; asthma; hepatitis; diabetes; kidney disease; neurologic problems; trauma; bone-joint problems; hearing, vision, and speech difficulties; and emotional and learning difficulties. In addition, it is important to inquire into the child's immunization status. The parents should be encouraged to bring the child's immunizations up to date if the following schedule has not been obtained: diphtheria, tetanus, pertussis (DPT), and trivalent polio vaccines at ages 2,4,6, and 18 months and between 4 and 6 years; and rubeola, rubella, and mumps vaccines by age 15 months.

3. Dental history. The most important question asked by the dentist will involve the explanation of why the patient (parent) is seeking dental care. This concern must be addressed and resolved by the dentist, even though it may not be perceived as a priority item, before compliance to other therapy and advice can be expected from the parent. The questionnaire should elicit if the child has been previously seen by another dentist and, if so, what the outcome was in terms of behavior displayed. The response to this question can significantly influence the selection of future behavior management modalities. Furthermore, if the parent was not satisfied with the previous care, the knowledge of what caused the dissatisfaction may lead to better dentist-child-parent relationships. Other features of a relevant dental history would include history of oral trauma and any oral habits such as lip, finger, thumb, or blanket sucking; nail and cheek biting; tongue thrusting; mouth breathing; jaw popping or clicking; and teeth grinding.

4. Home dental care. This section would include information on the child's fluoride history, oral hygiene practices, and dietary habits and could be applied to the implementation of an individualized preventative program. For example, the source of home drinking water should be determined, and the water should be analyzed if its fluoride content is uncertain. This information would be required if systemic fluoride therapy is to be prescribed. The brand of dentifrice should be determined, and substitution of a fluoridated dentifrice should be recommended where indicated. Also, the use of any prescribed or over-the-counter fluoride agent for systemic or topical application (drops, tablets, or rinses) must be validated. The frequency and timing of oral hygiene practices (toothbrushing and flossing) along with the identification of the individual responsible are valuable in establishing appropriate counseling. Information on the frequency and content of the diet, especially snack foods, may provide the direction for advice on nutrition and diet modification.

5. Social and behavioral history. Much of the child's response to dental care can be predicted through the careful gathering of information regarding child-parent interaction (child-rearing practices), past experiences, emotional and cognitive development, and family environment. Behavioral research has indicated the existence of a positive correlation between the display of apprehensive or disruptive behavior in the dental setting to a history or prior negative reactions to dental or medical care or knowledge of an existing dental problem. Furthermore, parental attitudes are an important variable, and knowledge of poor prior preparation of the child or low expectations or cooperative performance by the child superimposed by parental anxiety will be beneficial in anticipating potential management problems. In fact, if questioned, most parents will be very accurate in predicting the child's response to dental care and would be able to describe the child's behavior in such terms as calm, moody, shy, active, spoiled, defiant, fearful talkative, friendly, compulsive, high strung, suspicious, or cooperative. The health questionnaire should be expanded to include information on the child's special interests, such as hobbies and pets, and siblings. This information will help to establish communication with the child and alleviate apprehension.

Documentation of care: The patient record

The patient's dental record provides an accurate overview of the patient's involvement in the dental care system. The significance of accurate records is divided into four important areas: the patient's (parent's) consent to treatment; the patient's oral status at the onset of care; the patient's and parent's conduct during the course of care; and the termination of the dentist-patient (parent) relationship (Beyer, 1987).

Informed consent

Sufficient information must be given by the health professional to each parent or guardian so that the parent has a reasonable understanding of the proposed dental care for the child. This discussion should include acceptable alternatives, nonremote risks to care, consequences if proposed treatment is refused, and any referral to other health providers. These are the basic concepts of informed consent (Schultz, 1985).

Failure to obtain informed consent from the parent has legal consequences. Touching the child without parental consent constitutes a technical case of battery, even if the contact does not harm the child (Weber, 1987).

Blank, universal consent forms reviewed by someone else other than the dental professional is not generally considered informed consent (AAPD, l993). If standard consent forms are used, the attending dentist should review the form with the parent, and document the review process in the child's progress notes. *A standard consent form is not a substitute for a dentist-parent discussion.*

When a dental procedure is to be performed for a minor, the question arises whether the minor's consent is sufficient and , if not, who should give consent (Pozgar, 1983). Legally, the consent of a minor is ineffective. However, depending on state statutes, a minor may be considered a "mature" or "emancipated" minor; married, pregnant, or self-employed (Rozousky, 1984). An emancipated minor may seek dental care without parental consent.

Initial oral status

To provide quality care, the patient's record should include the following information (AAPD, 1993):

1. Complete dental, medical, and family histories.
2. Clinical assessments.
   a. Physical and behavioral. The patient's physical appearance and behavior at the onset of treatment should be recorded.
   b. Occlusal. The developing occlusion and growth and development of the orofacial complex are assessed.
   c. Hard tissue. Dental caries and any hard tissue abnormalities are evaluated.
   d. Soft tissue. The initial oral hygiene should be recorded with plaque and gingival scores or in-

dices. The prevention needs of the patient and parental attitudes should be documented.
   e. Radiographic. Radiographs enable the diagnosis of dental caries, sequela to dental caries, oral pathoses, and other anomalies. All radiographs should be of diagnostic quality.
3. Laboratory studies (if needed).
4. Consultation with other health providers, both verbal and written (recorded on the progress notes).
5. Diagnosis and treatment plan. From the clinical assessments, the diagnosis and treatment plan is formulated. The treatment plan should be:
   a. A logical step-by-step process to treat the dental health needs of the child.
   b. A means to prioritize the needs of the patient.

The parent must be informed of the needed care and the fee for the dental care. This relationship between the dentist and the parent is contractual—the treatment to be rendered and the fee for the service (Curtis et al, 1987). Again, because the health provider is dealing with a minor, the parent should sign the treatment plan or progress notes, agreeing to accept responsibility for the child's dental care and the fee for the care.

Patient's conduct during care

The dental record is an accurate statement of the parent's and patient's progress in the dental practice. The following should be charted (Beyer, 1987):

1. Poor parent-patient conduct, including frequently missed appointments; chronically poor oral hygiene, documented by plaque and gingival scores; missed recalled appointments; and failure to see recommended specialists.
2. Use of appropriate methods of behavior modification, including any specific management method and the result; and use of any therapeutic agents and their dosages, methods of administration, and effectiveness.

Termination of the dentist-patient (parent) relationship

When the patient leaves the practice, the question is "Who owns the patient's records?" In most states, the dentist is the legal owner of the records. However, the parent has the right to request a copy of the records. Plus, the parent has control of record access by third parties. The dentist should *never* release original records! Copies should be forwarded as indicated by the parent. Again, depending on the state, a reasonable fee can be charged for this service.

The dentist-patient relationship is based on a contract whereby the dentist is obligated to care for the child as long as the child's dental condition needs attention (Curtis et al, 1987). This relationship exists until both dentist and parent consent to terminate the relationship (Pozgar, 1984). Premature termination of dental care is often the subject of legal action for abandonment. The following elements are present in the legal description of abandonment (Pozgar, 1984):

1. Unreasonable discontinuance of dental care.
2. Discontinuance against the parent's will; a unilateral decision by the dentist.
3. Failure of a dentist to arrange emergency care by another dentist.
4. Discontinuing care may result in harm to the child.
5. Discontinuing dental care causes actual harm to the child.

If the parent decides to terminate the treatment, the record should show:

1. The date of the parent's decision.
2. Advice to the parent of any needed dental care with recommendations for future dental care.
3. An offer to sent a copy of the records to the new dentist.

Patients (parents) can be dismissed from the dental practice if specific problems arise (Beyer, 1987; Curtis et al, 1987):

1. Failure to keep appointments.
2. Lack of cooperation in the area of home care.
3. Failure to see recommended specialists.

If the dentist decides to terminate the relationship, because of failure to cooperate, the parent should be notified with a certified letter. The letter should include the following:

1. A brief reason for the termination
2. The date the relationship should end, usually 30 days from the date of notification.
3. A list of dentists in the area
4. An offer to forward copies of the records
5. An offer to provide emergency care for a reasonable period of time
6. An indication of the current dental status and any consequences of failure to complete the child's care

If termination is done properly, with proper documentation, parents will have no basis for charges of abandonment.

Summary

For each child in the practice, there should be an appropriate patient record. All entries in the child's record should be in ink, complete, clear, and legible, and signed by the attending dentist. The record should be an accurate overview of the child's progress in the dental care system (AAPD, 1993).

Behavioral assessment

The management of child behavior begins the moment the child enters the dental environment and continues until he or she leaves it. The patient's dental visit will have involved the collaboration of the dental operator and support personnel, each of whom has had a role in encouraging continued good behavior or in guiding or directing a patient whose behavior has been expressed in negative terms. These individuals must comprehend patient deportment in its various aspects and must become proficient in applying their skills to the management process.

Early in the era of dentistry for children successful management of behavior emerged from a small group of pediatric dentists who were dedicated and persistent in their efforts to render suitable dental care. Today, the aim and scope of effective patient management evolves from the orderly process of observation and study of the child's psychologic and sociologic involvement. The sociocultural and interpersonal aspects of pediatric patients are very much a part of the expanding predoctoral curriculum of behavioral dentistry.

Factors influencing behavior

Before the dentist can establish sound principles of diagnosis and the subsequent application of technical skills to control behavior, he or she must be familiar with those factors that influence behavior. They are growth and development, family and peer influences, past medical and dental experiences, and the dental office environment.

Growth and development

The child's development involves physical, intellectual, and emotional aspects of growth, and these aspects are exhibiting constant change in both magnitude and expanse.

A normal child's chronologic age plays a significant role in the growth and development patterns. In general, we may assume that the younger the child, the more likely the child may react negatively to dental intervention. The intellectual age of 3 years seems to be that point in developmental progress that signifies a maturational readiness to accept dental treatment (Ingersoll, 1982). At age 3, however, behavior may be interspersed with ambivalent expressions of negative or positive response. With further maturation, the responses become more dependably positive.

Sexual differences within the framework of growth and development are not particularly a consideration to variances in cooperative pattern.

A child's behavior may be attributed to some form of cranial damage rather than to other factors. A sizable number of children, because of prenatal or postnatal injury or disease, sustain cerebral trauma from which they recover without sequelae. There are, however, a number of children with histories of cranial trauma and clinical evidence of central nervous system damage. The child may show manifestations of central nervous system disorder, such as the seizures or motor disturbances common in patients with cerebral palsy.

On the other hand, there are children who appear physically normal but who demonstrate behavioral or sociologic problems. This type of patient may be referred to the dentist and labeled "unmanageable" with little realization by the referring person that the "behavior problem" may suggest some form of brain impairment. The autistic child is a prime example. Here is a child who is usually healthy in appearance but impaired by cognitive and language deficits (Dworkin, 1985). He or she demonstrates a limited capacity to comprehend and communicate verbally except in stressful situations. As Kopel (1977) relates, "They are withdrawn, apathetic, and unresponsive."

Family and peer influences

Psychosocial factors are probably the strongest influences on human behavior. Those within the family unit are particularly potent. Peer and institutional factors also shape behavior of individuals but to a lesser degree.

The parent's attitudinal structure, which molds, shapes, and directs child behavior in the early period of the offspring's development, is affected by the factors of socioeconomic position, cultural development, and ethnic background. From such sources emerge gradations of parenting ranging from the authoritative progenitor to the shy one. The parent who is personally distraught or depressed has difficulty parenting in an effective manner (Forehand and McMahon, 1981)

The socioeconomic status of the family unit directly affects its attitude toward the values of the dental health process. Those families with low income levels or below-average education have a tendency to attend dental needs when the symptoms dictate. Certain of these families harbor anxieties and fear of dental treatment, and children from these lower socioeconomic levels take on these fears and tend to be less cooperative. When, on the other hand, financial and educational means are ample, families value good dental health and are easily established into preventive programs. Too, cooperative behavior among their children is more prevalent (Ingersoll, 1982).

Though cooperative behavior does not appear related to race per se, ingrained cultural standards and ethnic orthodoxies have some bearing on the degree of acceptance of dental health measures. Their closed attitudes foster anxieties among the offspring, producing disparate behavior forms (Wright et al, 1983).

There is a mother-child interdependency that initiates at infancy and builds well into the preschool period (4 to 5 years). Should this interdependency overextend beyond its intended period, dual ambivalences may emerge between the mother and her child, with resultant maternal anxieties and the development of aberrant behavior patterns on the part of the offspring. Should the mother possess anxieties as a result of her own dental encounters or from fear for her child's first meeting with the dentist, that anxiety or fear can be transmitted to the offspring and is likely to produce a phobia of dentistry before the actual visit. Conversely, the mother may be cognizant of her influences on the child and manipulate them to sensible modeling in the presence of the child, thereby producing a behavior that is more positive toward the dental visit.

Internal family problems will influence child behavior. In the home beset with discord, the child can sense disharmony and may become emotionally frustrated and, thus, is more likely to be a management problem in the dental office. Similarly, a child from a single-parent or otherwise broken home may develop insecurities. The end result may be a behavior pattern that will not be conducive to a comfortable child-dentist relationship (Lenchner and Wright, 1975).

Still another area of family influence on child behavior is the sibling involvement. Older siblings can sabotage a child's adaptive behavior wittingly or unwittingly. By their actions they encourage the child to misbehave in the dental office. A child will model older siblings' behavior, good or bad.

The influence of peer association on child behavior is not as constant or concentrated as sibling exposure, but it can be a potential threat to the child who is witness to it. If the peer has had an undesirable dental experience or exaggerates his or her encounter to disconcerting proportions, the impressionable child can become a behavior problem.

Past medical and dental experiences

Past medical and dental experiences for the child do, in some instances, reflect unsatisfactory visits that produce management problems. Wright et al (1973) suggest that the emotional involvements wrought from past medical experiences and the child's generally poor attitude about medical office visits definitely shape and influence undesirable behavioral exhibitions in the child. McTigue (1984) points out that potentially uncooperative behavior may be related to fear sustained through a past, unpleasant dental experience. Inept handling of a child in the dental office produces unfavorable attitudes in the pediatric patient.

A study involving the child who had prior hospitalization and surgical intervention pointed out that the child with such an experience reacted more negatively at the first dental appointment (Martin et al, 1977). Interestingly enough, in the same study, it was shown that negative behavior was significantly related to maternal anxiety or a prediction on the mother's part of uncooperative behavior by her child.

Dental office environment

The dental office is a part of the child's experiential environment possessing people, things, and, hopefully, decoration. An office that reflects drabness or lack of warmth lends little to brightening a child's frame of mind or his or her subsequent attitude. Alpern (1975), in discussing etiologic sites for stress and emotion in the child, expressed the belief that an environment, such as the dental office, can manifest such exigencies.

The people in this environment are perhaps the most important factor. If each of the auxiliaries in the dental office operates independently of the other members, the opportunity for an efficient team function is destroyed. Healthy communication with the child patient is therefore hampered. While scheduling the child's initial appointment, the secretary may fail to employ the use of structured questions that might elicit clues from the parent as to past medical or dental experiences of the child. The receptionist who fails to note tell-tale patterns of reception room behavior does not afford the operating staff any additional insight that could be valuable in working with the child. The chairside assistant who converses with the child or others at inappropriate times breaks the communication link between the dentist and the patient. These types of inadequacies weaken the effectiveness of the dental team. Gruff remarks or a lack of concern on the dentist's part can crush any opportunity a child may have of displaying meaningful behavior or trusting the operator. A child who is exposed to an impersonal attitude and ominous sentences, such as "it will hurt some," "there will be some pain," and "it will just be a shot," or to the blatant display of fear-inspiring instruments cannot help but feel threatened. The mood and manner by which the dentist expresses himself or herself will exert greater influence on the child than what may actually be done.

The dentist and staff should contribute to positive influences with the dental office. Indirectly, the dental team can encourage positive family attitudes toward the dental visit and in so doing attenuate the negative remarks of those outside the family unit. Negative behavior, caused by a prior poor medical or dental experience, is influenced positively by wise family authority and behavioral retraining procedures used by the dental team.

Behavioral characteristics of the normal child

The dentist should learn to recognize characteristic behavior for a child at a given age and to identify any deviations from normal. In this way, he or she can more effectively work with the patient. The dentist knows that the child's behavioral pattern is influenced by psychomotor and emotional development as well as by environmental influences and personality traits, and to recognize these patterns and influences put meaning and vision in the hands of the operator and his or her personnel.

Stone and Church (1975) have segregated child development into five classifications: (1) infant, (2) toddler, (3) preschooler, (4) middle-years child, and (5) adolescent. Each of these classifications will be discussed from the objective of the child's or adolescent's dental needs and how best to meet them.

Infant

In the 15-month period of infancy, the neonate advances from relative helplessness to a positive, in-gear, ambulatory toddler. Erickson proposes that *infancy* is that period of life when the baby is informed about the world in which he or she is placed. Is it a good and acceptable place, or is it a locus of hurt and fickleness?

At about 6 months of age the baby begins to teeth and chew on anything in close approximation to the mouth. At this time maternal antibody protection is disappearing and minor illnesses begin to appear. The infant also experiences his or her first form of fear, referred to as *stranger anxiety,* wherein the baby displays apprehension on encountering persons outside the accustomed environment.

Another source of anxiety for the infant comes from the concept of trust or mistrust. When the baby's needs are met with reasonable promptness, basic trust is maintained at a high level. If there are unreasonable delays in attending the infant's demand for attention or feeding, a panic builds up and does not cease until that need is satisfied. This negative experience remains imprinted as a fiber of fear and distrust (Stone and Church, 1975).

The infant and parent each wields an influence over the other. The infant may demand cuddling and love or may resist it. This behavior will affect parental attitude. On the other hand, parental characteristics may modify the baby's behavior. The infant may have come at the wrong time in the marriage or may represent an end to the care-free times of youth. Stone and Church (1975) elaborate that "parents at times are not parents of good will." They are disturbed individuals shouldering unbearable pressure, only to let it out in abuse of their child, or are moralists who believe in their ordained right to drive sin and corruption from the child's body.

The abused or battered child may grow up retarded or intellectually substandard.

The main focus of parenting is to help the offspring develop proper habits. Watson (1975) stated that parents should "be objective and kindly firm." He believed in training the infant in regularity—regularity in feeding, sleeping, and eliminating—and from this regularity "the tiny baby will receive his [or her] first lessons in character building."

Fortunately, dental intervention for the infant is minimal. However, the factors that can cause dental need often arise out of regrettable circumstances. These factors may be emergencies precipitated by traumatic or pathologic situations. If moderate of major problems exist, dental treatment may best be achieved in the hospital using a general anesthetic. Should conscious sedation be the procedure of choice, the use of an anesthesiologist and the hospital setting is again a wise decision. Certain minor involvements requiring minimum time may be treated or provisionally treated in the dental office.

Toddler

The toddler represents a child ranging from 15 months to 2 years of age. He or she is still very much a baby, taking one or two naps daily, and yet is developing unbabylike skills. He or she readily displays an ambivalent nature, wanting to remain an infant one moment and yet grow up the next instant. The toddler is rapidly developing in cognitive and verbal skills, and self-awareness is moving to the forefront. Cooperative behavior and reasoning "why" are not in his or her inventory of accomplishments.

The toddler, considering the characteristics listed, is a child who is developing and growing in knowledge and motor skills but is still in immature individual. The child is incapable of perceiving why dental measures need to be accomplished or realizing the significance of cooperative behavior in the dental office. The behavioral characteristic will be reflective of the patterns observed. There are exceptions, and the dentist must allow for adjustments in behavior management to fit the individual child. The assessments are as follows:

1. Dental examination. Dental examination of the toddler may have to be done with the child in the parent's lap. Most examinations are easily accomplished, although the patient may whimper or move about. The toddler may sit alone in the dental chair.

2. Dental radiography. The toddler is usually not cooperative for radiographs. Occasionally a radiograph may be obtained with specialized techniques and the parent's help, perhaps with the child in the parent's lap, and the parent holding the film. Protective coverage should be provided for both individuals.

3. Minor dental caries. On rare occasions minor carious lesions may be excavated with spoon excavators and small enamel hatchets. A No. $^1/_4$ or $^1/_2$ round bur or a $33^1/_2$ inverted cone bur in a high-speed handpiece, and without a local anesthetic, might be meticulously used for an easily accessible lesion. The restoration may be a silver amalgam or a composite resin material. Such procedures are predicated on an emotionally well-behaved child, gentle touch, and the absence of discomfort.

4. Major dental caries. Carious involvement such as nursing bottle caries, will of necessity require moderate to extensive treatment procedures that are usually beyond normal behavior capabilities of the toddler.

5. Minor oral surgery. These types of procedures are usually achieved with conscious sedation or general anesthetic means.

6. Prophylactic measures. The toddler may tolerate a gently administered toothbrush prophylaxis with a pleasant-tasting prophylaxis paste.

Preschooler

The preschooler label designates the child 2 to 6 years of age. The preschooler "wears" his or her "personality" where it can be seen, thus making the child one whose behavior pattern is easily observed. He or she is more skilled in the use of words and symbols and more effective in interpersonal communications.

The preschoolers' behavior is influenced and shaped to a considerable degree by his or her immediate environment. Stone and Church (1975) have developed the following appraisal:

1. He or she is expanding the circle of acquaintances to people outside the immediate family.
2. Aggression and sympathy coexist in this individual. He or she may be very firm in opinion and expression but can be responsive to the needs of others.
3. His or her play is more role playing.
4. He or she adopts behavior of familiar individuals, complete with facial expressions, verbal mannerisms, and gestures.
5. The preschooler is developing a meaningful relationship with the immediate world. He or she readily identifies people and places, uses hand tools for his or her intended purposes, and has evolved a more cautious individuality.
6. The preschooler's idea of fantasy is dramatic. The illusion of the magician sawing the lady in half and putting her together is lost on him or her. The act is accepted as fact.
7. Pretense on the part of older people is often accepted as literal fact for the preschooler. Bizarre

storytelling and some bantering are accepted as actuality.

8. He or she will very likely create imaginary companions during this period.
9. The preschooler will often make apparent in drawings his or her emotional connotation.
10. Self-awareness for the preschooler is the identification of self. He or she inspects objectively the texture of the body, which is dry on the outside and wet on the inside with "lots of insides and blood."
11. Fears are both real and unreal and are the result of his or her self-awareness. The preschooler's fear of death develops from the realization that people die and that something can happen to him or her, too.
12. Time frames are unworkable and meaningless for the early preschooler, but at 5 years he or she has some hold on time and can project some plans over a number of days.
13. The preschooler does not have an adequate fix on the logic of space. If asked to plot a familiar area, such as the family home, the result will be an exaggerated drafting of the different areas.
14. Abstract thought is not yet a part of his or her reasoning ability.
15. Causal relations change sequentially with the increases in overall knowledge, intelligence, and thinking. At first, everything is animistic. All things, including rocks, water, wind, and trees are alive and have their own being. Next, he or she changes to artificialism, wherein all circumstances are originated by human intervention. An example is the child who views the ground covered with pine needles. The preschooler asks, "Why did they put them there?" His or her causal relations become more realistic with time.

The dentist's best approach toward cooperative behavior from the preschooler is to assess the following behavioral characteristics and apply them in the management scheme:

1. The readily observable personality traits displayed by the preschooler should be noted.
2. If the preschooler likes to verbalize, communication between the patient and the dentist should be employed to the utmost of its effectiveness.
3. The preschooler's imagination lends itself to physiognomic and euphemistic descriptions of dental procedures. Christen (1977) refer to euphemisms, or physiognomic usages, such as "Mr. Bumpy," alluding to the slowly turning bur when placed against tooth structure, or using "whistling Charlie" to describe the characteristic should of the high-speed handpiece.
4. Modeling has become important to the preschooler's learning during this period. The dentist and staff should use modeling in every conceivable situation.

5. Because of the preschooler's self-awareness and fears, particularly of pain and bleeding, the dentist and staff must be alert to avoid actions, words, or procedures that incite anxieties toward dental procedures.

Although immaturities are still evident for a 2- or 3-year-old child and may offer a problem in behavior for the dentist, the older preschooler will more likely present cooperative behavior.

Middle-years child

The stage from 6 to 12 years of age is a rather peaceful period of time compared with the hustle and bustle of the preschooler. It is the time of "the loose tooth." It is a time of moderately rapid physical growth; a time of reaching out for independent identity; a time for joining others of his or her own sex; a time of sexual growth latency; a time for scapegoating when disobedient; a time for fears, both realistic and imaginary; a time wherein the child locates in "time"; and a time of emotionalism and confusion.

Piaget divides this period of the middle years into two stages. The intuitive stage represents ages 4 to 7, overlapping Stone and Church's preschool years. The child's mind indulges in fancy. He or she understands only what is seen. An anesthetic syringe may pose a strong threat. By now the child possesses prelogical reasoning (Christen, 1977).

Piaget's second stage is the concrete operational stage. It ranges from 7 to 11 years of age. During this period the child learns conversation. His or her thinking becomes logical and reversible. The child can now reflect, reason, and understand logical relationships.

For the dentist and staff, this interval of the middle years contains minimal behavioral entanglement. Here is an individual who, for the most part, can accept reason. Anxiety can be dealt with in a reasonable way by staff personnel and the dentist.

Adolescent

Adolescence is a pause in the cycle of life. The individual is no longer a child but not yet an adult. Stone and Church (1975) designate this period as commencing at age 12 and continuing to full maturity. Piaget's formal operations stage extends from 11 to 15 years.

The adolescent's early development is marked by pubescence, which is the preadolescent period and is an interval of about 2 years, marked by a physical growth spurt, maturation of the primary and secondary sex characteristics, and varying changes in body proportions. Girls initially are ahead of boys in physical development and the maturation process, but boys begin to catch up around the second or third year of high school.

Puberty marks the arrival of sexual maturation. For girls it is designated by the first menses and for boys by a number of signs, the most notable being the presence of live spermatozoa in the urine.

The main point at issue for the adolescent is the identification of himself or herself for this new role. The individual has changed not only morphologically but also emotionally. There are new and different feelings and new potentials. The adolescent's environment has a different connotation, and he or she must seek a niche in this new society and thus prepare for the adult world. Self-awareness becomes intensified and results in a new push for independence.

According to Piagetian theory, an individual steps from the concrete operational stage cognitively bolstered with firm ideas and into the arena of formal operations. These concrete forms are modified into propositions and hypotheses by the adolescent to test other avenues of accomplishing designated projects (Phillips, 1975)

This new surge for independence directs the adolescent increasingly to peer groups with less family supervision and restraint and more privileges. He or she is concerned about peer status and where he or she is positioned in the world of the independent adult. Notwithstanding this independent attitude, the adolescent still welcomes adult intervention into problems over which he or she has questionable control.

The adolescent wants to be popular with everyone but selects his or her friends from a certain set. He or she has a large number of casual acquaintances from other sets. Most of his or her friends will be from within the particular set with which he or she most identifies.

The dentist and staff will find working for the adolescent a pleasant experience. The youngster will usually respond in an appreciative manner. There may be a period of time during pubescence when the individual may be a bit sensitive and moody, requiring diligent attention and patience on the part of the dental staff.

Behavioral classifications and behavioral patterns

Preappointment sociobehavioral assessment

Significant benefits are derived from social and behavioral information elicited from parents before a child's first visit to the dental office.

Advance information may be obtained in a number of ways. The most complete information comes from the family's response to a preappointment packet mailed before the initial visit. The packet contains information on office policy and practice philosophy, pertinent educational material, and a preappointment questionnaire to be completed and returned to the dental office. Another avenue for the information can be provided by the parent when the appointment is made by telephone or in person. The data collected should furnish information concerning who the child is, the composition of the family, where the family resides, the parental vocations, etc. The psychobehavioral history is the most important section for the dental team, and the knowledge gathered will benefit patient service (Fig 1-1). The support personnel are invaluable in acquiring subjective information about child-parent behavior in and about the dental office. The conversion of this information into workable data should provide the dental team with advance knowledge on the expectancies of the cooperative effort.

Categorical rating of behavioral patterns

A large number of studies since the 1960's have lent significant contribution to the classification of child behavior as it correlates with clinical diagnosis and patient management. Notably, behavior has been distinguished into patterns as related to their differences of clinical presentation.

Frankl et al (1962) introduced a behavioral rating instrument commonly referred to as the Frankl rating scale. It is one of the most reliable tools developed for behavioral measurement and is widely used by teaching institutions as well as the private sector of pediatric dentistry.

The device consists of a series of determinations numbered from 1 to 4. Each defines specific behavior (Table 1-1). Wright (1975) suggested that another item be added to the rating scale, permitting the dentist to record a behavioral base at the inception of dental treatment and to keep a progressive record of the child's behavioral responses. Too, it is clinically adaptable to any well-organized patient record system. Changes in patient behavior will be readily noted.

With the use of Wright's modification, a negative or positive symbol is placed opposite the appropriate rating (Table 1-1). The symbol is entered in the patient progress notes form as related to the behavior for that particular procedure. With the entrance of the appropriate sign adjacent to the performed treatment and the employment of a flow symbol ($\rightarrow$), the indication of behavioral change may be recorded for that treatment. Wright suggests that whatever part of a procedure brings about change in behavior be recorded in abbreviated form alongside (Table 1-2).

Patient behavioral ratings

Rating No. 1: Definitely negative (– –)

1. Refuses treatment
   a. Immature behavior: cannot reason or cope with situations
      Toddler or early preschooler
      The special child

1. How do you think your child has reacted to past dental or medical care?
   □ Very good   □ Moderately good   □ Moderately poor   □ Very poor

2. How do you think your child will react in our clinic?
   □ Very good   □ Moderately good   □ Moderately poor   □ Very poor

3. How would you rate your own anxiety or nervousness at the prospect
   of your child receiving dental care?
   □ Very good   □ Moderately good   □ Moderately poor   □ Very poor

4. Does your child believe that there is anything wrong with his/her teeth?   Yes   No

5. During the past year, has your child been aware of anyone who has
   had an unpleasant dental experience?   Yes   No

6. Which of the following best describes your child?
   □ Advanced in the learning process
   □ Progressing normally in the learning process
   □ Slow learner

7. Please check all words that best describe your child:
   □ Calm   □ Spoiled   □ Suspicious   □ Temper tantrums
   □ Moody   □ Sickly   □ Talkative   □ High-strung
   □ Shy   □ Defiant   □ Friendly   □ Cooperative
   □ Active   □ Fearful   □ Healthy   □ Compulsive

8. Does your child have any hobbies or special interests?   Yes   No

   If yes, please list _____

   _____

9. Does your child have any pets at home?   Yes   No

   If yes, please indicate type of pet(s) and name(s):

   _____

10. Are there other children in your family?
    If yes, please list below:

    First name: _____ Sex: _____ Age: _____

    First name: _____ Sex: _____ Age: _____

    First name: _____ Sex: _____ Age: _____

11. Is there any additional information we should know about your child that would allow us to better care
    for your child?

    If yes, please explain: _____

    _____

    _____

Fig 1-1 Sociobehavioral history patient information form (Division of Developmental Dentistry, University of Oklahoma, Oklahoma City).

b. Uncontrollable behavior: essentially a temper tantrum, suggestive of extreme anxiety
   Preschooler
c. Defiant behavior: active- or passive-type resistance; the "spoiled" child; stubbornness is also associated with this style of response.
   Middle-years child
2. Cries forcefully
   Uncontrollable behavior
   Late preschooler or middle-years child
3. Is extremely negative, associated with fear
   a. Uncontrollable behavior: may be exhibited, for example, in the "older" young person possess-ing deep-seated emotional problems
   b. Defiant behavior: includes passive resistance in the individual approaching adolescence

Rating No. 2: Negative (-)

1. Is reluctant to accept treatment
   a. Immature behavior
      Toddler or preschooler: too young in years
      The special child
   b. Timid behavior: seen in the child who is over-protected, exposed to few people (as observed in children from sparsely populated areas), or

Table 1-1   Behavioral scale of Frankl et al. with Wright's modification*

	Frankl behavior rating scale	Wright modification
Rating no. 1	Definitely negative Refusal of treatment; crying forcefully, fearful, extreme negativism	(−−)
Rating no. 2	Negative Reluctant, uncooperative, limited negativism, sullen, withdrawn	(−)
Rating no. 3	Positive Accepts treatment but may be cautious or reserved, follows directions	(+)
Rating no. 4	Definitely positive Good rapport, interested in dental procedures, laughs and enjoys	(++)

*Adapted from Wright (1975).

Table 1-2   Treatment progress notes using Wright's adaption of the Frankl ratings*

Procedure	Behavior[†]
Prevent I	(−)→(+)TSD
Prevent II	(++)
Tooth 85-MO Amalgam; Anes-carb/2%/; RD	(−) Inj (+) Rest
Tooth 74-Stainless Steel Crown; Anes-carb/2%/;RD	(−)→(+) Inj (−) Rest
Tooth 64-DO Amalgam; Anes-carb/2%/; RD	(+)→(−) Inj (−) Rest

*Adapted from Wright (1975).
†TSD = tell-show-do; Inj = injection; Rest = restoration; (→) = flow symbol indicating behavioral change; RD = rubber dam.

daunted by strange environments; this type of child may revert to uncooperative behavior if mismanaged
c. Influenced behavior: includes family and peer pressure
2. Displays evidence of slight negativism
   a. Timid behavior: must be taught confidence in himself or herself and the dentist
   b. Whining behavior
       Preschooler and middle-years child

Rating No. 3: Positive (+)

1. Accepts treatment
   a. Tense cooperative behavior: observed in all stages; follows the dentist's directions but may be hesitant and cautious
   b. Concertive behavior: responds harmoniously
   c. Whining behavior: may or may not be considered negative behavior. Wright (1975) makes an

interesting point on tolerance levels. Mental tolerance levels among clinicians are observable and demonstrable. One operator may interpret whining as a negative behavior because it is disturbing to him or her and staff. Another pays the behavior very little attention and accomplishes treatment as planned.
d. Timid behavior: follows the dentist's directions in a shy, quiet manner

Rating No. 4: Definitely positive (++)

1. Unique behavior: looks forward to and understands the importance of good preventive care

Dentist-patient relationship

Infant and toddler

When the infant or toddler is taken into the dental office, no attempt should be made to separate the child and parent. The parent's presence in the examining area produces a significant calming effect for a child who may otherwise be overwhelmed by strange people and surroundings.

Communication with the toddler will, at the most, be minimal or, more likely, one sided. Personnel should initiate conversation couched in language the child may comprehend but should not expect verbal response. In addition, the dentist and staff must ascertain whether the parent should hold or seat the child in the chair.

The infant or toddler makes the dental visit for one of three reasons: trauma of the oral structures, parental concerns, or carious lesions. In the event of trauma, the child will be emotionally upset and the parent concerned and anxious for the child. One can expect the behavior to be definitely negative (––) or negative (-). Occasionally the dentist may see a toddler exhibiting a positive (+) behavior, but any attempt to treat the injury usually ends on a negative note. The toddler is not capable of coping with trauma, and, if treatment is indicated, it will require a special management procedure or patient referral.

Quite often a parent will question some condition observed within the child's mouth. The concern may be a normal growth circumstance or, on occasion, an anomaly of one type or kind. The patient's behavior will vary between negative and positive. The oral assessment will be easily accomplished yet may be noisy.

When carious lesions are observed in a child 15 to 24 months of age, the treatment procedure best suited for that point in time becomes the main consideration and requires a thoughtful decision. Behavioral response will register as definitely negative and will require a special management procedure, such as a conscious sedation or general anesthetic regimen. Minor carious involvement may require a compromise approach to accomplish a restorative measure or a provisional procedure. The effort will require alert personnel and distraction to complete the task quickly and painlessly. With an incipient lesion and a child exercising a definitely negative response, regulated intervals of patient recall to observe the progress of the lesion may be the best procedure. As has been expressed many times to parents in instances such as this, "We are playing for time, perhaps 3 or 4 months. Understanding and behavior may be significantly improved." The parent appreciates this kind of concern for the child.

Understanding or managing the infant or toddler does not require a mastermind or magician. Proper management comes with a gentle, positive approach by the practitioner. One must realize there will be limitations to dental care rendered in the normal setting.

Preschooler

The preschooler has developed some self-autonomy and reaches out more to people beyond the family circle. With the increased interest in interpersonal relations, communication becomes a tool to use in the child's management. Behavioral shaping and reinforcement techniques are made effective through communication. Retraining procedures also depend on communication for effectiveness.

The early preschooler will still have some of the immaturities of toddlerhood, and, here again, the practitioner will be faced with problems of communication and coping. The philosophy of treatment and technical approach may be the same as for the toddler.

Between 3 and 3.5 years of age, the preschooler develops a more mature reasoning capacity. The child's awareness of self, space, and time are beginning to emerge, and the child quite often is a delight to work

with. It is not unusual that the child may have difficulty with emergence into the world of self-awareness and autonomy, which may offer obstacles to compatible behavior. It is here that the knowledge of behavioral management becomes most important.

Middle-years child and adolescent

The middle-years child and adolescent provide for a wide range of communication and understanding. There need be little consideration for compromise procedures because of uncooperative behavior. The establishment of effective communications and the use of adaptable behavior-control techniques work well for the average individual from these two categories.

Physical assessment

The physical assessment of a pediatric patient is best accomplished following an orderly sequence of steps and can be facilitated with a well-designed examination form for documenting the findings. The following is a list of items most often surveyed:

1. *General physical condition.* General physical appraisal is best accomplished before the patient is seated in the dental chair. Various fine and gross motor movements, including posture and gait, can be observed. Measurements of height and weight should be periodically performed and compared with norms or standards for that particular chronologic age and sex. Vital signs such as heart rate, blood pressure, temperature, and respiration rate should likewise be recorded. Deviations (greater than 2 standard deviations) from normal values should be confirmed and referred for appropriate medical consultation (Poole and Macko, 1984). Specific characteristics of the hands and fingers will help identify oral habits (eg, an isolated clean nail and wrinkled skin around the base of a digit), genetic anomalies (eg, shortened, curved, fused, or missing digits), and effects of systemic disease (eg, club fingers or cyanotic nail beds) (Currier, 1982). A more detailed discussion of physical growth and development follows later in this chapter.

2. *Head, neck, and face.* Important components include an evaluation of the skin, hair, eyes, and ears where structural abnormalities may be related to certain acquired disorders or developmental conditions and syndromes warranting further investigation. Lymph nodes should be palpated for tenderness. Facial asymmetry may implicate occlusal imbalance, and facial profile may help identify abnormal skeletal growth patterns. Likewise, the vertical component of the facial profile should be evaluated for the steepness of the mandibular angle. If the line of the mandibular plane (inferior border of the mandible) lies tangent to the oc-

ciput (posteroinferior portion of the skull), it would be considered normal. If the line intersects the skull, the mandibular plane is high and would result in an anterior vector of force favoring space closure in the dentition. The temporomandibular joints should be observed for limitation or deviation during movement, tenderness, and crepitation. Lips should be evaluated for color, texture, fullness, relative length, position during rest and swallowing, and evidence of trauma or pathologic lesions. Multiple scarring, bruising in different stages of healing, or a history of trauma inconsistent with the physical findings in the head and neck region warrant suspicion of child abuse. Speech must also be evaluated and compared with the maturational level of the child.

3. Intraoral soft tissue. The labial and buccal mucosa are examined first for relative height of frena attachments, abrasions, traumatic lesions (cheek biting), and ulcerations. The tongue and floor of the mouth are likewise examined for similar abnormalities. The hard and soft palates are observed and palpated for clefts and volopharyngeal incompetence. The size and condition of the tonsillar tissues and the quality and quantity of saliva should be noted. Finally, the gingiva is evaluated for color, form, and texture as well as for sulcus depth and width of attachment. Any abnormalities must be noted according to location. An assessment of plaque and calculus accumulation must be similarly scored.

4. Teeth. The presence or absence of every tooth should be determined along with an assessment of the sequence and timing of development and eruption according to chronologic age. Anomalies of number, size, shape, structure, texture, eruption, exfoliation, and position of the teeth are noted. All dental restorations and carious lesions should be charted by tooth number and surface. Examination of the supporting structures for evidence of pathologic conditions is essential. A comprehensive evaluation of the teeth requires a meticulous clinical examination supported by a radiographic survey appropriate for age and dictated by the clinical findings.

5. Occlusion. The occlusion should be evaluated in accordance with the three planes of space: sagittal (molar and canine classifications and overjet), transverse (crossbites and midline deviations), and vertical (overbite and open bite). The individual arches are observed for form, symmetry, and space (presence of diastemas or crowding).

Physical development

A persistent error in the physical evaluation of the growing child is the sole use of chronologic age as a measure of physical maturity. Four other developmen-

tal indicators of physical maturation are commonly used in the assessment of the growing child (Krogman, 1968). These indicators involve the dentition, bone, secondary sex characteristics, and height and weight. Height and weight are used to calculate morphologic age; attainment of secondary sexual maturity (eg, menarche) is used to determine circumpuberal age; and radiographic assessment of the hand-wrist bones is often used to appraise skeletal age. However, the dentition can be evaluated either radiographically for the degree of tooth formation or clinically for the degree of eruption to establish the dental age of the patient. Of these two methods, analysis of the degree of tooth formation is far superior to that of eruption. The analysis of eruption has limited use in determining dental age because of its variability and lack of an agreeable definition. Furthermore, arch length insufficiency and premature loss, ankylosis, infection, or endodontic treatment of primary teeth are local factors that influence the eruption of the succedaneous permanent teeth. In contrast, the formation rate of permanent teeth is affected by neither premature loss of their predecessors nor the degree of crowding present in the arch.

There are some positive, if not significant, correlations among the developmental indicators of physical maturation. Skeletal age is best associated with height and weight. Correlation coefficients among dental, skeletal, and chronologic ages show a moderate association. However, although both dental and chronologic age evaluations demonstrate significant correlations with other measures of development, neither demonstrates any universal advantage over the other.

The discussion is divided into the following phases of growth and development as defined by Lowrey (1973):

Growth period	Chronologic age
Prenatal	Conception to birth (40 weeks)
Infancy	Birth to 2 years
Early childhood (preschool)	2 to 6 years
Late childhood (prepubertal)	7 to 12 years
Adolescence (puberty)	13 to 20 years

Prenatal period

First trimester. The first trimester is a period of rapid differentiation and proliferation of cellular mass. At this time, the development of the embryo is influenced by complicated interactions between genetic predispositions and factors in the intrauterine environment. Sensitivity to various agents or genetic aberrations is greatest during this period. Severe insult can result in

Table 1-3 Amount of enamel completion found at birth in an infant of normal term*

Teeth	Enamel completion
Primary maxillary central incisors	Five sixths
Primary maxillary lateral incisors	Two thirds
Primary maxillary canines	One third
Primary maxillary first molars	Cusps united, occlusal surface completely calcified, plus one half to three fourths of the crown height
Primary maxillary second molars	Cusps united, occlusal surface incompletely calcified, plus one fifth to one fourth of the crown height
Primary mandibular central incisors	Three fifths
Primary mandibular lateral incisors	Three fifths
Primary mandibular canines	One third
Primary mandibular first molars	Cusps united, occlusal surface completely calcified
Primary mandibular second molars	Cusps united, occlusal surface incompletely calcified
Permanent maxillary and mandibular first molars	Sometimes a trace, mesiobuccal cusps first

*Adapted from Lunt and Law (1974a).

miscarriage and termination of the pregnancy. Congenital malformation can occur as a result of less severe insult from chemotherapeutic agents, radiation, infection, and mechanical trauma. Contact with viral diseases, such as rubella, during the first trimester has been associated with congenital heart disease, cataracts, deafness, and mental retardation.

The first week following conception is termed the *germinal period.* Differentiation of the ectoderm and endoderm occur during the second week, and mesodermal differentiation appears in the third week. The fourth week is marked by formation of the dental lamina and regular pulsation of the heart. By the sixth week, tooth buds of the primary teeth develop in the ectodermal tissue of the dental lamina, and invasion of the underlying mesodermal connective tissue begins to form the dental papilla. By the end of the first trimester, the fetus weighs 14 g (0.5 oz.) and is 7.5 cm (3 in.) in length. The lungs and a four-chamber heart are apparent, and the palatal processes have closed.

Second trimester. The second trimester is a period of rapid acquisition of functions and increasing maturation of the neuromuscular system spreading in a cephalocaudal direction. Hair, sweat, and sebaceous glands are present. Histodifferentiation of the enamel organ and dental papilla forms ameloblasts and odontoblasts, respectively. Crown calcification of the primary teeth begins by the 14th week for the incisors and first molars and by the 16th to 18th weeks for the canines and second molars. The sequence of calcification of the primary teeth occurs as follows: central incisor, first molar, lateral incisor, canine, and second molar.

At the same time as the calcification of the primary teeth, the tooth buds of the permanent incisors begin their development lingual to the primary teeth. In the 14th week, the fetus demonstrates swallowing movements, and the sucking reflex is present by the 20th week. By the end of the second trimester, the fetus weighs 1 kg (2.2 lb) and is approximately 35 cm (14 in.) in length.

Third trimester. The third trimester is a period that marks the beginning of fetal viability (minimum age at which the fetus can survive outside the uterus). Continued maturation of the organ systems and increased sophistication of functioning occurs during this period.

Infancy

Prenatal and postnatal growth is one continuous process, but the incident of birth and beginning of extrauterine existence is an important dividing point. At birth, the parasitic relationship of the fetus with the mother is terminated. The newborn must initiate respiration, changes in the circulatory system, maintenance of body temperature, and the establishment of digestion and excretion with dependence on an external source of nutrition. It is therefore easy to recognize why the neonatal period is the greatest period of risk to the infant's survival.

Average birth weight is 3.4 kg (7 to 7.5 lb). Ten percent of the infant's birth weight is lost but regained by the tenth day of life and tripled by the end of the first year. The formula for calculating normal weight (lb) during infancy is:

$$\text{weight (lb)} = \text{age (in months)} + 11$$

Average birth length is 50 cm (20 in.). A 50% increase will occur by the end of the first year.

Premature birth is defined as a gestational period of 37 weeks or less and may result in low birth weight. Premature birth should not be considered analogous to low–birth-weight infants, whose condition is more serious. Low–birth-weight infants are small-for-date in-

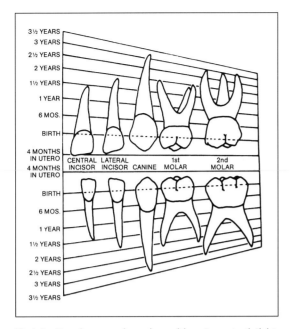

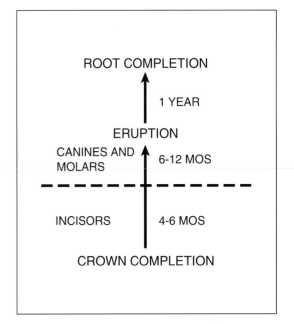

Fig 1-2 Development chronology of the primary teeth (labial view). Reprinted with permission from Pindborg, 1970.

Fig 1-3 Generalized time requirements for development of primary teeth.

Table 1-4 Sequence and timing of primary tooth eruption*

Primary teeth	Mean (range), in mo
Mandibular central incisors	8 (6–10)
Maxillary central incisors	10 (8–12)
Maxillary lateral incisors	11 (9–12)
Mandibular lateral incisors	13 (10–16)
Maxillary and mandibular first molars	16 (14–18)
Maxillary and mandibular canines	20 (16–23)
Mandibular second molars	27 (23–31)
Maxillary second molars	29 (25–33)

*Adapted from Lunt and Law (1974b).

Table 1-5 Sequence and timing of permanent tooth eruption

Permanent teeth	Mean, in years
Maxillary and mandibular first molars and mandibular central incisors	6–7
Maxillary central and mandibular lateral incisors	7–8
Maxillary lateral incisors	8–9
Mandibular canines	9–10
Maxillary and mandibular first premolars	10–11
Maxillary second premolars	10–12
Maxillary canines and mandibular second premolars	11–12
Maxillary and mandibular second molars	11–13

fants whose weight is 2.5 kg (5.5 lb) or less, regardless of the duration of gestation. This condition occurs in 7.6% of US births. Low birth weight results in a high incidence of infant mortality and an increased susceptibility to neurologic damage. The immature development of low–birth-weight infants renders them less equipped to cope with external insults. These infants are particularly prone to respiratory distress (hyaline membrane disease), hyperbilirubinemia (kernicterus), and anemia, as well as infection and secondary complications because of the immaturity of the immunologic system and imbalances in the electrolyte levels. Probably the most reliable indicator of the degree of maturation in the neonatal period is neurologic evaluation and changes in the electroencephalogram readings. The amount of enamel formed in an infant of normal term at birth is found in Table 1-3.

For the primary teeth, completion of enamel formation, or crown completion, occurs about 4 to 6 months before eruption for the eight incisors, which are the only teeth present at 1 year of age. For the remaining 12 primary teeth that erupt after 1 year of age, crown completion occurs approximately 6 to 12 months before eruption (Figs 1-2 and 1-3). Root completion occurs approximately 1 year following eruption. Eruption of the primary teeth occurs over approximately 2 years, from 8 to 30 months of age. The sequence and timing of eruption is found in Table 1-4.

Crown calcification of the permanent teeth begins at birth for the first molars, between 3 and 12 months for the anterior teeth, and between 1.5 and 3 years for the remaining posterior teeth, excluding third molars (Fig 1-4).

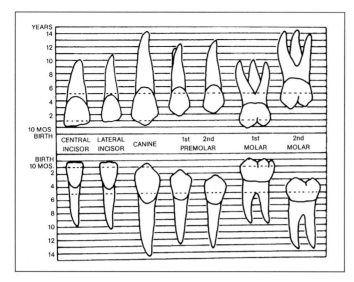

Fig 1-4 Development chronology of the permanent teeth (labial view). Reprinted with permission from Pindborg, 1970.

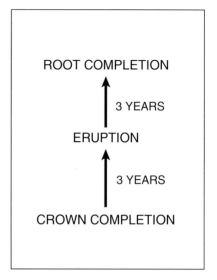

Fig 1-5 Generalized time requirements for development of permanent teeth.

Early childhood

Average weight gain is 4.5 lb (2 kg)/y. The formula for calculating normal weight for age during this period is:

$$\text{weight (lb)} = \text{age (years)} \times 5 + 17$$

Average height gain is 3 in. (7 cm)/y. By 3 years of age, the child has reached approximately one half his or her expected adult height. As the child grows, the head contributes proportionally less to the total body length, shrinking from one fourth of the total at birth to one twelfth at maturity.

Crown completion for each permanent tooth occurs approximately 3 years before eruption of that tooth. Therefore, the permanent incisors, first premolars, and first molars complete enamel formation during this period (Figs 1-4 and 1-5).

Late childhood

Average weight gain is 7 lb (3 kg)/y. The formula is:

$$\text{weight (lb)} = \text{age (years)} \times 7 + 5$$

Average height gain is 2.5 in. (6cm)/y. The formula is:

$$\text{height (in.)} = \text{age (years)} \times 2.5 + 30$$

Unique features affecting the general health of children during this period, such as the lymphatic tissues, are at the peak of their development, respiratory tract infections are common, and innocent "functional" heart murmurs reach their peak incidence.

Dental development is likewise unique in that this is the period of transition between primary and permanent dentitions. This transition is termed the *mixed dentition*. During this period all 20 primary teeth exfoliate, and 28 permanent teeth erupt. The most favorable sequence and timing of eruption for the permanent teeth is found in Table 1-5. As a rule, eruption of mandibular teeth usually precedes that of maxillary teeth and girls are more advanced than boys.

Root completion for each permanent tooth occurs approximately 3 years after eruption of that tooth (Figs 1-4 and 1-5).

Adolescence

Four events are characteristic of adolescence:

1. Onset of puberty (ability to procreate), which occurs in girls at 10 to 12 years of age and in boys after 12 to 14 years of age.
2. Marked physical growth, a growth spurt that occurs approximately 18 months following the onset of puberty.
3. Appearance of secondary sexual characteristics, such as menarche in girls, which occurs approximately 1 year after maximum growth spurt.
4. Intense emotional strain and adjustment.

References

Alpern, G. D. Child development: Basic concept and clinical considerations. In Wright, G. Z. Behavior Management in Dentistry for Children. Philadelphia: W. B. Saunders Co., 1975, pp. 38-39.

American Academy of Pediatric Dentistry (AAPD): Reference Manual, 1992-1993. Chicago: AAP 1993, pp. 83-85.

Beyer, D. G. The significance of charting in the defense of dentists. J. Mich. Dent. Assoc. 69:85, 1987.

Brady, W. F., and Martinoff, J. T. Validity of health history data collected from dental patients and patient perception of health status. J. Am. Dent. Assoc. 101:642, 1980.

Christen, A. Piagetian psychology: Some principles as helpful in treating the child patient. J. Dent. Child.44:40, 1977.

Currier, G. F. Data base collection and related considerations. In Stewart, R., et al. Pediatric Dentistry. St. Louis: The C.V. Mosby Co., 1982, pp. 857-871.

Curtis, J. W., Zarkowski, P., Feringa, S. D. Risk management: Protecting against litigation in dentistry. J. Mich. Dent. Assoc. 69:497, 1987.

Dworkin, P. H. Learning and Behavior Problems of Schoolchildren. Philadelphia: W.B. Saunders Co., 1985, pp. 160-162.

Forehand, R. S., and McMahon, R. J. Helping the Non-Compliant Child: A Clinician's Guide to Parent Training. New York: The Guilford Press, 1981, pp. 166-171.

Frankl, S. N., Shreve, F. R., and Fogels, H. R. Should the parent remain within the dental operatory? J. Dent. Child. 29:150, 1962.

Ingersoll, B. D. Behavioral Aspects in Dentistry. East Norwalk, Conn.: Appleton-Centry-Crofts, 1982.

Kopel, H. M. The autistic child in dental practice. J. Dent. Child. 44:302, 1977.

Krogman, W.M. Biological timing and the dentofacial complex. J. Dent. Child. 35:175, 328, 1968.

LeMasney, J.F. Medical history of children undergoing dental treatment in Ireland. Community Dent. Oral Epidemiol. 5:103, 1977.

Lenchner V., and Wright, G.Z. Nonpharmaco-therapeutic approaches to behavior management. In Wright, G. Z. Behavior Management in Dentistry for Children. Philadelphia: W. B. Saunders Co., 1975.

Lowrey, G. H. Growth and Development of Children. Chicago: Year Book Medical Publishers, Inc,. 1973, p. 13.

Lunt, R.C., and Law, D. B. A review of the chronology of calcification of deciduous teeth. J. Am. Dent. Assoc. 89:599, 1974a.

Lunt, R. C., and Law, D. B. A review of the chronology of eruption of deciduous teeth. J. Am. Dent. Assoc. 89:872, 1974b.

Martin, R. B., Shaw, M. S., and Taylor, P. P. The influences of prior surgical experience on the child's behavior at the initial dental visit. J. Dent. Child 44:35, 1977.

McTigue, D. J. Behavior management of children. In Spedding, R. H. Symposium on Pedodontics. Dent. Clin. North Am. 28:1, 1984.

Norheim, P. W., and Heloe, L. A. Differences between dental health data obtained by interview and questionnaires. Community Dent. Oral Epidemoil. 5:121, 1977.

Phillips, J. L., Jr. The Origins of Intellect—Piaget's Theory. 2nd ed. San Francisco: W. H. Freeman and Co., 1975.

Pindborg, J. J. Pathology of the Dental Hard Tissues. Philadelphia: W. B. Saunders Co., 1970.

Poole, A. E., and Macko, D. J. Pediatric vital signs: Recording methods and interpretation. Pediatr. Dent. 6:10, 1984.

Pozgar, G. D. Legal Aspects of Health Care Administration. Rockville, Md.: Aspen Publications, 1983.

Rozousky, F. A. Consent to Treatment: A Practical Guide. Boston: Little, Brown Co., 1984.

Shultz, M. M. From informed consent to patient choice: A new protected interest. Yale Law J. 95:219, 1985.

Stone, L. J., and Church, J. Childhood and Adolescence. 3rd ed. New York: Random House Inc., 1975.

Watson, J. B. Psychological care of infant and child. In Stone, L. J., and Church J. Childhood and Adolescence. 3rd ed. New York: Random House Inc., 1975.

Weber, R. D. Informed consent—a misunderstood basis of professional liability. J. Mich. Dent. Assoc. 69:163, 1987.

Wright, G. Z. Behavior Management in Dentistry for Children. Philadelphia: W. B. Saunders Co., 1975.

Wright, G. Z., Alpern, G. D., and Leake, J. L. The modificability of maternal anxiety as it relates to children's cooperative dental behavior. J. Dent. Child. 50:13, 1973.

Wright, G.Z., Starkey, P. E., and Gardner, D. E. Managing Children's Behavior in the Dental Office. St. Louis: The C. V. Mosby Co., 1983, pp. 42-45.

Questions

1. Health history questionnaires:
   a. Are not intended to provide a comprehensive medical assessment
   b. Focus attention on particular factors that might influence direction of dental care
   c. Cannot alone be designed to ensure validity and must be reviewed through personal interview
   d. Are structured to provide information on the personal history, medical history, dental history, behavioral history, and home dental care of the patient in an orderly and functional design
   e. All of the above

2. The sequence of calcification of the primary teeth during the second trimester where A = central incisor, B = lateral incisor, C = canine, D = first molar, and E = second molar is:
   a. A, B, C, D, E
   b. A, B, D, C, E
   c. A, C, B, D, E
   d. A, D, B, C, E
   e. None of the above

3. Eruption of the primary teeth occur over approximately a 2-year period from 8 to 30 months of age. Sequence of eruption follows which of the following patterns where A = central incisors, B = lateral incisor, C = canine, D = first molar, and E = second molar?
   a. A, B, C, D, E
   b. A, B, D, C, E
   c. A, C, B, D, E
   d. A, D, B, C, E
   e. None of the above

4. A 7-year old boy is seen in your office for dental care. Unfortunately, he has cerebral palsy. The mother gives a history of anoxia at birth, plus respiratory trouble for 3 weeks postnatally. Your oral examination and radiographs reveal several teeth with areas of hypoplasia. What teeth could be hypopolastic due to the anoxia and respiratory distress?
   a. All the primary teeth
   b. Primary first and second molars
   c. Primary centrals and laterals
   d. Primary canines
   e. First permanent molars
   f. b, d, and e
   g. b and c
   h. a and e
   i. b and e
   j. b, c, and d

5. Carlos, age 4, is in the reception area with his parent. It is his first dental visit. Carlos's behavior in the operatory will be primary influenced by factors in his environment. Which factor do you consider influential?
   a. Sibling influence
   b. How well the prospects of the dental visit were managed at home
   c. How much concern and care dental and staff personnel extend him

6a. According to Stone and Church's development classification, Carlos, age 4, would be classified developmentally as a(n):
   a. Toddler
   b. Preschooler
   c. Middle-years child
   d. Adolescent

6b. Based on this classification, do you expect Carlos to be:
   a. Fully cooperative
   b. Somewhat immature

7. Jimmy is just now 2 years old. Mother has him to the dentist to examine an area of oral development she is concerned about. Jimmy's reception room behavior is that of the active, happy, hustle-bustle type of preschooler. Most likely his behavioral response to the oral assessment will be:
   a. Definitely negative by the Frankl et al scale
   b. Negative by the Frankl et al scale
   c. Positive by the Frankl et al scale
   d. Positive toward modeling
   e. Positive to effective communication
   f. d,e
   g. c,e
   h. c,d

Chapter 2

Occlusal Assessment

Objectives

After studying this chapter, the student should be able to:
1. Assess the normal occlusal relationships of the primary, mixed and permanent dentitions.
2. Define terms used in assessing the occlusion of children.
3. Recognize the various arch forms in the primary and permanent dentitions.
4. Diagnose factors contributing to abnormal arch form development.
5. Discuss the ramifications of spacing and crowding in the primary and permanent dentitions.
6. Identify the canine and molar relationships in the primary, mixed, and permanent dentitions.
7. Describe the analytical methods available to assess potential growth patterns of the child.

The review of the facial profile and occlusion is an essential component of the overall assessment of the child. This extraoral and intraoral evaluation of the child begins with the primary dentition and continues through the transition (the mixed) dentition and the permanent dentition.

Deviation from the "normal" in tooth form, occlusion, and function in the presence of a dentofacial disharmony is considered a malocclusion. This includes single- or multiple-tooth malpositions, tooth-jaw size discrepancies, and severe skeletal abnormalities. A simple, but complete, system can be used to classify the three major classes of malocclusion:

1. Skeletal malocclusions are caused by abnormal maxillary and mandibular osseous relationships. These can be differences in size, shape, growth patterns, or proportions of the facial bony structures. Genetic patterns are a factor. This disharmony between the bones of the maxilla and mandible is the main factor in severe malocclusions.

2. Dental malocclusions are caused by a disparity within the dentition and the supporting alveolar bones structures: missing or extra teeth, or teeth of abnormal size.

3. Muscular malocclusions are caused by persistent abnormal malfunctions of the orofacial musculature. Thumb habits, lip sucking, or tongue thrusting are problems.

Clinical examination

The following is a step-by-step clinical examination method formulated to assess the developing occlusion of the child (Currier, 1992; AAPD, 1993).

Step 1: Facial view (Fig 2-1)

Viewing the child from both the front and the side, note the following:

1. Facial symmetry. Does the patient have a pleasing smile?
2. The facial profile. Is it straight, convex, or concave?
3. The size of the nose and chin.
4. The position of the lip at rest. Is the child a mouth breather? Is the child a tongue thruster with a hyperactive mentalis muscle? Is the upper lip short?

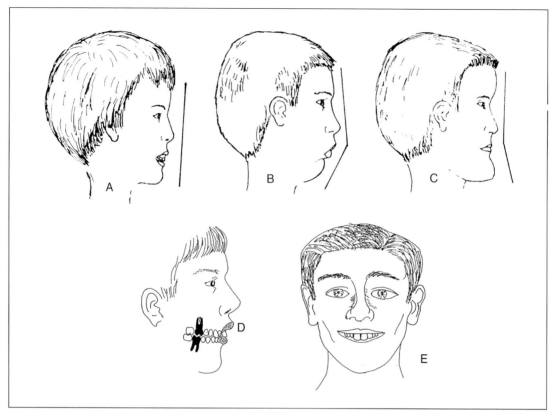

Fig 2-1   The facial profiles of children from the lateral and front views: *(A)* straight; *(B)* convex; *(C)* concave; *(D)* skeletal Class II profile; *(E)* frontal view of Class II profile showing maxillary overjet.

Step 2: Maxillary and mandibular arches

1. Arch form. Are the arches ovoid, square, or tapered? Are they symmetrically spaced? Is there crowding or spacing of teeth in the anterior or posterior segments?

   a. In the *primary dentition*, there is often generalized spacing of the anterior teeth. In the maxillary arch, this space can be mesial to the maxillary canine. In the mandibular arch, the space is distal to mandibular canine. These specific spaces are referred to as the *primate spaces*. In the primary dentition, lack of spacing can be caused by wider-than-average primary teeth or a narrow, smaller maxillary or mandibular arch.

   b. In the *permanent dentition*, teeth that are larger than average contribute to crowding. Large teeth with insufficient bone support often are caused by germination of fusion of teeth (Fig 2-2a). Factors causing spacing are malposed or smaller teeth or even congenitally missing teeth (Fig 2-2b).

2. Anomalies of position. (See Chapter 3 for an explanation of etiology. Chapter 23 describes treatment methods.)

   a. *Ectopic eruption*, usually of the permanent maxillary first molar, is a sign of maxillary arch length deficiency (Fig 2-2c).

   b. *Ankylosis* of primary molars and, rarely, permanent teeth can contribute to loss of arch length and form (Fig 2-2d).

   c. *Impaction* of permanent teeth, if not detected, can cause difficult corrective problems and alterations of arch length and form.

   d. *Over-retained* primary teeth or *supernumerary* teeth can disrupt the normal sequence of eruption of permanent teeth (Fig 2-2e).

3. Sequelae to dental caries.

   a. When *interproximal dental caries* is untreated, mesial drift of the primary molars reduces arch length. This lost arch length is difficult, if not impossible, to regain (Fig 2-2f).

   b. *Premature loss* of primary teeth to dental caries causes tipping and drifting of posterior permanent teeth (Fig 2-2g).

4. Sequelae to trauma. Is there space loss or change in arch length because of avulsed teeth (Fig 2-2h)?

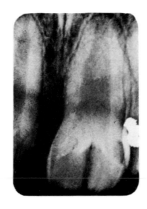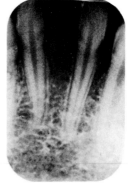

Fig 2-2a A geminated tooth in the permanent dentition exhibits a wider mesiodistal expanse and therefore demands more space in the arch.

Fig 2-2b Congenitally missing permanent mandibular central incisors. The spacing in this instance not only is an arch length factor but also is a cosmetic consideration.

Fig 2-2a   Fig 2-2b

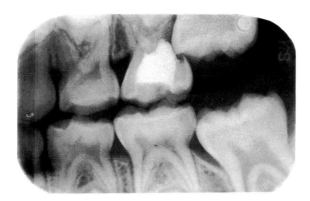

Fig 2-2c Ectopic eruption of a maxillary first permanent molar. Unless this is corrected by redirecting the permanent molar in a more normal eruptive pattern, valuable space will be lost.

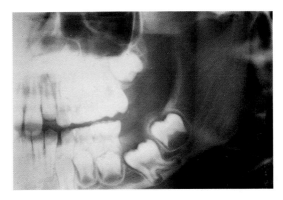

Fig 2-2d Ankylosis of a permanent first molar creates arch length and development problems.

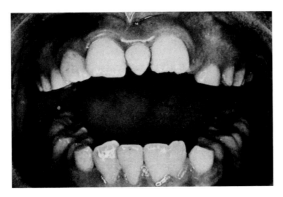

Fig 2-2e The mesiodens in this instance has created a lateral displacement of the permanent maxillary central incisors and a loss of arch length.

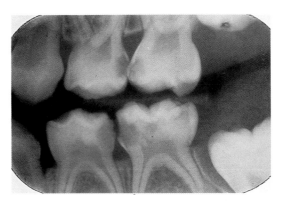

Fig 2-2f Because of interproximinal caries in the maxillary arch, the primary maxillary second molar has drifted mesially.

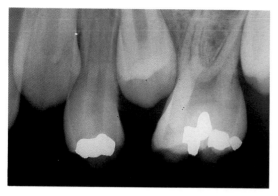

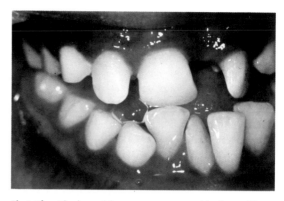

Fig 2-2g Premature loss of the primary second molar, without space maintenance, has resulted in mesial drift of the permanent first molar impacting the second premolar.

Fig 2-2h The loss of the permanent central incisor, without maintenance of the space, has caused space loss and a difficult choice of restoration.

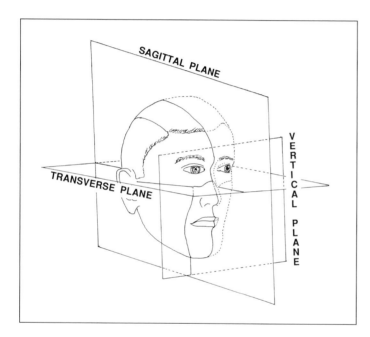

Fig 2-3a The orthogonal review of occlusion evaluates the face and occlusion in the transverse, sagittal, and vertical planes.

From the examination of the maxillary and mandibular arches, the examiner should be able to answer the following questions:

1. Is there a tooth-arch size discrepancy?
2. Are there factors adversely influencing arch size or length?
3. Do the maxillary and mandibular arches have "normal" growth patterns?

Step 3: Orthogonal review of occlusion (Bjork et al, 1964) (Fig 2-3a)

Transverse plane (Fig 2-3b)

1. Are the midlines in line with the middle of the face? View the child from the front. Is the midline of the maxillary or mandibular central incisor to the right or left of the midline of the face? Is there a functional shift of the mandible?
2. Does the patient have a posterior crossbite? A posterior crossbite is present when there is an abnormal buccolingual relationship of the primary or permanent molars. This can be unilateral or bilateral, including one or more teeth.

Sagittal plane

1. What is the overjet (in mm)? When the teeth are in occlusion, *overjet* is the distance between the labial surface of the maxillary incisor and the labial surface of the mandibular incisors (Fig 2-3c).
2. Are the anterior teeth in crossbite? Simple anterior crossbites are caused by abnormal inclinations of the maxillary anterior teeth. Or the mandibular incisors may be in a labial inclination (see Fig 2-3b).

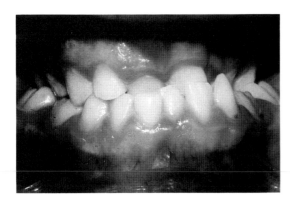

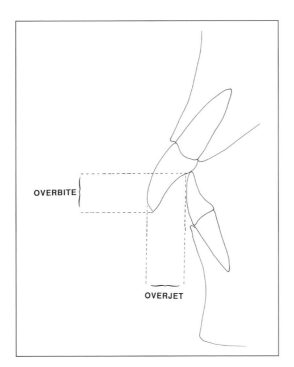

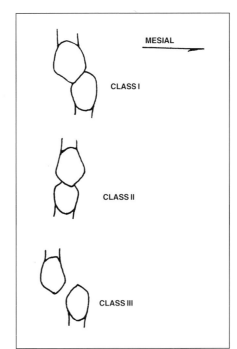

Fig 2-3b This child has anterior crossbite, bilateral posterior crossbites, and a midline deviation.

Fig 2-3c Overjet in the sagittal plane; overbite in the vertical plane.

Fig 2-3d Canine relationships.

3. What is the primary or permanent canine relationship?
   a. Class I relationship (Fig 2-3d):

      In the *primary dentition,* the cusp tip of the maxillary canine is in the embrasure between the mandibular canine and the mandibular first molar.

      In the *permanent dentition,* the cusp tip of the maxillary canine is the embrasure between the mandibular canine and the mandibular first premolar.
   b. Class II relationship:

      In the *primary dentition,* the cusp tip of the maxillary canine is in the embrasure between the mandibular canine and the mandibular lateral incisor.

      In the *permanent dentition,* the relationships are similar, substituting permanent for primary teeth.
   c. Class III relationship:

      In the *primary dentition,* the maxillary canine is distal to the embrasure between the mandibular canine and the mandibular first molar.

      In the *permanent dentition,* the maxillary canine is distal to the embrasure between the mandibular canine and mandibular first premolar.
   d. An "in-between" status can occur in the canine relationship in the primary and permanent dentitions; this is referred to as an end-to-end occlusion.

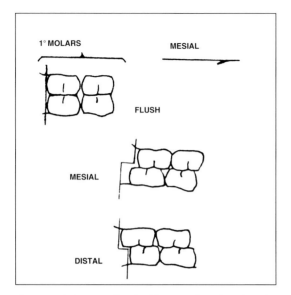

Fig 2-3e Primary molar classifications, based on the relationship of the distal surfaces of the primary second molar.

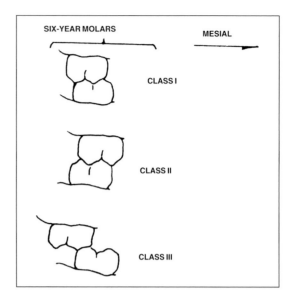

Fig 2-3f Classification of the permanent first molars.

Vertical Plane (Fig 2-3e, 2-3f)

1. What is the overbite? When the teeth are in occlusion, *overbite* is the distance the edges of the maxillary incisors close vertically past the edges of the mandibular incisors (see Fig 2-3c). Overbite is often expressed as the percentage of the mandibular crowns covered by the crowns of the maxillary incisors. If the overbite is excessive, with the mandibular incisors touching the hard palate, it is an *impinging* overbite.
2. Is there an open bite?
   a. An *anterior open bite* is the reverse of an overbite, with lack of occlusion of anterior teeth.
   b. A *posterior open bite* is the lack of occlusion of the posterior teeth. However, such an occlusion is rare.

Step 4: Oral habits

1. Do the parents express concern about the child's oral habits?
2. What habits are observed such as finger, thumb, or blanket sucking? lip sucking? nail biting? teeth grinding or bruxism? tongue thrusting? mouth breathing? Are the tonsils and adenoids present?
3. Does the child exhibit speech disorders? Does the child see a speech therapist?

Step 5: Temporomandibular joint

View the child from the front. Have the child open and close and note the following:

1. Is there a deviation of the mandible to the right or left?
2. Is there a "clicking" noise?
3. Does the patient have discomfort on opening and closing?

Additional aids to occlusal assessment

1. Completed clinical examination record
2. Current radiographs: bitewings; necessary periapicals; panoramic
3. Trimmed study casts
4. Boley gauge and flexible millimeter ruler
5. Mixed dentition analysis prediction charts

Use of radiographs

Bitewing radiographs. Note and record any interproximal carious lesions. Has there been arch length loss? Make special note of those carious lesions that may cause pulpal involvement.

Panoramic radiographs. Note any radiographic anomalies. Check for any evidence of oral pathoses. Are there impactions or malposed teeth? Are there any extra or missing teeth?

Analysis of the study casts

Study casts are used for additional data and not as a substitute for a thorough clinical assessment (Fig 2-4).

The study casts are trimmed in centric occlusion and studied systemically. The casts should be measured and observed for the following (Nanda, 1993):

1. Occlusion—both molar and canine relationships
2. Tooth alignment
3. Arch form
4. Midline alignment
5. Overbite and overjet
6. Posterior and anterior crossbites
7. General arch form and symmetry
8. Rotated or malposed teeth

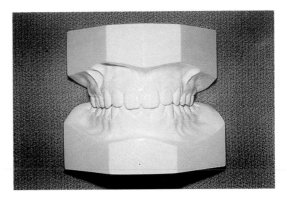

Fig 2-4 Properly, well-trimmed dental casts are an aid to occlusal assessment of the child.

The mixed dentition analysis

After completion of the dental cast review, depending on the age of the patient, a mixed dentition analysis can be completed. Inadequate space for permanent teeth is one of the most common causes of orthodontic problems. An early assessment of available space may permit early intervention or minimize the development of malocclusions. The objective of the mixed dentition analysis is to try to answer the question: "Is there enough room for the unerupted permanent teeth?" Evaluation of the size of the unerupted canines and premolars is an important factor in the assessment of the child's occlusion. The mixed dentition, which has both primary and permanent teeth, usually lasts from ages 6 to 12 years. Indications for a mixed dentition analysis are (1) premature loss of primary canines; (2) rotation or blocking of lateral incisors because of lost space; (3) ectopic eruption of permanent first molars; (4) distal terminal plane relationships; and (5) crossbites (Nanda, 1993).

The mixed dentition analysis is based on the following principles (Fields and Profitt, 1988):

1. The first permanent molars and permanent incisors and erupted.
2. The succedaneous permanent teeth are forming.
3. There is a size relationship between the unerupted permanent teeth and primary teeth.
4. There is size differential between the primary canines and molars and the succedaneous teeth. The mesiodistal widths of the primary canines and molars are greater than the widths of the permanent successors. Nance referred to this tooth size differential as the leeway space. This difference is estimated to be 0.9 mm per quadrant in the maxilla and 1.7 mm per quadrant in the mandible (Fig 2-5).

Methods for mixed dentition analysis

Hays Nance Analysis

Armamentarium
Dental casts

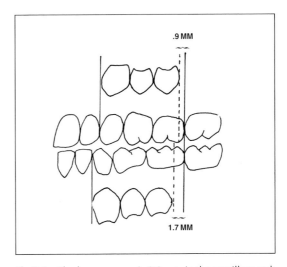

Fig 2-5 The leeway space is 0.9 mm in the maxillary arch and 1.7 mm in the mandibular arch.

Boley gauge, millimeter ruler
Periapical radiographs
Cephalometric radiograph with tracing and Tweed analysis

Procedure (Nanda, 1993)
1. Use the Boley gauge to record the maximum width of each permanent and primary maxillary and mandibular tooth from the permanent first molar. Record these dimensions on the Hays Nance form.
2. From the periapical radiographs, measure the maximum mesiodistal widths of the unerupted canines and premolars.
3. Use a radiographic measurement formula to correct for radiographic magnification and actual tooth size measurements.
4. A cephalometric analysis, using Tweed's analysis, is essential. This allows for correction of the protrusion of mandibular incisors.

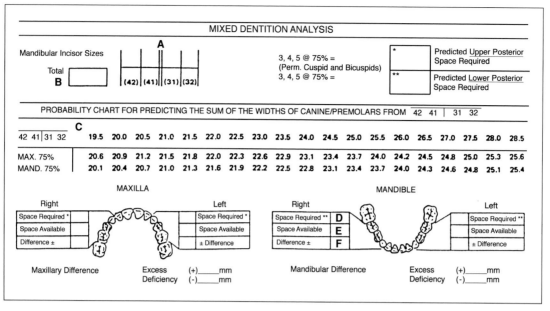

Fig 2-6 Example of a chart used to record data for the Moyers mixed dentition analysis. (From the University of Oklahoma, College of Dentistry, Department of Orthodontics.)

Advantages
1. It results in minimal error.
2. It can be performed with reliability.
3. It allows analysis of both arches.

Limitations
1. It requires a cephlometric radiograph, knowledge of the Tweed analysis, and an accurate tracing.
2. It is time consuming.
3. Complete-mouth radiographs are needed.

Moyers Analysis

Armamentarium
Dental casts
Boley gauge
Probability chart

Procedure (Moyers, 1973)
1. Measurements of the permanent mandibular incisors are used to predict the space needed for the maxillary and mandibular succedaneous teeth. Use a Boley gauge to measure the greatest mesiodistal width of each of the four mandibular incisors. The values are recorded on the mixed dentition analysis form (Fig 2-6A).
2. From step 1, total the mesiodistal widths of the mandibular incisors (Fig 2-6B). Use the prediction chart for the space available in the mandibular arch (Fig 2-6C). Using the probability chart (75% level), locate the value closest to the sum of the four mandibular incisors. This value gives a prediction of the sums of the widths of the canines and premolars (at the 75% level of confidence). Mark this value on the form as the mandibular space required for the right and left sides (Fig 2-6D).
3. On the study cast, determine and mark the midline of the mandibular arch.
4. Total the mesiodistal widths of the right mandibular incisors and set the Boley gauge to this value. Measure from the midline to the right side. Place one point of the gauge at the midline between the central incisors and let the other end lie along the line of the dental arch on the right side. Mark on the cast the precise point where the distal tip of the Boley gauge touched. Repeat the process for the left side.
5. Compute the amount of space available. Measure the distance from the point marked on the cast (step 4) to the mesial surface of the permanent first molar. Record that value (Fig. 2-6E) and calculate space difference (Fig. 2-6F).
6. Repeat the process for the maxillary arch using the prediction table for maxillary tooth size.

Advantages
1. It results in minimal error.
2. It is not a time-consuming procedure.
3. No special equipment is needed.
4. It can be used for maxillary and mandibular arches.

Limitations
1. The Moyer's analysis is a probability diagnosis.
2. The Moyer's analysis does not account for tipping of the mandibular incisor, either lingually or facially.
3. There is not a high correlation of size between different groups of teeth.

4. The maxillary tooth size is predicted from mandibular tooth size.

Hixon-Oldfather Analysis

Armamentarium
Boley gauge
Study casts
Periapical radiographs
Hixon-Oldfather prediction chart

Procedure (Staley and Kerber, 1980)
1. From the casts, on one side, measure the mesiodistal widths of the permanent mandibular central and lateral incisors.
2. From the periapical radiographs, measure the mesiodistal width of the unerupted first and second premolars.
3. Total the mesiodistal widths of the four (4) incisor teeth. Compare the measured value to estimated tooth size from the Hixon-Oldfather chart.
4. Repeat steps 1 to 3 for the other side of the arch.

Advantages
1. Only study casts and periapical radiographs are needed.
2. It has a coefficient of correlation of .87, or 75% reliability. It is a very accurate analysis.

Limitations
1. The technique can only be used for the mandibular arch.

Tanaka-Johnston Analysis

Armamentarium
Boley gauge
Study casts

Procedure (Tanaka and Johnson, 1974)
1. From the permanent first molar on one side, mark the distances on the casts in segments to the permanent first molar on the opposite side. Measure these segments over the contact points.
2. Add the measurements from step 1 to determine the total arch circumference.
3. Measure the mesiodistal widths of the mandibular central and lateral incisors.
4. Subtract this total from the arch circumference measurement.
5. Divide the sum of the widths of the mandibular incisors and add 10.5 mm.
6. This total gives the estimated size of the mandibular canine and the two premolars for one quadrant.
7. Double the total in step 6 for the canines and four premolars in the mandibular arch.
8. Subtract this dimension from the remaining space available in the arch to give a positive or negative for total arch space.

9. For the maxillary arch, repeat the process. However, instead of adding 10.5 mm to the widths of the mandibular incisors, add 11.0 mm to the sum.

Advantages
1. Improving on Moyer's analysis, it is a relatively accurate for children of European ancestry.
2. The technique involves simple, easily repeated procedures and minimal material needs.
3. It does not use prediction charts.

Limitations
1. There may be an error in the predicted size of the unerupted teeth if patients are not of northwestern European descent.

Summary

The clinical examination record plus data from cast analysis and radiographs can be used to make a preliminary assessment of the child's occlusal status. The data can be used to advise the parents of the child's growth potential and possible developmental problems; determine the need for further evaluation and additional data; and make a referral to a specialist specifically trained to manage the more complicated growth and development problems of the craniofacial complex.

Acknowledgment

Jack B. Austerman, DDS, MS, Department of Orthodontics, College of Dentistry, University of Oklahoma for reviewing this chapter.

References

American Academy of Pediatric Dentistry (AAP). Reference Manual. Chicago: AAP, 1993.

Bjork A., Krobs, A. A., and Solow, B. A method for epidemiological registration of malocclusion. Acta. Odontol. Scand. 22:27, 1964.

Currier, G. F. Working Manual for Didactic Orthodontics. Vol 1. Oklahoma City: Oklahoma University Press, 1992.

Fields, H. W., and Profitt, W. R. Diagnosis and treatment planning for orthodontic problems. Wei, S.H.Y. In Pediatric Dentistry. Philadelphia: Lea & Febiger, 1988.

Moyers, R. E. Handbook of Orthodontics. Chicago: Year Book Medical Publishers, Inc., 1973.

Nanda, R. S. Basics of Undergraduate Orthodontics. Oklahoma City: Oklahoma University Press, 1993.

Staley, R. N., and Kerber, P. E. A revision of the Hixon and Oldfather mixed-dentition prediction method. Am. J. Orthod. 78:296, 1980.

Tanaka, M. M., and Johnston L. E. The prediction of the size of unerupted canines and premolars in a contemporary orthodontic population. J. Am. Dent. Assoc. 88:798, 1974.

Questions

1. In the primary dentition, the primate space is located _____ to the canine in the maxillary arch, and if present, is located _____ to the canine in the mandibular arch.

2. The leeway space as determined by Nance refers to size differences between primary teeth and their successors. In the maxillary arch, this is _____ mm per quadrant, while in the mandibular arch this is _____ mm per quadrant.

3. In the primary dentition, the anatomic structure used to determine the molar relationship is:

   a. The mesiobuccal cusp of the primary second molar
   b. The distobuccal cusp of the primary first molar
   c. The distal plane of the primary second molars
   d. The mesiobuccal cusp of the primary second molar and the embrasure between the primary mandibular first and second molars.

4. What are the indications for a mixed dentition analysis?

   a. Ectopic eruption of permanent first molars
   b. Anterior and/or posterior crossbites
   c. Rotated or blocked out lateral incisors
   d. A distal relationship of the primary second molars
   e. All of the above

5. Evaluation of Susan, a 5-year-old child, reveals that the distal surface of the primary maxillary second molar is mesial to the distal surface of the primary mandibular second molar. This primary molar classification is referred to as:

   a. Class I
   b. Class II
   c. Class III
   d. Distal plane (or step)
   e. Mesial plane (or step)

Chapter 3

Radiographic Assessment

Objectives

After studying this chapter, the student should be able to:
1. Understand how to initiate and complete a radiographic survey for children.
2. Identify the type of film and specific survey for any child.
3. Use the indicated technique, dependent on the age of the child and caries activity, with the optimum number of films.
4. Be aware of the appropriate radiation safeguards to reduce unnecessary radiation exposure.
5. Review normal radiographs as well as those with errors in technique.

Radiographic examination of children should occur only after the following conditions are met:

1. Obtainment of previous radiographic history (to assess the availability of recent films from another dentist)
2. Clinical examination of the patient
3. Determination of appropriate number and size of films required
4. Placement of lead apron and thyroid collar on the patient (Sikorski and Taylor, 1984)

To increase the safety of the child, the dentist should not attempt retakes or duplicate views. It is essential that diagnostic radiographs be obtained on the first attempt.

Radiographs of acceptable diagnostic quality should meet particular standards. They should:

1. Follow the appropriate guidelines for the correct size, number, and type of film used at the appropriate time for the child's stage of occlusion.
2. Include the distal surface of the canine to the mesial surface of the most distal tooth for bitewing radiographs.
3. Include an unobstructed view of all contact areas (for bitewing radiographs) and periapical regions (for periapical radiographs).
4. Not be cone cut, overlapped, elongated, or shortened.
5. Be of proper exposure and should be correctly developed.

Radiographic indications and safety

A child with a low risk to dental caries may be defined as a normally healthy asymptomatic patient (no evidence of caries, trauma, anomalies, or malocclusion), exposed to optimal levels of fluoride (preferably since birth), performing daily preventive techniques, and consuming a diet with few exposures to retentive carbohydrates between meals.

The low-risk patient with closed proximal contacts should have posterior bitewing radiographs taken. If no caries is found, radiographs may be retaken every 12 months if the primary teeth are in contact or up to every 24 months if the permanent teeth are in contact. Bitewing radiographs may be taken more frequently if the child enters the high-risk category.

The child with a high risk to dental caries should have bitewing radiographs made as soon as the posterior primary teeth are in proximal contact. The age of the patient is not an important variable. If interproximal caries is detected, follow-up radiographs are indicated semiannually until the child is caries free and, therefore, is classified as having a low risk to dental caries (Fig 3-1) (Nowak et al, 1981; Nowak, 1982; AAPD, 1993).

Regardless of risk level, all pediatric patients should receive two panoramic radiographs—one at the early mixed dentition and one at the late mixed dentition—to diagnose undetected pathologic conditions. After eruption of the first permanent tooth, occlusal views should be taken.

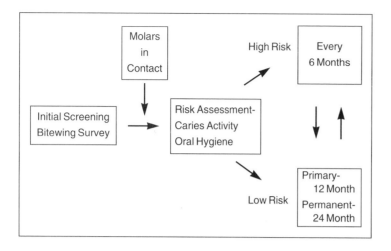

Fig 3-1 Radiographic indications.

If the patient is asymptomatic with open proximal contacts, radiographs can be delayed until the patient becomes symptomatic or reaches the appropriate age for occlusal or panoramic survey.

In 1988, a panel of various representatives from dentistry developed recommendations for radiologic examination of children and adolescents (Guidelines for Prescribing Dental Radiographs, 1988). These recommendations are based on three concepts (Table 3-1):

1. Categorize patients by type of visit: new patient or recall visit.
2. Define patients by dental status.
3. Categorize patients based on presence or absence of certain conditions.

The panel concluded that the use of the recommendations would result in fewer radiographs for the low-risk group. However, the high-risk group may have more radiographic exposures.

Postoperative radiographs will be taken only to (1) evaluate pulp treatment (periapically) and (2) diagnose new undetected carious lesions (bitewing radiographs) if a 6-month interval has occurred since the original treatment plan.

Myers (1984) listed the reasons why children are at a higher risk from radiation exposure than are adults:

1. The tissues of the child are in the growth period and are more sensitive to radiation.
2. Children have a longer life span with greater susceptibility to tumors.
3. The effects of radiation are cumulative.
4. Because of their smaller stature, children are closer to the central x-ray beam.
5. Because of carious activity, children may have an increased frequency of radiographs.

An excellent review of radiation safety for children has been presented by White (1982).

Child preparation and management

The importance of radiographs in dentistry for children needs no elaboration. It is important to realize that the taking of radiographs often is part of a child's first dental experience. If it is to be remembered as a pleasant experience, it must be done efficiently. Explain the procedure in terms the child can understand. Use such words as "picture" and "camera," not "roentgenogram" and "x-ray machine." In explaining to a young child, it is sometimes wise to bring the "camera" into contact with your own face to help dispel any fears the child may have. Allow the patients to inspect and touch the film packet before it is placed in the mouth. A good idea is to have the x-ray tube set at the needed angulation and placed next to the child's face, then all that remains is to gently insert the film.

Some tips to assist in the radiographic process are:

1. If a child has a tendency to reject the film, dampen (but do not saturate) the film packet. Such dampening takes away some of the taste of the packet.
2. Do not insert the packet directly but placed the film in a horizontal plane. Then, as the film is placed between the tongue and lingual surface of the teeth, it can be gently rotated into a vertical position. This approach works especially well with bitewing films (Fig 3-2a).
3. Before inserting the film, curve it slightly so that it does not impinge on the lingual tissue. Often it is also necessary to bend the lower anterior corner to prevent forcing the film into the floor of the mouth (Fig 3-2b). Such forcing is uncomfortable and may cause the patient to reject the film.

Table 3-1 Recommendations for radiologic dental examination of children and adolescents*

Patient category	Child		Adolescent
	Primary dentition (*prior to eruption of first permanent tooth*)	Transitional dentition (*following eruption of first permanent tooth*)	Permanent dentition (*prior to eruption of third molars*)
New patient† All new patients to assess dental diseases and growth and development	Posterior bitewing examination if proximal surfaces of primary teeth cannot be visualized or probed	Individualized radiographic examination consisting of periapical/occlusal views and posterior bitewings or panoramic examination and posterior bitewings	Individualized radiographic examination consisting of posterior bitewings and selected periapicals. A complete-mouth intraoral radiographic examination is appropriate when the patient presents with clinical evidence of generalized dental disease or a history of extensive dental treatment.
Recall patient† Clinical caries or high-risk factors for caries‡	Posterior bitewing examination at 6-month intervals or until no carious lesions are evident		Posterior bitewing examination at 6- to 12-month intervals or until no carious lesions are evident
No clinical caries and no high-risk factors for caries‡	Posterior bitewing examination at 12- to 24-month intervals if proximal surfaces of primary teeth cannot be visualized or probed	Posterior bitewing examination at 12- to 24-month intervals	Posterior bitewing examination at 18- to 36-month intervals
Periodontal disease or a history of periodontal treatment	Individualized radiographic examination consisting of selected periapical and/or bitewing radiographs for areas where periodontal disease (other than nonspecific gingivitis) can be demonstrated clinically		Individualized radiographic examination consisting of selected periapical and/or bitewing radiographs for areas where periodontal disease (other than nonspecific gingivitis) can be demonstrated clinically
Growth and development assessment	Usually not indicated	Individualized radiographic examination consisting of a periapical/occlusal or panoramic examination	Periapical or panoramic examination to assess developing third molars

*Adapted from Guidelines for Prescribing Dental Radiographs, publication No. N-80A, Eastman Kodak, 1988.

†Clinical situations for which radiographs may be indicated include:

A. Positive historical findings
1. Previous periodontal or endodontic therapy
2. History of pain or trauma
3. Familial history of dental anomalies
4. Postoperative evaluation of healing

B. Positive clinical signs/symptoms
1. Clinical evidence of periodontal disease
2. Large or deep restorations
3. Deep carious lesions
4. Malposed or clinically impacted teeth
5. Swelling
6. Evidence of facial trauma
7. Mobility of teeth
8. Fistula or sinus tract infection
9. Clinically suspected sinus pathosis
10. Growth abnormalities
11. Oral involvement in known or suspected systemic disease
12. Positive neurologic findings in the head and neck
13. Evidence of foreign objects
14. Pain and/or dysfunction of the temporomandibular joint
15. Facial asymmetry
16. Abutment teeth for fixed or removable partial prosthesis
17. Unexplained bleeding
18. Unexplained sensitivity of teeth
19. Unusual eruption, spacing, or migration of teeth
20. Unusual tooth morphology, calcification, or color
21. Missing teeth with unknown reason

‡Patients at high risk for caries may demonstrate any of the following:
1. High level of caries experience
2. History of recurrent caries
3. Existing restoration of poor quality
4. Poor oral hygiene
5. Inadequate fluoride exposure
6. Prolonged nursing (bottle or breast)
7. Diet with high sucrose frequency
8. Poor family dental health
9. Developmental enamel defects
10. Developmental disability
11. Xerostomia
12. Genetic abnormality of teeth
13. Many multisurface restorations
14. Chemo/radiation therapy

As you gain experience, you will develop your own ways of relating to child patients. Always remember to be kind, yet firm; always maintain a positive attitude and complete control of the situation. In taking radiographs of children, as in other procedures of dentistry for children, tell, show, and do.

Film sizes

The various sizes of film are shown in Fig 3-3.

Radiographic techniques

Occlusal views

Because the occlusal views of the primary dentition are the easiest to take, they should be taken first. The

ease of this initial procedure will reassure the patient, establish confidence, and encourage continuing cooperation.

Anterior occlusal films are used to:

1. Determine the presence, shape, and position of midline supernumerary teeth.
2. Determine impaction of canines.
3. Determine the presence or absence of incisors.
4. Assess the extent of trauma to teeth and anterior segments of the arches after accidents (Figs 3-4, 3-5, and 3-13 to 3-15).

Film sizes used are No. 2 for young children through the mixed dentition and anterior occlusal films for children in the late mixed dentition and permanent dentition.

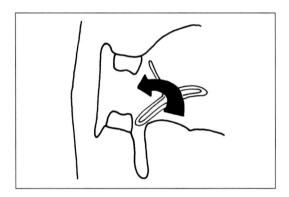

Fig 3-2a By rotating the bitewing radiograph, one can insert the film easily.

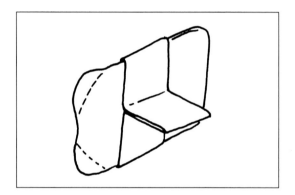

Fig 3-2b In a younger child it may be necessary to fold the film, reducing impingement on the soft tissue.

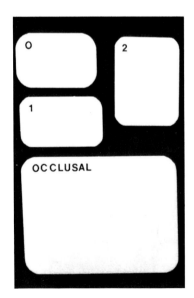

Fig 3-3 Size No. 0 is used for bitewing and periapical radiographs in young children. Size No. 1 is used in somewhat older children to take bitewing and periapical radiographs. Size No. 2 is used for anterior occlusal radiographs, periapical radiographs and bitewing survey in the mixed and permanent dentitions. The occlusal film is used for anterior occlusal views, complete quadrant views, and survey for the handicapped.

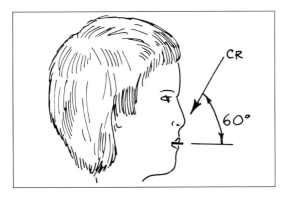

Fig 3-4 Maxillary occlusal radiograph. Seat the child with the occlusal plane parallel to the floor. Carry the film to the open mouth. Place it flat against the maxillary arch, with its long axis side to the side and the edge of the packet at the incisal edge of the teeth. Have the patient merely close the mouth to hold the film between the teeth. Direct the central x-ray beam at a 60° angle downward through the tip of the nose.

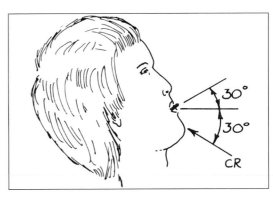

Fig 3-5 Mandibular occlusal radiograph. This film is the second film taken; the angle varies slightly from the maxillary projection. Place the film as in the maxillary arch (but with the shielded side toward the maxillary arch). Position the patient's head so that the occlusal plane is at a 30° angle to the floor. Direct the central ray 30° upward through the apices of the central incisors.

Periapical views of the molar area

For all four molar projections, the film is positioned to include the distal half of the canine (Fig 3-6 to 3-9, 3-17, and 3-18).

Periapical films are used to:

1. Determine root-end condition and environment in young permanent teeth.
2. Evaluate pulp treatment.
3. Detect developmental abnormalities, such as supernumerary, missing, or malformed teeth.
4. Discover pathologic changes associated with primary teeth (periapical rarefaction or internal resorption).
5. Detect alterations in the integrity of the periodontal membrane.
6. Diagnose pulp calcification or root resorption.
7. Analyze space in mixed dentition.

Film sizes used are No. 0 or 1 for younger children and No. 2 for older children.

Bitewing projections

Bitewing projections are usually considered the most difficult views to obtain (Figs 3-10 to 3-12, and 3-16).

Bitewing films are used to:

1. Detect incipient interproximal caries.
2. Determine pulp chamber configuration and depth of carious lesions.
3. Record the width of spaces created by premature loss of primary teeth.

4. Determine the presence or absence of premolar crowns.
5. Determine the relation of the occlusal plane to possible tooth ankylosis.
6. Direct the central beam between the contacts of the primary teeth, not perpendicular to the midline.

Film sizes used are No. 0 or 1 for the younger child and No. 2 for older children.

Canine projections

The techniques described for the occlusal views can be used for the canine projections. Place the film so that the incisal edge of the canine is in the center of the edge of the short axis of the film. For the maxillary canine, direct the central ray toward the ala of the nose at a vertical angulation of 55°, with the occlusal plane parallel to the floor.

For the mandibular canine, elevate the patient's chin so that the occlusal plane forms an angle of 30° with the floor. Direct the central ray upward through the apex of the canine at an angle of 30°. This approach provides a good view of the entire tooth and all its periapical structures, although the view is slightly foreshortened.

Additional surveys

Panoramic radiography is used for handicapped patients and as a substitute for a complete periapical survey, with less accumulative radiation (Figs 3-19, 3-27, and 3-35).

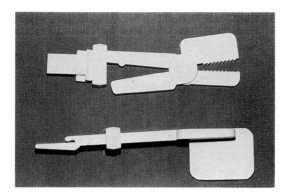

Fig 3-6 The periapical view of each molar area is taken with the aid of the Rinn Snap-A-Ray. This device holds the film and provides a stable surface the patient can bite.

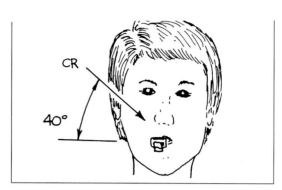

Fig 3-7 Maxillary molar radiograph. Seat the patient with the occlusal plane parallel to the floor. Place the film in the holder and crease the film anteriorly to conform to the curve of the palate. Have the child bite on the plastic platform that holds the film in the mouth. Direct the central ray 40° downward through a point directly below the pupil of the eye.

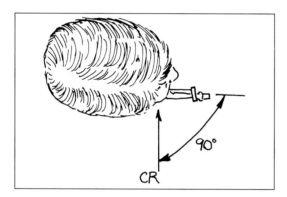

Fig 3-8 The handle of the plastic holder projects from the mouth and provides a reference for establishing the horizontal angulation.

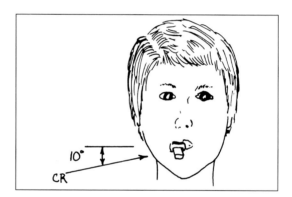

Fig 3-9 Mandibular molar radiograph. Use the Rinn Snap-A-Ray as in the maxillary projection but direct the film downward against the mandibular teeth. Crease the anterior corner of the film to avoid impinging on the floor of the mouth. Direct the central ray at a -10° angle to meet the center of the packet. As in all four molar projections, position the film to include the distal half of the canine.

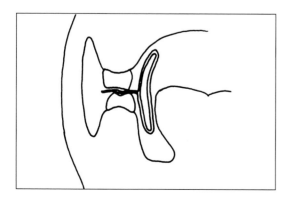

Fig 3-10 A bite-tab is used, and the patients holds the film in the mouth by biting on the projection of the tab.

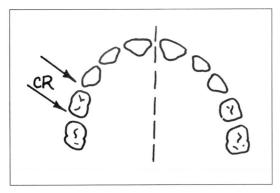

Fig 3-11 The horizontal angulation can be visualized directly by having the patient "smile" while biting on the tab, thus exposing to view the tab and the buccal surfaces of the teeth.

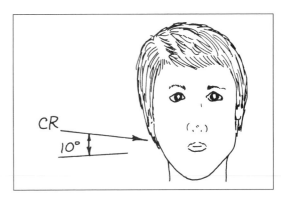

Fig 3-12 Direct the beam vertically at an angulation of 10° through the center of the packet.

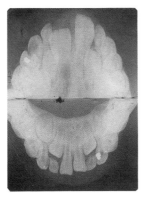

Fig 3-13 Combined occlusal film. Take the large anterior occlusal film. Fold it in half with the lead lining inside. Place the film with the folded portion in the patient's mouth. Position the patient as described for the maxillary anterior view. After exposing the maxillary view, position the patient for the mandibular radiograph, leaving the film in the patient's mouth. Expose the radiograph.

Radiographic diagnosis

Normal findings

Being able to identify normal radiographic landmarks and typical everyday findings in the primary, mixed, and permanent dentitions is the basis for treatment planning in dentistry for children. Following are examples of radiographs of children in the primary, mixed, and early permanent dentitions. Normal radiographic findings are listed by letters corresponding to the letters on the radiographs.

Figures 3-14 to 3-18 represent a radiographic survey of a 3-year-old child. Figure 3-19 is an example of the panoramic view of a child in the primary dentition. The letters illustrate normal anatomic landmarks. Figures 3-20 to 3-27 represent the normal findings of a child in the early mixed dentition. Figures 3-28 to 3-35 are of a child in the early permanent dentition.

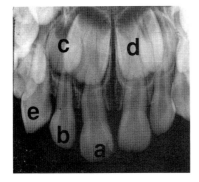

Fig 3-14 Anterior occlusal view shows the maxillary *(a)* primary central incisor, *(b)* primary lateral incisor, *(c)* permanent lateral incisor, *(d)* permanent central incisor, and *(e)* primary canine.

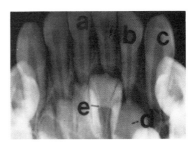

Fig 3-15 Mandibular occlusal view reveals the *(a)* primary central incisor, *(b)* primary lateral incisor, *(c)* primary canine, *(d)* permanent lateral incisor, and *(e)* permanent central incisor and developing root structure.

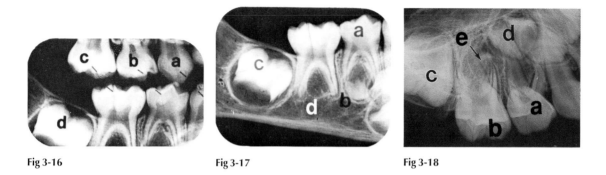

Fig 3-16   Fig 3-17   Fig 3-18

Fig 3-16   Bitewing views are used as the "cavity detecting" film. This bitewing radiograph extends from the distal of the canine to the mesial of the permanent first molar (if erupted): *(a)* primary canines, *(b)* primary first molars, *(c)* primary second molars, and *(d)* developing permanent first molar.

Fig 3-17   The mandibular periapical radiograph is used to check pulp treatment, the developing dentition, and other anomalies: *(a)* primary first molar, *(b)* first premolar in early development, and *(c)* permanent first molar in early development. Note that the second premolar *(d)* has really not given any indication of development. There still is hope at this age.

Fig 3-18   Maxillary periapical view: *(a)* primary first molar, *(b)* primary second molar, *(c)* developing permanent first molar, and *(d)* developing first premolar. Note that the maxillary second premolar *(e)* has not yet developed.

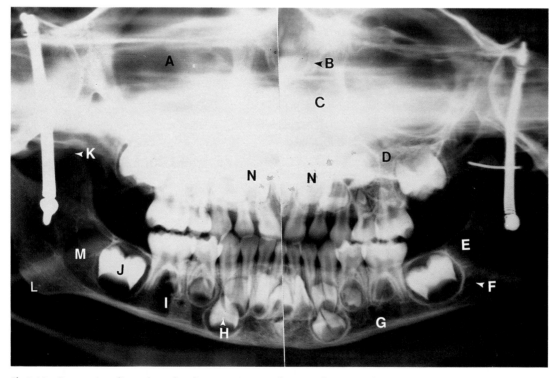

Fig 3-19   Panoramic radiograph used to diagnose missing and extra teeth, gross pathoses, and development of the dentition; diagnosis of caries is difficult. *(A)* Orbit, *(B)* conchae, *(C)* nasal cavity, *(D)* maxillary sinus, *(E)* crypt of permanent second molar, *(F)* mandibular canal, *(G)* mental foramen, *(H)* developing permanent mandibular canine, *(I)* permanent mandibular second premolar, *(J)* first permanent mandibular molar, *(K)* coronal process, *(L)* angle of the mandible, *(M)* artifact, and *(N)* succedaneous maxillary incisors.

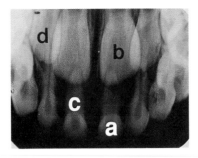

Fig 3-20

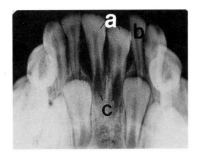

Fig 3-21

Fig 3-20   Maxillary occlusal radiograph shows the maxillary *(a)* primary central incisors, *(b)* permanent central incisors, *(c)* nasopalatine fissure, and *(d)* permanent lateral incisors.

Fig 3-21   Opposing mandibular occlusal radiograph of *(a)* permanent central incisor; *(b)* primary lateral incisor; and *(c)* open apices of permanent central incisors, which are normal for this age.

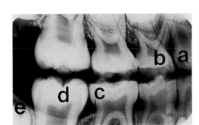

Fig 3-22

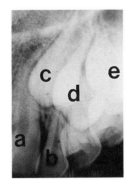

Fig 3-23

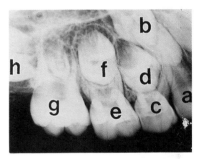

Fig 3-24

Fig 3-22   The bitewing radiograph defines the following: *(a)* primary canine, *(b)* primary first molar, *(c)* cervical burnout of primary mandibular second molar, *(d)* erupted permanent molar, and *(e)* developing crown of permanent mandibular second molar.

Fig 3-23   The canine view is important at this stage of development. The canine has a tendency to become horizontally impacted; to correct this is a major undertaking. Note the missing permanent lateral incisor. Maxillary canine radiograph shows *(a)* permanent maxillary central incisor, *(b)* primary lateral incisor, *(c)* permanent canine, *(d)* permanent first premolar, and *(e)* permanent second premolar.

Fig 3-24   Maxillary periapical radiograph of a 6-year-old child shows *(a)* primary canine, *(b)* permanent canine, *(c)* primary first molar, *(d)* permanent first premolar, *(e)* primary second molar, *(f)* developing second premolar, *(g)* developing first molar, and *(h)* developing permanent second molar. Interest should be focused on *d* and *f*. The first and second premolars are developing at this age.

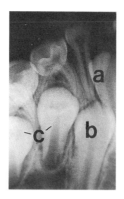

Fig 3-25

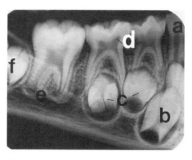

Fig 3-26

Fig 3-25 Mandibular canine view. The mandibular canines do not tend to become impacted as do their maxillary counterparts. They still should be checked periodically. *(a)* Erupting lateral incisor, *(b)* unerupted canine, and *(c)* permanent first and second premolars.

Fig 3-26 Mandibular periapical radiograph showing the *(a)* primary canine, *(b)* permanent canine, *(c)* permanent premolars, *(d)* primary molars, *(e)* open apices of permanent first molars (normal for this age), and *(f)* developing permanent second molars.

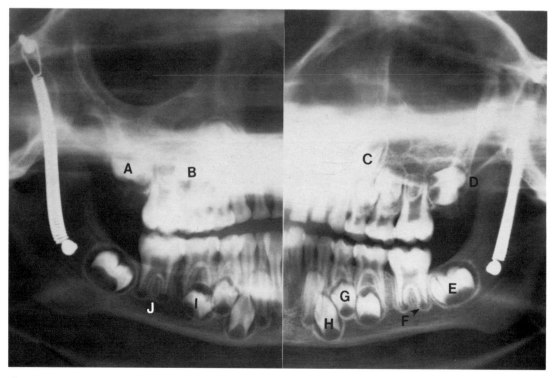

Fig 3-27 Excellent panoramic radiograph of the mixed dentition. Note the developing teeth—the erupted mandibular incisors and permanent first molars. This is the time to begin to watch the position of the canines to intercept impactions, a difficult situation (even for the orthodontist). *(a)* Permanent maxillary second molar, *(b)* permanent maxillary second premolar, *(c)* permanent maxillary canine, *(d)* maxillary tuberosity with the permanent maxillary second molar, *(e)* permanent mandibular second molar, *(f)* open apices of permanent first molar, *(g)* permanent mandibular first premolar, *(h)* permanent mandibular canine, *(i)* permanent mandibular second premolar, and *(j)* skull artifact.

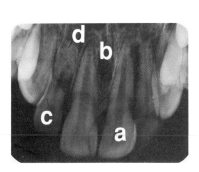

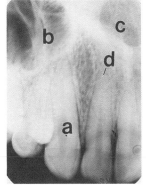

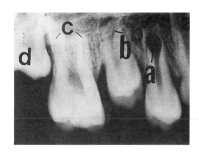

Fig 3-28

Fig 3-29

Fig 3-30

Fig 3-28 Maxillary occlusal radiograph of a 12-year-old patient reveals *(a)* permanent central incisor, *(b)* nasopalatine fissure, *(c)* permanent lateral incisor, and *(d)* apices closed on both central and lateral incisors.

Fig 3-29 View of the canine area. The permanent canine has erupted into normal position: *(a)* canine, *(b)* antrum, *(c)* nares, and *(d)* curved apex of the lateral incisor.

Fig 3-30 Maxillary periapical view: *(a)* open apex of the canine; *(b)* apices open on both premolars, second premolars, which are in the process of erupting; *(c)* apices of the permanent first molar are closed; *(d)* permanent second molar erupting.

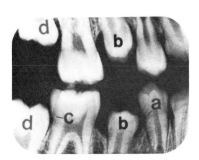

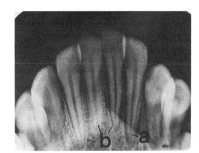

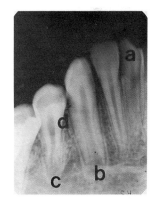

Fig 3-31

Fig 3-32

Fig 3-33

Fig 3-31 Bitewing radiograph shows *(a)* cervical burnout on the mandibular first premolar, *(b)* opposing second premolars erupting, *(c)* some cervical burnout on mandibular first molar, and *(d)* both maxillary and mandibular permanent second molars erupting.

Fig 3-32 Mandibular occlusal view showing the erupting permanent incisors. It is important to note *(a)* the curved root of the lateral incisor and *(b)* all apices closed on the maxillary incisors.

Fig 3-33 Canine view of a 12-year-old child: *(a)* a fractured central incisor, *(b)* open apex of the canine, *(c)* apex is open on first premolar, and *(d)* some cervical burnout on the canine.

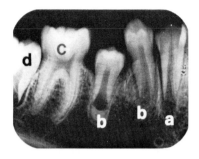

Fig 3-34 *(a)* Apex open on the canine; *(b)* apices open on both premolars; *(c)* permanent molar fully developed, apices closed; and *(d)* erupting second molar, open apices.

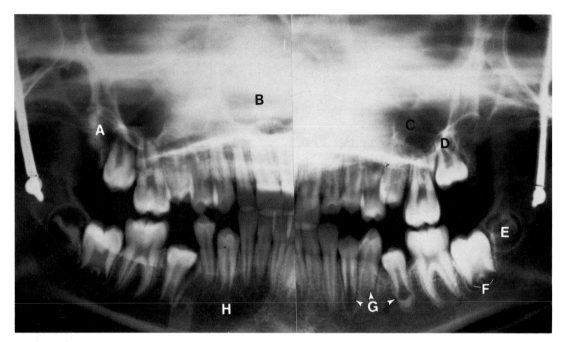

Fig 3-35 Panoramic radiograph of the permanent dentition showing the maxillary canines are ready to erupt into good alignment. The third molars are beginning to develop. As the child matures, the third molars need to be observed for impaction potential. *(a)* Developing maxillary molar, *(b)* nasal cavity, *(c)* maxillary sinus, *(d)* erupting maxillary second molar, *(e)* developing mandibular third molar, *(f)* open apices of second molar in process of erupting, *(g)* apices open on mandibular canine and first and second premolars, and *(h)* artifact.

Errors in radiographic technique

Figures 3-36 to 3-44 illustrate some common errors in the use of radiographic techniques. The description with the figures also includes some remedies for the errors.

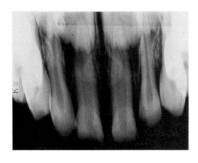
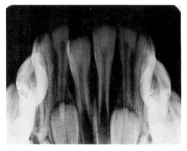

Figs 3-36a and b These maxillary and mandibular occlusal radiographs are elongated. The elongation of the images is the result of a faulty positive vertical angulation. This angulation should be at 60°. The other cause is that the child's occlusal plane is not parallel to the horizontal. Often elongation results from a combination of both causes.

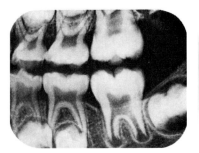 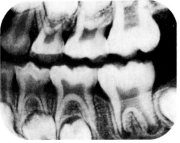 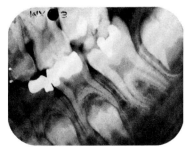

Fig 3-37   Fig 3-38   Fig 3-39

Fig 3-37   The bitewing radiograph has been extended beyond the distal surface of the permanent first molar. As a result, the distal portion of the primary canine cannot be seen. The function of the bitewing radiograph is to view interproximal caries from the canine to the mesial surface of the permanent first molar.

Fig 3-38   The contacts of the teeth are overlapped. As a result, the areas to be viewed for caries are obscured. The central ray and the head of the x-ray were not directed through the contacts but perpendicular to the midline of the patient. The horizontal angulation was incorrect.

Fig 3-39   This bitewing radiograph shows a more-than-adequate view of the mandibular arch and an inadequate view of the maxillary arch because *(1)* the occlusal plane is not parallel to the floor; *(2)* the angulation of the x-ray head was at –10° (the correct setting is +10°); or *(3)* the child bit down on the bite-tab, causing the film packet to be disoriented.

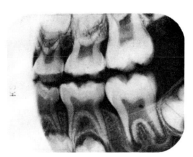 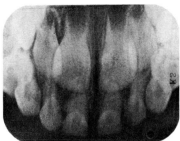 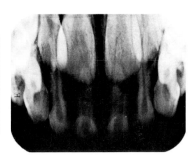

Fig 3-40   Fig 3-41   Fig 3-42

Fig 3-40   Radiograph illustrating a common malady, cone cutting. The head of the x-ray was positioned so that the film was not exposed.

Fig 3-41   This film is too light, and it has a grainy appearance. Probable causes include *(1)* underexposure, *(2)* an error in development, and *(3)* weak developer solution. The grainy appearance may also be a result of faulty processing technique.

Fig 3-42   Notice how dark this radiograph is due to overexposure to radiation. Other causes can be attributed to improper film processing, such as overdeveloping or poor developer-fixer solutions.

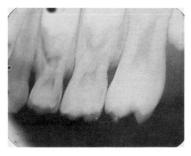 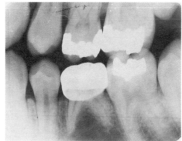 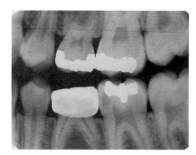

Fig 3-43   Fig 3-44a   Fig 3-44b

Fig 3-43   The elongated roots of the primary molars and the permanent first molar are a result of the wrong horizontal angulation. The indicated angulation for this view is 40°.

Fig 3-44a   Clinical example of use of a distorted bitewing. Check the above bitewing radiograph, specifically the mandibular first permanent molar. Because of the error in angulation, active caries was missed on the mesial surface.

Fig 3-44b   Six months later the caries has encroached the pulp and an indirect pulp cap is now indicated. An error in technique plus an error in diagnosis equals a more involved and unnecessary procedure.

Radiographic diagnosis of dental anomalies

The purpose of the following series of radiographs is to illustrate common clinical anomalies in children (Figs 3-45 to 3-73). The practitioner should be able to recognize anomalies prevalent in children, evaluate the influence of the anomaly on oral growth and function, and then plan subsequent treatment. Anomalies of the oral cavity are prevalent in about 5% of all children. These anomalies occur more often in the primary dentition. They are seen more often in boys than in girls. Anomalies are divided into six categories related to deficient or excessive development during the embryonic stages of tooth development:

1. Number of teeth: disturbances in the initiation-proliferation stage
2. Shape of teeth: disturbances in the morphodifferentiation stage
3. Color of teeth: disturbances in the apposition or calcification stage
4. Structure or texture of teeth: disturbances in the apposition or calcification stage
5. Eruption or exfoliation of teeth: disturbances in the eruption stage of tooth development
6. Position: disturbances in the eruption stage of tooth development

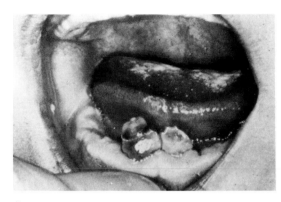
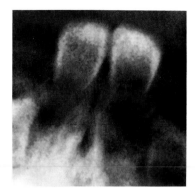

Fig 3-45   **Fig 3-46**

Fig 3-45 Natal teeth. These natal teeth are primary supernumerary teeth, whereas neonatal teeth are primary teeth that have erupted prematurely. Many times, however, the terms refer only to the time of eruption, natal (at birth) and neonatal (first year of life) and not to whether the tooth is supernumerary or primary. Both usually contribute to nursing problems and because of their hypoplastic development endanger the infant with possible aspiration. Quantitative enamel, dental, and root defects usually preclude restorative procedures in favor of extraction.

Fig 3-46 Neonatal teeth. The two neonatal teeth in this radiograph are precociously erupted primary incisors. Because of the lack of root development, surgical removal is indicated.

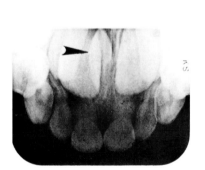
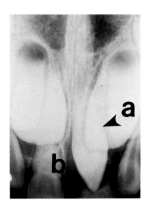
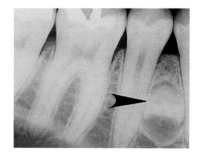

Fig 3-47   **Fig 3-48**   **Fig 3-49**

Fig 3-47 A supernumerary tooth exists in the midline. Sometimes called a *mesiodens*, it is often detected by use of the occlusal radiograph. It is not apparent clinically. Supernumerary teeth occur more often in the permanent dentition than in the primary dentition. The estimates range from 2.7% to 3.1% of all children (Grahnen and Lindahl, 1961; Castaldi, 1966). The treatment in this instance should be removal. An excellent review of the literature related to the etiology, diagnosis, and treatment of supernumerary teeth has been reported by Primosch (1981).

Fig 3-48 Often a midline supernumerary *(a)*, or mesiodens, will cause a disturbance in eruption. Note the premature resorption of the primary central incisors *(b)*. The primary incisor was removed, as was the supernumerary tooth. There is some controversy as to the timing of the removal of supernumerary teeth. Some recommend early removal (Rotberg and Kopel, 1984); others recommend a compromise based on the shape, type, and stage of eruption of the supernumerary tooth (DiBase, 1971).

Fig 3-49 The second most common area of occurrence for supernumerary teeth is the premolar area. This extra tooth is between the two premolars. Careful removal is indicated.

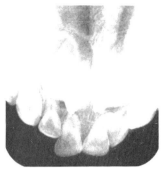

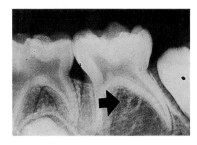

Fig 3-50

Fig 3-51

Fig 3-50 Two supernumerary teeth are present. The one on the left is somewhat difficult to see. Clinically, supernumerary teeth can retard eruption of the permanent central incisors. Also, irregularities in the permanent incisors can occur and result in the need for follow-up orthodontic care.

Fig 3-51 Excluding permanent third molars, the tooth most often congenitally missing is the second premolar. The second premolar is most often missing in the mandible of girls. The primary tooth often remains in function for a number of years. However, in those instances where the tooth is lost, the space can be closed either orthodontically or restored with a fixed prosthetic appliance. Such individuals frequently have multiple second premolars missing. Often a familial tendency for missing teeth exists.

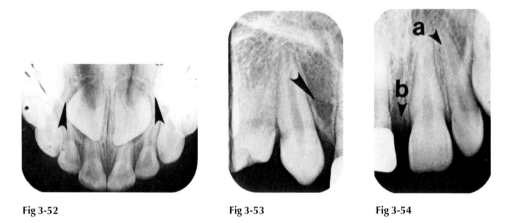

Fig 3-52

Fig 3-53

Fig 3-54

Fig 3-52 Another reason for the routine use of anterior occlusal radiographs is to detect congenitally missing lateral incisors. This view is not conclusive but gives a hint that the area normally occupied by the lateral incisors is devoid of tooth structure. Supplemental periapical radiographs of the canine region are now indicated. When this situation is diagnosed, the treatment alternatives are (1) to maintain the space of the missing teeth and replace them with fixed prosthetic appliances or (2) to close the spaces orthodontically and recontour the canines to appear similar to the lateral incisors. Each patient has to be evaluated according to individual occlusion and orthodontic status before a treatment plan is determined.

Fig 3-53 From the anterior maxillary occlusal radiograph, it was suspected that a permanent lateral incisor might be missing. Note that the lateral incisor is missing there is a radiolucent area that gives the appearance of a cyst. It is not uncommon for globulomaxillary cysts to exist in this area.

Fig 3-54 On the opposite side, there is a lateral incisor, but it is peg shaped. The permanent canine (a) has erupted into the oral cavity. Note the diastema (b) between the central incisors.

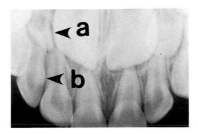
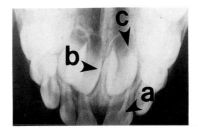

Fig 3-55

Fig 3-56

Fig 3-55   This anterior view illustrates a peg-shaped lateral incisor *(a)*. There are five primary incisors. An extra primary lateral incisor is present *(b)*.

Fig 3-56   A common anomaly of shape occurring in the primary dentition is fusion *(a)*. Fused teeth are two separate buds that fuse with a common dentin union. These teeth have individual root canals. This child also has a supernumerary tooth *(b)* and a congenitally missing lateral incisor *(c)*.

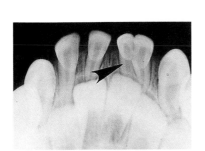
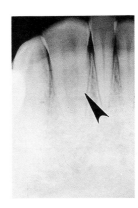
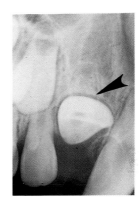

Fig 3-57

Fig 3-58

Fig 3-59

Fig 3-57   An anomaly similar to fusion is concrescence, which is a cemental union of two separate teeth with individual root canals and pulp structure. This example is somewhat between fusion and concrescence with a small amount of dentin union and a greater percentage of common cementum. These anomalies are usually of academic interest only but can cause orthodontic, esthetic, and periodontal problems (Milazzo and Alexander, 1982).

Fig 3-58   When there are a single root and pulp canal but a crown size equal to that of two teeth, the term *gemination* is used. Gemination is the result of an unsuccessful attempt of an individual tooth bud to divide into two separate teeth.

Fig 3-59   When there is a sharp or abnormal curvature of the crown or root, dilaceration of the tooth is evident. Trauma to the developing tooth causes an aberrant formation. Dilaceration is common in children with cleft palate, especially where the cleft area includes the maxillary alveolar ridge. Andreasen (1971) evaluated 207 permanent teeth with a history of trauma to the primary dentition. Approximately 25% of the permanent teeth demonstrated some form of dilaceration. Intrusion of the primary tooth was the major cause of dilaceration. The clinical solution to dilaceration can involve oral surgery, orthodontics, or prosthodontics, or a combination of the three.

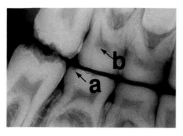

Fig 3-60

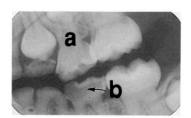

Fig 3-61

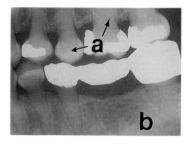

Fig 3-62

Fig 3-60　The radiograph shows a defect in enamel formation, amelogenesis imperfecta. There are many types, all of which are inherited. This patient is one of four children in a family of five with the disease. The father also has amelogenesis imperfecta. Note the thin enamel *(a)* and the somewhat increased amount of dentin *(b)*. The pulp chambers are somewhat smaller because of the increased amount of dentin. Both primary and permanent teeth are involved.

Fig 3-61　Dentinogenesis imperfecta is a dominant-inherited disturbance of dentin that is non–sex-linked. Note the lack of pulp chambers *(a)*, bulbous crown forms *(b)*, short roots, and the spontaneous periapical abscess. These children usually have a low caries rate. Both the primary and permanent teeth are involved in this patient.

Fig 3-62　Radiograph of the parent of the child in Fig 3-61. Note the absence of a pulp chamber *(a)*, the bulbous crowns, and a periapical abscess on the mesial root of the first permanent molar *(b)*. Fortunately there is little abrasion.

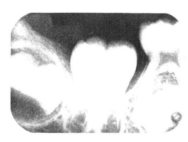

Fig 3-63

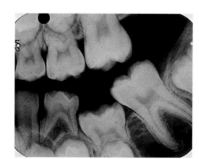

Fig 3-64

Fig 3-63　The permanent first molar demonstrates idiopathic internal resorption before eruption. Referred to in the past as *preeruptive caries*, the lesion is not related to caries. Treatment consists of removing the areas of resorption as soon as possible, doing an indirect pulp cap if needed, and allowing the tooth to erupt into the mouth. A permanent restoration is then placed.

Fig 3-64　The main diagnostic criteria for ankylosis (infraocclusion) is that the tooth begins to fall below the plane of occlusion. By some mechanism, there seems to be an attachment of cementum to the adjacent alveolar bone. Note the arch length loss caused by the tipping of the permanent first molar. Treatment here should be extraction and a space maintainer.

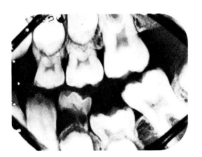

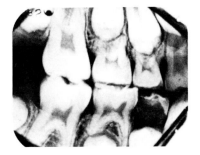

Fig 3-65a   **Fig 3-65b**

Figs 3-65a and b   The primary mandibular second molar has become ankylosed with subsequent space loss. Also note idiopathic internal resorption of the right and left mandibular first primary molars. Again, treatment is removal of the ankylosed tooth plus the two primary first molars. A space maintainer is indicated. Histologically, ankylosis occurs on the inner root surface of the primary teeth and is an attempt at repair by a hard tissue resembling bone; the process of root resorption is within normal limits (Kurol and Magnusson, 1984). Maxillary molars may become ankylosed first, resulting in more severe infraocclusion. Primary mandibular first molars are less of a problem, and primary mandibular molars and maxillary first and second molars have a greater tendency for infraocclusion (Messer and Cline, 1980). Children with ankylosis reportedly have a higher incidence of crossbites (Kula et al, 1984).

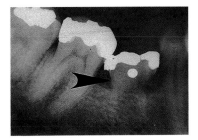

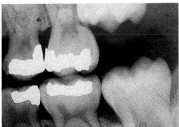

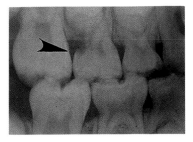

Fig 3-66   **Fig 3-67**   **Fig 3-68**

Fig 3-66   This bitewing survey of an adult shows an ankylosed primary second molar and a congenitally missing second premolar. Because of the lack of eruption, there is a lack of alveolar bone growth around the primary second molars. Extraction and replacement with a fixed prosthetic appliance is the treatment of choice.

Fig 3-67   Eruption out of position, or ectopic eruption, is seen here. Contributing factors theorized to cause this defect include *(1)* maxillary tuberosity size, *(2)* larger tooth size to bone size, *(3)* abnormal eruption path of the permanent first molar, and *(4)* abnormal eruptive tooth position (Pulver, 1968). This patient needs to have the permanent first molar moved distally. It has been suggested that ectopic eruption may have some familial tendency, with siblings having a higher prevalence of ectopic eruption than the normal population (Kurol, 1982).

Fig 3-68   Note the area of external resorption on the distal surface of the primary maxillary second molar. The permanent maxillary first molar was held in position, but jumped from beneath the primary second molar. Clinicians refer to this as a *jump type* of ectopic eruption.

53

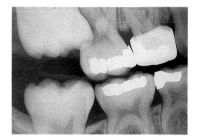

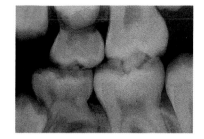

Fig 3-69   **Fig 3-70**

Fig 3-69 When the permanent maxillary first molar is held in position, it is often referred to as a *hold type* of ectopic eruption. In this instance, treatment was not begun, and 6 months later the primary second molar had to be extracted. An orthodontic appliance is now needed to move the permanent maxillary first molar to a distal position, which is normal for this age. In a study of ectopic eruption by Bjerklin and Kurol (1981), ectopic eruption *(1)* occurred in 4.3% of their sample, *(2)* was irreversible in 41% of the children (hold type), *(3)* could be determined in 90% of the children by age 7, and *(4)* was seen in more boys than girls.

Fig 3-70 The first premolar is trapped under the mesial marginal ridge of the primary second molar. Note the resorption of the mesial root. The plan should be to remove the primary second molar and maintain the space until the second premolar erupts.

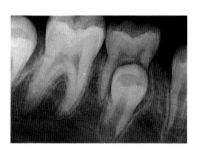

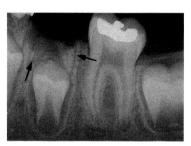

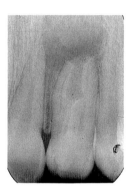

Fig 3-71   **Fig 3-72**   **Fig 3-73**

Fig 3-71 For some reason, yet unknown, primary teeth will have normal resorption of one root but lack of resorption of another. The permanent tooth is deviated from its normal path, possibly resulting in impaction or malalignment. Treatment consists of extraction and observation of the eruption of the second premolar into normal alignment.

Fig 3-72 It is not uncommon, especially in children with chronic caries and irregular dental care, to find retained root tips. The distal root of the primary second molar has been retained, causing some periapical pathosis and subsequent bone loss. Removal of the offending root tip is the treatment of choice.

Fig 3-73 Dens invaginatus, or dens in dente, is caused by an invagination of the enamel organ. It occurs in 3% to 5% of the population and most frequently in the maxillary lateral incisor area. This radiograph is an example of a more extreme invagination occluding the coronal portion of the pulp and extending half of the way into the pulp canals. Histologically, the enamel and dentin may be defective in the invaginated area.

References

American Academy of Pediatric Dentistry (AAPD). Oral Health Policies for Children. III. Dental Radiographs for Children. Chicago: AAPD, 1993.

Guidelines for Prescribing Dental Radiographs, publication No. N-80A, Eastman Kodak, 1988.

Myers, D. R. Dental radiology for children. Dent. Clin. North Am. 28:37, 1984.

Nowak, A. J. Radiation exposure in pediatric dentistry: An introduction. Pediatr. Dent. 3:380, 1982.

Nowak, A. J., et al. Summary on the conference on radiation exposure in pediatric dentistry. J. Am. Dent. Assoc. 103:426, 1981.

Sikorski, P. A., and Taylor, K. W. The effectiveness of the thyroid shield in dental radiology. Oral Surg. Oral Med. Oral Pathol. 58:225, 1984

White, S. C. Radiation safety for children. Int. Dent. J. 32:259, 1982.

Additional readings

American Association of Dental Schools. Position paper on ionizing radiation. May 22, 1979.

American Dental Association Council on Dental Materials, Instruments, and Equipment. Biological effects on radiation from dental radiology. J. Am. Dent. Assoc. 105:275, 1982.

Bawden, J. W. The use of radiographs in pediatric dentistry: The challenge of the eighties. Pediatr Dent. 3(2):455, 1982.

Bean, L. R., and Akerman, W. Y. Jr. Intraoral or panoramic radiography? Dent. Clin. North Am 28(1):47, 1984.

Bean, L. R., and Devore, W. F. Comparison of gonodal dosage of dental x-radiation using various types of lead protective aprons. Oral Surg. 28:505, 1969.

Bean, L. R., and Isaac, H. K. X-ray and the child patient. Dent. Clin. North Am. 13:13, 1973.

Berkman, M. D. Pedodontic radiographic interpretation. Dent. Radiogr. Photogr. 44:27, 1971.

Goepp, R. A. Risk/benefit considerations in pedodontic radiology. Pediatr. Dent. 3:437, 1982.

Kula, et al. An occlusal and cephalometric study of children with ankylosis of primary ,molars. J. Ped. 8(2):146, 1984.

Langlais, R. P., and Kasle, M. J. Intraoral Radiographic Interpretation. vol. 1. Philadelphia: W. B. Saunders Co., 1978.

Nowak, A. J., and Miller, J. W. High-yield pedodontic radiology. Gen. Dent. 33:45, 1985.

Myers, D. R., Barenie, J., and Bell, R. A. Requirements for supplemental periapical radiographs following No. 0 and No. 2 bitewings. Pediatr. Dent. 6:235, 1984.

Valachonic, R. W., and Lurie, A. G. Risk-benefit considerations in pedodontic radiology. Pediatr. Dent. 2:128, 1980.

White, S. C. Radiation in pediatric dentistry: Current standards in pedodontic radiology with suggestions for alternatives. Pediatr. Dent. 3:441, 1982.

Questions

1. A 7-year-old has a large space between the permanent central incisors. A supernumerary is suspected. The choice of film to detect its presence is:

   a. Panoramic
   b. Anterior maxillary occlusal
   c. Periapical
   d. Any one of the above
   e. None of the above

2. A 7-year-old visits your office. This visit is the child's first appointment with the dentist. The optimum initial survey(s) is (are):

   a. A 12-film survey plus two bitewing radiographs
   b. Two bitewing radiographs plus a panoramic radiograph
   c. Maxillary and mandibular occlusal radiographs plus two bitewing radiographs
   d. An eight-film survey, two occlusal radiographs, two bitewing radiographs, and four periapical radiographs
   e. Twenty films plus a panoramic radiograph
   f. a,d,e
   g. d,e
   h. b,c
   i. c,d,e
   j. a,b

3. Match the central ray angulations with the proper film projections (use choices f. to j. for all five questions).

		Choices
a. Bitewing _____		f. +40°
b. Maxillary molar _____		g. −30°
c. Mandibular molar _____		h. +60°
d. Mandibular occlusal _____		i. +55°
e. Maxillary occlusal _____		j. None of the above

4. An 18 month old fractures two primary maxillary central incisors. The best diagnostic survey you could use is:

   a. Panoramic radiograph plus two bitewing radiographs
   b. Two anterior occlusal radiographs
   c. Two bitewing radiographs plus two occlusal radiographs
   d. An eight-film survey
   e. Two bitewing radiographs

5. A 6-year-old has returned for a 6-month recall. At the previous appointment the child had bitewing radiographs taken, revealing no dental caries. Your choice of radiographic survey at this appointment is:

   a. Two bitewing radiographs
   b. Two bitewing radiographs plus a panoramic radiograph
   c. Two bitewing plus two occlusal radiographs
   d. A 12-film survey
   e. None of the above

Chapter 4

Soft Tissue Assessment

Objectives

After studying this chapter, the student should be able to:
1. List the characteristics of healthy periodontium found in children.
2. Discuss the influence of permanent tooth eruption on the periodontium.
3. Describe common gingival problems and diseases, including chronic gingivitis, pericoronitis, acute necrotizing ulcerative gingivitis, gingival hyperplasia, and gingival recession, and their respective treatments.
4. Diagnose and treat prepubertal and early-onset periodontitis.
5. List several systemic diseases associated with periodontitis in children.
6. Outline steps in the surgical intervention of mucogingival problems associated with orthodontic therapy, including surgical exposure of unerupted teeth, free gingival graft, surgical crown extension, supra-alveolar fibrotomy, and frenectomy.
7. Differentiate and treat common oral lesions and infections in children.

Soft tissue assessment of the pediatric dental patient involves a thorough knowledge of the normal size, shape, color, and texture of the oral soft tissue structures. A standardized approach to the examination and evaluation of the oral soft tissues generally precedes examination of the hard tissues (dentition) and the occlusion and must be carefully documented in the patient's record. The oral structures that must be evaluated are the lips, buccal mucosa, gingiva, hard and soft palates, tonsils, and pharynx. The periodontium, or supporting structures of the teeth, will be discussed first.

Characteristics of healthy periodontium

Gingiva

For the purposes of this discussion, description of the gingiva will be divided into three zones: papillary, marginal, and attached (Zappler, 1948) (Fig 4-1).

Papillary gingiva

The influence of cervical dental morphology on papillary and marginal gingival configuration is illustrated

in Fig 4-2 for both primary and permanent teeth. The zone lying beneath the interproximal contact area and between the dental papillae is known as the *interdental col*. Because of its location, morphology, and lack of keratinized epithelium, this area is particularly vulnerable to bacterial growth and secondary tissue invasion.

However, in the primary dentition, interdental spacing is common. Without the development of interproximal contacts, col formation will not occur. Instead, so-called interdental saddle areas are present where spacing occurs, resulting in a well-keratinized surface (Fig 4-3). This feature may contribute to the lower prevalence of periodontal lesions in children because the saddle areas are less vulnerable to the development and progression of the inflammatory process (Ruben et al, 1971).

Marginal gingiva

Marginal gingiva includes the gingival crevice or sulcus and the free gingival margin. Sulcus depth around primary teeth is comparatively greater than that found around permanent teeth, with mean values ranging from 1.4 mm (Chawla, 1973) to 2.1 mm (Rosenblum, 1966). The free gingival margin is thicker and rounder around the primary teeth than in the permanent dentition. Morphologic characteristics of primary teeth, such as the cervical bulge and underlying constriction at the cementoenamel junction, contribute to the thick, rounded form of the free marginal gingiva. This

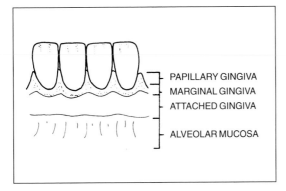

Fig 4-1 The gingival tissues can be divided into three zones: papillary, marginal, and attached.

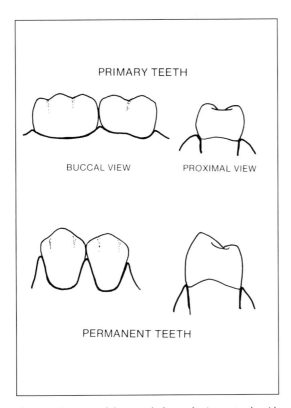

Fig 4-2 Because of the morphology of primary teeth with their broad, flat, and low contact areas, the papillae is comparatively shorter and rounder than its counterpart in the permanent dentition. In addition, the prominent cervical bulge on the buccal and lingual surfaces of primary teeth causes the underlying gingival margin to be rounder than the knife-edged gingival margin associated with permanent teeth, whose morphology is not as accentuated.

form is in contrast to the knife-edged margin found with permanent teeth (see Fig 4-2). Because of the edema produced by gingivitis, the rolled marginal gingiva may be more accented in children (Fig 4-4). The marginal gingiva is also very flaccid and retractable, a condition verified on clinical examination with an air syringe. The diminished rigidity and increased retractability of the marginal gingiva around primary teeth have several causes (Ruben et al, 1971):

1. *Immature connective tissue composition.* The collagen bundles are less differentiated and more hydrated; its polypeptide chains are not as tightly cross-linked. Also, there is a lower ratio of collagen to ground substance in the connective tissue, making it less rigid.
2. *Immature gingival fiber system.* The gingival fiber system, particularly the circular and groups A and B fibers, are incompletely differentiated in their arrangement, leading to a less organized state.
3. *Increased vascularization.* Increased blood flow during this dynamic period of gingival metabolism promotes tissue hydration and fluid transfer into the sulcus.

Attached gingiva

Because of the thinner, less keratinized epithelium with its greater vascularity, the attached gingiva appears less dense and redder (darker pink) than it appears in the adult. In patients with dark complexions, the affinity of melanin pigmentation for the attached gingiva makes the zone more easily identifiable (see Fig 4-3). The attached gingiva is more flaccid because it has lesser connective tissue density and its texture is less stippled. The incidence of stippling in children is 35% (Soni, 1963). The width of the attached gingiva is comparatively greater than that found in adults. The mean width ranges between 1 and 6 mm compared with that around the permanent dentition (mean width of 1 to 9 mm) and appears to remain fairly constant with age (Bowers, 1963).

Two unique anatomic characteristics are found in the attached gingiva in children: the interdental cleft and the retrocuspid papilla. Interdental clefts are normal anatomic features found in the interradicular zone underlying most interdental saddle areas (see Fig 4-4). The retrocuspid papilla is found approximately 1 mm below the free gingival groove on the attached gingiva lingual to the mandibular canine. This feature, which bears no clinical importance, unless mistaken for a fistulous tract, occurs in 85% of children examined (Easley and Weis, 1970) and apparently decreases in prevalence with age.

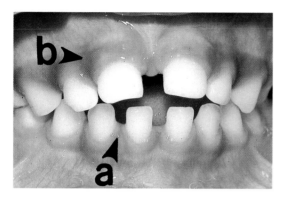

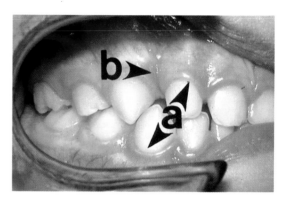

Fig 4-3 Interdental saddle area and attached gingiva. (a) Interdental spacing, common in the primary dentition, results in the formation of gingival saddle areas that are more resistant to the initiation of periodontal disease than are cols formed in areas of proximal dental contact. (b) The zone of attached gingiva is clearly illustrated in patients with dark complexion because of the affinity of melanin pigmentation for this area.

Fig 4-4 Marginal gingiva and interdental cleft area. (a) inflammation of the marginal gingiva (gingivitis) accents the normally rounded margin found in healthy gingiva around primary teeth. (b) Interdental cleft formation is a common occurrence underlying most interdental saddle areas and is a normal anatomic finding.

Alveolar mucosa

Thin epithelium and an absence of keratin makes the alveolar mucosa redder than the pink gingiva. This tissue has an abundance of elastic fibers and is readily movable. Its width increases with chronologic age and dental eruption.

Periodontal membrane

The periodontal space is wider and less dense (fewer fibers/unit area) in children.

Alveolar bone

The alveolar bone of children has been characterized as less calcified, more vascular, and having fewer but thicker trabeculae. Also, there appear to be larger marrow spaces, thinner lamina dura, and flatter interdental crests. The majority of these features indicate the dynamic and transitional metabolic state of young and maturing bone.

Influence of permanent tooth eruption on the periodontium

During eruption of the permanent teeth, there are two phases: active and passive (Gottlieb and Orban, 1933).

Active eruption

Active eruption is the eruption that occurs until contact with the tooth's functional antagonist is made. Histologically, as the erupting tooth enters the oral cavity, the gingival tissue that surrounds it is composed of reduced enamel epithelium (odontogenic origin). This layer is replaced by an epithelial cuff that is transitional until the stratified squamous epithelium of oral origin migrates into its position. The periodontal fibers remain parallel and disoriented until contact with the opposing tooth is made.

Passive eruption

Passive eruption occurs when the sulcular epithelium changes in position from enamel to cementum attachment after occlusion is established. This process occurs over a 10-year period, resulting in increased crown height (approximately a 1.5-mm addition) and decreased sulcular depth with age (Volchansky and Cleaton-Jones, 1974). Recently erupted permanent teeth have greater sulcus depth (Fuder and Jamison 1963) than established permanent teeth (mean depth of 1.8 mm). Passive eruption stabilizes when an individual is between 16 and 18 years of age.

Gingival diseases and conditions

Chronic gingivitis

Chronic gingivitis is the most common gingival problem in children. It may be localized or generalized and is insidious and painless. Changes in gingival color, contour, and texture may be apparent (Fig 4-5).

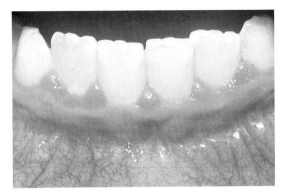

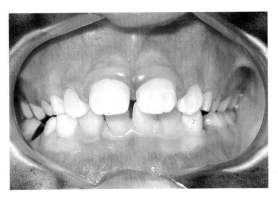

Fig 4-5 Gingivitis. Chronic nonspecific gingivitis in children is usually limited to the marginal and papillary gingiva. Tissue edema secondary to the inflammation produces swollen interdental papillae and generalized redness. Often the inflammation results in a change in gingival color, contour, and texture. Spontaneous hemorrhage is evident in more severe cases, but the condition is reversible when proper oral hygiene maintenance is instituted.

Fig 4-6 Eruption gingivitis. Eruption gingivitis is the result of plaque accumulation superimposed on the absence of contour and embrasure protection of the gingiva normally provided by a fully erupted tooth.

The local factor that contributes most to its development is the accumulation of plaque (Ranney et al, 1981). The signs of the disease, however, are more easily attributed to host response rather than solely to the effects of bacterial enzymes or cytotoxins. Calculus formation may play a role, but its prevalence increases with age and thus may be more important in older children (Everett et al, 1963; Suomi et al, 1971). Other factors of a traumatic origin may also be significant. These include eruption, exfoliation, carious teeth, food impaction, malocclusion, orthodontic appliances, mouth breathing, and faulty restorations (Fig 4-6). For example, there is a significant association between improper marginal extension of stainless steel crowns and gingivitis (Myers, 1975), probably due more to the entrapment of plaque than to the irritation potential of the crown margin. However, systemic factors in the formation of gingivitis must not be overlooked. These factors include the influence of hormones, malnutrition, chronic illness, and medications. The prevalence of gingivitis in children varies greatly according to the study examined (Table 4-1).

This variation reflects differences in the criteria selection of the examiners rather than any population differences. The subjective nature of the clinical assessment, even when the same criteria are used between different examiners, is a problem (Poulsen, 1981). For example, the commonly used Gingival Index (GI) developed by Löe (1967) for the evaluation of gingival inflammation is very subjective (Table 4-2). What is apparent is that the prevalence of gingivitis is low in young children and dramatically increases in prevalence as children grow older. Marked increases are obvious during the period of dental eruption and puberty in children (Massler et al, 1950; Parfitt, 1957; Carter and Wells, 1960). The termination of the mixed

Table 4-1 Prevalence of gingivitis in children

Investigator	Age range (y)	Prevalence (%)
Brucker (1943)	4–16	8
Stahl and Goldman (1953)	6–15	28
Carter and Wells (1960)	6–12	50
Jamison (1963)	5–14	75

Table 4-2 Criteria for scores in the Gingival Index

Score	Criteria
0	Absence of inflammation
1	Mild inflammation—slight change in color and texture
2	Moderate inflammation—redness, edema, and bleeding on pressure
3	Severe inflammation—marked redness, edema, ulceration, and spontaneous bleeding

dentition ushers in a slight decline in the prevalence and severity of gingivitis in children. By 15 years of age, 40% of the population has evidence of loss of periodontal attachment (Poulsen, 1981).

Treatment of gingivitis is accomplished by maintenance of sound oral hygiene practices, because gingivitis has been shown to be a reversible process (Löe et al, 1965; Theilade et al, 1966). When oral hygiene is suspended in humans, gingivitis will develop in 15 to 21 days. As plaque accumulates, definite changes occur in the oral flora ecology. Gram-positive cocci and small rods are early inhabitants. They are later replaced by fil-

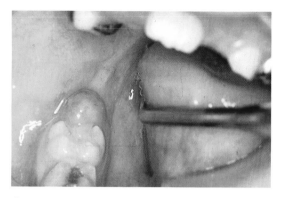

Fig 4-7 Pericoronitis. Pericoronitis is a gingival disturbance associated with active dental eruption. The causative factor is the accumulation of debris under an operculum of tissue that rests across the occlusal surface. The entrapment of the debris results in inflammation and infection. Treatment may require antibiotics, irrigation, and excision.

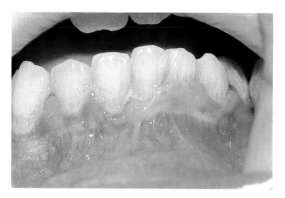

Fig 4-8 Acute necrotizing ulcerative gingivitis. This condition may result in punched-out dental papilla, gingival recession, pseudopockets. Lack of proper oral hygiene attention contributed to the condition present here.

amentous forms and spirochetes. With the resumption of oral hygiene, gingivitis will resolve in 7 days, and the oral flora will return to its original composition.

The ultimate unanswered question is whether adult periodontitis has a childhood origin. The fact that periodontitis is a progressive process and that, epidemiologically speaking, there appears to be a transition from childhood gingivitis to adult periodontitis, gives support to this hypothesis. However, no direct cause-and-effect relationship has been found in humans. If a natural transition exists, one would expect to find more cases of incipient marginal periodontitis in children than are reported. In fact, gingivitis rarely progresses to periodontitis in prepubertal children and seems to be lymphocyte dominated rather than plasma cell dominated as in adults (Ranney, 1981).

Thus, periodontal disease may be a biphasic phenomenon (Massler, 1958) that in children is transient but acute (overt, rapid response to both irritation and healing) and in adults is progressive and chronic. But, if there are differences in the disease process between children and adults, what is the cause? Several possible factors related to the limited involvement of periodontal disease in children have been proposed.

First, the greater metabolic activity in children, in whom anabolism is dominant over catabolism (Robinson, 1951; Kelsten, 1955), may offer the periodontium greater resistance to breakdown or, when it does occur, may enhance concurrent repair.

Second, the oral flora is different in children. The late establishment of spirochetes and *Bacteroides melaninogenicus*, which have been associated with the development of gingivitis in children (deArugo, 1964; Maltais et al, 1978), may delay the onset of periodontal disease in children. The late establishment of these pathogens in the gingival sulcus is related to the absence of heme and α_2-globulin, necessary for their growth (Socransky and Manganiello, 1971).

Third, the composition and metabolism of plaque found in children may be responsible for its reported lower irritation potential. When preschoolers withheld oral hygiene practices for 27 days, no increase in the degree of gingivitis occurred (Mackler and Crawford, 1973). This response is in direct contradiction to the findings of a similar study of adults (Löe et al, 1965). When the study was repeated, the results were confirmed (Cox et al, 1974). They found that healthy preschool children with a Plaque Index four times that of adults had only one fourth the Gingival Index.

Several reasons for the delayed development of gingivitis in children have been proposed. There appears to be a slight decrease in the leukocytic migratory rate in children (Cox et al, 1974; Longhurst et al, 1977; Matsson, 1978). This lower tissue response may be a reflection of a lack of antibody or cellular hypersensitivity (low levels of immunoglobulin specific for plaque bacteria), or perhaps less gingival permeability to bacterial antigen (Cox et al, 1974). More significantly, the vascular inflammatory response may be more retarded in children. The retarded vascular inflammatory response is reflected in the decreased amount of gingival exudate and bleeding found in children (Matsson, 1978). Thus, the difference in the propensities of children and adults to develop gingivitis may be a result of the inability of gingival plaque in children to affect the inflammatory response of the vasculature to the same degree as in adults.

In summary, periodontal disease in children is a well-defined, restricted, inflammatory state that remains limited in severity; in the adult, periodontal disease is chronic and progressive, perhaps because the tissues are no longer able to contain the inflammatory process structurally, reparatively, or immunologically (Ruben et al, 1971).

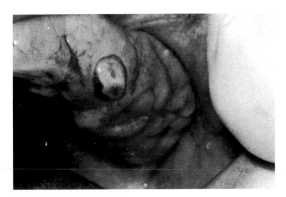

Fig 4-9a Severe gingival hyperplasia secondary to the administration of phenytoin for control of seizures.

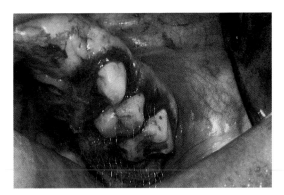

Fig 4-9b The hyperplastic condition is treated with a gingivectomy procedure for esthetic and functional reasons.

Acute periocoronitis

During gingival emergence of a tooth, an operculum of tissue may rest across the occlusal surface (Fig 4-7). This operculum attracts debris, which may lead to inflammation and infection. Regional lymphadenopathy, fever, and trismus may result. Treatment may require antibiotics, irrigation, and excision.

Acute necrotizing ulcerative gingivitis (ANUG)

Formerly referred to as *Vincent's infection*, ANUG occurs in 2.5% of the adolescent population. Etiology is of bacterial origin (*Borrelia vincentii*, a spirochete, and *Prevotella [Bacteroides] intermedia*) and occurrence may be related to malnutrition, systemic illness, and stress. Acute necrotizing ulcerative gingivitis is characterized by the formation of a gray pseudomembrane with ulcerated and necrotic interdental papillae (Fig 4-8). Fever malaise, acute gingival pain, and a prominent fetid odor are common. These lesions respond dramatically, within 48 hours, to oral cleansing and mouth rinsing with diluted hydrogen peroxide or other oxidizing agents (Jimenez and Baer, 1975; Loesche et al, 1982).

Gingival fibromatosis and hyperplasia

Gingival fibromatosis is an autosomal-dominant hereditary condition; gingival hyperplasia, in contrast, is acquired. Gingival hyperplasia occurs in 40% to 50% of children taking phenytoin (Dilantin) for seizure control. Approximately 30% of these lesions warrant excision. The hyperplastic tissue is thought to be an exaggerated response to plaque and therefore can be partially controlled with institution of good oral hygiene practices. However, in some cases, a gingivectomy procedure may be required for esthetic or functional reasons in patients taking phenytoin (Figs 4-9a and b).

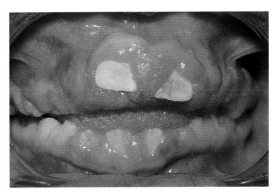

Fig 10 Gingival hyperplasia associated with cyclosporine therapy. The firm, fibrous, gingival enlargement is fibroepithelial in nature, most evident in the interdental areas, and limited to the keratinized portions of the tissue. Generally, it is granular in appearance but may become edematous and smooth because of secondary inflammation.

Drug-induced gingival hyperplasia has received much attention lately. Besides phenytoin, other drugs such as cyclosporine (Fig 4-10), a powerful immunosuppressant drug used in organ transplantation, and nifedipine, an antihypertensive drug used in the treatment of cardiac angina and arrhythmias, have been reported to produce gingival hyperplasia (Butler et al, 1987). Proposed mechanisms for drug-induced gingival hyperplasia include inflammation from bacterial plaque, increased sulfated glycosaminoglycans, immunoglobulins, gingival fibroblast phenotype population differences, epithelial growth factor, collagenase activation, folic acid, and disruption of fibroblastic cellular sodium/calcium flux (Brown et al, 1991). The prevalence of gingival hyperplasia associated with cyclosporine therapy is as high as 70% and children have a higher predisposition than adults. Since a correlation exists between plaque accumulation and severity of the hyperplasia, strict oral hygiene practices supplemented with chlorhexidine rinses may be beneficial.

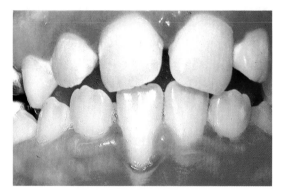

Fig 4-11 Gingival recession. Gingival recession most commonly occurs with mandibular central incisors in children. The causative factor most often cited is insufficient arch length, resulting in insufficient width of attached gingiva.

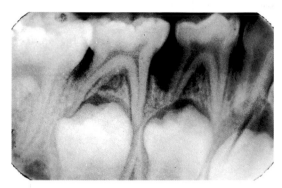

Fig 4-12 Prepubertal periodontitis. A severe and rapid form of periodontal destruction found in children with underlying systemic disease or defects in neutrophil adherence or chemotaxis. These conditions render the afflicted individuals more susceptible to virulent and putative periodontal pathogens. Treatment often involves antibiotic therapy and local debridement of the affected sites or extraction of the affected teeth.

There is some evidence that cyclosporine-induced gingival hyperplasia is clinically reversible on cessation of drug therapy (Daley et al, 1986).

It has also been shown that generalized moderate hyperplastic gingivitis will develop within 1 month after placement of orthodontic appliances, even in patients who have demonstrated perfect tooth-cleaning ability (Zachrisson and Zachrisson, 1972). However, these gingival changes are transient. Following appliance removal, sulcus depths return to normal, and no permanent tissue damage is evident.

Gingival recession

Recession of gingival tissue from the cementoenamel junction results in loss of attachment, which promotes the advancement of periodontal disease. The incidence of gingival recession of 3 to 5 mm (considered irreversible) in children aged 9 to 12 years is reported to be 6.5% (Parfitt and Mjör, 1964). Mandibular central incisors are most commonly affected (Fig 4-11). The main etiologic factor appears to be insufficient space for eruption, resulting in ectopic eruption, rotation, and, in some cases, crossbite (Powell and McEniery, 1982). The traumatic occlusion caused by crossbite compounds the problem. Other aggravating factors, such as plaque accumulation, high frenulum attachment on the marginal gingiva, food impaction, and mechanical abrasion, should also be evaluated. The treatment of choice is orthodontic correction and placement of an autogenous free gingival graft where the attached gingival width is less than 1 mm and the patient has demonstrated prior ability to maintain adequate oral hygiene practices.

Prepubertal periodontitis

Prepubertal periodontitis was classified by Page et al (1983) into two types: localized and generalized. Localized prepubertal periodontitis usually has an onset of 4 years of age in healthy children. Bone loss is rapid at the affected sites but significant plaque accumulation and gingival inflammation are absent (Fig 4-12). Functional abnormalities in leukocyte chemotaxis have been reported in the neutrophils or the monocytes, but not both (Watanabe, 1990). Progress of the disease may be altered by local debridement, antibiotic therapy, and improved oral hygiene. The affected sites harbor elevated percentages of certain virulent periodontal pathogens, such as *Actinobacillus actinomycetemcomitans, Provotella (Bacteroides) intermedia*, and *Porphyromonas (Bacteroides) gingivalis.*

Generalized prepubertal periodontitis, unlike the localized type, occurs in children with persistent infections and delayed wound healing. The alveolar bone destruction is more rapid and it occurs in the presence of severe gingival inflammation and clefting. Functional abnormalities occur in both neutrophils and monocytes in the same patient. The generalized type has been associated with leukocyte-adhesion deficiency involving a defect in the surface glycoprotein of the neutrophil. Leukocyte-adhesion deficiency is an autosomal-recessive condition resulting in increased susceptibility to bacterial infections. Generalized prepubertal periodontitis seems refractory to antibiotic therapy, and extraction of the affected teeth may be the only treatment.

Prepubertal periodontitis involving primary teeth will advance to periodontitis of the permanent dentition. The diagnosis of prepubertal periodontitis may be difficult to make in the absence of laboratory studies or solely on the patient's clinical history and appearance, because some patients may have undiagnosed underlying systemic diseases such as hypophosphatasia, agranulocytosis, or functional neutropenias (AAPD, 1991).

Early-onset periodontitis

Early-onset periodontitis is now the accepted term for both types of juvenile periodontitis, localized and generalized. The disease affects adolescents and young adults who are otherwise healthy (AAPD, 1989). These two distinct types of inflammatory periodontitis are distinguishable clinically, radiographically, and microbiologically. The localized type, formerly called *periodontosis* (Baer, 1971), appears to be self-limiting and affects mainly the permanent first molars and incisors in adolescents. Bone loss is rapid (three to four times the rate found in adult periodontitis) and is not commensurate with the amount of local irritants present, such as plaque and calculus. Susceptible individuals have both functional defects involving the neutrophils, which exhibit faulty chemotaxis, and highly virulent strains of *Actinobacillus actinomycetemocomitans* and *Bacteroides* species.

Generalized juvenile periodontitis, also referred to as *severe periodontitis* and *rapidly progressive periodontitis*, appears more commonly in young adults and involves the entire permanent dentition. Also, unlike the localized type, generalized juvenile periodontitis occurs in the presence of marked gingival inflammation and gross plaque accumulations. Subgingival plaque from the affected sites harbors high percentages of *Porphyromonas (Bacteroides) gingivalis*.

Early-onset periodontitis, when diagnosed early, responds to mechanical debridement of the affected sites in conjunction with antibiotic therapy to promote an environment conducive to healing. Among the suggested antibiotic regimens are tetracycline, 1 g/d for 14 to 21 days (Slots and Rosling, 1983) or amoxicillin, 1 g/d, plus metronidazole, 750 mg/d for 7 days (Van Winkelhoff et al, 1992). Refractory periodontitis may be more susceptible to other antibiotics such as augmentin, clindamycin, or ciprofloxacin (Genco, 1991).

Systemic disorders associated with periodontitis

Periodontitis is extremely rare in children. One should suspect the existence of the following systemic disturbances when periodontal destruction is diagnosed in children (Baer and Benjamin, 1974; Dorfman et al, 1976; Goepferd, 1981; AAP, 1991).

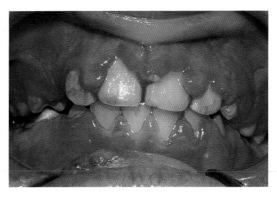

Fig 4-13 Leukemia. Acute gingival enlargement and spontaneous hemorrhage result from leukocytic infiltrate and thrombocytopenia. Gingivitis that is refractory to standard therapy should alert the clinician to suspect an underlying systemic disease.

Leukemia

This neoplastic disease results in abnormal and uncontrolled proliferation of immature leukocytes, usually the agranulocytic types, such as lymphocytic and monocytic leukocytes. Blood count is diagnostic. Gingival enlargement and ulceration may result from the leukocytic infiltration of the gingival tissue (Fig 4-13). Gingival changes can also occur as a result of chemotherapeutic agents used to combat the disease. Leukocytic infiltration results in thinning of lamina dura and destruction of the periodontal ligaments, which results in tooth migration.

Cyclic neutropenia

This autosomal-dominant disorder is characterized by rhythmic reduction of polymorphonuclear neutrophils in 21-day cycles. Severe ulcerative gingivitis and alveolar bone loss around primary teeth, permanent teeth, or both, may be present. Other hematologic disorders that can cause periodontitis in children include sickle cell anemia, aplastic anemia, and thalassemia.

Hypophosphatasia

This autosomal-recessive disorder is characterized by low serum alkaline phosphatase and reciprocal change in urine phosphoethanolamine levels. Premature mobility and loss of primary teeth are common, affecting the incisors more than the molars (higher prevalence in uniradicular primary teeth). Acementogenesis, dentinal dysplasia, and enlarged pulp chambers also occur.

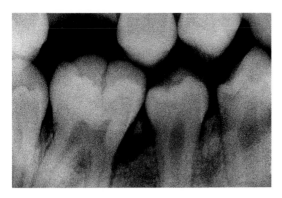

Fig 4-14   Localized periodontal defect associated with a retained primary root tip. This 15-year-old patient with type I diabetes mellitus presents with the classic three-wall, arc-shaped osseous defect usually seen in localized juvenile periodontitis.

Papillon-LeFevre syndrome

This autosomal-recessive disorder manifests in hyperkeratosis palmoplantaris (palms of hands and soles of feet) and premature loss of both primary and permanent teeth.

Histocytosis X

This disease is a nonlipid reticuloendotheliosis marked by multiple hard and soft tissue lesions containing histiocytes and eosinophils. There are three clinical entities: *(1)* Letterer-Siwe disease, which is the most severe form and affects mostly infants; *(2)* Hand-Schüller-Christian disease, which affects children older than 3 years and involves mostly bony sites; and *(3)* eosinophilic granuloma, which is the most benign variant, affecting older children. Oral manifestations are present in only one third of the patients. These manifestations include necrotic gingivitis, bony loss in the bifurcation of molars, and radiolucent lesions of the mandible and skull.

Acrodynia

This acquired disease, also called *Pink's* or *Swift's disease,* is a result of excessive exposure to mercury. It is marked by desquamation of skin, glossitis, and premature eruption and exfoliation of teeth.

Vitamin D–resistant rickets

This sex-linked dominant disorder is resistant to vitamin D therapy because renal tubular malresorption, not the lack of vitamin D, results in low serum phosphate. This disorder is also known by other names, such as *refractory rickets* or *low phosphate diabetes.*

Diabetes mellitus and chronic granulomatous disease

Diabetes mellitus and chronic granulomatous disease have been reported to cause periodontal changes (Fig 4-14). Recently, a survey of 263 persons with juvenile diabetes, 11 to 18 years old, indicated that 10% demonstrated early-onset periodontitis. (Cianciola et al, 1982).

Down's syndrome

A genetic condition arising from trisomy chromosome 21, Down's syndrome results in mental retardation and many orofacial manifestations. Down's syndrome children are more susceptible to hepatitis, upper respiratory infections, leukemia, and periodontal disease, all of which are probably related to a specific immune defect involving T lymphocytes.

Mucogingival considerations in orthodontics

Surgical exposure of unerupted teeth

Prevention of gingival recession during orthodontic movement is essential. Generally, a gingivectomy procedure to expose the labial surface of an unerupted tooth for direct bonding is sufficient treatment provided the following conditions are present: *(1)* sufficient attached tissue apical to site, *(2)* no bony covering, and *(3)* close proximity of the tooth to the plane of occlusion.

If these conditions are not present, flap surgery is indicated (Figs 4-15 to 4-18). Flap surgery is accomplished in the following manner (Vanarsdall and Corn, 1977; Shiloah and Kopczyk, 1978):

1. Provide adequate space for movement of tooth into proper arch alignment prior to surgery.
2. Make horizontal incision over the edentulous space.
3. Make two slightly converging vertical releasing incisions from the alveolar mucosa to the horizontal incision, allowing the apical base of the flap to be wider (to ensure adequate blood supply to the flap).
4. Release a partial-thickness flap to uncover the crown surface. Do not interfere with the cementoenamel junction because of future dentogingival attachment requirements.
5. Apically position and suture the flap at a minimum of 3 mm incisal to the cementoenamel junction of the exposed crown.

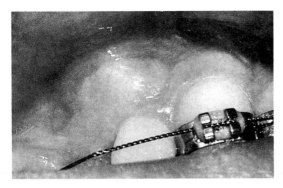

Fig 4-15 In this clinical situation, insufficient attached gingiva is apical to an unerupted maxillary canine before its surgical exposure and orthodontic extrusion.

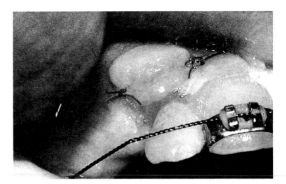

Fig 4-16 An apically repositioned flap is completed to elevate sufficient keratinized tissue above the crown and sutured in place.

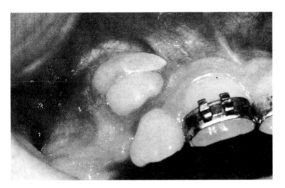

Fig 4-17 Ten days following the procedure, the labial surface is ready for a direct-bonded orthodontic bracket.

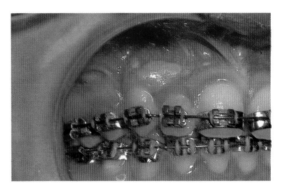

Fig 4-18 Following completion of the orthodontic movement of the canine into the arch, there is sufficient keratinized gingival tissue above the crown to help prevent recession.

6. Place a pack and leave it in position for 7 to 10 days.
7. Remove the pack and place the direct-bonded bracket. Sufficient attached gingiva is now apical to the crown to ensure its location following orthodontic movement of the tooth into the arch.

Treatment of gingival recession

To withstand the frictional and tensional forces placed on it, the attached gingiva must have a minimum width of 1 mm (Ochsenbeim and Maynard 1974). To ensure an adequate width of keratinized gingival tissue, the autogenous free gingival graft is preferred over the laterally positioned flap in children (Maynard and Ochsenbein, 1975). Before surgery, removal of local irritation and inflammation with plaque control must be accomplished. The graft should be placed before orthodontic correction to prevent further risk of attachment loss (Maynard and Ochsenbein, 1975) (Figs 4-19 to 4-22).

Surgical crown extension

Following orthodontic treatment, surgical crown extension may be esthetically desirable. By performing a gingivectomy to the bottom of the existing gingival crevice, a mean increase in crown height of 1 mm will occur, with regeneration of 44% of the original crevice depth in 5 weeks (Monefeldt and Zachrisson, 1977). Healing occurs by coronal proliferation, not apical migration. Net gain in crown height can be predicted to be 40% to 50% of initial crevice depth.

Supra-alveolar and gingival crest fibrotomy

During orthodontic movement, the transeptal and circumferential gingival fibers resist movement and become distorted. The resulting tension contributes to relapse and ultimate treatment failure. Severance of these fibers after orthodontic treatment will relieve these tensile forces and allow reattachment free of tension (Crum and Andreasen, 1974). These fibers are cut by placement of a scalpel into the gingival crevice, extending the incision to or below the alveolar crest

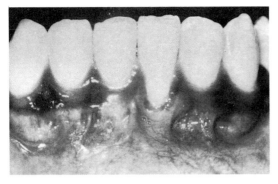

Fig 4-19 In this clinical situation, mandibular central incisor demonstrates extensive gingival recession, resulting in inadequate attached keratinized gingival tissue.

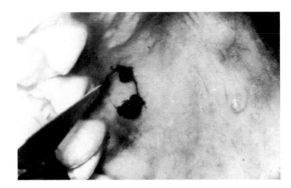

Fig 4-20 The patient's palatal tissue is anesthetized, and an adequate-sized section of tissue is excised from the donor site.

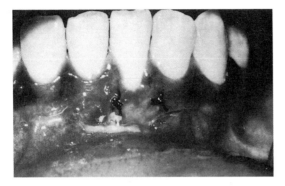

Fig 4-21 The recipient site is prepared before the suturing of the autogenous graft at that site. A periodontal pack is placed over the site for 1 week.

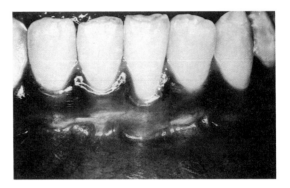

Fig 4-22 Results 1 year later confirm the presence of sufficient attached tissue and a slight reduction in the severity of the recession.

around the entire crown circumference. Studies have indicated that this treatment does not affect future periodontal health of the tooth (Hansson and Linder-Aronson, 1976). However, retention is still required to allow for periodontal ligament and osseous adjustment to the orthodontic movement.

Labial frenulotomy

A hypertrophied labial frenum results from an excess of fibrous connective tissue in the frenum that often transverses from the lip to the lingual papilla with extension into the intermaxillary suture and median palatal raphe (Fig 4-23). It generally does not affect nursing, speech, or alveolar growth in the infant and young child. As the primary teeth erupt, and with alveolar bone growth, the frenum attachments migrate superiorly from the alveolar ridge. If it persists after the eruption of the anterior permanent teeth, a median incisal diastema, a maxillary median alveolar cleft, and resultant malocclusion and periodontal problems may develop. Entrapment of epithelial rests may prevent com-

plete fusion of premaxilla. Often, eruptive movement of the permanent anterior teeth causes closure of this diastema, making frenulotomy and treatment by orthodontic closure unnecessary.

Ankyloglossia

Hypertrophied lingual frenum results from fibrous connective tissue that extends from a higher than normal attachment on the mandibular alveolar ridge and ventral tip of the tongue along the midline raphe and may restrict movement (ankyloglossia) (Fig 4-24). This defect rarely causes nursing or speech problems, probably because of immediate adaptation by the infant. Early surgical correction is contraindicated because of reported postsurgical bilateral infection of the submandibular glands. It is unlikely that this hypertrophic frenum will cause residual occlusal and periodontal problems. Frenulotomy should be based on these residual dental problems and not on speech problems from supposed unrestricted articulatory tongue movements because these are not significant.

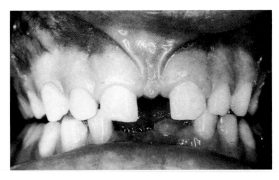

Fig 4-23 Hypertrophic labial frenum. Hypertrophic labial frenum results from excess fibrous connective tissue in the frenum that transverses from the lip to the lingual papilla with extensions into the intermaxillary suture and median palatal raphe. It generally does not affect nursing, speech development, alveolar growth, or eruption of the primary dentition.

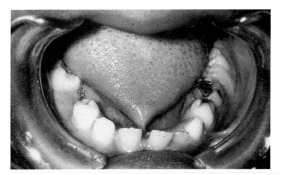

Fig 4-24 Hypertrophic lingual frenum. Hypertrophic lingual frenum results from excess fibrous connective tissue that extends from a higher-than-normal attachment on both the mandibular alveolar ridge and ventral tip of the tongue along the midline raphe. It may restrict tongue movement (ankyloglossia).

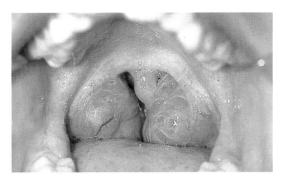

Fig 4-25 Hyperplastic tonsillar tissue.

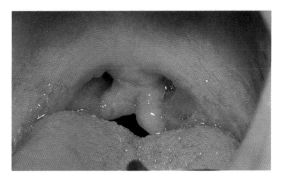

Fig 4-26 Bifid uvula.

Hypoplastic tonsils

Hyperplastic tonsillar tissue is noninflammatory, hyperplastic tissue in the tonsillar area that is often confused with pharyngotonsillitis (Fig 4-25). The enlarged tonsillar tissue may approximate the midline and may impinge on the uvula. Hyponasal speech, feeding difficulties, and anterior tongue trusting secondary to this disturbance may necessitate tonsillectomy.

Bifid uvula

A bifid uvula indicates the probable presence of a submucosal cleft which can be further confirmed by the palpable notching of the posterior portion of the hard and soft palates and a zona pellucida or thin, translucent membrane covering the cleft (Fig 4-26).

Oral lesions and infections

The following is a list of oral lesions and infections in children that might be encountered in dental practice (Sanger, 1978):

1. White lesions and infections
   Inclusion cysts
   White sponge nevus
   Geographic tongue (migratory glossitis)
   Candidiasis
   Lichen planus
   Focal hyperkeratosis associated with smokeless tobacco
2. Vesicular-desquamative lesions and infections
   Herpetic gingivostomatitis
   Herpangina
3. Ulcerative lesions
   Recurrent aphthous stomatitis
   Traumatic ulcers
4. Pigmented lesions
   Nevus and ephelis
5. Compressible lesions
   Eruption cyst
   Hemorrhagic cyst
   Gingival parulis
   Mucous retention phenomenon (mucocele)
   Hemangioma
   Lymphangioma
6. Nonhemorrhagic soft tissue lesions
   Congenital epulis

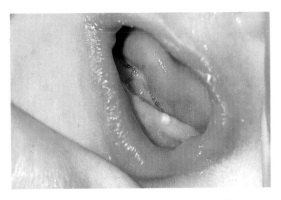

Fig 4-27 Inclusion cyst. Inclusion cysts, frequently encountered in the neonate, are one or multiple freely mobile, circumscribed, nodular, white lesions. This small, superficial, keratin-containing cyst is referred to as a *dental lamina cyst* when present on the crest of the alveolar ridge. The lesions are asymptomatic and nonexpansive, and exfoliate spontaneously within a few weeks after appearance. Therefore, they require no treatment except parental counseling.

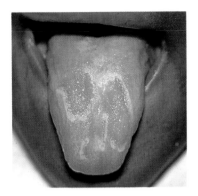

Fig 4-28 Geographic tongue. Migratory glossitis, or geographic tongue, has desquamative areas on the dorsal and lateral aspects of the tongue. The desquamative areas (lacking filiform papillae) heal but reappear in other locations, contributing to its migratory characteristic. It has no known etiology.

Table 4-3 Differential diagnosis of inclusion cysts based on their location and content*

Location	Content	Infant	Child/ Adolescent
Midpalate	Squamous epithelium	Epstein's pearls	Medial palatine cyst
Side of ridge	Mucous gland remnants	Bohn's nodules	Mucocele
Crest of ridge	Odontogenic epithelium	Dental lamina (eruption) cyst	Dentigerous cyst

*Adapted from Fromm (1967).

7. Hemorrhagic soft tissue lesions
   Peripheral giant cell reparative granuloma
   Pyogenic granuloma
8. Papillary lesions
   Papilloma
   Verruca vulgaris (wart)

A more complete list with delineation can be found in the numerous oral pathology reference texts. The lesions and infections are delineated by clinical appearance, behavior, or both and should aid the clinician in problem-oriented diagnosis and treatment (Bhasker and Jacoway, 1966b; Gardner, 1964; Robinson, 1956; Wright et al, 1984).

White lesions and infections

Inclusion cysts. Inclusion cysts are one or more white, freely mobile, circumscribed nodular lesions encountered in 75% of newborns. They are small, superficial, keratin-containing cysts that are classified according to content and location as (1) Epstein's pearls when they appear along the palatal midline and contain squamous epithelium, (2) dental lamina cysts when they appear on the crest of the alveolar ridge as a preeruption phenomenon and contain odontogenic epithelium (Fig 4-27), and (3) Bohn's nodules when they appear along the buccal and lingual aspects of the alveolar ridge and contain mucous gland remnants. The lesions usually are multiple and asymptomatic, do not increase in size, and are spontaneously exfoliated within a few weeks and therefore require no treatment. The lesions appear to have similar counterparts in the child and adolescent as median palatine cysts, dentigerous cysts, and mucous retention cysts (Fromm, 1967) (Table 4-3).

White sponge nevus. A white sponge nevus is a childhood genokeratosis characterized by diffuse, spongy, and patchy white lesions present of the buccal mucosa, usually bilaterally, and occasionally on the tongue and other mucosal areas. The lesions may be confused with those of hereditary benign intraepithelial dyskeratosis, lichen planus, and monilial infection; a biopsy is necessary for definitive diagnosis. The lesions are inherited as an autosomal-dominant condition. No treatment is necessary. Variable involvement of the esophageal, anal, vulval, and vaginal mucosa may be expected.

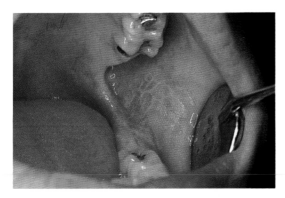

Fig 4-29 Lichen planus. Oral lichen planus presents as asymptomatic white striae, usually on the buccal mucosa but sometimes on the tongue, gingiva, and palate. It is a common, chronic inflammatory mucocutaneous disease of adults but is rarely seen in children.

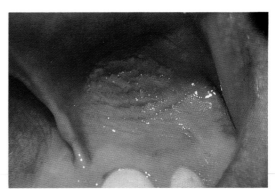

Fig 4-30 Focal hyperkeratosis associated with smokeless tobacco. The white wrinkled lesions in the mucobuccal fold occur in the immediate area where the tobacco is habitually placed by an adolescent with a smokeless tobacco habit.

Geographic tongue (migratory glossitis). Geographic tongue, or migratory glossitis is characterized by migratory desquamative areas on the dorsal and lateral margins of the tongue (Fig 4-28). Erosion and loss of the filiform papillae are seen in the desquamative area circumscribed by white keratotic hypertrophic filiform papillae. The tongue may appear then to have both white and red lesions. The migratory nature of the lesions makes for definitive diagnosis. The lesions appear in childhood and may last for years, with an incidence of 1% to 2% of the population; girls are more commonly affected. The lesions may also accompany a host of other dermatologic conditions. The lesions are benign, and no treatment is necessary. Glossodynia is a persistent symptom (Redman, 1970).

Candidiasis. Fungal infections occur frequently in infants 5 to 7 days after birth and appear in the classic form as multiple, small, white, curdlike patch lesions that may be easily removed from the mucous-exposing areas of erythema and ulceration, which readily bleed. The buccal, labial, and gingival mucosa as well as the tongue and palate are often simultaneously involved. The infection is caused by a yeastlike fungus *Candida* (formerly *Monilia*) *albicans.* Lesions contain desquamated epithelial cells, keratin, fibrin, necrotic tissue, food debris, inflammatory cells, bacteria, and a heavy infiltration of fungal hyphae. Definitive diagnosis is often made by clinical features and cytology, and culture is rarely necessary. Symptoms may be mild, but the infant may exhibit some difficulty in nursing and irritability. Recurrence of the condition is rare. The condition may be transmitted from the mother's vagina or from contamination in the nursery. Infants with systemic disease or those receiving antibiotics, steroids, or cytotoxins are more susceptible and less amenable to treat-

ment. The physician should eliminate topical or parenteral antibiotics and corticosteroids where possible before therapy for oral lesions is instituted. When systemic disease or predisposing factors are present, nystatin can be used topically. Suspensions of nystatin (Mycostatin) (100,000 to 200,000 units/mL) in an adhesive vehicle or clotrimazole troches may be applied several times daily until the infection is eliminated. Chronic infections involving areas outside the mouth are difficult to treat and should be aggressively treated by a physician.

Lichen planus. Lichen planus is a chronic inflammatory mucocutaneous disease, often presenting in a reticular form, that is characterized by the presence of numerous interlacing keratotic lines (Wickham's striae) that produce a lacy pattern (Fig 4-29). The primary target is epithelial basal cells, whose damage is related to a cell-mediated immune process in which the severity of the disease parallels the patient's stress level. Corticosteriods are used to treat the disease because of their ability to modulate inflammation and the immune response.

Focal hyperkeratosis associated with smokeless tobacco. The increasing use of smokeless tobacco by US youth has been related to both peer pressure and media advertising (Creath et al, 1988). The white lesions of the oral mucosa develop in the immediate area, usually the mandibular mucobuccal fold, where the tobacco or snuff is habitually placed by the user. The epithelium will have a granular or wrinkled appearance but generally remains asymptomatic (Fig 4-30). Treatment consists of counseling the patient to discontinue the habit and biopsy of persistent or suspicious areas because of the potential for malignant transformation.

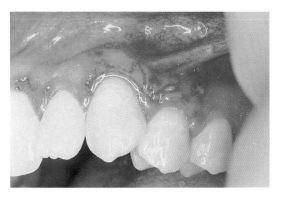

Fig 4-31 Primary herpetic gingivostomatitis. Primary herpetic gingivostomatitis, characterized by acute, marginal gingivitis and involvement of primarily mucous membranes with vesicular-ulcerative lesions, is a herpes simplex viral disease usually of type I. It is self-limiting, with a duration of 7 to 14 days, does not cause scarring, is usually accompanied secondarily by fever, malaise, and anorexia, and is treated symptomatically and supportively. Fluids should be encouraged to prevent dehydration. Antibiotics and cortcosteriods are ineffective.

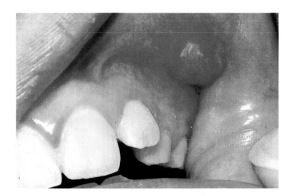

Fig 4-32 Recurrent aphthous ulceration—minor type. Recurrent aphthous ulcerations, or canker sores, are characterized by rapid development of highly sensitive craters with a grayish membrane surrounded by an indurated zone of inflammation in the mucobuccal fold of the mucous membrane. The lesions, larger than those of herpetic origin, are thought to be of bacterial origin and appear with few secondary systemic symptoms. Treatment is usually palliative, but, in severe cases, tetracycline suspension has been effective.

Vesicular-desquamative lesions and infections

Herpetic gingivostomatitis. Herpetic gingivostomatitis is a viral infection characterized as a generalized acute marginal gingivitis with involvement of primarily mucous membranes with vesicular-ulcerative lesions (Fig 4-31). Two known types of herpes simplex infections specific to the two herpes simplex viruses (HSV) exist, HSV type I and HSV type II. Herpes simplex virus type I is generally responsible for the majority of oral and pharyngeal infections, meningoencephalitis, and dermatitis above the waist, whereas HSV type II is generally responsible for the majority of infections in the neonatal period and dermatitis below the waist. Herpes simplex virus type II infections of the newborn are probably related to contact of the newborn with maternal HSV type II vaginal infection. Herpes simplex virus type I rarely occurs before the age of 6 months because of the presence of circulating antibodies in most infants from their mothers.

The presence of neutralizing antibodies to this virus in 70% of the population indicates the widespread prevalence of this disease in infants and young children (Cohen, 1964). The peak incidence appears to be around 2 years of age (Brooke, 1973). Incubation period is 4 to 5 days. There is a prodromal period of 1 to 2 days featuring malaise, fever, discomfort, and gingival inflammation. Then yellowish or white vesicles (1 to 2 mm in diameter) appear, rupture, and leave very painful erosions.

Adjacent erosions coalesce to form larger irregular ulcers. Symptoms include fever (99°F to 104°F; 37.3°C to 40°C,) anorexia, malaise, and lymphadenopathy. Secondary bacterial infection may occur. Duration of

the disease is from 10 to 14 days and is self-limiting. Because little can be done to change its course, treatment is supportive. Forced fluids may be required to prevent dehydration and maintain proper electrolyte balance (Lennette and Magoffen, 1973). Bland diet with multiple vitamin therapy has been suggested, with application of a mild topical anesthetic before feeding. A mixture of diphenhydramine (Benadryl) elixir and kaolin-pectin (Kaopectate) in equal parts may be helpful as a mouthwash before meals to reduce soreness. Antipyretics and analgesics will help control fever and pain. Only about 1% of those infected will display the severe, acute manifestations of this disease. The remainder will have subclinical infections. The virus may remain dormant intracellularly and, if activated, will produce recurrent lesions.

Recently, a number of virus-specific drugs have been developed but with limited and inconsistent success in alleviating HSV infections. Oral acyclovir is recommended for severe systemic infections or in the immunocompromised child. Topical 5% acyclovir ointment may be helpful in reducing the duration of secondary lesions at the first sign of symptoms. Acyclovir interrupts viral replication through inhibition of DNA polymerization.

Herpangina. Herpangina, or aphthous pharyngitis, is a viral disease characterized by the appearance of small vesicular-ulcerative lesions in the anterior faucial pillars, soft palate, and tongue. Before the appearance of the vesicular lesions, there may be pharyngitis, fever, headache, vomiting, prostration, and abdominal pain. A generalized gingivitis and stomatitis may be present

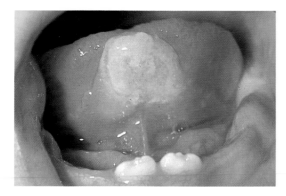

Fig 4-33 Traumatic ulcerative lesions. Ulcerative lesions are common in children and are usually identified as Riga-Fede's disease when present on the lingual frenum and ventral tip of the tongue and as pterygoid ulcers (Bednar's apthae) when present near the greater palatine foramen. Ulceration is usually caused by natal-neonatal teeth or attempts at birth to clear the oral cavity of foreign matter. Extraction of natal-neonatal teeth may be necessary, but most often treatment is supportive because the ulcers are self-limiting and heal spontaneously.

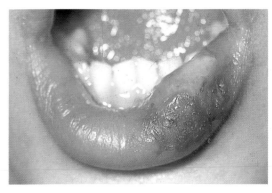

Fig 4-34 Traumatic lip biting. Frequently after anesthesia of the mucosa on a young child unaccustomed to the loss of such sensory sensation, biting of the mucosa of the lips and vestibule will result in gross ulceration, loss of tissue, and possible scarring. Proper instruction to the patient after anesthesia is essential in the prevention of this traumatic lip bite.

along with regional lymphadenopathy. The disease is caused by different strains of coxsackie viruses A and B. Infants and young children may be affected numerous times during the summer season because of the different strains of coxsackie viruses A and B. A differential diagnosis should include primary herpetic gingivostomatitis and hand-foot-mouth disease. The disease is contagious and common among school-aged children. Treatment may consist of a palliative mouth rinse of antihistamine elixir with kaolin-pectin in a 50:50 mixture. The infection is self-limiting and recovery occurs in less than 1 week.

Ulcerative lesions

Recurrent aphthous stomatitis. Aphthous ulcers (canker sores) may occur as singular or multiple lesions. They are shallow and flat, have a central white fibrinous pseudomembrane, and are surrounded by an erythematous halo (Fig 4-32). Etiologic factors are varied, but delayed hypersensitivity, autoimmune responses to oral epithelium, and streptococci organisms are commonly implicated. The lesions tend to occur during periods of stress, and the frequency of the recurrence and multiplicity is extremely varied. Because no vesicles form before ulceration, the lesions should be easily distinguished from typical viral lesions. A prodromal sensation of burning followed by the appearance of a highly sensitive ulcerative crater is typical. Treatment is usually palliative and supportive. In extreme cases topical steroid preparations may be applied two to three times per day. Tetracycline suspension is also helpful if

a streptococcal etiology is suspected. A dose of 125 mg of tetracycline suspension is rinsed in the mouth for 2 minutes and then swallowed four times per day for 5 to 7 days. No food is taken for 1 hour after each dose. An excellent review of the etiology, pathogenesis, diagnosis, and treatment of aphthous ulcerations is highly recommended to the interested reader (Antoon and Miller, 1980).

Traumatic ulcers. Traumatic ulcers occur commonly in children as a result of a variety of self-inflicted or iatrogenic dental insults. They are often classified according to location.

Pterygoid ulcers (Bednar's aphthae) are superficial, traumatic abrasions of the palatal mucosa near the greater palatine foramen resulting from attempts to clear the mouth of foreign matter at birth. Abrasion of the mucosa covering the pterygoid processes results in the stripping of this area, which is then covered with necrotic membrane. Treatment is supportive since ulcers are self-limiting and heal spontaneously.

Riga-Fede disease is an ulcerative lesion occurring on the lingual frenum and ventral tip of the tongue of newborns and infants (Fig 4-33). It may be caused by natal and neonatal teeth. The lesion is an ulcerative response to local irritation. Treatment includes removal of the irritation source and supportive therapy until the lesion disappears.

Lip biting after the administration of mandibular block anesthesia occurs in young children not familiar with the loss of sensory perception in the lip. Failure to warn the child to refrain from lip biting can result in a traumatic ulceration (Fig 4-34).

Pigmented lesions

The oral mucosa of blacks and many dark-skinned whites is often speckled with diffuse and multifocal brownish pigmentations. These are not lesions per se but mere accumulations of melanin granules in the basal cell layer resulting from racial evolution. These should be considered normal variations in these individuals. In whites without pigmented skin, the presence of these pigmentations may indicate systemic disease, such as Addison's disease, neurofibromatosis, or heavy metal ingestion.

Nevus and ephelis. Nevi are plaque or dome-shaped sessile nodules that may occur on the oral structures with blue or black pigmentation. More commonly they are nonpigmented. They appear during childhood, reach a given size, and persist into adulthood. Common sites are the palate, buccal mucosa, and lips. Nevus types include junctional, compound, intramucosal, blue, and spindle cell nevi differentiated by tissue involvement. An ephelis is a common freckle appearing on the lips as a brown macule of varying size that lacks nevus cells. Because of the possibility that a junctional nevus in an adult may evolve into a malignant melanoma, all pigmented lesions in children and adolescents in which nevus is a possibility in the differential diagnosis should be excised and submitted for histologic evaluation.

Compressible lesions

Eruption cyst. An eruption cyst is a bluish, translucent, elevated, compressible, dome-shaped lesion of the alveolar ridge associated with an erupting primary or permanent tooth (Fig 4-35). Transillumination will help differentiate it from a bluish opaque eruption hematoma, which results from spontaneous bleeding into the gingival tissue during eruption. An eruption cyst is a soft tissue dentigerous cyst in which the associated tooth carries the cystic lesion to the alveolar ridge. They may be seen occasionally on a radiograph and are painless unless secondarily infected. The cyst may be punctured, marsupialized, or "deroofed" (removal of a portion of the tissue overlying the crown), which facilitates eruption. If left untreated, the cyst may rupture spontaneously. Delay in eruption may occur with these cysts, but this delay is temporary. On rare occasions, displacement of the erupting tooth may occur (Clark, 1962; Seward, 1973).

Hemorrhagic cyst. This bluish, asymptomatic lesion is found overlying some erupting teeth (Fig. 4-36). The swelling is due to accumulation of tissue fluid, blood, or both in the dilated follicular sac around the erupting crown. Treatment is not indicated, although incision is sometimes performed.

Gingival parulis. Intraoral drainage from an abscessed tooth is created by a fistulous tract that, if blocked, results in a swelling termed *parulis* (Fig 4-37).

Mucous retention phenomenon (mucocele). The mucous retention phenomenon, or mucocele, is a pseudocystic subepithelial lesion formed subsequent to traumatic injury and breakage of a minor salivary duct with resultant pooling of extraductal mucin and inflammatory cells in the mucosal pseudocyst (Fig 4-38). As a dome-shaped lesion it has a bluish fluid-containing appearance, especially if superficially located on the buccal mucosa and lip. Blood may also enter the pseudocystic space with resultant hemorrhagic appearance. If it occurs in the floor of the mouth, the lesion is referred to as a *ranula* (Fig 4-39). A history of paroxysmal swelling and collapse in response to gustatory activity and antecedent trauma is common. The lesion should be excised with inclusion of underlying salivary tissue to minimize recurrence.

Hemangioma and lymphangoima. Hemangiomas and lymphangiomas may be congenital or early neonatal. Hemangiomas are smooth, purplish red, compressible lesions that are partly elevated and partly submerged and will blanch under pressure. Oral hemangiomas are classified as capillary, cavernous, and juvenile. Capillary hemangiomas consist of numerous, diffuse capillaries that penetrate the mucosa, especially of the lips and cheeks (Fig 4-40). Cavernous hemangiomas consist of few or numerous blood-containing spaces that occupy the area, especially the tongue. Juvenile hemangoimas consist of numerous small vessels that infiltrate the site, especially the salivary glands and lip musculature.

Oral hemangiomas have limited growth and will generally hemorrhage if traumatized. Superficial lesions can be removed by excision or fibrosed by the induction of sclerosing solutions. Spontaneous regression often follows biopsy or traumatization. Therefore, surgical treatment is usually postponed unless growth is rapid and alters function.

Oral lymphangiomas are commonly seen on the tongue. Superficial lesions may be small clusters of compressible excrescences on the mucosa, whereas deep-seated lesions may produce diffuse enlargement of the tongue and obliterate its normal surface architecture and, in severe cases, cause macroglossia. Oral lymphangiomas consist of large lymph-containing spaces that, when superficial, lie immediately under the epithelium. Lymphangiomas are treated only by excision.

Lymphangioma of the soft tissues, usually found in the neck of infants and children, is classified as cystic hygroma, which may develop as a large, soft, pliable, singular mass, becoming pendulous. The mass may be present at birth and will require total surgical removal during early childhood.

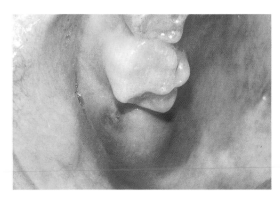

Fig 4-35 Eruption cyst. The eruption cyst is a bluish, transparent, elevated, compressible, dome-shaped lesion of the alveolar ridge associated with eruption of a primary or permanent tooth. Transillumination will help differentiate it from a bluish opaque eruption hematoma that results from bleeding into gingival tissues during eruption. Eruption cysts may be dentigerous cysts.

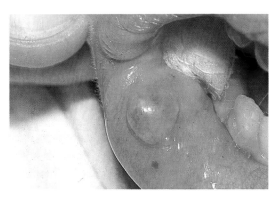

Fig 4-36 Eruption hematoma. The eruption hematoma is a bluish, opaque, asymptomatic lesion that may be found underlying an erupting tooth (in this case a permanent first molar). The swelling is due to accumulation of fluid in the dental follicular sac and is self-limiting on rupture during gingival emergence.

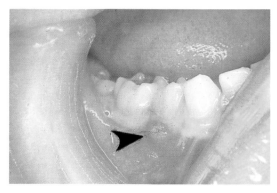

Fig 4-37 Gingival parulis. Chronic abscess formation at nonvital teeth may result in a gingival parulis (arrow) adjacent to the infected tooth. The parulis represents a fistulous tract through which purulent exudate drains.

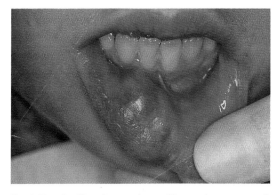

Fig 4-38 Mucous retention phenomenon. Mucous retention phenomenon, or mucocele, the most common lip swelling in children, is caused by trauma to a minor salivary duct resulting in the accumulation of mucus in the soft tissue and proliferation of granulation tissue. Although the lesion may rupture spontaneously, recurrences are high unless the lesion is totally excised.

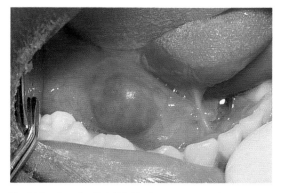

Fig 4-39 Ranula. Sialolith blockage or traumatic severance of a salivary duct may result in a cyclic, sometimes painful, swelling in the lateral floor of the mouth that appears as a fluctuant, bluish-white elevation.

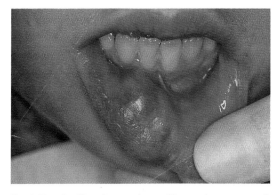

Fig 4-40 Capillary hemangioma. Hemangiomas are reddish-blue lesions that blanch when compressed and represent a congenital vascular malformation.

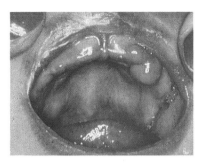

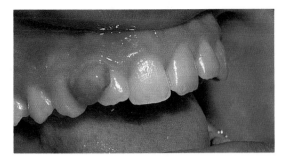

Fig 4-41 Congenital epulis. This lesion, originally thought to be congenital but which may also be neonatal, usually appears as a single, elevated, smooth, nonhemorrhagic, benign soft tissue growth of the mucosa of the maxilla or, rarely, of the mandible. It is commonly described as a congenital epulis of the newborn. It is more common in girls, occurs sporadically, is classified as an embryonic hamartoma, and often requires surgical excision with low recurrence rate.

Fig 4-42 Peripheral giant cell reparative granuloma. This lesion is a firm, benign tumor of gingival tissue and is capable of eroding underlying bone.

Nonhemorrhagic soft tissue lesions

Congenital epulis. The lesion, which was originally thought to be congenital but which may also be neonatal, usually appears as a single, elevated, pedunculated, smooth, nonhemorrhagic tumor of the mucosa of the maxilla or, rarely, of the mandible (Fig 4-41). It is a benign tumor commonly occurring sporadically in females and classified as an embryonic hamartoma. Although histologically similar to a granular cell tumor, the epulis has different pathogenesis and unknown etiology. Conservative surgical excision is recommended, and few recurrences are reported. This tumor should not be confused with the rare melanotic neuroectodermal tumor of infancy, which is a radiolucent benign tumor of neural crest cells involving the developing primary dentition areas of the maxilla. The clinically evident soft tissue mass resembles an epulis. Biopsy and surgical curettage are usually required for this tumor because sarcomatous change is possible (Fuhr and Krough, 1972; Brekke and Gorlin, 1975; Lopez, 1976).

Hemorrhagic soft tissue lesions

Peripheral giant cell reparative granuloma. The peripheral giant cell reparative granuloma is a bluish, aggressive, firm, benign tumor of the gingival tissue (periosteum) surrounding primary or permanent teeth (Fig 4-42). The tumor is capable of eroding underlying bone. Consistent with reactive gingival tumor, it is commonly found in the hormonally developing or pregnant woman. Treatment includes scaling and curettage of the area and surgical excision of the tumor to the periosteum. If this is not adequately accomplished, recurrence is common (Giansanti and Waldron, 1969; Eversole et al, 1972)

Pyogenic granuloma. The pyogenic granuloma is a reactive gingival tumor that appears as growth of granulation tissue, generally at the dental papillae, and results from chronic irritation. The tumor is often encountered in the young pregnant woman and is classified as a pregnancy tumor. Treatment includes scaling and curettage of the area and surgical excision of the tumor. In the pregnant patient, recurrence is common, and surgical treatment should be postponed until after delivery (Eversole et al, 1972; Bhaskar and Jacoway, 1966a).

Papillary lesions

Papilloma. A papilloma is a white pedunculated broad-based, cauliflowerlike lesion that may be encountered anywhere in the oral cavity. The lesion is slow growing and painless. It can be easily excised and seldom recurs.

Verruca vulgaris (wart). Verruca vulgaris, or wart, is a white, papillary lesion usually seen on the vermillion border of the lip. It is virally induced by a papova virus. The lesion is slow growing and painless. It also can be easily excised and seldom recurs.

References

American Academy of Periodontology (AAP). Proceedings of the World Workshop in Clinical Periodontics. Chicago: AAP, 1989, pp. 123-124.

American Academy of Periodontology (AAP). Periodontal Diseases of Children and Adolescents. Chicago: AAP Research, Science and Therapy Committee, 1991,

Antoon, J.W., and Miller, R.L. Aphthous ulcers—A review of the literature on etiology, pathogenesis, diagnosis, and treatment. J. Am. Dent. Assoc. 101:803, 1980.

Baer, P.N. The case of periodontosis as a clinical entity. J. Periodontol. 42:516, 1971.

Baer, P.N., and Benjamin, S.D. Periodontal disease in children and adolescents. Philadelphia: J.B. Lippincott Co., 1974.

Bhaskar, S.N., and Jacoway, J.R. Pyogenic granuloma clinical features, incidence, histology and result of treatment: Report of 242 cases. J. Oral Surg. 24:391, 1966a.

Bhasker, S.N., and Jacoway, J.R. Oral lesions in infants and newborns. Dent. Clin. North Am. 10:421, 1966b.

Bowers, G.M. A study of the width of attached gingiva. J. Periodontol. 34:201, 1963.

Brekke, R., and Gorlin, R.J. Melanotic neuroectodermal tumor of infancy. J. Oral Surg. 33:858, 1975.

Brooke, A.H. Acute herpetic gingivostomatitis in children. J. Dent. Child, 40:12, 1973.

Brown R.S., et al. On the mechanism of drug-induced gingival hyperplasia. J. Oral Pathol. Med. 20:201, 1991.

Brucker M. Studies on the incidence and cause of dental defects in children. III. Gingivitis. J. Dent. Res. 22:309, 1943.

Butler, R.T. et al. Drug-induced gingival hyperplasia: Phenytoin, cyclosporine, and nifedipine. J. Am. Dent. Assoc. 114:56, 1987.

Carter, W.J., and Wells, J.E. Epidemiology of gingival disease in Kansas City, MIssouri, school children. Midwest Dent. 36:21, 1960.

Chawla, H.S. Clinical evaluation of depth of gingival sulcus of primary teeth. J. Ind. Dent. Assoc. 45:175, 1973.

Cianciola, L.J., et al. Prevalence of periodontal disease in insulin-dependent diabetes mellitus (juvenile diabetes). J. Am. Dent. Assoc. 104:653, 1982.

Clark, C.A. A survey of eruption cysts in the newborn. Oral Surg. 14:917, 1962.

Cohen, M.M. Recognition of periodontal disease in children. J. Dent. Child. 31:7, 1964.

Cox, M.O., et al. Oral leukocytes and gingivitis in primary dentition. J. Periodont. Res. 9:23, 1974.

Creath, C.J., et al. The prevalence of smokeless tobacco use among adolescent male athletes. J. Am. Dent. Assoc. 116:43-47, 1988.

Crum, R.E., and Andreasen, G.F. The effect of gingival fiber surgery on the retention of rotated teeth. Am. J. Orthod. 65:626, 1974.

Daley, T.D., et al. Clinical and pharmacologic correlations in cyclosporine-induced gingival hyperplasia. Oral Surg. Oral Med. Oral Pathol. 62:417-21, 1986.

deAraugo, W.C., and MacDonald, J.B. The gingival crevice microbiota of preschool children. J. Periodontol. 35:285, 1964.

Dorfman, J.S., Lentz, J.D., and Currier, G.F. Pediatric periodontics. Va. Dent. J. 53:48, 1976.

Easley, J.R., and Weis, R.W. Incidence of the retrocuspid papilla. J. Dent. Child. 37:523, 1970.

Everett, F.G., Tuchler, H., and Lu, K.H. Occurrence of calculus in grade school children in Portland, Oregon. J. Periodontol. 34:54, 1963.

Eversole, L.R., Sabes, W.R., and Rovin, S. Reactive lesions of the gingiva. J. Oral Pathol. 1:30, 1972.

Fromm, A. Epstein's pearls, Bohn's nodules, and inclusion cysts of the oral cavity. J. Dent. Child. 34:275, 1967.

Fuder, E., and Jamison, H. Depth of the gingival sulcus surrounding young permanent teeth. J. Periodontol. 34:457, 1963.

Fuhr, A.H., and Krough, P.H. Congenital eupulis of the newborn: Centennial review of the literature and report of a case. J. Oral Surg. 30:30, 1972.

Gardner, A.F. Tumor and tumor-like lesions of oral cavity in infants and children. J. Dent. Child. 31:42, 1964.

Genco, R.J. Using antimicrobial agents to manage periodontal disease. J. Am. Dent. Assoc. 122:31, 1991.

Giansanti, J.S., and Waldron, C.A. Peripheral giant cell granuloma: Review of 720 cases. Oral Surg. 27:787, 1969.

Goepferd, S.J. Advanced alveolar bone loss in the primary dentition. A case report. J. Periodontol. 52:753, 1981.

Gottlieb, B., and Orban, B. Active and passive continuous eruption of teeth. J. Dent. Res. 13:214, 1933.

Hansson, C., and Linder-Aronson, S. Periodontal health following fibrotomy of the supra-alveolar fibers. Scand. J. Dent. Res. 84:11, 1976.

Jamison, H.C. Prevalence of periodontal disease of the deciduous teeth. J. Am. Dent. Assoc. 66:207, 1963.

Jimenez, L.M., and Baer, P.M. Necrotizing ulcerative gingivitis in children: A 9 year clinical study. J. Periodontol. 46:715, 1975.

Kelsten, L.B. Periodontal and soft tissue diseases in children. J. Dent. Med. 10:67, 1955.

Lennette, E.H., and Magoffen, R.L. Virologic and immunologic aspects of major oral ulcerations. J. Am. Dent. Assoc. 87:1055, 1973.

Löe, H. The gingival index, the plaque index, and the retention index systems. J Peridontal 38;610, 1967.

Löe, H., Theilade, E., and Jensen, S.B. Experimental gingivitis in man. J. Periodontol. 36:177, 1965.

Loesche, W.J. et al The bacteriology of acute necrotizing ulcerative gingivitis. J. Periodontol. 53:223-30, 1982.

Longhurst, P., Johnson, N.W., and Hopps, R.M. Differences in lymphocyte and plasma cell densities in inflamed gingiva from adults and young children. J. Periodontol. 48:705, 1977.

Lopez, J. Melanotic neuroectodermal tumor of infancy: Review of literature and report of case. J. Am. Dent. Assoc. 93:1159, 1976.

Mackler, S.B., and Crawford, J.J. Plaque development and gingivitis in the primary dentition. J. Periodontol. 44:18, 1973.

Maltias, B., et al. Association of gingivitis with the incidence of Bacteroides melaniogenicus in children. J. Dent. Res. 57:216, 1978 (abstract No. 567).

Massler, M. Co-report: Periodontal disease in children. Int. Dent. J. 8:323, 1958.

Massler, M., Schour, I., and Chopra, B. Occurrence of gingivitis in suburban Chicago school children. J. Periodontol. 21:146, 1950.

Matsson, L. Development of gingivitis in preschool children and young adults. J. Clin. Periodontol. 5:24, 1978.

Maynard, J.G., and Ochsenbein, C. Mucogingival problems, prevalence and therapy in children. J. Periodontol. 46:543, 1975.

Monefeldt, I., and Zachrisson, B. Adjustment of clinical crown height by gingivectomy following orthodontic space closure. Angle Orthod, 47:256, 1977.

Myers, D. A clinical study of the response of the gingival tissue surrounding stainless steel crowns. J. Dent. Child. 42:281, 1975.

Ochsenbein, C., and Maynard, J.G. The problem of attached gingiva in children. J. Dent. Child. 41:263, 1974.

Page, R.C., et al. Prepubertal periodontitis. I. Definition of a clinical entity. J. Periodontol. 54:257, 1983.

Parfitt, G. A five-year longitudinal study of the gingival condition of a group of children in England. J. Peridontol. 28:26, 1957.

Parfitt, G.J., and Mjör, I.A. A clinical evaluation of local gingival recession in children. J. Dent. Child. 31:257, 1964.

Poulsen, S. Epidemiology and indices of gingival and periodontal disease. Pediatr. Dent 3:82, 1981.

Powell, R.N., and McEniery, T.M. Longitudinal study of isolated gingival recession in the mandibular central incisor region of children aged 6-8 years. J. Clin. Periodontol. 9:357, 1982.

Ranney, R.R. Pathogenesis of gingivitis and periodontal disease in children and young adults. Pediatr. Dent. 3:89, 1981.

Redman, RS. Prevalence of geographic tongue, fissured tongue, median rhomboid glossitis, and hair tongue among 3,611 Minnesota school children. Oral Surg 30:390, 1970.

Robinson, H.G. Periodontitis and periodontosis in children and young adolescents. J. Am. Dent. Assoc. 43:709, 1951.

Robinson, H.G. Oral neoplasms of children. Pediatr. Clin. North Am. 3:885, 1956.

Rosenblum, F. Clinical study of the depth of the gingival sulcus in the primary dentition. J. Dent. Child. 33:289, 1966.

Ruben, M.P., Frankl, S.N., and Wallace, S. The histopathology of periodontal disease in children. J. Periodontol. 42:473, 1971.

Sanger, R.G. The mouth of the newborn and infant: Oral conditions and clinical significance. In Moss, S.J. Pediatric Dental Care: An Update for the Dentist and for the Pediatrician. New York: American Academy of Pedodontics, Medcom, Inc., 1978, pp. 6-12.

Seward, M.H. Eruption cyst: An analysis of its clinical features. J. Oral Surg. 31:31, 1973.

Shiloah, J., and Kopczyk, R. Mucogingival considerations in surgical exposure of maxillary impacted canines: Report of a case. J. Dent. Child. 45:79, 1978.

Slots, J., and Rosling, B.G. Suppression of the periodontopathic microflora in localized juvenile periodontitis by systemic tetracycline. J. Clin. Periodontol. 10:465, 1983.

Socransky, S.S., and Manganiello, S.D. The oral microbiota of man from birth to senility. J. Periodontol. 42:485, 1971.

Soni, N.N., Silberkweit, M., and Hayes, R.L. Histological characteristics of stippling in children. J. Periodontol. 34:427, 1963.

Stahl, D.G., and Goldman, H.M. The incidence of gingivitis among a sample of Massachusetts school children. Oral Surg. 6:700, 1953.

Suomi, J.D., et al. Oral calculus in children. J. Periodontol. 42:341, 1971.

Theilade, E., et al. Experimental gingivitis in man, II. A longitudinal clinical and bacteriological investigation. J. Periodont. Res. 1:1, 1966.

Vanarsdall, R.L., and Corn, H. Soft-tissue management of labially positioned unerupted teeth. Am J. Orthod. 72:53, 1977.

Van Winkelhoff, A.J., et al. Microbiological and clinical results of metronidazole plus amoxicillin therapy in *Actinobacillus actinomycetemcomitans*-associated periodontitis. J. Periodontol. 65:52, 1992.

Volchansky, A., and Cleaton-Jones, P. The position of the gingival margin as expressed by clinical crown height in children age 6-16 years. J. Dent. 4:116, 1974.

Watanabe, K. Prepubertal periodontitis: A review of diagnostic criteria, pathogenesis, and differential diagnosis. J. Periodont. Res. 25:31, 1990.

Wright, J.M., et al. A review of the oral manifestations of infections in pediatric patients. Pediatr. Infect. Dis. 3:80, 1984.

Zachrisson, S., and Zachrisson;, B. Gingival condition associated with orthodontic treatment. Angle Orthod. 42:26, 1972.

Zappler, S.E. Periodontal disease in children. J. Am Dent. Assoc. 37:333, 1948.

Questions

1. The prevalence of gingivitis in children:

   a. Is rare (less than 10%) under the age of 5
   b. Increases during the period of the mixed dentition
   c. Reaches a peak at puberty
   d. Varies greatly according to the study examined and the criteria used
   e. All of the above

2. According to the study "Experimental gingivitis in man" (Löe et al, 1965):

   a. Total suspension of oral hygiene practices resulted in the development of gingivitis in 5 days
   b. Only the type, not the number, of oral flora cultured changed
   c. Filamentous forms and spirochetes were early colonizers of the gingival crevice
   d. Gingivitis resolved in 7 days following the resumption of oral hygiene practices
   e. All of the above

3. When the attached gingiva of primary teeth is compared with that of permanent teeth, it is noted that:

   a. The color is redder
   b. The epithelium is thinner and less keratinized
   c. The texture is less stippled
   d. The width is comparatively greater, although mean values are somewhat less
   e. All of the above

4. A 2.5-year-old girl complains of a sore mouth for the last 2 days. The patient has painful cervical lymphadenopathy and a temperature of 38.8° C (102°F). Oral examination reveals numerous yellow-gray vesicles with red margins on the palate, tongue, and gingiva. Which of the following disease conditions is most likely?

   a. Rubella measles
   b. Erythema multiforme
   c. Candidiasis
   d. Herpetic gingivostomatitis
   e. Acute necrotizing ulcerative gingivitis

5. A neonate has asymptomatic, multiple, nodular, white lesions along the midpalatal raphae. What is your diagnosis?

   a. Primary herpetic lesions
   b. Bohn's nodules
   c. Epstein's pearls
   d. Dental lamina cysts
   e. Mucous retention cysts

6. A child has a very sore ulceration of the lower lip. There is no previous history of obvious trauma, and it has appeared to spontaneously occur several hours after receiving dental treatment. What is your diagnosis?

   a. Erosive lichen planus secondary to stress of the dental appointment
   b. Allergic stomatitis to some dental material used
   c. Aphthous ulcer secondary to stress
   d. Traumatic ulcer secondary to administration of local anesthetic
   e. Riga-Fede's disease without any direct association to the treatment rendered

7. On examining the soft tissues, you come across a highly sensitive ulceration located in the mucobuccal fold between the mandibular canine and lateral incisor. It has a grayish membrane surrounded by an indurated zone of inflammation and has been present for only a few days. What is your diagnosis?

   a. Pemphigus vulgaris
   b. Aphthous ulcer
   c. Lichen planus
   d. Eruption cyst (permanent canine)
   e. Mucocele

Chapter 5

Hard Tissue Assessment

Objectives

After studying this chapter, the student should be able to:
1. Identify various dental anomalies of color and texture.
2. Cite etiologic factors influencing the formation of dental caries in children and the interacting relationships of those factors.
3. Discuss the prevalence of dental caries in the primary dentition and in the permanent teeth of the mixed dentition.
4. Describe the distribution of dental caries in children according to tooth type and surface and those factors contributing to its pattern.
5. Describe the clinical development of a carious lesion.
6. Identify differences in the rates of caries progression of primary and permanent teeth.

Anomalies of color and texture

Both intrinsic and extrinsic discoloration of the teeth can occur from a number of different genetic and acquired conditions (Eisenberg and Bernick, 1975). Extrinsic staining of the teeth is superficial and easily removed. Such discolorations are often the result of beverage and food use, iron supplementation, and poor oral hygiene practices. Intrinsic staining can be caused by blood-borne pigments resulting from several conditions (eg, hyperbilirubinemia, porphyria, and erythroblastosis fetalis), drug administration (eg, tetracycline) (Fig 5-1) and a variety of causes resulting in enamel defects (hypomineralization or hypoplasia).

Enamel defects are produced by disruptions in the histodifferentiation, apposition, and mineralization stages of dental development. Environmentally induced enamel defects are found in patients with a negative family history and have an identifiable causative insult and a localized distribution that is horizontal in pattern and corresponds to the timing of the insult at the stage of dental formation (Jorgenson and Yost, 1982). The insult may be related to localized trauma and/or metabolic changes (Figs 5-2 and 5-3). The prevalence of macroscopic enamel defects in primary anterior teeth has been reported to be as high as 41% (Needleman et al, 1991). Hypoplastic enamel defects occurred most commonly on the middle third of the

labial surface of maxillary incisors and correspond frequently with the "neonatal line" believed to emanate from transient neonatal hypocalcemia. Hypoplastic defects on the labial surface of primary canines most likely are caused by localized trauma during development as a result of pressure exerted against the cortical bone. Labial hypoplasia found on primary canines is more susceptible to dental caries formation (Duncan et al, 1988).

In a recent review of enamel hypoplasia in primary teeth, Seow (1991) correlated birth prematurity and low birth weight to the occurrence of enamel hypoplasia. She theorized that the pathogenesis of the condition was associated with osteopenia at birth. In addition, local trauma secondary to placement of laryngoscope and/or orotracheal tubes in prematurely born children has also been cited as a contributory factor.

Enamel defects of genetic origin are found in children with a positive family history and have an unidentifiable nature of insult and a wide distribution in a vertical pattern (Jorgensen and Yost, 1982). Inherited types of enamel hypoplasia are rare and commonly identified as a specific type of amelogenesis imperfecta. These types have been classified as hypoplastic (Fig 5-4), hypocalcification (Fig 5-5), and hypomaturation (Fig 5-6).

Dental fluorosis is observed in areas where water has high fluoride concentrations, and its severity (Fig

5-7 and 5-8) is directly proportional to that concentration. The mechanism of fluoride-induced enamel changes remains unclear but the disturbance occurs during the mineralization stage of crown formation.

Etiology of dental caries

The development of dental caries in children is governed by a complex of etiologic factors. The relative influence of each factor is not completely understood and apparently varies considerably among individuals. Although there is a genetic component to caries formation, heredity plays only a minor role. Dental caries is largely an acquired disease affected by environmental conditions. Four major factors must interact simultaneously to create a carious lesion. They are *(1)* susceptible tooth, *(2)* plaque, *(3)* substrate, and *(4)* time (Keyes, 1969) (Fig 5-9). Each one of these factors and its role in predisposing an individual to caries formation are discussed separately.

Susceptible tooth

Obviously, a susceptible tooth surface must first be present in the oral environment. Beyond its mere presence, several factors will increase the particular susceptibility of an individual tooth to the initiation of caries. First, aberrant anatomic and morphologic configurations, such as deep pits and grooves and broad, flat proximal contact areas, will greatly increase its susceptibility. Second, abnormal position within the den-

tal arch, resulting in poor alignment and crowding, will decrease its accessibility to hygienic measures and will allow it to accumulate quantities of plaque. Third, deficiencies during matrix formation or mineralization resulting in hypoplasia or hypocalcification, respectively, and inadequate incorporation of fluoride into the enamel surface during maturation will produce a surface texture and content less resistant to solubility and demineralization. Last, posteruption age is a factor because newly erupted teeth are less mature and thus more vulnerable to attack by caries.

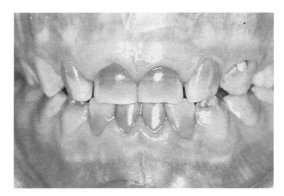

Fig 5-1 Tetracycline discoloration. When tetracyclines are prescribed for pregnant women, especially during the last trimester, the children's primary teeth, and possibly the permanent first molars, may be stained gray brown. Tetracycline does cross the placental barrier, and studies have suggested that the risk of tetracycline staining in the fetus begins after 29 weeks in utero. Tetracyclines intrinsically stain the teeth by becoming incorporated into developing tooth structure. This 7-year-old, who has a history of cystic fibrosis, received tetracycline immediately after birth.

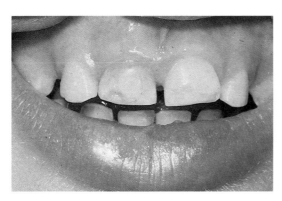

Fig 5-2 Enamel defects. This 4 year old has prenatal enamel hypoplasia. The insult to enamel development probably occurred during the fourth through sixth months of fetal development. Note the primary right central incisor has a blackish color. The primary incisor has a history of trauma. A radiograph would probably show a degenerating pulp with some bone loss or root resorption.

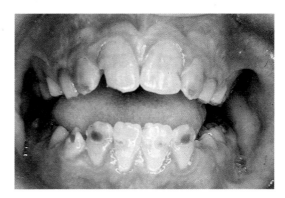

Fig 5-3 Enamel defects. This child has multiple enamel defects of both the hypocalcified and hypoplastic varieties. Hypocalcified enamel is represented by the mild white bands near the incisal edge of the maxillary central incisors. At 18 months, there was a history of an acute systemic disease. This event probably resulted in the hypoplastic involvement of the maxillary and mandibular incisors. The discoloration of the defects is a result of secondary extrinsic staining.

Plaque

For any disease process, there must be not only a host but also an agent. In the case of dental caries, the host is the susceptible tooth, and the agent is cariogenic bacteria organized in a colony termed *plaque.* On smooth surfaces, the principal offending agent in plaque formation is *Streptococcus mutans,* which has the ability to produce a sticky extracellular polysaccharide called *dextran.* Through the manufacture of dextran, these bacterial colonies are able to multiply and adhere in direct contact with the surface. Provided

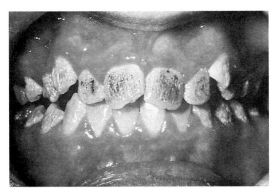

Fig 5-4 Hypoplastic type of amelogenesis imperfecta. Amelogenesis imperfecta is divided into three developmental groups—hypoplastic, hypocalcification. and hypomaturation— with many subtypes and modes of inheritance. The hypoplastic types are attributed to defects in which all or localized portions of the enamel do not reach normal thickness. Clinically, the enamel is very hard and does not flake easily. Complete coverage of the involved teeth is often necessary, but acid etching with a composite resin veneer may also be used.

that the other two interacting factors, substrate and time, are present, the conditions will be conducive to the initiation of a carious lesion. *Streptococcus mutans* has also been shown to have a direct relationship to occlusal caries formation as well as to caries on smooth surfaces in children as young as 5 years (Street et al, 1976). Furthermore, there is a direct increase in growth of this organism as increasing numbers of primary teeth erupt, and the most frequent site of early colonization appears to be in proximal contact areas of molars (Catalanotto et al, 1975). The ecology of the plaque flora changes from aerobic types to facultative anaerobic organisms with maturity. When the lesion has progressed well into dentin, another cariogenic species of bacteria, *Lactobacillus acidophilus,* is often cultured. Therefore, in general terms, *S mutans* is responsible for the initiation of a carious lesion either by adherence to the surface by means of dextran production, or by mechanical retention in pit and fissure areas, whereas *L acidophilus* is more responsible for the progression of the lesion in the subsurface areas.

Substrate

Because dental caries is a disease of bacterial origin, studies confirm that it has an infectious and transmissible nature (Keyes, 1960). However, the inoculation of cariogenic bacteria into the oral environment will not, in itself, induce caries formation. A source of substrate must be available for the metabolism of the bacteria. Refined carbohydrates, especially in the form of sucrose, are the substrate of choice of cariogenic bacteria. Sucrose is metabolized by the bacteria to produce dextran. In addition, fermentable carbohydrates, such

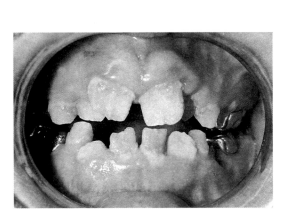

Fig 5-5 Hypocalcification type of amelogenesis imperfecta. Hypocalcified amelogenesis imperfecta types are attributed to defects in calcification of the enamel matrix resulting in enamel of normal thickness but with a soft, cheesy consistency that may be lost soon after eruption or may be easily removed with an instrument. These types are more frequent and must be treated with complete coverage restorations.

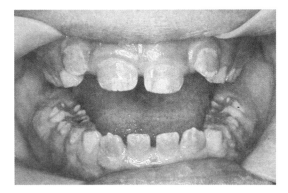

Fig 5-6 Hypomaturation type of amelogenesis imperfecta. Hypomaturation amelogenesis imperfecta types are attributed to defects in enamel maturation or mineralization, resulting in enamel of normal thickness, but softer with a brown-yellow-white appearance and approaching the radiodensity of dentin. These types are often confused with fluorosis. These types must also be treated with complete coverage restorations.

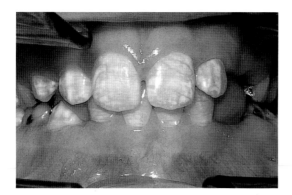

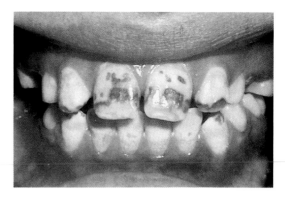

Fig 5-7 Dental fluorosis. These teeth have a milder form of dental fluorosis. Note the symmetric appearance of the white bands around the incisors. When the fluoride content in the water exceeds 1.5 ppm, a few fluoride-induced opacities may occur. With the increase of fluoride ion content, there is an increase in the severity of the fluorosis. The defect is thought to be related to a disturbance in the function of ameloblasts during calcification of the tooth matrix.

Fig 5-8 Dental fluorosis. These teeth have a more extreme form of fluorosis. The child grew up in west Texas, where there is a naturally occurring high fluoride content. This severely mottled enamel shows a brown staining and some pitting with abrasion. These teeth can be bleached with some success. The use of a composite resin veneer for the labial surfaces is a good compromise.

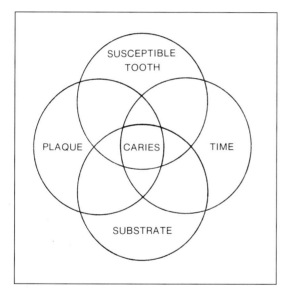

Fig 5-9 The four major interacting variables in the formation of dental caries in children.

as sucrose, are converted by the bacteria into acid. It is this acid production, provided that the pH is sufficiently low, that will result in demineralization of the enamel. However, this process of demineralization may be initially reversed or lessened in severity by various components in saliva. Increased salivary secretory flow rate and the buffering capacity of bicarbonate in the saliva will help lessen the effects of the bacterial acid production. Other minerals within the saliva, such as fluoride, calcium, and phosphorous, contribute to the remineralization of the surface. Thus, the process of dental caries formation is chronic and influenced by the last of the variable factors—time.

Time

It is well documented that the occurrence of dental caries in children is based not on the quantity of fermentable carbohydrates consumed but rather on the consistency and frequency of consumption (Gustafsson et al, 1954). Dietary habits, therefore, play an extremely important role. Because the pH of plaque remains at a cariogenic level up to 30 minutes following consumption of carbohydrates, repeated consumption in the form of between-meal snacks may result in an almost constant assault of acid on the surface. In fact, a direct relationship between caries prevalence in children and the frequency of between-meal snack consumption has been shown (Weiss and Trithart, 1960; Steinman and Woods, 1964). In addition, bedtime dietary habits have been indicted (Palmer, 1971).

In infants, the use of prolonged, nonnutritional bottle feeding or sweetened comforters as pacifiers, particularly during sleep, can produce devastating effects on the dentition (Winter et al, 1971; Ripa, 1988). During sleep, the protective effect of saliva is minimal because the flow rate is greatly reduced. The contents of the bottle (milk, sweetened liquid, etc) stagnate around the teeth, resulting in rapid destruction of the maxillary incisors and first molars (Fig 5-10). Only the protection afforded by the lower lip, eruption sequence, and termination of the habit saves the remaining teeth (Snawder, 1974). This phenomenon has been termed *nursing caries* or *baby bottle tooth decay* (Johnsen, 1988). Nursing caries can likewise result from demand breast feeding. Fortunately, this condition is rare and must be associated with prolonged, intense feeding practices (Hackett et al, 1984). After an extensive review of the literature, Ripa (1988) concluded that the prevalence of nursing caries in the United States is no higher than 5%.

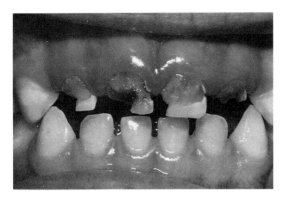

Fig 5-10 Rapid carious destruction of maxillary incisors because of nursing caries.

Table 5-1 Dental caries experience of preschool children in fluoride-deficient areas

Chronologic age (y)	Caries prevalence* (%)
1	5
2	10
3	50
5	75

*Percent of population having one or more carious teeth.

Nursing caries syndrome is often a problem of overindulgence found in children of small, intact families (Johnsen, 1984). *S mutans* is the causative agent of the condition. It colonizes the teeth immediately after eruption and is reported to be of maternal origin. Recent reports have confirmed the maternal transmission of *Streptococcus mutans* to the infant's mouth, especially when the mother possesses dense salivary reservoirs of the organism (Berkowitz, 1985).

Parents are often eager to have the affected incisors restored to proper function and esthetics. Prevention of this condition, however, goes beyond transfer of information through parent education. Interestingly, one third of surveyed parents admitted awareness of the potential hazard but chose this destructive feeding practice because of overriding concerns such as pacification (Johnsen, 1984). Differential diagnosis of nursing caries must include caries secondary to enamel hypoplasia.

Often, enamel hypoplasia of the incisors is misdiagnosed as nursing caries. Enamel hypoplasia is best differentiated by its symmetric circular outline involving the incisal edge that follows the pattern of enamel deposition (Johnsen, 1984). In some cases there is a concurrent history of prematurity or low birth weight. Once nursing caries is properly diagnosed according to the history of feeding practices, it is best to recommend substitution of water for the cariogenic substrate. The parents should anticipate that the transition will

create vocal resistance and some sleepless nights until full acceptance by the infant occurs. Future preventive measures must be directed at children treated for nursing caries, because recent studies have revealed that these children are at higher risk for development of future dental caries (Johnsen et al, 1986; Greenwell et al, 1990).

Epidemiology of dental caries

Prevalence

Primary dentition

Numerous studies have reported on the prevalence of dental caries in the primary dentition. The prevalence during preschool years is of particular interest because the magnitude and impact of this disease at such a young age is a shocking revelation. Table 5-1 is a compiled summary of surveys taken in fluoride-deficient communities (Toverud et al, 1953; Hennon et al, 1969; Winter et al, 1971) and simplified to account for differences in methodologic design.

By age 3, the age at which some dentists recommend a child's first dental visit, the number of carious surfaces may range between three and six if the child resides in a low-fluoride area (Hennon et al, 1969; Winter et al, 1971; Holm and Arvidsson, 1974). In general, preschool children exhibit an "all or none" phenomenon in the prevalence of dental caries in that most appear either caries rampant or caries free (Johnsen et al, 1984).

There exists much debate as to whether the degree of the caries experience found in the primary teeth corresponds to the future caries experience in the permanent teeth of the same individual. Some studies report this concept (Hill et al, 1967; Zadick, 1976; Klein, et al, 1981) and others do not (Adler, 1968; Holm, 1978). More probably, the caries experience found in primary teeth may not be a good indicator of future caries experience in the permanent teeth because of the multifactorial nature of the disease.

Mixed dentition

During the mixed dentition, 6 to 12 years of age, caries in the permanent teeth progresses at a steady and rapid rate. The annual caries increment for the school-aged child was calculated to be one new carious tooth per year (Klein et al, 1938). However, a more recent survey suggested that the current annual rate is one half that previously reported (Kelley and Scanlon, 1971). Although this result is encouraging because it indicates improvement in the delivery of preventive dental services (Table 5-2), independent comparison and adjustment for methodologic differences between these two studies revealed that the rate in the latter was underestimated (Glass, 1973).

Nevertheless, the current caries prevalence for school-aged children is at an unprecedented low level (Graves and Stamm, 1985; Hicks et al, 1985). A survey completed in 1982 revealed a dramatic 50% decline in caries prevalence since 1972 for Indiana schoolchildren (Stookey et al, 1985). National caries surveys for children aged 5 to 17 years have shown marked increases in caries-free individuals since the early 1970s. These surveys revealed that 36% of US schoolchildren were caries free (Brunnelle and Carlos, 1982) and that a 13% increase in caries-free children has occurred since 1971 (NIH, 1981). Although the trend of decreasing caries prevalence among US schoolchildren has continued, the prevalence of caries-free US schoolchildren decreases with chronologic age (Table 5-3). As with preschool children, there is an uneven distribution pattern (20% of the children account for 50% of the total caries prevalence), warranting the identification of high-risk patients.

Diagnosis and distribution

Clinical diagnosis is accomplished by visual and tactile examination of the dental surface with a sharp dental explorer. An area is defined as carious when the explorer resists withdrawal after insertion with moderate to firm pressure and when, in addition, there is softness at the base of the area, opacity, discoloration, loss of translucency, or all of these compared with the condition of adjacent tooth structure.

The pattern of distribution for caries formation in primary teeth varies greatly according to the patient's chronologic age and the tooth surface and type. In the primary dentition (preschooler), the occlusal surface is the most susceptible to carious attack, attributable to its anatomy of pits and fissures. However, with the eruption of the permanent first molars at age 6, the normal developmental spaces of the primary dentition begin to close (Fig 5-11). With space closure and the formation of contact areas, the incidence of proximal caries greatly increases. One study indicated that teeth with proximal space less than 0.5 mm had ten times the prevalence of caries of those teeth with open contacts (Parfitt, 1956). By age 8, the prevalence of proximal caries equals that of the occlusal surface (Parfitt, 1955). However, it should not be inferred that susceptibility to occlusal caries mandates the prevalence on proximal surfaces or vice versa, because these lesions are similar but independent of each other in development (Parfitt, 1956). One study revealed that 48% of 4 to 6 year olds without signs of clinical caries demonstrated proximal lesions on radiographic examination (Stecksen-Blicks and Wahlin, 1983). Proximal lesions develop slightly gingival to the contact area, and early diagnosis is accomplished only by radiographic examination.

Table 5-2 Mean number of decayed, missing, and filled teeth (DMFT) among US children in the mixed dentition

Chronologic age (y)	DMFT*	DMFT†
6	0.5	0.2
12	6.0	2.8

*Klein et al (1938).
†Kelley and Scanlon (1971).

Table 5-3 Caries-free schoolchildren according to age

Age (y)	Caries free (%)	
	1979–1980*	1986–1987**
6	90	94
8	56	75
10	38	56
12	27	42
15	15	22
17	11	16

*NIH, 1981
**NIH, 1989

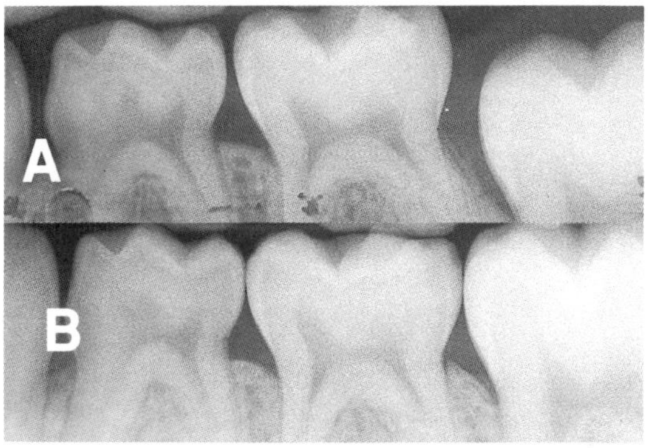

Fig 5-11 Normally occurring developmental interproximal spaces of the primary dentition in a 6 year old (A) closes following eruption of the permanent first molar (B). This event contributes to the dramatic rise in prevalence of proximal caries in children of this age.

When the relative susceptibility of proximal surfaces in the primary dentition is analyzed, a general trend of increased caries incidence in a distal direction occurs. In other words, the canine-first molar contact is much less susceptible than the first molar-second molar contact (Volker and Russell, 1973). However, the adjacent surfaces of each contact area, as well as its contralateral site, have remarkably similar caries experience. The highly significant correlation between the adjacent surfaces has been attributed to the transmissible nature of caries enhanced by the existence of similar anatomic conditions. Since symmetry of attack is expected, the detection of proximal lesions in one quadrant should encourage the clinician to look very critically for similar lesions in other quadrants (Kennedy, 1976) (Fig 5-12). The equal frequency of proximal caries on adjacent sites in primary molars requires time to develop, but generally the lesions do not appear simultaneously because of differences in eruption sequence. For example, the mesial lesion on a second molar will lag in development from the distal lesion on a first molar by an interval of 18 months, which corresponds to the 18 months' interval between their eruption times (Parfitt, 1956) Figs 5-13 and 5-14). Similarly, the distal surface of the primary second molar remains relatively caries immune for 4 years until contact is made with the mesial surface of the erupting permanent first molar (Volker and Russell, 1973). Once contact is made, the development of a lesion on the distal surface of the primary second molar can infect the mesial surface of the permanent first molar (Fig 5-15). If left untreated, the caries can spread to the dis-

tal surface of the second premolar following its eruption.

Bitewing radiographs are absolutely required to detect proximal lesions in primary molars. However, diagnostic radiographs must be free of proximal overlap (Fig 5-16). Proximal molar lesions, detected only by radiographic examination, of preschool children in nonfluoridated communities have been reported to be 68% (Murray and Majid, 1978) and 75% (Hennon et al, 1969). In other words, almost three fourths of all posterior carious lesions in children would go undetected if only a clinical examination were conducted. The inability to clinically detect incipient proximal lesions is attributed to the low, broad, and flat contact areas of primary molars that defy accessibility to probing. In fact, the dentist's inability to detect proximal lesions by probing increases with the patient's age; 32% of such lesions in 4-year-olds expands to 91% in 6-year-olds (Stecksen-Blicks and Wahlin, 1983). The detection of incipient proximal lesions is essential be-

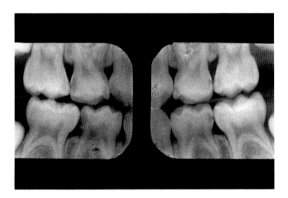

Fig 5-12 This patient demonstrates bilateral surface symmetry between left and right sides and proximal carious involvement of varying severity between the primary molars.

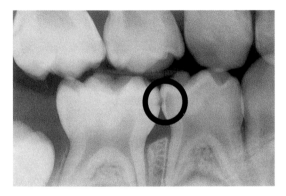

Fig 5-13 This patient demonstrates adjacent surface symmetry. The distal surface of the primary first molar reveals carious advancement into dentin, whereas involvement of the mesial surface of the second molar lags in development, being confined to enamel.

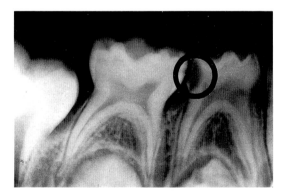

Fig 5-14 This radiograph illustrates a more advanced condition than that found in Fig 5-13. Note how the lesion spreads along the dentinoenamel junction on penetration through the enamel and the close proximity of its advancement to the pulp.

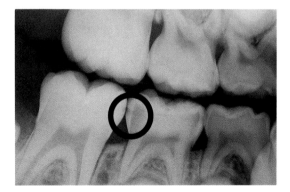

Fig 5-15 The infectious spread of a carious lesion from the distal surface of a primary second molar to the mesial surface of a permanent first molar demonstrates the necessity for restoration of primary teeth.

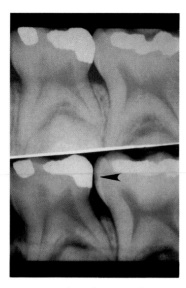

Fig 5-16 Interproximal overlapping will conceal the initiation of an incipient carious lesion *(arrow)*. Therefore, diagnostic radiographs must be free of overlap in the contact areas.

Table 5-4 Surfaces of primary teeth most commonly affected by dental caries formation*

Teeth	Mandibular	Maxillary
Second molar	Occlusobuccal	Occlusolingual
First molar	Occlusobuccal	Occlusal
Canine	Buccal	Buccal
Lateral incisor	Mesial	Mesial
Central incisor	Mesial	Mesial

*Adapted from Hennon et al (1969).

cause of the rapid rate of progression of such lesions in primary teeth (to be discussed later), and the comparatively short distance between the external surface and pulp dictates that these lesions be considered for restoration. In addition, such incipient areas of demineralization, appearing as radiographic etches of enamel, frequently exhibit histologic penetration into the dentin (Darling, 1959; Dwyer et al, 1973). For these reasons, restoration of radiographic proximal enamel etches in primary molars is both justifiable and recommended following assessment of the exfoliation time, the child's previous level of care or caries incidence, the anticipated response to preventive services, and the regularity of dental visits (Kennedy, 1976).

As previously mentioned, the surface anatomy of the tooth corresponds to the susceptibility of caries formation. For these reasons, second molars have greater caries prevalence than first molars, and the mandibular molars are more vulnerable than maxillary molars (Volker and Russell, 1973). Table 5-4 lists the specific surfaces found to be more commonly affected (Hennon et al, 1969).

The distribution of carious sites in young permanent teeth is affected by the same conditions that affect the primary teeth. The surface anatomy plays an extremely influential role. For this age group, the order of susceptibility (most to least) of teeth to carious attack is as follows (Berman and Slack, 1972): *(1)* first molar, *(2)* second molar, *(3)* premolars, *(4)* maxillary anterior teeth, and *(5)* canines and mandibular incisors. As with primary teeth, there is a high association of adjacent carious sites, and the bilateral occurrence of carious attack on the same surface sites of posterior molars has been calculated to be 80% or higher (Berman and Slack, 1973; Powell et al, 1977).

Rate of progression

The carious lesion initially develops in enamel, with decalcification occurring several micrometers below the surface. The external surface remains intact because it is bathed in the remineralizing fluids of the saliva. This initial stage, characterized by slight demineralization, loss of enamel translucency, and clinical appearance as a white-spot enamel opacity, is termed an *incipient lesion* (Fig 5-17). Eventually, the matrix support is lost, and a clinically detectable lesion is evident, characterized by a soft, yellow discoloration that resists withdrawal of the dental explorer.

Once the carious process penetrates the enamel surface, it will spread rapidly along the dentinoenamel junction (see Fig 5-13). The destruction of the supporting dentin layer eventually will cause collapse of the enamel layer with obvious cavitation (see Fig 5-14). The caries will continue to spread toward the pulp, and the infection will ultimately result in necrosis and abscess formation. However, the initial radiographic site of a chronic abscess formation in primary molars differs from that in permanent molars. Unlike abscess formation in permanent molars, where the first changes will be noticed in the periapical region, chronic abscess formation of primary molars most commonly occurs as an interradicular rarefaction with maximum intensity at the bifurcation area (Winter, 1962) (Fig 5-18 to 5-21). It is postulated that the presence of accessory root canals or areas of macroscopic root resorption encouraged by a thin and porous pulp chamber floor accounts for this finding (Moss et al, 1965).

This condition leads to an aberrant communication of the pulp with the interradicular tissues. Clinically, the infection will spread through the buccal soft tissue, forming a parulis or gingival sac containing the purulent exudate (Fig 5-19). This parulis will eventually rupture, leaving a draining fistulous tract. If the infection is severe and occurs during the critical stages of crown formation for the underlying premolar, the formation or calcification (or both) of the premolar may be sufficiently altered to result in defective enamel formation (Fig 5-20).

The rate of spread by a carious lesion through the tooth is more rapid in primary teeth. It was shown that

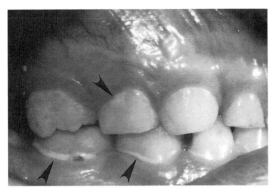

Fig 5-17 Cervical demineralization *(arrows)* is a sign of acute susceptibility to dental caries formation.

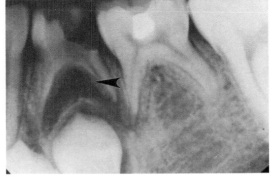

Fig 5-18 Interradicular radiolucency *(arrow)* initiating at the bifurcation of primary molars, is radiographic evidence of chronic abscess formation due to necrotic pulpal tissue arising from a carious exposure.

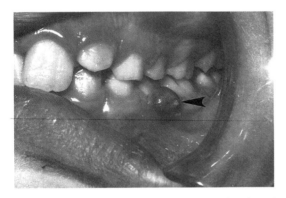

Fig 5-19 A parulis *(arrow)* located on the buccal surface of the gingiva is clinical evidence of chronic abscess formation of the adjacent tooth. Radiographic examination (see Fig 5-18) should confirm the diagnosis.

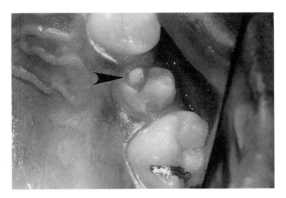

Fig 5-20 Defective enamel formation *(arrow)* of a premolar can result from chronic abscess formation of the preceding primary molar because the developing premolar is located within the bifurcation area of the primary molar.

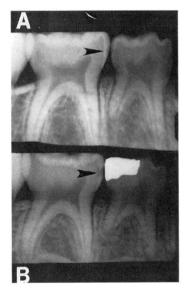

Fig 5-21 Evidence in support of the rapid advancement of carious lesions in primary teeth is demonstrated by the fact that radiographic enamel caries *(A)* has progressed well into dentin 1 year later *(B)*.

46% of the incipient proximal carious lesions in primary molars became clinically detectable within 1 year (Murray and Majid, 1978). Furthermore, radiographic analysis revealed that 69 of 71 "enamel-only" lesions progressed to dentin within 1 year (Fig 5-21). However, for permanent teeth, the average time required for spread of caries through the enamel is 2 to 3 years, with progression occurring faster in less accessible areas but slower in older individuals (Marthaler, 1967; Zamir et al, 1976 Sharav et al, 1978). The thinness of enamel and its lower degree of mineralization most probably account for the more rapid progression of caries in primary teeth (Mortimer, 1970). The phenomenon of arrested (nonprogressing) caries is also more prevalent in the permanent teeth. Over a 3-year period, proximal incipient caries in permanent teeth failed to show progression in 27% (Zamir et al, 1976) and 50% (Berman and Slack, 1973) of the cases examined. Nevertheless, the finding that 28% of incipient occlusal lesions become clinically detectable within 6 months justifies the need for periodic recall (Volker and Russell, 1973).

Summary

Several trends concerning caries formation in children can be noted. Caries formation occurs most commonly on adjacent and bilateral surfaces. Posterior teeth are more affected than anterior teeth, with mandibular molars more susceptible than maxillary. In addition, the onset and rate of progression of dental caries is more rapid, insidious, and potentially dangerous in primary teeth than in permanent teeth. Thus, early detection and treatment of carious lesions in primary teeth are essential.

References

Adler, P. Correlation between dental caries prevalence at different ages. Caries Res. 2:79, 1968.

Berkowitz, R. J. Streptococcus mutans and dental caries in infants. Compend. Cont Educ. Dent. 6:463, 1985.

Berman, D.S., and Slack, G.L. Susceptibility of tooth surfaces to caries attack. Br. Dent. J. 134:135, 1973.

Brunnelle, J.A., and Carlos, J.P. Changes in the prevalence of dental caries in US school children, 1961-1980. J. Dent. Res. 61:1346, 1982.

Catalanotto, F.A., Shklair, I.L., and Keene, H.J. Prevalence and localization of streptococcus mutans in infants and children. J. Am. Dent. Assoc. 91:606, 1975.

Darling, A.I. The pathology and prevention of caries. Br. Dent. J. 107:287, 1959.

Duncan, W., Et al. Labial hypoplasia of primary canines in black Head Start children. J. Dent. Child. 55:423, 1988.

Dwyer, D. M., Berman, D.S., and Silverstone, L.M. A study of approximal carious lesions in primary molars. J. Int. Assoc. Dent. Child. 4:41, 1973.

Eisenberg, E., and Bernick, S. Anomalies of the teeth with stains and discolorations. J. Prev. Dent 2:7, 1975.

Glass, R.L. Caries prevalence in children from the United States J. Dent. Res. 52:1161, 1973.

Graves, R.C., and Stamm, J.W. Decline of dental caries: What occurred and will it continue? J. Can Dent. Assoc. 51:693, 1985.

Greenwell, A., et al. Longitudinal evaluation of caries patterns from the primary to the mixed dentition. Pediatr. Dent. 12:278, 1990.

Gustafsson, B.E., et al. The Vipeholm dental caries study. The effect of different levels of carbohydrates intake on caries activity in 436 individuals observed for five years. Acta Odontol. Scand. 11:232, 1954.

Hackett, A.F., et al. Can breastfeeding cause dental caries? Hum. Nutr. 38:23, 1984.

Hennon, D.K., Stookey, G.K., and Muhler, J.C. Prevalence and distribution of dental caries in preschool children. J. Am. Dent Assoc. 79:1405, 1969.

Hicks, M.J. et al. The current status of dental caries in the pediatric population. J. Pedod. 10:57, 1985.

Hill, I.N., et al. Deciduous teeth and future caries experience. J. Am. Dent Assoc. 74:430, 1967.

Holm, A.K. Dental health in a group of Swedish 8 year olds followed since the age of 3. Community Dent. Oral Epidemiol. 6:71, 1978.

Holm, A.K., and Arvidsson, S. Oral health in preschool Swedish children. I. Three year old children. Odontol. Rev. 25:81, 1974.

Johnsen, D.C. Dental caries patterns in preschool children. Dent. Clin. North Am. 28:3, 1984.

Johnsen, D.C. Baby bottle tooth decay: A preventable health problem in infants. Update Pediatr. Dent. 2:1, 1988.

Johnsen, D.C., et al. Caries progression reconstructed for children in the primary dentition. J. Dent. Res. 63:182, 1984.

Johnsen, D.C., et al. Susceptibility of nursing-caries children to future approximal molar decay. Pediatr. Dent. 8:168, 1986.

Jorgenson, R., and Yost, C. Etiology of enamel dysplasias. J. Pedod. 6:315, 1982.

Kelley, G., and Scanlon, R. Decayed, missing and filled teeth among children. Department of Health, Education and Welfare publication No. 72-1003, 1971 In decayed, missing and filled teeth among children. J. Dent. Child. 38:47, 1971.

Kennedy, D.B. Paediatric Operative Dentistry. Bristol, England: John Wright & Sons, Ltd., 1976.

Keyes, P.H. Infectious and transmissible nature of experimental dental caries. Arch. Oral Biol. 1:304, 1960.

Keyes, P.H. Present and future measures for dental caries control. J. Am. Dental Assoc. 79:1395, 1969.

Klein, H., Palmer, C., and Knutson, J. Studies on dental caries. I. Dental status and dental needs of elementary school children. Pub. Health Rep. 58:751, 1938.

Klein, H., et al. Caries prevalence of the primary dentition at age seven: An indicator for future caries prevalence in the permanent dentition. Pediatr. Dent. 3:184, 1981.

Marthaler, T.M. Epidemiological and clinical dental findings in relation to intake of carbohydrates. Caries Res. 1:222, 1967.

Mortimer, K.V. The relationship of deciduous enamel structure to dental disease. Caries Res. 4:206, 1970.

Moss, S.J., et al Histologic study of pulpal floor of deciduous molars. J. Am. Dent. Assoc. 70:372, 1965.

Murray, J.J., and Majid, Z.A. The prevalence and progression of approximal caries in the deciduous dentition in British children. Br. Dent. J. 145:161, 1978.

National Institutes of Health (NIH), The prevalence of dental caries in US children. 1979-80. NIH publication No. 82-2245, 1981.

National Institutes of Health (NIH). Dental caries in United States children, 1986-1987. NIH publication No. 89-2247, 1989.

Needleman, H., et al Macroscopic enamel defects of primary anterior teeth—types, prevalence, and distribution. Pediatr. Dent. 13:208, 1991

Palmer, J.D. Dietary habits at bedtime in relation to dental caries in children. Br. Dent. J. 130:288, 1971.

Parfitt, G.J. The distribution of caries on different sites of the teeth in English children from age 2-15 years. Br. Dent. J. 99:423, 1955.

Parfitt, G.J. Conditions influencing the incidence of occlusal and interstitial caries in children. J. Dent. Child. 23:31, 1956.

Powell, E., et al Effect of population size on the occurrence of bilateral caries symmetry. J. Dent. Res. 56:B72, 1977 (AADR abstract No. 83).

Ripa, L. Nursing caries: A comprehensive review. Pediatr. Dent. 10:268, 1988.

Seow, K. Enamel hypoplasia in the primary dentition: A review. J. Dent. Child. 58:441, 1991.

Sharav, Y., Fisher, D., and Zamir, T. The influence of location on the rate of spread of human approximal dental caries. Arch. Oral Biol. 23:603, 1978.

Snawder, K.D. The nursing bottle syndrome and related problems. In Goldman, H.M. Current Therapy in Dentistry. Vol. 5. St. Louis: The C.V. Mosby Co., 1974.

Stecksen-Blicks, C., and Wahlin, Y.B. Diagnosis of approximal caries in pre-school children. Swed. Dent. J. 7:179, 1983.

Steinman, R.R., and Woods, R.W. Heredity, environment, diet and caries in children. J. South. Calif. State Dent. Assoc. 32:163, 1964.

Stookey, G.K., et al Prevalence of dental caries in Indiana school children: Results of 1982 survey. Pediatr. Dent. 7:8, 1985.

Street, C.M., Goldner, C.M., and LeRiche, W.H. Epidemiology of dental caries in relation to Streptococcus mutans on tooth surfaces in 5 year old children. Arch. Oral Biol. 21:273, 1976.

Toverud, G. et al Survey of the literature of dental caries. Washington, D.C.: National Academy of Sciences- National Research Council publication No. 225, 1953.

Volker, J.F. and Russell D.L. The epidemiology of dental caries. In Finn, S.B. Clinical Pedodontics. 4th ed. Philadelphia: W.B. Saunders Co., 1973.

Weiss, R.L., and Trihart, A.H. Between meal eating habits and dental caries experience in preschool children. Am. J. Public Health 50:1097, 1960.

Winter, G.B. Abscess formation in connection with deciduous molar teeth. Arch. Oral Biol. 7:373, 1962.

Winter, G.B., et al The prevalence of dental caries in preschool children aged 1-4 years. Br. Dent. J. 130:271, 1971.

Zadik, D. Caries experience in primary and permanent dentition of the same individuals. J. Dent. Res. 55:1125, 1976.

Zamir T., Fisher, D. Fishel, D., and Sharav, Y. A longitudinal radiograph study of the rate of spread of human approximal dental caries. Arch. Oral Biol. 21:423, 1976.

Questions

1. The principal causative agent in the initiation of dental caries is:

   a. Poor oral hygiene
   b. Insufficient fluoride exposure
   c. *Lactobacillus acidophilus*
   d. Fermentable carbohydrates
   e. *Streptococcus mutans*

2. A 2-year-old girl comes to your office with selective carious destruction of the maxillary first molars and incisors. To aid in your diagnosis and to assist in fostering dental education of the parents regarding this condition, what question should you ask them?

   a. Was there a developmental disturbance during the second trimester of pregnancy?
   b. Is there a familial tendency for this condition to occur?
   c. Was the child given a bottle at night to encourage sleep?
   d. How often are the child's teeth cleaned?
   e. Does the child live in a fluoridated area?

3. Which of the following statements is false regarding the epidemiology of dental caries in the primary dentition?

   a. Approximately 50% of all 3-year-olds have at least one carious surface
   b. Mandibular incisors are the least susceptible teeth to carious formation
   c. Second molars are more susceptible to carious formation than first molars
   d. Occlusal surfaces are more susceptible to carious formation than proximal surfaces
   e. Maxillary molars are more susceptible to carious formation than mandibular molars.

4. During the examination of a 9-year-old child, which permanent tooth surface would have the highest prevalence of caries?

   a. Labial surface of the canines
   b. Mesial surface of the central incisors
   c. Occlusal surface of first molars
   d. Occlusal surface of second premolars
   e. Lingual surface of lateral incisors

5. Examination of a 10-year-old reveals multiple carious lesions. According to statistics gathered on the epidemiology of dental caries, what would you predict the order of sequence for caries formation on a primary mandibular second molar would be if 1 = mesial, 2= occlusal, and 3= distal surface:

   a. 1,2,3
   b. 1,3,2
   c. 2,3,1
   d. 2,1,3
   e. 3,2,1

Chapter 6

Oral Hygiene Education

Objectives

After studying this chapter, the student should be able to:
1. Develop an individualized program of oral health care for the child patient.
2. Understand the use of preventive techniques commonly prescribed.
3. Explain the methods employed to motivate patients to practice proper oral hygiene.
4. Cite the instructions given for toothbrushing and flossing and the modifications rendered according to the child's age.
5. Describe a practical method for oral hygiene instruction and dental prophylaxis in the office.
6. Discuss guidelines for nutritional counseling and diet modification.
7. Outline approaches to the prevention of dental disease in infants.

Because dental caries and periodontal disease are largely preventable, increased emphasis on prevention should be the goal of every dental practice. The development of a successful preventive program hinges on the establishment of open communication between the patient and the entire dental staff. The patient's attitude toward maintaining dental health must be freely discussed, and the potential benefits must be freely discussed, and the potential benefits derived from the patient's participation in the preventive program must be fully understood. The goals and responsibilities of all parties involved must likewise be jointly agreed on. As dentists, we have a moral and professional obligation to give parents and patients information about home care, diet, fluoride therapy, and the influences of these factors on dental health. The patient's (or parent's) obligation is to accept this information, remove plaque, alter diet, and use fluorides.

No single preventive approach or program can be tailored to fit the needs of all patients. Rather, the most effective preventive programs, like treatment plans, are individualized to meet the patient's needs once they have been identified. The individualized program must also meet the patient's level of motivation and ability to complete the task.

In Chapter 5, the etiology of dental caries was presented in terms of four interacting factors: susceptible tooth, plaque, substrate, and time. It is the intention of this chapter to concentrate on each of the factors separately in terms of currently available techniques and philosophies used to reduce their influence on dental caries formation. However, it must be remembered that the prevention of a multifactorial disease such as dental caries must never rely on the elimination of only one of the etiologic factors. Preventive measures used to control periodontal disease in children are also incorporated into this discussion because the two processes have a common causative agent (plaque) and similar methods of reducing its virulence. However, because dental caries is the major dental health problem in children, emphasis is given to this special concern (Keyes, 1969).

This chapter contains a number of educational aids. You probably will not use all of these aids in your practice because a prevention program that motivates one dentist and one patient may fail with others. Avoid becoming an irrational disciple or a prevention crusader. Instead, regard preventive dentistry as the keystone of an excellent dental practice.

Susceptible tooth

Any means that increases the resistance of a susceptible tooth to caries formation will be a valuable preventive measure. Such measures in children are aimed at improving the structural integrity of the tooth. The more effective and proven means of accomplishing this differ according to the kind of surface to which they are directed. For example, smooth surfaces are best protected by systemic fluoride ingestion during formation (preeruption) and by topical fluoride application during maturation (posteruption), whereas pit and fissure surfaces are best protected by sealant application. For best overall results, these agents should be used in combination. These preventive methods have contributed so greatly to the reduction of dental caries in children that special attention is directed to them in Chapters 7 and 8, respectively.

Plaque

To a major extent, dentistry owes its existence to plaque. If treatment of traumas, genetic defects, and developmental anomalies (probably 5% of all treatment rendered) are excluded, all other procedures are a direct result of plaque accumulation. Consider further that one third of all malocclusions are related to premature loss of primary teeth to caries. Therefore, it becomes evident that removal of plaque (plaque control) should be the primary focus of every preventive program. Before the dentist can discuss the methods and techniques of plaque removal, the patient must be motivated to participate in the care of his or her teeth. Attainment of patient compliance in an oral hygiene education program is the most difficult challenge facing delivery of preventive dental care.

Oral hygiene education and patient motivation

There is a theory that those patients most susceptible to dental disease are also the ones most resistant to prevention. There is great concern as to what percentage of the population is willing to make a commitment to plaque removal. Patients must become aware of the necessity for proper oral hygiene maintenance (through education), and they must become motivated strongly enough to develop an interest in active involvement. Then, through active involvement, the practice can become a daily habit. A major difficulty is overcoming the socioeconomic and cultural factors influencing patients' dental health practices. Patient education, in itself, is insufficient; merely possessing knowledge does not guarantee that it will be used. It is a dubious assumption to expect to motivate patients to improve their oral hygiene merely by acting on their level of knowledge and their attitude toward dental health. The evaluation of a preventive program must be based on behavioral outcome, not knowledge (Heloe and Konig, 1978).

There are several methods of patient education, but there is considerable variation in the impact each method has on the duration of maintenance of the im-

proved oral hygiene levels. An excellent review that compares the various educational approaches has been conducted (Melcer and Feldman, 1979). The review can be summarized as follows:

1. Patient education will promote improved oral hygiene for only a short period of time following the teaching period.
2. Regression to baseline values in performance tends to occur as the period of time lengthens after instruction is terminated.
3. One teaching session will not alter performance.
4. Disclosing materials will provide motivation for a period of only a few weeks.
5. Closely supervised teaching on a multiple-visit basis, allowing for periodic reinforcement, is the best approach.

Thus, repetitive stimulus is probably required to sustain patient motivation. The need for periodic reinforcement is supported by another study showing that retention of health education material is poor in parents of children undergoing treatment (Gillig, 1969). Written material in combination with illustrated slides proved effective in educating the parents initially, but, when they were retested after 6 weeks, the results demonstrated that little, if any, information was retained.

Certainly the educator's attitude and effective timing in the delivery of dental health instruction will influence the level of patient motivation obtained. The motivation of the patient is a reflection of the instructor's own attitude and approach. The instructor's genuine enthusiasm about the effectiveness of habitual oral hygiene practices is most likely to influence patients to carry out their obligation diligently. Moveover, the timing of the instruction, when it is presented, is important to obtain patient interest. In this regard, instruction before prenatal and infant care classes has produced promising results. However, the usual approach of presenting a pretreatment caries control program may be an example of poor timing because efforts may not effectively reach the patient. Doyle (1974) suggests that the preventive program phase be delayed until after treatment is completed. The dentist can then teach the patient how to prevent the problems from recurring. He argues that most patients' chief compliant or problem is self-oriented and demands resolution. The patient's overriding concerns will restrict all paths of effective communication if the dentist imposes his or her own priorities, such as a preventive control program, on the patient before treatment is rendered.

Educational aids

Most available educational aids offered to patients are used to motivate them. Many visual aids are available

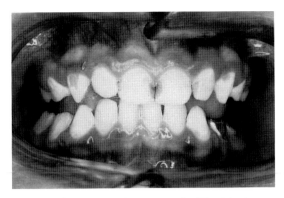

Fig 6-1a Plaque accumulation is usually difficult for the parent and child to identify.

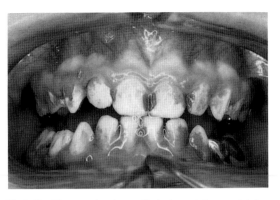

Fig 6-1b The use of a plaque-disclosing solution containing a red dye provides easy identification of plaque and may be used to assess the effectiveness of prior cleaning.

for office use, and take-home leaflets can be dispensed for later reinforcement. Other aids the clinician may use are disclosing solution, plaque index, and caries activity testing. Dietary analysis in the form of a food diary also is a motivational aid, but it is discussed separately in a later section.

Disclosing solution and plaque index

Disclosing solution is an invaluable aid for the identification of plaque and the effectiveness of plaque removal (Arnim, 1963). The solution normally employs an erythrosin dye that stains plaque a bright red. This acts as a diagnostic tool to show the amount and location of the plaque on the tooth and may be used at home to evaluate the effectiveness of cleaning. (Figs 6-1a and b).

Depending on the patient's ability to cooperate, the solution can be swished in the mouth or topically applied with a cotton tip applicator. Tablets are available for older children, who can be instructed to chew the "sugarless, red candy" thoroughly. Individually packaged solutions and tablets for home use are available. At least 1 minute must elapse before the teeth are examined for plaque, to allow the noncariogenic mucinous bacteria to be flushed off the teeth. Advise the parent that the staining process should not be done at a sink and that the disclosing tablet should not be called a "tablet" or "pill." To do so may cause the child to expectorate, staining the clothing and the sink. Such an experience is likely to discourage use of the tablet.

When the staining process is used in conjunction with a plaque index, it becomes an effective evaluation tool. A plaque index is a method of scoring the amount and location of the plaque on the teeth using a scoring sheet or diagram. Many different types of indexes are available to record plaque, but the important factor is that the index be used often as a means of recording patient progress through the program.

Caries activity testing

A number of tests have been developed in an attempt to predict the patient's cariogenic potential, but direct correlations between oral bacteria and future caries formation have been difficult to achieve. It seems that these tests fail chiefly because they measure only one of the major variables in the etiology of caries. The tests are probably most useful for monitoring the patient's progress after proper oral hygiene levels have been attained (Sims, 1970). Two common types of tests are used: the modified Snyder caries activity test and the *Lactobacillus* count. The modified Snyder caries activity test is a colorimetric method for determining the amount of acids formed in a carbohydrate medium by oral microorganisms collected in saliva. In other words, it measures the acidogenic potential but is limited in predictive value because these salivary microorganisms may not be representative of those in plaque. The indicator is bromcresol green, which changes from blue-green to yellow in the presence of acids.

This test is a practical way to monitor patient motivation and to measure the effectiveness of the caries control program. The procedure for using the modified Snyder caries activity test is as follows:

1. Have the patient drool unstimulated saliva into a tube of Snyder medium, just covering the surface of the medium. If it is difficult to collect the sample (as with young children), rub a cotton swab on the facial surfaces of the teeth or dip the swab into the saliva under the tongue. Stab the swab into the agar to a depth just under the surface. Leave the swab in the medium, break off the end of the stick, and cap the tube.
2. Incubate the tube at 37°C. Observe and record color change for 3 days (24, 48, and 72 hours).
3. Note the color. The production of acid is detected by an indicator—bromcresol green—that changes from blue-green (pH 4.7 to 5.0) to green (pH 4.2 to

Table 6-1 Interpretation of the modified Snyder caries activity test

Caries activity	Result after incubation for		
	24h	48h	72h
Marked	Positive		
Moderate	Negative	Positive	
Slight	Negative	Negative	Positive
Negative	Negative	Negative	Negative

4.6) to yellow (pH 4.0 or lower). Yellow indicates a positive test. The final result is obtained within 72 hours. The significance of the results are shown in Table 6-1.

Both speed and volume of acid production are indicated and serve as a point of reference in comparison testing for interpretation. "Improved" would be slower or less color change when compared with previous results. "Worse" would be faster or more pronounced color change when compared with previous results.

Toothbrushing—Home care

The toothbrush is the most popular device for oral hygiene use in our country. Although there are many designs, no specific type has been shown to be superior to others with respect to the ability to remove plaque (Heifetz, 1977; Newbrun, 1985). However, in general, recommendations have tended to favor small toothbrushes with soft, multitufted nylon bristles. Toothbrushes come in varying sizes to accommodate individual needs.

Electric toothbrushes have no clear advantage over manual types (Owen, 1972). However, electric toothbrushes may have one distinct advantage over the conventional type when used by children. This advantage is the novelty effect, which might influence children to brush better and longer. It is uncertain how long this novelty effect lasts.

It does not matter how an individual brushes his or her teeth as long as they get clean. In other words, the diligent application of the brush is more important than the technique itself. Studies show that children devote 75% of their brushing time (average duration equals 1 minute) to the labial surfaces of anterior teeth and occlusal surfaces of mandibular molars (Kimmelman and Tassman, 1960; Rugg-Gunn and MacGregor, 1978; Kleber et al, 1981). The most frequently missed areas are lingual surfaces of the teeth and the side of handedness. The duration of toothbrushing significantly influences a child's effectiveness in plaque removal (Honkala et al, 1986). The duration of toothbrushing practice needs to be emphasized in oral hygiene education.

To encourage acceptance of toothbrushing and to improve its effectiveness, the child should be taught the method that is most comfortable to him or her. It has been shown that the preferred method of toothbrushing by children without formal instruction is the horizontal method (Rugg-Gunn and MacGregor, 1978; Sundell and Klein, 1982). Since there is little difference in effectiveness between the various methods of removing plaque (Newbrun, 1985), the horizontal (scrubbing) stroke should be encouraged in children. Although damage to gingival tissue by the horizontal scrubbing method is considered by some to be a potential hazard, research does not support this suggestion (Sangnes and Gjermo, 1976).

Generally, children younger than age 9 years have not developed the conceptual ability and dexterity to remove plaque effectively. Although instruction does improve skills, there are strong age-related factors between the development of motor skills and the ability to brush effectively for both preschool (Simmons et al, 1983) and school-aged (Sundell and Klein, 1982) children. It is recommended that parents assume the primary role and responsibility for cleaning the teeth of their children younger than 9 years of age. The recommended position for this method is to have the child stand in front of the parent and tilt his or her head back. The parent uses one forearm to support the head while using the fingers to retract the lips. The other hand does the brushing while the child watches in a mirror (Starkey, 1961). The brushing method suggested for parents using this technique is the horizontal scrub method because this has been shown to be the most comfortable and effective (Sangnes, 1974). Motivating parents to assume this responsibility is difficult. Interviewed mothers stated that the most frequent problem at home was getting their children to brush but that they rarely inspected the thoroughness of the brushing other than asking if it was done (Linn, 1976).

Recommendations for the frequency of toothbrushing vary greatly. However, no research is available to support any single regimen. Naturally, the quality of cleaning is more important than the frequency of its performance (Bellini et al, 1981). It seems appropriate that patients be encouraged to brush their teeth after meals and before going to bed. If cleaning is limited to once a day, the preferred time is before bedtime because the decreased salivary flow during sleep encourages plaque demineralization of enamel.

Toothbrushing—Office care

Dental prophylaxis is a routine office procedure normally completed on a semiannual basis. It is a time-honored practice that has a high level of patient acceptance. Periodic dental scaling and polishing is recommended to prevent periodontal disease in adults. However, in children, this practice is highly questionable for a number of reasons. First, extrinsic stain and calculus formation is relatively rare in children. The routine user of a rubber cup and abrasive paste to clean and polish teeth without stain is unwarranted. Second, it used to be thought that the acquired pellicle that formed over the enamel surface prior to plaque colonization was a barrier to fluoride uptake of the enamel. Since the acquired pellicle penetrated the enamel surface, a pumice prophylaxis was required for its removal. However, research indicates that the removal of the acquired pellicle is not necessary prior to topical fluoride application for optimal uptake (Tinanoff et al, 1974). Third, attempts to polish teeth with an abrasive paste are detrimental to prevention of smooth-surface caries in children because it removes the outer surface level of enamel (up to 4 um) which is the most fluoride-rich area of the tooth. Because of this surface fluoride loss, less fluoride is ultimately retained in the enamel following topical fluoride application than would occur without prior pumice prophylaxis (Tinanoff et al, 1974). Even when a fluoridated paste is used, the final result would be detrimental if not followed by a topical fluoride application. This adverse effect is especially demonstrable on initial areas of enamel demineralization, termed *white-spot enamel opacities* (Zuniga and Caldwell, 1969). Thus, little is gained and, under certain circumstances, caries protection is reduced if a rubber cup pumice prophylaxis is performed on children.

The obvious benefit gained with a professional prophylaxis is plaque removal, but certainly the same result could be accomplished with a less abrasive method. We suggest that the use of supervised toothbrushing with a fluoridated prophylaxis paste is sufficient for plaque removal before topical fluoride application. Besides not removing the fluoride-rich surface layer, a toothbrush prophylaxis is more educational for the patient. The time normally devoted to performing a rubber cup prophylaxis can be used for patient instruction and motivation while simultaneous removal of plaque occurs.

The key to motivating a patient toward daily, conscientious plaque control is getting the patient to understand that he or she is in control of the consequences. Rather than creating a passive reliance on the therapist, encourage the patient to participate in the process actively. The negative effect on patient behavior created by a professional prophylaxis is caused by the impression that patients cannot adequately clean their teeth because periodically they must receive a professional cleaning. This contradictory and somewhat demeaning approach has no value in the delivery of preventive services to children. To facilitate the development of a program using prophylaxis in the dental office, you should designate a separate, private area within the office that has the decor and feeling of a home environment. In addition, a closet or cabinet should be designed to hold the toothbrushes of children participating in the program for ready access during each child's recall visit.

Because the treatment pattern and oral health habits of parents have an early and distinct influence on the dental health of their children (Heloe and Konig, 1978), efforts to affect the oral hygiene habits of children should be simultaneously directed at the parents to be successful. While performing a toothbrush prophylaxis on a child, have the parent actively participate in the process. To demonstrate and reinforce the brushing technique, the oral hygiene educator should clean one side of the child's mouth while the child and parent observe the process. To maximize the learning process, the child and parent could be asked to clean the remaining teeth under the instructor's supervision and guidance. Bullen et al (1988) demonstrated that parental involvement is a key element in preventive dentistry. Their study revealed that parental proficiency in toothbrushing improves the plaque scores of preschool children.

It appears that with increased frequency of brushing, there is a corresponding improvement in the oral hygiene status (Barenie et al, 1973). However, increased frequency of brushing does not have a major effect on caries reduction (Barenie et al, 1973). Any minor reduction achieved in the caries experience is most likely related to the increased exposure of the fluoride in the dentifrice rather than to a direct improvement in the oral hygiene level (Leske et al, 1976). It is probable that only a few highly motivated, well-instructed individuals reach and maintain the required oral hygiene efficiency necessary to prevent caries.

Several studies indicate that oral hygiene instruction and self-performed practice in proper toothcleaning techniques reduce the prevalence of plaque and gingivitis but have little effect on dental caries reduction (Bellini et al, 1981; Axelsson and Lindhe, 1981). The same results have been reported for supervised tooth cleaning (Horowitz et al, 1977; Silverstein et al, 1977), but repeated professional tooth cleaning does appear to enhance caries reduction in some studies (Bellini et al, 1981; Axelsson and Lindhe, 1981). In summary, toothbrushing as a means to prevent dental caries in children should not be overemphasized, but its positive effect on gingival health should be stressed.

Flossing

Since it has been shown that brushing cleans only the dental smooth surfaces, floss must be used to clean the interproximal surfaces (Axelsson, 1981). Unwaxed floss will cut plaque off the teeth better, but, where there are rough restorations, sharp teeth, or stainless steel crowns, it is probably more practical to use waxed floss. Floss holders are of great benefit while the parent or child is being trained to use dental floss (Fig 6-2).

Although the use of dental floss holders facilitates cleaning efforts for the parent, the efficacy of its use depends on the level of dexterity and the anatomy of the interproximal surface (Newbrun, 1985). Care must be

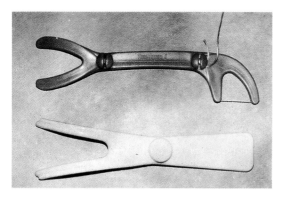

Fig 6-2 Examples of two types of floss-holding devices, used to overcome the difficulty with intraoral access and the manual dexterity of the operator. They must be used with care to prevent tissue damage and pain.

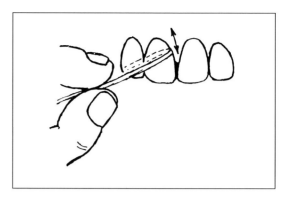

Fig 6-3 Wrap about 45 cm (18 in.) of floss around the middle fingers, guide the floss interproximally beyond the contact area with the index fingers. Move the floss back and forth against the tooth surface beneath the free gingival margin. Repeat movement on adjacent tooth surface before removing the floss back through the contact area.

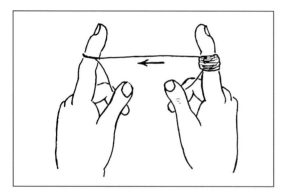

Fig 6-4 Gather up the used floss onto one middle finger and unwind fresh floss from the middle finger of the opposite hand. Use fresh floss sections periodically.

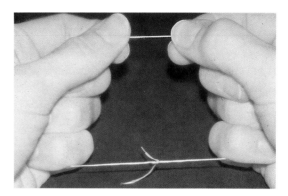

Fig 6-5 An alternate technique employs the tying of the two loose ends of floss together with a knot. This technique provides sufficient tension without the need to wrap the floss around the fingers.

exerted not to hurt the child or inflict tissue damage when a floss holder is used. Many parents feel that the use of a floss holder increases the possibility of hurting the child and that better control of the floss is rendered by using their fingers (Wright, 1980).

For preschool children, flossing may not be required since proximal contacts between teeth are often lacking. As the developmental spacing closes with the eruption of permanent teeth, the parent should assume responsibility for flossing, concentrating on the interproximal surfaces of the molars. Parents should be taught to floss a young child's teeth while the child lies in a supine position. Toothbrushing may also be practiced in this position. Children older than 9 years of age can begin to learn the flossing technique and assume responsibility for this practice over time (Wright, 1980). The procedure for flossing is described in Figs 6-3 to 6-5.

One study has demonstrated that children 8 to 11 years old require a minimum of 10 days of concentrat-ed training to become effective in plaque removal (Terhune, 1973). This is related to the level of eye-hand coordination, which improves with chronologic age. Preliminary evidence suggests that unlike supervised brushing, supervised flossing in school may produce a significant reduction in caries. Wright et al (1979), in a 20-month study, found a 50% reduction in the incidence of proximal caries in primary teeth when compared with contralateral controls, and the magnitude of the effect increased the longer the flossing was continued.

Oral irrigation

Oral rinsing, whether performed manually or with the aid of a mechanical device, will not remove plaque from the tooth surface (Newbrun, 1985). However, this method is effective in removing large deposits of debris and is recommended to patients who have fixed orthodontic appliances. It should be emphasized to the patient that oral irrigation should be a supplement to, not a substitute for, other means of oral hygiene.

Chemotherapeutic agents

Because patient motivation toward the goal of proper oral hygiene maintenance is difficult to obtain, research has been directed toward other means of prevention that do not require mechanical removal of plaque and that would require less patient cooperation and dexterity. These methods employ various direct means of inhibiting plaque growth (Keyes, 1969). For example, dextranase, an enzyme that inhibits plaque growth by stimulating the breakdown of dextrans, has been studied on a limited basis. Inhibition of dextran by dextranase should prevent adherence of plaque to the tooth surface. However, because clinical testing has not been promising and the daily concentration required for effective use may be unsafe, dextranase has not received sufficient support for continued use as an antiplaque agent in its present form.

Another direction of research in this area is the investigation of antimicrobial agents, which, because of their bacteriostatic or bactericidal effects, inhibit plaque growth and colonization. Daily rinses of such agents as vancomycin and chlorhexidine have shown good short-term benefits. However, continued use on a long-term basis provides less beneficial effects while increasing the risk of resistant strain development. In addition, some agents cause discoloration of tissue and mucosal sloughing.

A final method worth considering is the development of an effective caries vaccine program. The immunization of animals with bacterial antigens to produce an antibody reaction against plaque formation is in the experimental stages. There are, however, many problems to be overcome with this approach. First a specific antigen must be developed for each of the cariogenic strains known to exist. Second, large amounts of antigen must be administered because it is diluted in saliva and lost when swallowed. Third, one approach uses direct injection of an antiglucosyltransferase antibody into the parotid gland, but this approach would probably have poor patient acceptance. Finally, a more acceptable approach for the patient is ingestion of a capsule containing attenuated *Streptococcus mutans* cells. However, there is some danger with this approach because of the production of serum antibody response thought to contribute to autoimmune cardiac and renal tissue lesions. These complications may be avoided if an effective means of inducing a strictly oral secretory response in humans could be perfected (Messer, 1978).

Substrate

It is clear that dental plaque plays a dominant role in the initiation of dental caries and gingivitis in children. It is also known that plaque growth is controlled by the availability of its nutrient supply. Fermentable carbohydrates (sugar), particularly in the form of sucrose, appear to be the substrate of choice by cariogenic microorganisms. Since nearly one fourth of the average American diet is made up of sugar and the average American consumes approximately 45 kg (100 lb) of sugar every year, there is abundant availability of this nutrient supply for growth of cariogenic bacterial colonies. A further difficulty in control arises from the fact that nearly two thirds of the amount is consumed from foods to which sugar has been added before the consumer purchases it. Presweetened cereals and pastries are two examples. Many food products not thought of a containing sugar do, in fact, contain large amounts of it. One brand of ketchup, for example, is approximately one-fourth sugar. Some salad dressings are nearly one-third sugar. Sugar is used in the making of bakery goods, soft drinks, desserts and candies, almost all fruit drinks, soups, pot pies, frozen TV dinners, and some canned and most frozen vegetables (MHD, 1979).

Sugar is a fermentable carbohydrate. It is found in several forms—fructose, lactose, and sucrose. Fructose occurs naturally in fruits and vegetables. Because it is broken down more slowly in the mouth than other forms of sugar, it is not a serious problem in dental caries. Approximately 3% of our sugar intake is in the form of fructose. Lactose is the sugar found naturally in dairy products. It, too, makes up only 3% of our sugar intake. Sucrose, the most common form of sugar, makes up approximately 94% of our sugar intake. Sucrose is metabolized by cariogenic microorganisms to produce *(1)* extracellular polysaccharides (dextran) for adherence to the dental smooth surfaces and *(2)* acid, which initiates the demineralization process. Therefore, any means by which the availability of fermentable carbohydrates can be reduced will contribute to the prevention of caries and gingivitis in children. Current methods of prevention are based on diet modification and supplementation.

The modification of a family's diet is difficult to achieve. The selection of food types by a family is influenced by individual preference, tradition, past experiences, social pressures, daily schedules, and income (Nizel, 1972a). All of these factors probably have a stronger impact on the food choices of a family than any desire to prevent dental disease. Nevertheless, nutritional counseling to achieve dietary modifications may succeed with some highly motivated individuals or families within the general population. It is to this population that our efforts should be directed.

First day	Second day	Third day

Breakfast
1 bowl Rice Crispies
    with 2 tsp sugar
1 glass Tang
1 Blueberry Pop Tart
	Breakfast
	1 bowl Trix
	    with 2 tsp sugar
	2 slices cinnamon toast
	1 glass orange juice
		Breakfast
		1 bowl Fruit Loops
		    with 2 tsp sugar

Lunch 1 hamburger 1 bag potato chips 1 glass milk	**Lunch** 2 hot dogs 1 glass chocolate milk 1 Twinkie	**Lunch** 2 tacos 1 bowl soup 1 Coke
Dinner 1 slice roast beef mashed potatoes—2 scoops 1 serving corn 1 glass milk 1 dish jello	**Dinner** 1 chicken leg 1 baked potato 1 serving peas 1 slice white bread 1 glass milk 1 slice cake	**Dinner** 1 beef patty 1 serving french fried potatoes 1 serving beans 1 glass milk 1 dish ice cream
Extras: 2 chocolate chip cookies 1 Dr. Pepper 1 stick bubble gum	*Extras:* 1 bag taco chips 1 Coke	*Extras:* 3 oatmeal cookies 1 peanut butter and jelly sandwich 1 Dr. Pepper

Fig 6-6   Three-day dietary diary.

Dietary diary

Nutritional counseling should focus primarily on the balance and adequacy of the present diet using the four basic food groups; identifying the cariogenic foods in the diet, with emphasis on frequency of consumption and retentiveness of the food; guiding the patient in making suggestions as to appropriate substitutes through your recommendations; and providing follow-up evaluations for reinforcement (Nizel, 1972b). An educational aid available for the analysis of a patient's diet is the 3-day food intake diary. Following is the procedure for recording and analyzing the 3-day food intake diary.

Method

1. Instruct the patient to write down everything he or she eats and drinks, except water, for 3 days (Fig 6-6). In the case of young children, the parent will keep the record.
2. To assure that the patient or parent understands how to fill out the diary correctly, ask what the patient ate for breakfast that day. Most patients will reply, "Cereal and toast." If this response is entered on the record simply as "cereal" and "toast," the information is of little or no value. Therefore, ask the patient what kind of cereal was eaten, how much, whether there was milk on the cereal, and how much, whether there was sugar on the cereal, and how much. Enter all this information in the dairy while the patient (or parent) observes exactly how the recording is done. The patient (or parent) is then much more likely to return a history that contains useful information.
3. After recording the breakfast history, ask whether the patient ate anything after breakfast and before the noon meal. Record anything eaten between meals.
4. After the patient (or parent) understands how the diary is completed, dispense a blank form with the following instructions

   (A) Please record in detail everything you eat or drink. This includes between-meal snacks, candies, gum, as well as regular meals over a 3-day period to include one weekend day or holiday.

   (B) The following should be included: *(1)* kind of food (chicken, apple, bread, etc); *(2)* approximate amount in household measures, 1 cup (8 oz), 1 T (tablespoon), 1 average serving; *(3)* preparation (raw, cooked, fried, etc); *(4)* number of teaspoons of sugar or sugar products eaten, as well as milk added to cereal, beverages, or other foods.

   (C) Specific information on the time and frequency that between-meal snacks are eaten is essential.

Table 6-2 Snack foods

Good snacks		Bad snacks	
Peanuts	Apples	Cookies	Candy
Walnuts	Oranges	Cake	Caramel popcorn
Popcorn	Bananas	Pie	Ice Cream
Celery	Plums	Sweet rolls	
Radishes	Cantaloupe	Crackers (graham or soda)	
Cucumber slices	Watermelon	Gelatin desserts	
Pickles	Deviled eggs	Peanut butter sandwiches	
Cheese wedges	Hard-boiled eggs	Anything sticky, sweet or starchy	
Meat slices (ham)		(eg, white bread)	

Table 6-3 Sugar contents of foods

Food	Size	Amount of sugar (tsp)
Chocolate cake, two-layer, icing	1 average piece	15
Apple pie	1 medium piece	12
Doughnut (plain)	1 average	4
Gelatin (Jello)	$\frac{1}{2}$ cup	4
Jelly	1 level tablespoon	$2\frac{1}{2}$
Chocolate fudge	$1\frac{1}{2}$-inch square	4
Chewing gum (including Dentyne)	1 stick	$\frac{1}{2}$
Hard candy	1 piece	$\frac{1}{3}$
Marshmallow	1 average	$1\frac{1}{2}$
Ice cream	1 cone or bar	5 or 6
Chocolate milk	1 cup (5 oz)	6
Soft drinks	6-oz bottle	4
Candy bar	5 oz	20

Analysis

1. Emphasize that the purpose of the record is not to criticize the patient's eating habits but to help prevent tooth decay.
2. With a red pencil, underline in the diary all foods containing carbohydrate (sugar).
3. Mark a large red X beside any of the underlined foods that are a sticky consistency.
4. Note whether the recorded breakfast consisted mostly of carbohydrate foods and very little protein.
5. Explain in simple terms how the teeth decay.
6. Go over the record with the patient and point out which foods produce decay. A record well marked with red pencil is very effective in focusing the parent's attention of the amount of sweet food eaten.
7. If much sweet food is eaten between meals, point out that such snacks increase tooth decay. Explain that decay can be greatly reduced by leaving out between-meal eating entirely or by substituting fresh fruit, nuts, or salted popcorn. (Parents will also be interested to know that the avoidance of between-meal snacks may overcome most of the meal-time problems they may be experiencing with their child.)

8. Point out that a breakfast consisting only of cereal (especially the sugar-coated kinds) with milk and sugar will increase tooth decay. A much better breakfast would be an egg, ham, milk, and whole-wheat toast.
9. Explain the need for toothbrushing or for rinsing the mouth vigorously with water any time sweet food is eaten.
10. Point our that artificial sweeteners can be substituted in making desserts.

Specific recommendations as to appropriate snack foods should be provided and reinforced with a handout that can be placed in the kitchen as a continual reminder. Examples of appropriate suggestions or food facts should include some of the information found in Tables 6-2 through 6-4. Sucrose substitutes, such as sorbitol, mannitol, Xylitol, cyclamate, aspartame, and saccharin have been studied and experimentally used in humans. Chewing gums containing sorbitol, mannitol, and Xylitol are beneficial in neutralizing plaque acid by stimulation of salivary flow and promotion of enamel remineralization. There are only a limited number of foods identified as anticariogenic (not causing plaque pH to fall below 5.5 after ingestion) and are thus targeted as strongly recommended snack foods.

Table 6-4 Meal patterns

	Include	Avoid
Breakfast		
Eggs	Any style (bacon or sausage, if desired)	French toast and syrup
Bread or cereal	Whole-grain or enriched cooked cereal with butter and milk	Dry cereals with sugar or sugar-coated cereals, syrups, jams, jellies, buns, pastries, or sweet rolls
Fruit/citrus	Whole fruit, fresh, frozen or unsweetened canned juice	Adding sugar to fruit
Milk	Plain or buttermilk	Chocolate or other flavored and sweetened milk
Lunch		
Soups or juice	Fresh or canned	
Sandwich	Toasted or dark bread, meat, fish, fowl, egg, or cheese	Raisin or cinnamon bread, jams, jellies, or honey filling
Salads	Any combination	
Milk	Plain or buttermilk	Any flavored milks or soft drinks
Desserts	Raw apples, oranges, tangerines, or other fruits in season	Cakes, cookies, pies, pastries, bananas ice cream, raisins, figs, dates, or other dried fruits
Dinner		
Soup or juice	Fresh or canned	
Meat or fish	Beef, lamb, pork, veal, fowl, or fish (liver at least once weekly)	
Vegetables	One or two portions, especially green or yellow, potatoes	Candied sweet potatoes or glazed vegetables
Salads	Any combination	
Desserts	Raw apples, oranges, tangerines	Same as lunch
Milk	Plain or buttermilk	Any sweetened milks or soft drinks
Beverage	Coffee, tea, or water	

Anticariogenic snack foods have been identified as eggs, cheese (blue, brie, aged cheddar, gouda, monterey jack, mozzarella, swiss), ham, peanuts, and walnuts (Schachetle and Harlander, 1984). Consideration has also been given to the contribution of fats and proteins in the reduction of caries. These food groups may have an effect on the enamel surface, saliva, and plaque metabolism and pH (Alfano, 1979).

To encourage the development of good food habits, make the following recommendations to your patients:

1. Serve a variety of foods; don't make meals monotonous or unappetizing.
2. Emphasize foods that require chewing; don't select soft or sticky foods.
3. Make mealtime enjoyable and pleasant; don't fuss.
4. Let appetite gauge how much to eat; don't force.
5. Consider food preference (if they meet dental needs); don't be impractical.
6. Brush teeth immediately after eating, or rinse, swish, and swallow; don't allow food debris to remain in the mouth.
7. Always brush at bedtime.

Time

It is well documented that the formation of caries on children is regulated more by the frequency of sucrose consumption than by the actual quantity consumed. As the frequency of between-meal snacks increases, so will the child's caries rate. However, increased consumption of carbohydrates during regular meals will not significantly alter the caries rate (Mack, 1949). This result suggests that the eating of cariogenic foods should be confined to mealtimes, if they are consumed at all. Studies in institutions where the diet has been strictly regulated to reduce the amount and frequency of carbohydrate consumption have reported up to a 75% decrease in the caries incidence of the confined residents (Hartles and Leach, 1975).

It is obvious that a patient's willingness to limit carbohydrate consumption will produce beneficial effects on his or her caries activity. However, the pressures of contemporary lifestyles on dietary habits and patterns and the ever-increasing availability of convenience foods makes it difficult for individuals to adhere to a strict regimen of noncariogenic foods and a daily routine of three complete meals without snacking. One survey of 1,494 American families indicated that the average child (aged 5 to 12 years) consumed 1.37

Table 6-5 Summary of caries control methods and agents

Factor	Method	Agent
General	Patient education and motivation	Disclosing solution Plaque index Caries activity tests Diet diary Audiovisual materials Handouts
Susceptible tooth	Improve resistance	Fluorides Sealants
Plaque	Removal	Toothbrushing Flossing
	Inhibition	Vancomycin Chlorhexidine Vaccine
Substrate	Sugar substitution	Sorbitol Xylitol
	Diet modification	Anticariogenic foods
Time	Diet modification	Decrease frequency and consistency of snack consumption

snacks per day but that these snacks contributed significantly to the total daily nutritional intake (15% or more) of these children (Morgan and Leveille, 1979). This finding contradicts the common belief that most snacks consumed by children are of poor nutritional quality. There is need, however, to continue research efforts to develop snack foods with a reduced potential for cariogenicity. It is an unrealistic and insensitive approach to insist that patients totally eliminate sugar from their diet. Instead, dentists should suggest alternative patterns of consumption during meals rather than total abstinence from sugar intake.

The influence of time in the formation of dental caries in children is a variable factor. Caries formation is a chronic process and its rate of progression is affected by the intensity, duration, and frequency of acid attack on the enamel surface and the local environment's ability to resist demineralization or to remineralize the affected surface. Time also plays a role as an expression of the tooth's posteruptive dental age. The less mature the enamel surface is in terms of its exposure to the oral fluids, the more susceptible it is to caries formation. Therefore, recently erupted teeth are the most vulnerable to caries attack.

Summary

Many methods are available to prevent dental caries in children (Table 6-5). However, the approach to prevention should not be a universal application of these methods to all patients but rather a selective, individualized approach to accommodate each patient's needs. Because of the complex, multifactorial etiology of dental caries, the discovery of a simple and direct means of prevention is unlikely. More effort must be concentrated on developing methods of predicting those individuals who are at highest risk so that the delivery of preventive services can be maximized in that direction. This task, in itself, is not easy because of the wide variation among individuals in dietary patterns and preferences; plaque pathogenicity; salivary buffering, immunologic, enzymatic, and cleansing potential; tooth resistance; and oral hygiene practices. The clinical paradox of one child who has rampant caries in spite of optimal fluoride exposure, low sucrose exposure, and good oral hygiene and another child who is caries free in spite of no orientation or exposure to preventive concepts or attitudes is ample proof of the influence of individual variation on dental caries formation and the magnitude of a problem that defies a simple solution.

Preventive care for the infant

Many articles have discussed the establishment of preventive programs for the oral health care of infants (Cheney and Cheney, 1974; Nowak et al, 1976; Sanger, 1977; Nowak, 1980; Goepferd, 1987). These articles have focused attention on the need for early intervention of preventive measures, especially dental

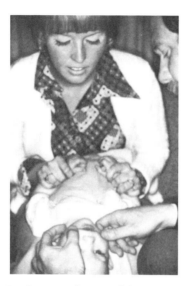

Fig 6-7 For direct visualization of the intraoral structures during the examination procedures, the infant should be placed in the supine position with his or her legs wrapped around the parent's waist and the head cradled and extended over the knees. Stability is obtained by having the parent holding the infant's hands down and maintaining control of the legs with the elbows. With the child cradled in the parent's lap, oral hygiene can be accomplished by wrapping a moist washcloth around the index finger and simply wiping the infant's mouth and teeth free of debris after eating.

health education for parents, to minimize the incidence of oral diseases during infancy. It is recognized that the best opportunity to obtain the attention of parents is during the child's perinatal period when motivation and interest are probably at their highest level. Surveys of expectant and nursing mothers indicate that many are misinformed or inadequate in their practice of proper dental health habits and that information disseminated at this time may encourage acceptance of new attitudes and practices (Blinkhorn, 1981; Doshi, 1985; Lee, 1984).

Because preventive dental health programming should be included along with the initial dental examination, most pediatric dentists recommend that the infant be seen as soon after birth as is convenient for the family, and this appointment should be followed with subsequent visits at regular intervals for reinforcement. The procedures provided during these visits should include but not be limited to the following (Sanger, 1977):

1. Thorough examination of the infant's mouth with close inspection for any abnormalities
2. Discussion with the parents about the growth and development of the dentition, with special reference to the normal timing and pattern of primary tooth eruption.

3. Discussion of fluoride supplementation and prescription, where indicated
4. Discussion of diet and feeding habits to prevent nursing caries
5. Discussion of sucking habits and use of pacifiers
6. Discussion or oral trauma and precautions for its avoidance
7. Demonstration of recommended oral hygiene practices

Oral examination

Figure 6-7 illustrates the technique recommended for proper positioning of parent, infant, and dentist during the oral examination. By the use of digital palpation and tongue blade manipulation, it is possible to examine the infant in this position. This same technique may be used at home to provide oral hygiene measures. The mouth of the infant although simple in appearance, is a rather complex organ system. Unlike the edentulous mouth of the adult, which is subject to degenerative changes, the mouth of the infant is continually developing into a more sophisticated organ system and is in a very dynamic relationship with other developing organ systems. Anatomic structures of the infant's mouth are unique, characteristic, and transitory for this period. The lips of the infant exhibit a prominent line of demarcation at the vermillion border or junction of the skin and mucous membrane. The skin may appear smooth and pink and will cover the outer third of the lip surface. The mucous membrane may appear wrinkled and mildly purplish and may be slightly elevated, moist, and glistening.

A few days after birth, the mucous membrane exhibits a superficially furrowed appearance with dry surface and gradually separates the outer layer of cornified epithelium from the underlying mucus to form crusts known as sucking calluses that are, in turn, shed and replaced by new calluses. This process most commonly occurs near the midline or central portion of the lips and often persists for several weeks after birth.

The maxilla and palate are separated from the upper lip by a shallow sulcus, which is interrupted by a midline labial frenum and two lateral frenums (Fig 6-8). The lip shows a definite division from the visual aspect into an outer smooth zone, the pars glabra, and an inner zone characterized by fine villi, the pars villosa. The pars villosa, near the midline, is prominent and forms the tuberculum of the upper lip, which connects the upper lip to the labial frenum. During prenatal development, this tuberculum extended across the alveolar ridge, joined the palatine papilla, and formed the tectolabial frenum. With prenatal alveolar process growth, the tectolabial frenum separated from the palatine papilla and became the labial frenum. The palatine (incisive) papilla contains the oral components of the nasopalatine ducts, which are blind ducts of varying lengths. The palatal rugae are irregular and asymmetric ridges that transverse the anterior part of the palate. Posterior palatal morphology and color may vary depending on the underlying submucous layer containing fatty and glandular components. The palate will end posteriorly with the uvula medially and with the palatine tonsils and arch laterally. The alveolar ridge peaks anteriorly and then flattens as it approaches the molar region. A protuberance in the molar region is the pseudoalveolar ridge, which gradually disappears with growth of the alveolar process. Until this happens, a pseudoalveolar groove extends along the medial borders of the ridge as it approximates palatal mucosa. The shape of the ridges correspond to the shape of the teeth, with the labiolingual dimension of the ridge slightly greater than that of the teeth it encompasses. Areas of individual tooth buds can be seen in regular arrangement on the alveolar ridges. There may be on the free margin a membranous fringelike tissue with a serrated edge extending as much as 1 mm above the alveolar tissue, which may persist for a few weeks or more.

The tongue differentiates little from that of the adult. Various types of papillae can be visualized in the anterior dorsal region, with the lingual follicles and the foramen cecum in the posterior dorsal region. The foramen cecum marks the oral termination in the tongue of the thyroglossal duct, a transitory duct extending from the tongue to the thyroid as it made its prenatal descent to the throat region. The ventral surface of the tongue is smooth, glistening and free of papillae, and lingual vessels are easily seen. The floor of the mouth is characterized by superficial vessels covered by thin, less specialized mucosa under which are located the sublingual glands. A tissue fold transversing the base of the tongue (sublingual fold), containing minor sublingual gland ducts and the submandibular (Wharton) duct, meets near the lingual frenum to form the sublingual carbuncles. The lingual frenum connects the anterior base of the tongue with the lingual mucosa and mandibular alveolar ridge.

The mandibular alveolar ridge likewise peaks anteriorly and flattens posteriorly (Fig 6-9). It joins the floor of the mouth and labial sulcus, which is interrupted by a labial frenum and minor lateral frenums. The labial frenum connects the lower lip to the alveolar ridge at the midline. As the primary tooth erupts in the alveolar process, a glistening, reddened bulge outlining the underlying crown may be seen on the alveolar ridge. As the crown of the primary tooth pierces the alveolar mucosa, the semilunar contour of the marginal gingiva and sulcus become apparent. This gingiva may initially appear red and edematous. Systemic effects of tooth eruption include dehydration, increased salivation, skin eruptions, and gastrointestinal disturbances (Galili, 1969; Seward, 1972a; Tsamtsouris and White; 1977, Carpenter, 1978).

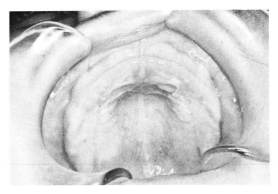

Fig 6-8 Normal maxillary arch and palate (infant). The maxillary arch and palate of the infant, although similar in gross appearance, is unlike the edentulous mouth of the adult, Unlike the edentulous adult maxillary ridge, that of the infant peaks anteriorly and flattens as it approaches the molar region, with a pseudoalveolar ridge disappearing as growth of the alveolar process and eruption of primary teeth commence. The labial frenum in the infant extends across the anterior ridge to the palatine (incisive) papilla and continues to do so until eruption of the primary anterior teeth.

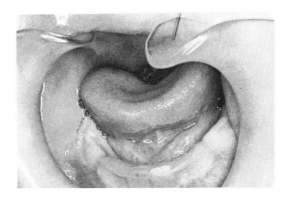

Fig 6-9 Normal mandibular arch (infant). The mandibular alveolar ridge likewise peaks anteriorly and flattens posteriorly. Tissue folds transversing the base of the tongue (sublingual fold) are very prominent, contain minor sublingual glands and ducts and the submandibular (Wharton) duct, and meet at the lingual frenum to form the sublingual carbuncles. The tongue differs little from that of the adult.

Natal or neonatal teeth

Natal teeth are present at birth, whereas neonatal teeth erupt soon after birth (Kates et al, 1984). Most natal and neonatal teeth are of normal primary complement. The mandibular incisor region is the most prevalent location. Natal teeth appear to be attached to a pad of soft tissue above the alveolar ridge, whereas neonatal teeth appear to be covered by mucosa. The condition is probably attributed to a superficial position of the formation of the tooth germ involved. Natal teeth may resemble normal primary teeth. In many instances, however, they are poorly developed, small, conical, yellowish brown opaque, and have hypoplastic enamel and dentin, poor texture, and poor, if any, root development. Natal and neonatal teeth, lacking root structure, will usually prematurely exfoliate during infancy, presenting a potential hazard for aspiration.

Both natal and neonatal teeth may present nursing problems, contribute to ulcerative lesions, and endanger the infant with possible aspiration. Radiographic analysis of the tooth and alveolar area should be performed and a differential diagnosis attempted on the tooth. If extraction is indicated, parent counseling is essential to avoid any confusion later regarding the extraction of a primary tooth. Loss of an early erupted primary tooth is definitely more desirable than the possibility of tooth aspiration by the infant. Even if teeth are not mobile and extraction is not planned, the teeth are generally nonrestorable because of quantitative enamel and dentin defects. Where possible, extraction should be avoided until after the tenth postnatal day to avoid excessive hemorrhage.

Less frequently, one or more primary teeth will prematurely erupt during infancy. Eruption is not complete, and therefore no problems are encountered with these teeth. These teeth should remain unless problems arise. Natal or neonatal teeth appear to occur sporadically, whereas early incomplete eruption of primary teeth may be familial.

Teething

Teething occurs most commonly during 4 to 10 months of age at the time of primary incisor eruption. Symptoms often associated with teething are irritability (most prevalent), restlessness, drooling, disturbed sleep, decreased food consumption, increased fluid intake, diarrhea, fever, and rash. Among those symptoms, the occurrence of diarrhea, fever, and rash indicate systemic involvement. There is much divergence of opinion as to whether local irritation causes these systemic manifestations. It is argued that the eruption of primary incisors and the secondary systemic manifestations are merely coincidental. In one study, a review medical records indicated that 40% of the children of this age erupt teeth without any symptoms (Carpenter, 1978). Other studies have shown a relationship between fevers of unknown origin and the occurrence of dental eruption. Recently, King et al (1992) reported a correlation between teething symptoms and the presence of herpes simplex virus without evidence of oral infection. In any case, it is impossible to prove cause and effect. What can be dangerous is the sometimes casual attitude of attributing fever or gastrointestinal or respiratory tract problems to the simultaneous occurrence of tooth eruption without seeking consultation. Failure to consult or to examine other possible etiologic factors may delay recognition of serious illnesses, such as pneumonia, meningitis, and septicemia (British Medical Journal, 1975). It is also convenient to attribute such problems to teething to avoid recognition or management of developmental changes and behavioral maladjustments. Irritability and restlessness may be the result of parental mismanagement of sleeping habits or changes in the child's attachment preferences (separation anxiety) and feeding habits (Honig, 1975). These factors could reduce the child's resistance to infections, which is compounded by the fact that the child's circulating maternal antibodies (a key immunologic defense mechanism) are decreasing at 6 months of age.

Treatment for teething is symptomatic and palliative (Seward, 1972b; Tsamtsouris and White, 1977). Reassuring the parents is helpful. Fever, if present, should be treated with acetaminophen. If the fever is persistent, the child should be referred to a pediatrician. Use of a chewable object and topical anesthetics will help relieve local irritation.

References

Alfano, M.C. Understanding the role of diet and nutrition in dental caries. In Alfano, M.C. Changing Perspectives in Nutrition and Caries Research. New York: Medcom, Inc. 1979.

Arnim, S.S. The use of disclosing agents for measuring tooth cleanliness. J. Periodontol. 34:227, 1963.

Axelsson, P. Concept and practice of plaque-control. Pediatr. Dent. 3:101, 1981.

Axelsson P., and Lindhe, J. Effect of oral hygiene instruction and professional toothcleaning on caries and gingivitis in schoolchildren. Community Dent. Oral Epidemiol. 9:251, 1981.

Barenie, J., Ripa, L.W., and Leske, G. The relationship of frequency of tooth brushing, oral hygiene, gingival health, and caries experience in school children. J. Public Health Dent. 33:160. 1973

Bellini, H.T., et al. Oral hygiene and caries. A review. Acta Odontol. Scand. 39:257, 1981.

Blinkhorn, A.S. Dental preventive advice for pregnant and nursing mothers—Sociological implications. Int. Dent. J. 31:14, 1981.

British Medical Journal. Teething myths (editorial). Br. Med. J. 4:64, 1975.

Bullen, C, et al. Improving children's oral hygiene through parental involvement. J. Dent. Child. 54:125, 1988.

Carpenter, J.V. The relationship between teething and systemic disturbances. J. Dent. Child. 45:381, 1978.

Cheney, H.G., and Cheney, V.A. The dental hygienist as a health educator in prenatal care. Dent. Hyg. 48:150, 1974.

Doshi, S.B. A study of dental habits, knowledge and opinions of nursing mothers. J. Can. Dent. Assoc. 51:429, 1985.

Doyle, W.A. Preventive program for children. In Goldman, H.M. Current Therapy in Dentistry. Vol. 5. St. Louis: The C.V. Mosby Co., 1974.

Galili, G. Eruption of primary teeth and general pathologic conditions. J. Dent. Child. 26:51, 1959.

Gillig, J.L. Retention of health information. J. Dent Child. 36:56, 1969.

Goepferd, S. An infant oral health program: The first 18 months. J. Dent Child. 53:8, 1987.

Hartles, R.L., and Leach, S.A. Effect of diet on dental caries. Br. Med. Bull. 31:137, 1975.

Heifetz, S.B., Bagramian, R.A., and Suomi, J.D. Programs for the mass control of plaque: An appraisal. J. Public Health Dent. 37:3, 1977.

Heloe, L.A., and Konig, K.G. Oral hygiene and educational programs for caries prevention. Caries Res. 12 (suppl. 1):83, 1978.

Honig, P.J. Teething—Are today's pediatrician's using yesterdays notions? J. Pediatr. 87:415, 1975.

Honkala, E., et al. Effectiveness of children's habitual toothbrushing. J. Clin. Periodontol. 13:81, 1986.

Horowitz, A.M., Suomi, J.D., and Peterson, J.K. Effects of supervised dental plaque removal by children: Results after third and final year. J. Dent. Res. 56:2, 1977 (IADR abstract).

Kates, G., et al. Natal and neonatal teeth: A clinical study. J. Am. Dent. Assoc. 109:441, 1984.

Keyes, P.H. Present and future measures for dental caries control. J. Am. Dent. Assoc. 79:1395, 1969.

Kimmelman, B.B., and Tassman, G.C. Research in designs of children's toothbrushes. J. Dent. Child. 27:60, 1960.

King, D, et al. Herpetic gingivostomatitis and teething difficulty in infants. Pediatr. Dent. 14:82, 1992.

Kleber, C.J., et al. Duration and pattern of toothbrushing in children using a gel or paste dentifrice. J. Am. Dent. Assoc. 103:723, 1981.

Lee, A.J. A survey of dental knowledge, attitudes and behavior of expectant parents. J. Can. Dent. Assoc 50:145, 1984.

Leske, G.S., Ripa, L.W., and Barenie, J. Comparison of caries prevalence of children with different daily toothbrushing frequencies. Community Dent. Oral Epidemiol. 4:102, 1976.

Linn, E.L. Mother's involvement in children's oral hygiene. J. Am. Dent. Assoc. 93:398, 1976.

Mack, P.B. A study of institutional children with particular reference to the caloric value as well as other factors of the diet. Soc. Res. Child. Dev. 13:62, 1949.

Melcer, S., and Feldman, S. Preventive dentistry teaching methods and improved oral hygiene—A summary of research. Clin. Prev. Dent. 6:7, 1979.

Messer, L.B. The current status cariology. Oper. Dent. 3:60, 1978. 3:60, 1978.

Minneapolis Health Department (MHD). Child Health News—Sugar. Minneapolis, Minn.: MHD, 1979.

Morgan, K. J. and Leveille, G.A. Frequency and composition of children's snacks. In Alfano, M.C. Changing Perspectives in Nutrition and Caries Research. New York: Medcom, Inc., 1979.

Newbrun E. Chemical and mechanical removal of plaque. Compend. Cont. Educ. Dent. 6:110, 1985.

Nizel, A.E. Nutrition in Preventive Dentistry, Science and Dentistry. Philadelphia: W.B. Saunders Co., 1972a.

Nizel, A.E. Personalized nutrition counseling. J. Dent. Child., 39:353, 1972b.

Nowak, A.J. The infant patient: Initial appointment management. In McDonald, R., et al. Current Therapy in Dentistry. Vol. 8. St. Louis: The C.V. Mosby Co., 1980.

Nowak, A.J., et al. Prevention of dental disease from nine months in utero to eruption of the first tooth. J. Am. Soc. Prev. Dent. 6:6, 1976.

Owen, T.L. A clinical evaluation of electric and manual toothbrushing by children with primary dentition. J. Dent Child. 39:15, 1972.

Rugg-Gunn, A.J., and MacGregor, I.D.M. A survey of toothbrushing behavior in children and young adults. J. Periodont. Res. 13:282, 1978.

Sanger R.G. Preventive dental health program for the infant. Dent. Hyg. 51:408, 1977.

Sanger, R.G., and Bystrtom, E.B. Breast feeding: Does it affect oral facial growth? Dent. Hyg. 56:44, 1982.

Sangnes, G. Effectiveness of vertical and horizontal toothbrushing techniques in the removal of plaque. J. Dent. Child. 41:119, 1974.

Sangnes, G., and Gjermo, P. Prevalence of oral soft and hard tissue lesions related to mechanical toothcleansing procedures. Community Dent. Oral Epidemiol. 4:77, 1976.

Schachtele, C.F., and Harlander, S.K. Will the diets of the future be less cariogenic? J. Can. Dent. Assoc. 50:213, 1984.

Seward, M.H. General disturbances attributed to eruption of the human primary dentition. J. Dent. Child. 39:178, 1972a.

Seward, M.H. The treatment of teething in infants. Br. Dent. J. 123:33, 1972b.

Silverstein, S., Gold, S., and Heilbron, D. Effect of supervised deplaquing on dental caries, gingivitis and plaque. J. Dent. Res., 56:2, 1977 (IADR abstract).

Simmons, S., et al. Effect of oral hygiene instruction on brushing skills in preschool children. Community Dent. Oral Epidemiol. 11:193, 1983.

Sims, W. The interpretation and use of Snyder tests and lactobacillus counts. J. Am. Dent. Assoc. 80:1315, 1970.

Starkey, P. Instructions to parents for brushing the child's teeth. J. Dent Child. 28:42, 1961

Sundell, S.O., and Klein, H. Toothbrushing behavior in children: A study of pressure and stroke frequency. Pediatr. Dent. 4:225, 1982.

Terhune, J.A. Predicting the readiness of elementary school children to learn an effective dental flossing technique. J. Am. Dent Assoc. 86:1332, 1973.

Tinanoff, N., Wei, S., and Parkins, F. Effect of a pumice prophylaxis on fluoride uptake in tooth enamel. J. Am. Dent. Assoc. 88:384, 1974.

Tsamtsouris, A., and White, G.E. Controversy, teething as a problem of infancy. J. Pedod. 4:305, 1977.

Wright, G.Z. The flossing technique: Can it be effective in reducing caries and gingivitis in children? In McDonald, R., et al. Current Therapy in Dentistry, vol. 8. St. Louis: The C.V. Mosby Co., 1980.

Wright, G.Z. Banting, D.W. and Feasby, W.H. The Dorchester dental flossing study: Final report. Clin Prev. Dent. 1:23, 1979.

Zuniga, M.A., and Caldwell, R.C. Pastes on normal and "white spot" enamel—The effect of fluoride containing prophylaxis pastes. J. Dent. Child. 36:345, 1969.

Questions

1. Which of the following practices is most effective in motivating a willing patient toward prolonged oral hygiene improvement?

   a. Patient education through personal instruction supplemented with take-home pamphlets for re-inforcement

   b. The use of disclosing agents to monitor progress

   c. An enthusiastic and positive approach expressed by the therapist providing the instruction

   d. Patient education provided before treatment is rendered

   e. Supervised patient education on a multiple-visit basis allowing for periodic reinforcement

2. Which of the following statements concerning toothbrushing in children is correct?

   a. The responsibility for toothbrushing is assumed primarily by the parent until the child is 6 years old

   b. There is no direct correlation between frequency of toothbrushing and oral hygiene status

   c. There is no direct correlation between frequency of toothbrushing and gingival health

   d. There is no direct correlation between frequency of toothbrushing and prevalence of caries

   e. Oral irrigation is an effective substitute for toothbrushing

3. Which brushing technique is recommended for cleaning children's teeth because it is comfortable to use and readily acceptable to both the parent and child?

   a. Up-and-down technique

   b. Bass technique

   c. Modified Stillman technique

   d. Horizontal scrub technique

   e. No one method is superior over another

4. Which of the following reasons support using a toothbrush prophylaxis instead of a rubber cup prophylaxis as a routine dental office procedure for children?

   a. To remove stain

   b. To remove plaque

   c. To remove the acquired pellicle that acts as a barrier to subsequent fluoride uptake

   d. To stress to patients the importance of assuming responsibility for cleaning their own teeth and reinforcing their ability to do so

   e. To prevent removal of the fluoride-rich enamel surface, especially in areas of initial demineralization

   f. a.b.d.

   g. b,d,e

   h. a,b,c,d,

   i. b,c,d,e

   j. All of the above

5. What problems were cited as contributing to the denial of using a dental caries vaccine in human populations?

   a. There may be pain upon its injection into the parotid salivary gland.

   b. Injection of live *S mutans* to stimulate antibody formation may result in abscess formation.

   c. A large amount of antigen must be administered because it is diluted in saliva and swallowed.

   d. Ingestion of attenuated *S mutans* cells may contribute to autoimmune cardiac and renal tissue lesions.

   e. a,c

   f. b,d

   g. a,c,d

   h. b,c,d

   i. All of the above

Chapter 7

Fluoride Therapy

Objectives

After studying this chapter, the student should be able to:
1. Discuss the mechanism by which fluoride inhibits dental caries formation.
2. Describe the metabolism of fluoride with reference to absorption, distribution, excretion, and chronic and acute toxicity.
3. Discuss individually the vehicles used in systemic and topical fluoride administration and their relative effectiveness in terms of caries reduction.
4. Explain current recommendation regarding prenatal fluoride supplementation.
5. Cite protocol for prescribing postnatal fluoride supplements.
6. Describe the management of acute fluoride toxicity.
7. Demonstrate several modes of in-office topical fluoride application.
8. Outline appropriate agent, concentration, dosage, and interval of use for various vehicles of at-home topical fluoride application.

When systematically ingested, topically applied, or both, fluoride will confer on the tooth a greater resistance to carious destruction. The degree to which this is accomplished will depend on the child's dental age at administration, the concentration, duration, and frequency of application, and the type of vehicle used for administration.

Metabolism and mechanism of action

When ingested, fluoride is absorbed into the plasma from the gastrointestinal tract. Peak plasma fluoride occurs within 1 hour of ingestion. Salivary and gingival crevicular fluoride levels reflect elevations in plasma concentration and provide additional topical effects on the teeth. Plasma fluoride is deposited in bone where a steady state of equilibrium of eventually achieved. Bone is the body's major reservoir for fluoride deposition and reflects the net balance between uptake and withdrawal. Developing teeth are likewise recipients of fluoride uptake. The remaining plasma fluoride is excreted in urine and to a lesser degree in sweat. The fluoride that remains unabsorbed is lost in feces.

The mechanism by which fluoride inhibits cariogenesis have not been completely identified or understood. Although some are only speculative, there appear to be several interrelated modes of action (Brown and Konig, 1977). First, fluoride ions act on the hydroxyapatite crystal in enamel, substituting themselves for the hydroxyl ions, forming fluorapatite. This chemical substitution

$$Ca_{10}(PO_4)_6(OH)_2 + 2F \rightarrow Ca_{10}(PO_4)_6F_2 + 20H$$

Hydroxyapatite   Fluorapatite

forms a more resistant surface layer to acid dissolution by promoting remineralization, improving crystallinity, and decreasing solubility of the enamel. Second, fluoride ions act on cariogenic bacteria by inhibiting glycolysis (fermentation of sugars into acid) and plaque colonization through suppression of salivary protein adsorption onto the enamel and by a direct antibacterial effect (Moss and Wei, 1976).

Further studies have shown that there is a direct relationship between the fluoride concentration of the enamel surface and the caries protection afforded by it (Mellberg, 1977). There are two critical periods for fluoride incorporation into the enamel surface. These periods are during the terminal stages of crown formation and when the crown undergoes preeruptive maturation in the dental sac while being bathed in tissue fluids. The longer the enamel surface is in contact with the tissue fluids, the greater the concentration of fluoride incorporated into it.

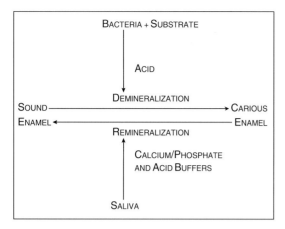

Fig 7-1 The dynamic equilibrium of the carious process in enamel.

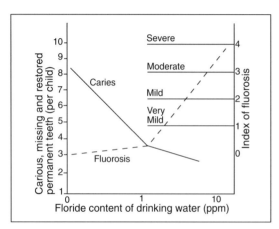

Fig 7-2 With increasing levels of fluoride concentration in the drinking water (more than 1 ppm of fluoride), the occurrence of fluorosis greatly increases without a proportional decrease in caries prevalence (Hodge and Smith, 1954). Therefore, the optimal fluoride concentration in the drinking water to produce the maximal level of caries prevention without the risk of fluorosis is 1 ppm of fluoride.

In regard to topical effects, the presence of fluoride in the saliva interacts at several stages of the carious process to inhibit progression or enhance reversal through three important mechanisms. First, fluoride has antibacterial properties at low plaque pH through the formation of hydrofluoric acid, which interferes with enzymes involved with glycolysis. Second, fluoride inhibits dissolution of calcium and phosphate in the enamel subsurface of an incipient carious lesion during an acid challenge (demineralization). Third, fluoride enhances remineralization by helping calcium-phosphate precipitates at the enamel surface to recrystallize into a more acid-resistant surface. Remineralization occurring after demineralization makes the enamel surface increasingly more resistant to caries progression over time. The inhibition of demineralization and enhancement of remineralization are now

considered the primary factors in fluoride's role as a cariostatic agent. The dynamic equilibrium occurring at the enamel surface of an incipient carious process (Fig 7-1) is therefore modified by the presence of salivary fluoride in plaque at the external enamel surface and by its presence greater than 10 mm beneath the surface.

There are basically two methods used in fluoride therapy: systemic and topical. These methods can be used singularly or in combination and employ several different vehicles for administration: water, tablets, drops, pastes, gels, and solutions.

Systemic fluoride therapy

Water fluoridation

Perhaps dentistry's greatest contribution to the improvement of children's health throughout the world is the discovery and utilization of fluoride as a caries-preventive measure. The development and testing of this agent are of historic and scientific merit. Excellent reviews of this topic are available (Backer-Dirks, 1974; Backer-Dirks et al, 1978) and are summarized here.

In 1931, the discolored and pitted "mottled enamel" observed in certain regions of the world was found to be the result of defective enamel calcification caused by excessive amounts of fluoride in the drinking water. Concentration in excess of 2 ppm of fluoride were considered sufficient to cause defective enamel. Although this condition, termed *dental fluorosis*, was unacceptable cosmetically, it did provide apparent beneficial effects in terms of a lower caries prevalence. When the US Public Health Service conducted epidemiologic surveys of this phenomenon, it concluded that teeth formed in the presence of approximately 1 ppm of fluoride in the drinking water exhibited fewer caries but no clinical signs of dental fluorosis. With increasing levels of fluoride concentration in the drinking water, fluorosis dramatically increased in prevalence without a proportional decrease in caries prevalence (Hodge and Smith, 1954) (Fig 7-2). Therefore, the 1-ppm fluoride concentration was considered optimal in the benefits it provided.

These observations became the basis for several community experiments in which fluoride was added to the deficient water supplies of Grand Rapids, Michigan; Evanston, Illinois; and Newburgh, New York. The results of these and other such experiments over a 15-year period confirmed that the benefit derived from continuous exposure to optimally fluoridated water since birth in terms of percent caries reduction ranged between 50% and 70%. Fluoride therapy instituted at 6 years of age produced a caries reduction of between 20% and 45%. Therefore, the benefits derived from fluoridated water are proportional to the duration of exposure. These benefits are cumulative and extend into adult life if continued. Discontinuation of fluoridated water programs has resulted in a return to previous levels of carious activity and is therefore not recommended.

Epidemiologic studies also have revealed that the potential for the formation of dental fluorosis is influenced not only by the concentration of fluoride in the drinking water but also by the amount of water consumed daily. Because water consumption is proportional to the temperature level of the area (resident of warmer climates consume more water), adjustments in the water fluoride level according to climate were deemed necessary. Optimal levels of fluoridation are therefore determined by the mean annual maximum daily air temperature of the community. Accordingly, a community located in a cold climate would receive higher levels of fluoride (up to 1.2 ppm), whereas those in warmer climates would receive less (adjusted down to 0.7 ppm) (Moss and Wei, 1976) (Table 7-1).

Commonly used compounds for communal water fluoridation are sodium fluoride, hydrofluosilic acid, and sodium silicofluoride.

Although the protective effect of fluoridation is great, it is not uniform for each tooth type. Anterior teeth receive far greater protection than the posterior teeth. This discrimination is best explained by the selective ability of fluoride to resist caries formation on smooth enamel surfaces far greater than it can on pit and fissure surfaces of the posterior teeth.

Not only has water fluoridation been proved effective, but it has also been demonstrated to be safe and economical. Extensive comparisons of morbidity and mortality statistics between fluoridated and nonfluoridated communities have failed to detect any differences in health that could be attributed to fluoride. Furthermore, there is little debate over the benefit of reduced dental costs derived from less frequent dental treatment needs when the estimated cost of fluoridation for 1 year is 15 cents per person. From the standpoint of dental health benefits, safety, and economics, water fluoridation has been shown to be the single most effective method of preventing dental caries. In addition, its use requires no cooperative efforts from the beneficiaries.

Supplemental fluoride therapy

Although water fluoridation is extremely effective and economical, only about 49% of the US population receives its benefits (DHEW, 1977). Those individuals who do not receive optimally fluoridated water, either because they reside in an area without communal water supplies or there is public opposition to fluoridation, may receive its benefits through supplemental therapy, provided that they live in a fluoride-deficient area. If fluoride supplements are conscientiously given in the recommended manner, dental caries protection will approach that derived from consuming optimally

Table 7-1 Recommended adjustment in optimal fluoride level according to air temperature of the community

Average annual maximum daily air temperature		Recommended optimal fluoride level (ppm)
°C	°F	
10.0–12.1	50.0–53.7	1.2
12.2–14.6	53.8–58.3	1.1
14.7–17.7	58.4–63.8	1.0
17.8–21.4	63.9–70.6	0.9
21.5–26.2	70.7–79.2	0.8
26.3–32.5	79.3–90.5	0.7

Table 7-2 Cost-benefit ratios for various fluoride treatments in nonfluoridated communities*

Method	Ratio
Water fluoridation	1:65
Weekly mouth rinse (school)	1:25
Daily mouth rinse (home)	1:8
Daily tablet (school)	1:5
Daily tablet (home)	1:3.5
Semiannual topical gel (office)	1:0.5

*Adapted from Moss and Wei (1976).

fluoridated water (Driscoll and Horowitz, 1978). However, the cost and inconvenience will be considerably more. For a comparison of the cost effectiveness of various fluoride treatments in nonfluoridated communities, consult Table 7-2.

Additional drawbacks in supplemental fluoride therapy are patient compliance and reliance. A recent survey of reasons given by parents for discontinuing supplemental therapy to their children indicated that inconvenience, not expense, was the source of their dissatisfaction (Newbrun, 1978). Although this problem is discouraging, it is felt that improvement in compliance might occur through proper patient selection according to their expressed interest and motivation. Periodic recall (every 6 months) to refill the prescription would help to encourage and reinforce its usage.

Prenatal fluoride therapy

It is apparent that fluoride will cross the placental barrier, but whether it reaches the fetus with sufficient concentration to provide anticaries protection is the subject of much debate. The placenta does act as a regulator, and the fluoride concentration that reaches the fetus is considerably lower than that found in the maternal circulation (Hennon, 1977). It is uncertain whether prenatal fluoride supplementation in addition to postnatal fluoride gives any additional benefits. As stated previously, the critical period for fluoride ingestion is between the final stages of crown formation and the beginning of gingival emergence (eruption) when the greatest concentration of surface fluoride is incorporated into the enamel. This period, with respect to primary teeth, occurs during the first 2 years of life. A number of studies have reported caries reduction in primary teeth of approximately 50% to 80% when fluoride supplementation was begun before 2 years of age and continued for a minimum of 3 to 4 years (Binder et al, 1978). Other studies have indicated that the effect of fluoride ion on primary teeth is mostly, if not entirely, postnatal (Katz and Muhler, 1968; Pritchard, 1969).

The use of prenatal fluoride therapy continues to be a controversial topic. Although recent reports have claimed beneficial results (Glenn, 1981), others have raised significant questions regarding their design and interpretation (Driscoll, 1981). Therefore, it is not currently recommended that pregnant women ingest supplemental fluoride for the benefit of their unborn children. In light of the questioned effectiveness, not safety, the FDA removed prenatal fluoride supplements from the market in 1966.

Postnatal fluoride therapy

There are several alternatives to community fluoridation during the postnatal period for individuals living in fluoride-deficient areas. A fluoridator may be installed at home. It gives excellent caries protection but is expensive to install and maintain. Fluoridators can be installed in schools at considerably less cost per person while delivering the same level of caries protection. Because children attend school only 180 days per year, it is recommended that the fluoride level of the drinking water be adjusted up to 4.5 times the normal optimal concentration to receive the same benefit.

Fluoride tablets, rinses, and drops are alternative methods of delivering supplemental fluoride therapy. One tablet of 2.2 mg of sodium fluoride yields 1 mg of fluoride ion, which, when dissolved in 1 L of distilled water, produces a 1-ppm concentration. When chewed and swished, the tablets provide excellent topical effects, and, when swallowed, they deliver the desired systemic effect. Although bone acts as a reservoir to maintain a somewhat constant fluoride serum level, the single daily dose probably does not confer on the developing teeth the same level of caries resistance as would be provided by multiple daily dosages of fluoridated water.

In evaluating the dietary sources of fluoride for children, Singer and Ophaug (1981) concluded that many infants receive less than an optimum daily intake of fluoride. Because human breast milk and cow's milk products are lacking in fluoride, fluoride supplementation is recommended under those dietary restrictions.

On the other hand, some commercially prepared infant formulas contain greater-than-optimum fluoride concentrations (Adair and Wei, 1978; Singer and Ophaug, 1981; van Wyk et al, 1985). There is evidence that bottle-fed infants on formula diluted with optimally fluoridated water receive approximately 150 times more fluoride than breast-fed infants (Ekstrand et al, 1984). In fact, breast-fed infants have a negative fluoride balance. The variation in fluoride concentration among various infant diets may have contributed to the finding that fluorosis is more prevalent in bottle-fed than breast-fed children (Walton and Messer, 1981). Clearly the differences in dietary fluoride intake in infants has made prescribing fluoride supplements confusing and risky.

However, the decision to supplement an infant's diet has been simplified because, as of January 1979, all infant formulas produced in the United States had to be standardized to contain less than 0.1 ppm of fluoride. Therefore, infants residing in fluoridated communities where nutrient intake is primarily breast milk, cow's milk, or formula should be supplemented with fluoride until the child begins drinking the communal fluoridated water or unless formula used is diluted from this source (Kula and Tinanoff, 1982).

Before any prescription for supplemental fluoride therapy, the dentist must ascertain the natural fluoride content of the individual's drinking water. This determination is best accomplished through submission of a water sample to the state department of health or local agency providing such services.

An alternative to agency testing of the water sample is an in-office analysis with a miniature colorimeter (DR-100 Colorimeter, Hach Co). It is a simple and accurate method of comparing a standard fluoride solution to the sample using a colored reagent and light meter.

Water analysis for fluoride is especially important where well water is the source of drinking water. Groundwater lies in water-yielding geologic formations called *aquifers* beneath the earth's surface. The closer the aquifer is to bedrock, the higher the fluoride concentration of the water. Since both bedrock and aquifers vary in depth, it is impossible to predict fluoride concentration based on well depth alone. A well may tap into any aquifer depending on its depth, and thus water samples taken from surrounding wells may differ in fluoride concentration (Davis, 1985). Therefore, a sample must be analyzed from the individual source and periodically reevaluated.

After analysis is completed, the Council on Dental Therapeutics of the American Dental Association (ADA) recommends that supplements be prescribed only if less than 60% of the recommended optimal fluoride concentration for that climatic area is found (Driscoll and Horowitz, 1978). For example, a prescription should be written only if the fluoride analysis reveals less than 0.6 ppm for a 1-ppm area or less than 0.4 ppm for a 0.7-ppm area.

Table 7-3 Current[†] and proposed[‡] daily fluoride supplement dosage (mg F/d*) recommendations

Current Age (y)	Proposed Age (y)	Fluoride content of drinking water (ppm)		
		<0.3	0.3–0.6	>.06
Birth to 2	0.5 to 3	0.25	0.00	0
2 to 3	3 to 6	0.50	0.25	0
3 to 14	6 to 16	1.00	0.50	0

*2.2 mg of sodium fluoride contains 1 mg of fluoride.
†American Dental Association, 1977.
‡American Academy of Pediatric Dentistry, 1994.

Table 7-4 Sample prescriptions for daily supplemental fluoride therapy.

Note: Since few pharmacies carry more than one or two brands, it is best to write prescriptions in generic form to ensure obtainability (Kula and Tinanoff, 1982).

Example 1: Tablets

For a child age 7 years in a fluoride-deficient area (<0.3 ppm of F)
Ŗ: Sodium fluoride tablets 2.2 mg NaF (1 mg of F)
Disp.:   120 chewable tablets
Sig.:   Chew one tablet daily after brushing and flossing at bedtime. Swish between teeth and swallow. Refill three times (1-year supply).

Example 2: Rinse

For a child age 7 years in a fluoride-deficient area (<0.3 ppm of F)
Ŗ: Acidulated phosphate fluoride liquid (1 mg of F/5 mL)
Disp.:   250 mL
Sig.:   After thorough brushing and flossing at bedtime, rinse 1 teaspoonful (5 mL) around and between teeth for 1 minute, and then swallow, daily.

Example 3: Drops

For an infant age 2 years in a fluoride-deficient area (<0.3 ppm of F)
Ŗ: Sodium fluoride drops (0.125 mg of F/drop)
Disp.:   30 mL
Sig.:   Place two drops daily on tongue or inside cheek at bedtime.

Example 4: Vitamin-fluoride drops

For an infant age 2 years in a fluoride-deficient area (<0.3 ppm of F) and requiring multivitamin supplements
Ŗ: Multivitamin–sodium fluoride drops (0.25 mg of F/mL)
Disp.:   50 mL
Sig.:   Dispense 1 mL daily into mouth.

Calculated dosage for fluoride supplementation not only must be adjusted according to existing natural fluoride levels in the drinking water but must also be adjusted according to chronologic age (Table 7-3). Chronologic age roughly reflects the child's body mass. Young children obviously intake and use less fluoride than older children. Generally speaking, children between the ages of 6 and 15 years get the maximum dosage adjusted to the water fluoride level (Table 7-4). Children between the ages of 3 and 6 years receive one half this dose. However, there is controversy about when therapy should begin in the birth-to-3-years age group. It should be understood that recommended dosages are somewhat arbitrarily determined because they are based on estimates of total fluoride intake for children at various ages. The supplemental dosage must be adjusted to ensure maximum caries protection without the risk of producing subsequent fluorosis and should begin at birth (Driscoll and Horowitz, 1978).

In 1977, the dosage schedule for supplemental fluoride for infants was revised. In the pioneer research responsible for its revision, children were given 0.5-mg fluoride tablets daily from birth to 3 years of age, then 1.0 mg of fluoride daily between 3 and 10 years of age in a nonfluoridated community (Aasenden and Peebles, 1974). The results indicated that test subjects had a 80% caries reduction over control subjects not receiving supplemental fluoride. But a 14% incidence of moderate fluorosis (twice as high as found in optimally fluoridated communities) was also reported. Because the fluorosis occurred on teeth calcified during the first year of life, the 0.5-mg fluoride tablet daily was considered excessive for infants. To reduce the potential for fluorosis, a lower dosage of 0.25 mg of fluoride has been recommended for infants between birth and 3 years of age.

Because differences of opinion do exist on the matter, additional research is needed to establish the optimal dosage regimen for infant fluoride supplementation. In the meantime, the following recommendation is made for infants living in a fluoride-deficient area: Dissolve 1 mg of fluoride into 1 L (approximately 1 qt) of water used as a source for all drinking and food preparation, or use 0.25-mg fluoride drops daily (Table 7-4). Table 7-3 provides the regimen recommended by both the ADA (1977) and the American Academy of Pediatrics (1979). These recommendations represent improvements in our understanding of fluoride's metabolism and mechanism of action sustained by continued research efforts and responsible reevaluation of therapeutics.

Clear evidence now exists that the prevalence of dental fluorosis has increased in the United States in both fluoridated and nonfluoridated communities (Pendrys, 1991). Many additional sources of fluoride are now available in the diet of children during the first 7 years of life and are likely contributing to this trend. Potential fluoride risk factors appear to impact most at the early maturational phase of enamel formation beginning at 2 to 3 years of age. Scientific evidence is accumulating to support a reduction and simplification in the fluoride supplement dosage schedule. These modifications might include dosage by weight rather than age or by delaying the chronologic age threshold by which an increasing dose is recommended (Table 7-3). Likely in the near future, consensus will be achieved on a modified fluoride dose schedule. In 1992, the American Academy of Pediatric Dentistry agreed that any practitioner who wished to minimize the risk for fluorosis could consider halving the fluoride dosage for low-caries-risk children less than 6 years of age.

Because of problems with patient compliance whenever supplements are prescribed, it has been suggested that the addition of multiple vitamins to the fluoride supplement would enhance usage and interest in the regimen (Hennon et al, 1972)., However, this combination should be discouraged unless the child's physician feels the patient would benefit from a multiple-vitamin diet supplementation. Only if both fluoride and vitamins are needed should this method be used. Another problem with vitamin-fluoride supplementation is that the fluoride administration usually needs to be continued beyond the period required for vitamin supplementation. The multivitamin-fluoride supplement is manufactured in different concentrations of fluoride (0.25, 0.50, and 1.0 mg) so as not to adversely affect the vitamin dosage required (Table 7-4).

Acute toxicity

Concern over potential toxicity warrants the need for careful professional judgment in prescribing fluoride modalities (Feigal, 1983). An acute lethal dose of fluoride has been estimated to be 36 mg/kg of body weight. To ensure minimum toxicologic risk, the recommended maximum one-time dosage of fluoride to be prescribed is 264 mg of sodium fluoride (120 mg of fluoride ion). A 4-month supply of 120 1-mg tablets is considered safe if accidental poisoning might occur.

Common symptoms of acute toxicity are nausea, vomiting, hypersalivation, and abdominal pain due to irritation of the gastrointestinal tract through formation of hydrofluoric acid (Heifetz and Horowitz, 1984). Fluoride is itself, therefore, an effective emetic if ingested in excess. A method to calculate the amount of fluoride swallowed from the different vehicles used and a summary of the emergency protocol for overdose has been developed (Bayless and Tinanoff, 1985). If accidental overdose does occur, it is recommended to induce vomiting and administer syrup of ipecac or milk as an antidote to help bind the fluoride ion. A recent review of records at two Australian hospitals during a 6-year period revealed 20 cases of acute fluoride toxicity (Monsour et al., 1984). A contribution to the prevalence of toxicity is that fluoride tablets are multicolored and flavored, therefore having great appeal to the child.

Topical fluoride therapy

Many vehicles are used to deliver topical fluorides. These include gels, mouthrinses, prophylaxis pastes, and dentifrices. Whether self-applied or applied in an office procedure, these methods exhibit varying abilities to inhibit caries formation in children (Brudevold and Naujoks, 1978). Because of the differences found between the methods of application and the agents used, the vehicles are discussed separately. Since topical fluorides are manufactured in many flavors, it is good practice to taste the agent you intend to use before applying it to your patient's teeth. Through this practice, you will avoid imposing a bad-tasting experience on your patients if the agent fails to have an agreeable flavor.

Topical fluoride therapy is best used as a supplement to systemic fluoride therapy and not as a substitute. Optimal benefits will be provided if topical fluoride is used in a multiple-regimen approach of frequent applications over a prolonged period because of the additive or cumulative action of fluoride on the enamel. Topical fluoride application for low-risk patients (negligible caries rate) residing in optimally fluoridated areas may not be considered useful when analyzed from a cost-benefit viewpoint (Heifetz, 1978). Generally speaking, topical fluorides are given in high con-

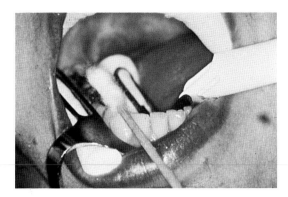

Fig 7-3 Topical fluoride application using cotton tip applicator and cotton roll holder for isolation.

centration with low frequency of application (semiannual office use) or in low concentration with high frequency of application (daily home use). Discussion here is based on office procedures; home fluoride therapy is discussed later.

Office therapy

Gels

Fluoride gels have the advantage of being easier to apply, especially if used with trays, than the solution form. The consistency of the gel allows better adherence to the teeth but may not penetrate interproximal areas as well as solutions. Because there is no difference between the clinical effectiveness of a solution versus a gel, the gel form is more extensively used because of its ease of application.

Several agents are available in gel form for topical application. However, the two agents most studied and recommended for treatment are stannous fluoride (8% to 10% fluoride ion) and acidulated phosphate fluoride (APF, 1.23% fluoride ion in 0.1% orthophosphoric acid). The recommended application frequency is semiannually for either agent. The effectiveness of each agent in terms of percent caries reduction is similar, and caries-reduction values vary according to the fluoride level of the drinking water: 30% to 50% (suboptimally fluoridated area) to 20% to 25% (optimally fluoridated area).

Stannous fluoride can be astringent and disagreeable to taste. Pigmented staining of teeth has also been reported in areas of demineralized enamel and margins of restorations. On the other hand, APF is better tasting and more stable. Storage must be in a plastic container, and the recent manufacturing change in pH from 3.5 to 5.0 has enhanced its shelf life. The low pH enhances enamel fluoride uptake, and the presence of the phosphate ions helps to suppress enamel dissolu-

tion. Acidulated phosphate fluoride has been shown to produce longer-lasting benefits in terms of caries reduction following termination of treatment than any other agent. Therefore, APF is the preferred agent when one is selecting a topical fluoride gel.

A new thixotropic gel is unique in that under tray pressure it flows like a liquid into tight areas such as interproximal contacts; then, when pressure is removed on tray removal, the liquid turns into a gel that clings to the enamel surface.

Methods of topical fluoride application using a gel vary from a seemingly simple cotton roll isolation with cotton tip applicators to the more complex air membrane tray with paper inserts (Wei and Wefel, 1977). The cotton roll holder method is bulky and messy, requiring constant monitoring (Fig 7-3). Custom-fitted wax trays or mouth guards consume much time in preparation and retain the gel poorly but adapt well to extreme malocclusion. Disposable polystyrene trays without paper inserts are messy and frequently overflow. However, these trays are well contoured, soft, pliable, and comfortable (Fig 7-4). Another disposable method combines a foam liner directly into the polystyrene tray but is limited in size selection, and the foam liner requires excessive amounts of fluoride to soak it (Figs 7-5 and 7-6). A procedural description of the cotton roll holder method is found in Figs 7-7 to 7-10. A procedural description of the tray method is found in Figs 7-11 to 7-13.

Extensive investigation into the amount of fluoride gel retained and subsequently swallowed from topical applications as performed in the dental office has recently been conducted. These studies indicate that substantial systemic absorption of fluoride may occur with peak plasma levels in excess of that capable to produce fluorosis. There is no existing clinical evidence, however, that fluorosis can be caused by routine semiannual office fluoride therapy (Ripa, 1991). When APF gel was painted on under cotton roll isolation, an average of 17.4 mg of fluoride was retained (47% of applied dose) in the oral cavity (LeCompte and Whitford, 1982). However, tray systems with some form of absorptive liner to hold the fluoride in position resulted in significantly less oral retention than previously demonstrated (LeCompte and Doyle, 1982; LeCompte and Rubenstein, 1984). Furthermore, a thixotropic gel was shown to have less retention than an APF gel (LeCompte and Rubenstein, 1984). As would be expected, expectoration following completion of topical application will significantly reduce the amount of intraoral fluoride retained (LeCompte and Doyle, 1982; LeCompte and Rubenstein, 1984). In fact, expectoration for 30 to 60 seconds after topical fluoride application was even more effective in eliminating excess fluoride than suction devices placed during application, but both methods are highly recommended (LeCompte and Doyle, 1985; Eisen and LeCompte, 1985). The viscosity of the gel selected may also be an important factor in reducing the amount of

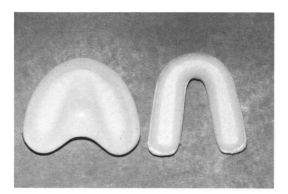

Fig 7-4　Disposable polystyrene trays.

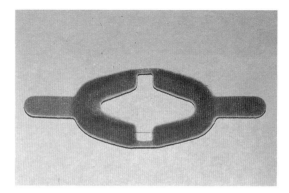

Fig 7-5　Disposable foam-lined trays are comfortable to the patient but may require excessive amounts of fluoride.

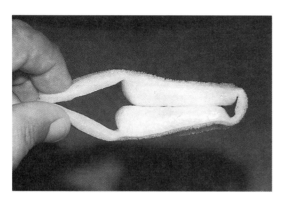

Fig 7-6　The folding over of these trays allows for simultaneous treatment of both arches comfortably.

fluoride retained following topical application because lower-viscosity gels would be expected to flow easier, resulting in stimulation of salivary flow and swallowing. Research has demonstrated that intermediate- and high-viscosity gels are best in reducing retained fluoride—even better than absorptive tray liners (Eisen and LeCompte, 1985). In conclusion, the following recommendations are expended from those cited by Heifetz and Horowitz (1984) as the preferred technique to reduce acute fluoride toxicity from tray applications:

1. Use appropriate-sized, absorptive liner trays.
2. Select an intermediate- or high-viscosity APF gel.
3. Dispense a minimum amount (0.5 to 1.0 tsp) into the tray.
4. Apply a suction device during and after application.
5. Seat the patient upright and warn the patient not to swallow.
6. Never leave the patient unobserved during treatment.
7. Encourage expectoration following treatment.

Prophylaxis paste

Dental prophylaxis is a routine office procedure. When performed, the prophylaxis should be completed with a fluoridated paste. However, the use of a fluoridated paste without subsequent application of topical fluoride gel is likely to produce little effect on caries reduction (Brudevold and Naujoks, 1978). Little caries reduction occurs because the professional prophylaxis, which uses a rubber cup with abrasive pumice cleaners, removes up to 4 μm of surface enamel (Vrbic et al, 1967). Because the surface enamel is the most fluoride-rich area on the tooth, a significant loss of fluoride may occur. The fluoride concentration gradient of enamel dramatically decreases with increasing depth from the outer surface (Mellberg, 1977). High fluoride concentration rarely exists below 30 to 50 μm from the surface. Because fluoride penetration beyond this depth is accomplished only by multiple applications of high-potency preparations (Mellberg, 1977), it is perhaps not coincidental that below this depth initial demineralization and carious formation are first observed.

It was once believed that the acquired pellicle that forms over the enamel surface before plaque colonization was a barrier to enamel fluoride uptake. Because the acquired pellicle often penetrated up to 3 μm into the enamel surface, a pumice prophylaxis was recommended for it removal.

Recent studies have revealed data that suggests a review of this long-accepted procedure (Ripa, 1984). Studies on the diffusion of fluoride solutions through pellicle and plaque have demonstrated that such layers do not prevent the uptake of fluoride into enamel. Several in vivo studies indicated that enamel receiving different topical fluoride treatments with some form of prior prophylaxis retained similar amounts of incorporated fluoride (Tinanoff et al. 1974; Steele, et al, 1982; Houpt et al, 1983). Bruun and Stoltze (1976) reported that teeth cleaned with a rubber cup without paste and teeth with 5-day plaque deposits demonstrated similar fluoride concentrations following topical therapy.

Figs 7-7 to 7-10   Cotton roll isolation method for applying topical fluoride.

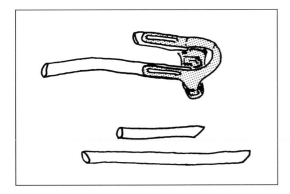

Fig 7-7   Place the appropriate cotton roll holder on the side of the mouth to be isolated (holders are designed for right and left sides).

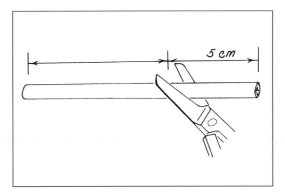

Fig 7-8   Cut a 5-cm (2-in.) segment from a cotton roll at an angle. Insert the segment so that it extends from the midline to the retromolar area on the lingual side of the mandibular teeth. With the remainder of the cotton roll, isolate the buccal aspect from the maxillary midline to the mandibular midline.

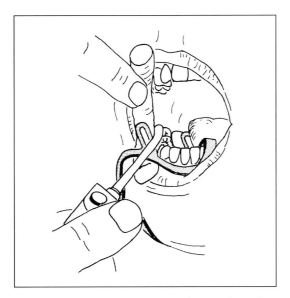

Fig 7-9   Isolate the half of the mouth to be treated. Dry thoroughly; excess saliva inhibits the uptake of fluoride. A dry, isolated field aids in determining whether the gel has been placed properly.

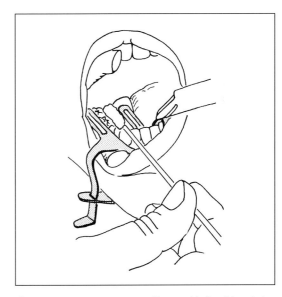

Fig 7-10   Saturate a cotton applicator with fluoride gel. Apply the gel to all exposed tooth surfaces, and use a suction device to remove excess gel and saliva. Apply for 2 to 4 minutes. Wipe off excess, and floss interproximally. Repeat the procedure for the opposite side. Instruct the patient not to rinse or eat for 30 minutes after treatment but encourage expectoration.

These studies present evidence for the elimination of prior rubber cup prophylaxis with pumice as a routine procedure when professional topical fluoride applications are performed (Ripa, 1984).

Therefore, professional prophylaxis is not prerequisite to topical fluoride applications unless extrinsic stain requires removal. Because extrinsic staining is not common in children, supervised toothbrushing with a fluoridated prophylaxis paste is sufficient. Aside

from not removing the fluoride-rich surface layer, a toothbrush prophylaxis is more educational for the patient. The time normally devoted to delivering a pumice prophylaxis can be used for patient instruction and motivation while simultaneous removal of plaque occurs (Primosch, 1980).

Many fluoridated prophylaxis pastes are available, but significant caries reduction by this technique alone should not be anticipated. The expected caries inhibi-

Figs 7-11 to 7-13 Tray method for applying topical fluoride.

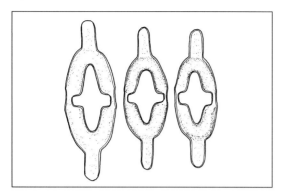

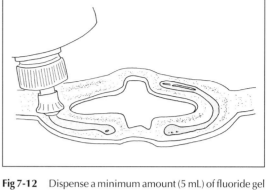

Fig 7-11 Select the proper tray size by trying any of the three sizes in the mouth.

Fig 7-12 Dispense a minimum amount (5 mL) of fluoride gel into the absorptive liner of the tray.

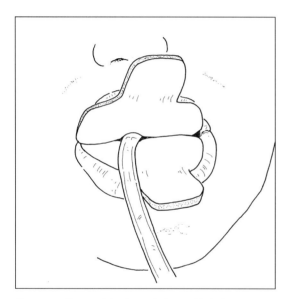

Fig 7-13 Clean and dry the teeth thoroughly before inserting trays. Treat both arches simultaneously and insert the saliva ejector between the trays to remove excess gel and saliva. Patient acceptance of fluoride treatments will be greatly enhanced if some form of diversion is provided. For example, the child may be given a puzzle or coloring book during treatment. Remove trays after 2 to 4 minutes of application. Warn the patient not to swallow or rinse, but encourage expectoration.

tion is generally considered to be in the magnitude of 10% to 20%. A major consideration in selection of a paste should be its flavor.

Home therapy

Three types of fluoride preparations are designed for home use: dentifrice, mouth rinse, and gel. Generally, the use of a fluoridated dentifrice should be routinely recommended. Gels or mouth rinses are usually recommended for those patients with greater susceptibility to rampant caries. Self-application is economical and will probably become the method of choice for the delivery of topical fluorides (Horowitz, 1973). However, unless closely supervised, self-application at home can produce less desirable results. Supervised mouth rinse programs in public schools show a great promise (Horowtiz, 1973).

Dentifrices

Dentifrice application provides the user with a pleasant-tasting means of applying an abrasive to remove plaque and stains. The addition of fluoride provides some, but limited, anticaries benefits in the range of 15% to 20% caries reduction (von der Fehr and Moller, 1978). In spite of the impressive amount of scientific literature, there is insufficient evidence to provide definite statements regarding the relative effectiveness of various formulas.

The incorporation of amine fluoride is strictly a European venture. It is felt that the detergent action of these organic compounds could enhance the fluoride effect and that the long-chain alkyl amines may possess antiplaque activity. On the other hand, the incorporation of stannous fluoride into a dentifrice is mostly an American venture. The first product accepted by the ADA comprised 0.4% stannous fluoride and a calcium pyrophosphate abrasive (Crest, Procter and Gamble). A 0.76% sodium monofluorophosphate dentifrice (0.1% fluoride ion) (Colgate, Colgate-Palmolive Co) appears to be better than stannous fluoride because there is no staining problem, the pH is close to neutral, it is a stable and compatible compound, and in comparative studies it is been proved more effective in reducing caries (von der Fehr and Moller, 1978) All commercial dentifrices currently approved by the ADA are formulated with fluoride.

It may be desirable not to recommend the use of a fluoridated dentifrice for children less than 3 years of age because they are likely to swallow some of the fluoride paste used. In addition, the foam created by the dentifrice will interfere with the parent's field of vision during the cleansing and might make the child more uncomfortable and less cooperative.

The potential for chronic fluoride toxicity in infants ingesting dentifrice has raised concerned that such practices could result in fluorosis of the permanent dentition. The exact amount of fluoride ingested is dependent on the amount of dentifrice used and the age of the child. A recent survey of parents revealed that dentifrice use began in 75% of the infants before 18 months of age but that the quantity dispensed varied greatly (Dowell, 1981). The amount of dentifrice required to cover the bristles of a toothbrush is approximately 2g, which yields 2 mg of fluoride. Barnhart et al (1974) measured mean ingestion of fluoride per toothbrushing at 0.30 mg for 2 to 4 year olds, 0.13 mg for 5 to 7 year olds, and 0.07 mg for 11 to 13 year olds.Recently, Ripa (1991) calculated from the literature that the average fluoride retention per brushing was 0.1 mg F. Although no significant difference was reported in the prevalence of fluorosis between children who brushed with fluoridated dentifrice and a placebo dentifrice during the age of permanent enamel formation (Houwink and Wagg, 1979), it is highly recommended that unsupervised use of dentifrice in preschool children be restricted and that only a pea-sized portion of dentifrice be dispensed (Heifetz and Horowitz, 1984).

Mouth rinses

Indications for the use of mouth rinses include rampant caries, orthodontic therapy, salivary depression caused by pathologic conditions or medications, jaw fixation, and dental hypersensitivity. The effectiveness of mouth rinses is directly related to its frequency of application. Continuous exposure is essential for maintenance of the anticarious benefit. Once mouth rinse therapy is withdrawn, the caries increment returns to normal (Birkleland and Torell, 1978). Sodium fluoride is the agent of choice for mouth rinse therapy. Caries reduction with sodium fluoride rinses has been reported to be 40% Acidulated phosphate fluoride rinses provide only a 20% to 30% caries reduction. Recommended dosage is 0.2% sodium fluoride weekly or 0.05% daily, rinsing for 1 to 2 minutes.

Sodium fluoride (0.05%) mouth rinses are now available over the counter in most supermarkets and drugstores without a prescription. It is recommended that the manufacturer's instructions be followed closely, such as swishing 10 mL at bedtime after thorough tooth cleaning and then expectorating (not swallowing).

Based on a study by Ericsson and Forsman (1969), preschool children ingested on the average 0.4 mg of fluoride per rinse because of inadequate swallowing reflexes. It was later confirmed that children younger than 6 years of age commonly swallow the entire contents of the rinse (Wei and Kanellis, 1983). Therefore, daily usage of fluoride mouth rinses in preschool children should be restricted to limit the risk of fluorosis. In addition, a few rinses contain 6% alcohol, which may be objectionable.

Gels

High-concentration APF gels intended for semiannual office application should never be recommended for daily use at home (Ekstrand et al, 1981). Instead, a 0.5% APF gel or 0.4% stannous fluoride gel applied on a toothbrush should be recommended (Table 7-5). Older children can use the same agents dispensed in custom-made mouth guards or trays. Caution must be exercised if used during odontogenesis of the permanent incisors because significant oral fluoride retention has been demonstrated (McCall et al, 1983). Brush-on gels can result in three times the oral fluoride retention of rinses (Bell et al, 1985). When identical amounts (2 g) of home fluoride gels are used, the 0.5% APF brush-on gel will yield five times the fluoride concentration of that delivered by either the 0.4% stannous fluoride or any commercial dentifrice. Because of concern over potential chronic toxicity of fluoride treatments resulting in fluorosis, Tables 7-6 and 7-7 are provided for a relative comparison between commonly used office and home fluoride treatments.

Multiple fluoride therapy

For patients to receive the maximum degree of dental caries protection (up to 75% caries reduction), multiple fluoride therapy must be instituted. Additional benefits are provided when different fluoride methods are used in combination. These methods include (1) communal water fluoridation or its equivalent through use of supplemental fluoride therapy, (2) semiannual prophylaxis with topical fluoride, and (3) daily use of a fluoridated dentifrice.

A study of the benefits of multiple fluoride therapies was recently reported for a school-based, teacher-supervised program in a fluoride-deficient rural community (Horowtiz et al, 1984). After 8 years of using a 0.2% sodium fluoride weekly rinse, a 1.0-mg fluoride daily tablet, and 0.1% fluoridated dentifrice, test subjects had a 49% caries reduction (86% on proximal surfaces) compared with similar-aged controls.

In summary, several generalizations regarding topical fluoride therapy can be made, regardless of which agent is used (Brudevold and Naujoks, 1978). First, the caries-reducing effect is greater in newly erupted teeth. Newly erupted teeth are less mature structurally (surface fluoride level of 800 ppm) than are teeth with a longer history of exposure to oral fluids (surface levels of 1,500 to 2,000 ppm). Because an enamel surface fluoride level of 1,000 ppm is required for caries resistance, newly erupted teeth are more vulnerable to the carious process and should therefore receive topical fluoride applications shortly after emergence. Second, the effectiveness of topical fluorides in terms of percent caries reduction is of the same order for both primary and permanent teeth. Third, regardless of the fluoride history, topical treatments confer added protection to the caries-susceptible individual.

Table 7-5   Sample prescriptions for home use of topical fluorides

Example 1: Brush-on gel

R: Acidulated phosphate fluoride (0.5%) gel
Disp.:   24-mL drops
Sig.:   Apply with brush at bedtime after thorough tooth cleaning, expectorate, but do not rinse.

Example 2: Brush-on gel

R: Stannous fluoride (0.4%) gel
Disp.:   50-g tube
Sig.:   Same as above

Table 7-6   Chart of fluoride therapy*

Class	Type	Amount	Total mg
Office gel	2% NaF	5 mL/arch	50
	8–10% SnF$_2$	5 mL/arch	100–125
	1.23% APF	5 mL/arch	61.5
Home gel	0.5% APF	6 g/trays	30
		2 g/brush	10
	0.4% SnF$_2$	6 g	6
		2 g	2
Prophylaxis paste	9% SnF2·ZrSiO$_4$	2 g	45
	1.2% APF·SiO$_2$	2 g	24
Dentifrice	0.2% NaF	2 g	2
	0.4% SnF$_2$	2 g	2
	0.76% MFP	2 g	2
Rinse	0.05% NaF	7–10 mL	1.75–2.5
	0.2% NaF	7–10 mL	0.7–1.0
	0.1% SnF$_2$	7–10 mL	1.75–2.5

*Courtesy of Dr James Wefel, University of Iowa, Iowa City, Iowa.

Table 7-7   Relative strengths of fluoride agents

| Concentration and type | Strength | | |
	mg F/mL	%F ion	ppm
1.23 % APF gel	12	1.23	12,000
2.0% NaF gel	9	0.9	9,000
1.1% NaF gel	5	0.5	5,000
0.4% SnF$_2$ gel	1	0.1	1,000
0.24% NaF dentifrice	1	0.1	1,100
0.05% NaF rinse	0.2	0.02	220
Hydrofluosiliac acid in water	0.001	0.0001	1

References

Aasenden, R., and Peebles, T. Effects of fluoride supplementation from birth on human deciduous and permanent teeth. Arch. Oral Biol. 19:321, 1974.

Adair, S., and Wei, S. Supplemental fluoride recommendations for infants based on dietary fluoride intake. Caries Res. 12:76, 1978.

American Academy of Pediatrics. Committee on Nutrition. Fluoride supplementations: Revised dosage schedule. Pediatrics 63:150, 1979.

American Dental Association Council on Dental Therapeutics. Fluoride compounds, accepted dental therapeutics. 37th ed. Chicago: The American Dental Association, 1977.

Backer-Dirks, O. The benefits of water fluoridation. Caries Res. 8 (suppl. 1):2, 1974.

Backer-Dirks, O., Kumzel, W., and Carlos, J. Caries-preventive water fluoridation. Caries Res. 12 (suppl. 1):8, 1978.

Barnhart, W.E., et al. Dentifrice usage and ingestion among four age groups. J. Dent. Res. 53:1317, 1974.

Bayless, J.M., and Tinanoff, N., Diagnosis and treatment of acute fluoride toxicity. J. Am. Dent. Assoc. 110:209, 1985.

Bell, R.A., et al. Fluoride retention in children using self-applied topical fluoride products. Clin. Prev. Dent. 7:22, 1985.

Binder, K., Driscoll, W., and Schutzmannsky, G. Caries-preventive fluoride tablets program. Caries Res. 12 (suppl. 1):22, 1978.

Birkeland, J.M., and Torell, P. Caries-preventive fluoride mouthrinses. Caries Res. 12 (suppl 1):38, 1978.

Brown, W., and Konig, K. Cariostatic mechanisms of fluoride. Caries Res. 11 (suppl. 1):1, 1977.

Brudevold, F., and Naujoks, R. Caries-preventive fluoride treatment of the individual. Caries Res. 12 (suppl. 1):52, 1978.

Bruun, C., and Stoltze, K. In vivo uptake a fluoride by surface enamel of cleaned and plaque-covered teeth. Scand. J. Dent. Res. 84:268, 1976.

Davis, I. Testing well water for prescribing fluoride supplements. J. Mich. Dent. Assoc. 67:77, 1985.

Department of Health, Education, and Welfare (DHEW) Fluoridation Census 1975. Atlanta: Center for Disease Control, April, 1977.

Dowell, T.B. The use of toothpaste in infancy. Br. Dent. J. 150:247, 1981.

Driscoll, W.S. A review of clinical research on the use of prenatal fluoride administration of prevention of dental caries. J. Dent. Child. 48:109, 1981.

Driscoll, W.S., and Horowitz, H.S. A discussion of optimal dosage for dietary fluoride supplementation. J. Am. Dent. Assoc. 96:1050, 1978.

Eisen, J.J., and Le Compte, E.J. A comparison of oral fluoride retention following topical treatments with APF gels or varying viscosities. Pediatr. Dent. 7:175, 1985.

Ekstrand, J., et al. Pharmacokinetics of fluoride gels in children and adults. Caries Res. 15:213, 1981.

Ekstrand, J., et al. Fluoride balance studies on infants in a 1 ppm water fluoride area. Caries Res. 18:87, 1984.

Ericsson, Y., and Forsman, B. Fluoride retained from mouthrinses and dentifrices in preschool children. Caries Res. 3:290, 1969.

Feigal, R.J. Recent modifications in the use of fluoride for children. Northwest Dent. 62:19, 1983.

Glenn, F. The rationale for the administration of a NaF tablet supplement during pregnancy and postnatally in a private practice setting. J. Dent. Child. 48:118, 1981.

Heifetz, S.B. Cost-effectiveness of topically applied fluorides. In The Relative Efficiency of Methods of Caries Prevention in Dental Public Health, Proceeding of a Workshop. Ann Arbor: University of Michigan Press, 1978.

Heifetz, S.B., and Horowitz, H.S. The amounts of fluoride in current fluoride therapies: Safety consideration for children. J. Dent. Child. 51:257, 1984.

Hennon, D.K. Prenatal and post-natal fluoride supplements: Are they effective? In Goldman, H.M. et al. Current Therapy in Dentistry. vol. 6 St. Louis: The C.V. Mosby Co., 1977.

Hennon, D.K., Stookey, G.K., and Muhler, J.C. Prophylaxis of dental caries: Relative effectiveness of chewable fluoride preparations with and without added vitamins. J. Pediatr. 80:1018, 1972.

Hodge, H., and Smith, F. Some public health aspects of water fluoridation. In Shaw, J. Fluoridation as a Public Health Measure. Washington, D.C.: American Association for the Advancement of Science, 1954.

Horowitz, H.S. A review of systemic and topical fluorides for the prevention of dental caries. Community Dent Oral Epidemiol. 1:104, 1973.

Horowitz, H.S., et al. Eight-year evaluation of a combined fluoride program in a nonfluoride area. J. Am. Dent. Assoc. 109:575, 1984.

Houpt, M., et al. The effect of prior toothcleaning on the efficacy of topical fluoride treatment. Clin. Prev. Dent. 5:8, 1983.

Houwink, B., and Wagg, B.J. Effect of fluoride dentifrice usage during infancy upon enamel mottling of the permanent teeth. Caries Res. 13:231, 1979.

Katz, S., and Muhler, J. Prenatal and post-natal fluoride and dental caries experience in primary teeth. J. Am. Dent Assoc. 76:305, 1968.

Kula, K., and Tinanoff, N. Fluoride therapy for the pediatric patient. Pediatr. Clin. 29:669, 1982.

Le Compte, E.J., and Doyle, T.E. Oral fluoride retention following various topical application techniques in children. J. Dent. Res. 61:1397, 1982.

Le Compte, E.J. and Doyle, T.E. Effect of suctioning devices on oral fluoride retention. J. Am. Dent. Assoc. 110:357, 1985.

Le Compte, E.J., and Rubenstein, L.K. Oral fluoride retention with thixotropic and APF gels and foam-lined and unlined trays. J. Dent Res. 63:69, 1984.

Le Compte, E.J., and Whitford, G.M. Pharmacokinetics of fluoride from APF gel and fluoride tablets in children J. Dent Res. 61:469, 1982.

McCall, O.R., et al. Fluoride ingestion following APF gel application. Br. Dent. J. 155:333, 1983.

Mellberg, J.R. Enamel fluoride and its anticaries effects. J. Prev. Dent. 4:8, 1977.

Monsour, P.A. et al. Acute fluoride poisoning after ingestion of sodium fluoride tablets. Med. J. Aust. 141:503, 1984.

Moss, S., and Wei, S. Fluorides: An Update for Dental Practice. New York: Medcom, Inc., 1976.

Newbrun, E. Problems of compliance in fluoride-supplementation therapy. In Moss, S. Pediatric Dental Care. New York: Medcom, Inc., 1978.

Pendrys, D. Dental fluorosis in perspective. J. Am. Dent. Assoc. 122:63, 1991.

Primosch, F.E. The role of rubber cup prophylaxis: A reevaluation of its use in pediatric dental patients. Dent. Hyg. 54:525, 1980.

Pritchard, J.L. The pre-natal and post-natal effects of fluoride supplementation on West Australian school children aged 6-8. Aust. Dent. J. 14:335, 1969.

Ripa, L.W. Need for prior tooth cleaning when performing a professional topical fluoride application: Review and recommendation for change. J. Am. Dent. Assoc. 109:281, 1984.

Ripa, L.W. A critique of topical fluoride methods (dentifrices, mouthrinses, operator- and self-applied gels) in an era of decreased caries and increased fluorosis prevalence. J. Public Health Dent. 51:23, 1991.

Singer, L., and Ophaug, R. Dietary sources of fluoride for infants and children. In Stewart, R., et al. Pediatric Dentistry. St. Louis: The C.V. Mosby Co., 1981.

Steele, R.C., et al. The effect of tooth cleaning procedures on fluoride uptake in enamel. Pediatr. Dent. 4:228, 1982.

Tinanoff, N. Wei, S., and Parkins, F. Effect of a pumice prophylaxis on fluoride uptake in tooth enamel. J. Am. Dent. Assoc. 88:384, 1974.

van Wyk, P.J., et al. Dietary fluoride intake and fluoride supplementation in infants. J. Dent. Assoc. S. Afr. 40:179, 1985.

von der Fehr, F. R., and Moller, I.J. Caries-preventive fluoride dentifrices. Caries Res. 12 (suppl. 1):31, 1978.

Vrbic, V., Brudevold, F., and McCann, H. Acquisition of fluoride by enamel from fluoride pumice pastes. Helv. Odontol. Acta 11:21, 1967.

Walton, J.L., and Messer, L.B. Dental caries and fluorosis in breast-fed and bottle fed children. Caries Res. 15:124, 1981.

Wei, S., and Kanellis, M.J. Fluoride retention after sodium fluoride mouthrinsing by preschool children. J. Am. Dent. Assoc. 106:626, 1983.

Wei, S., and Wefel, J. Topical fluorides in dental practice. J. Prev. Dent. 4:25, 1977.

Questions

1. Topical fluoride applications act to reduce the incidence of dental caries in all of the following ways except by:

   a. Enhancing the coalescence of susceptible enamel pits and fissures
   b. Making the enamel more resistant to acid demineralization through improving crystallinity and decreasing solubility
   c. Promoting remineralization of surface enamel
   d. Having a direct antibacterial effect on plaque
   e. Inhibiting glycolysis in the bacterial plaque

2. What is the recommended range of fluoride concentration in a communal water supply that delivers optimal benefits in caries reduction without producing clinically significant evidence of dental fluorosis?

   a. 0.1 to 0.5 ppm
   b. 0.7 to 1.2 ppm
   c. 0.9 to 1.1 ppm
   d. 1.0 to 1.2 ppm
   e. 1.2 to 2.0 ppm

3. The caries-inhibiting benefit of optimally fluoridated drinking water is proportional to the duration of its exposure. What is the average reduction in dental caries in the permanent dentition produced after 15 years of exposure to optimally fluoridated water since birth?

   a. 10%
   b. 30%
   c. 45%
   d. 60%
   e. 80%

4. What factors must be considered when calculating the dosage for prescribing a fluoride supplement?

   a. The patient's age and previous caries history
   b. The patient's age and oral hygiene status
   c. The patient's age and fluoride concentration of the drinking water
   d. The patient's medical history and willingness to comply
   e. The patient's caries history and fluoride concentration of drinking water

5. What is the recommended daily dose of fluoride for a 3-year-old child whose drinking water contains less than 0.3 ppm of fluoride?

   a. 0.25 mg
   b. 0.5 mg
   c. 1 mg
   d. 2 mg

Chapter 8

Sealants and Preventive Resin Restorations

Objectives

After studying this chapter, the student should be able to:
1. Discuss the epidemiology of occlusal caries in children.
2. Comprehend the anatomic differences between normal and etched enamel surfaces.
3. Appreciate the historic development and current rationale for occlusal sealant use in children.
4. Understand the factors influencing enamel acid etching and mechanical bonding of the sealant.
5. Recite selection, application, and evaluation criteria for sealant materials.
6. Discuss the limitations of sealant usage and inherent problems of the technique.
7. Justify the use of preventive resin restorations.
8. List the types of preventive resin restorations.
9. Outline the steps employed in the placement of preventive resin restorations.

Debate continues regarding the efficiency of the application of pit and fissure sealants as a preventive dental caries measure in children. However, in a multimethod approach to prevention, occlusal sealants are considered an effective caries-reducing agent when proper patient selection and application techniques are followed (Horowitz, 1982; Silverstone, 1982; Ripa, 1973, 1983, 1985; Weintraub, 1989).

Prevalence of occlusal caries in children

The prevalence of occlusal caries in children is a significant dental health problem. Although caries rates in children are declining, there appears to be a disproportionate reduction according to tooth surface, resulting in a relative increase in the percentage of pit and fissure caries (Brunelle and Carlos, 1982). According to the National Dental Caries Survey (1979 to 1980) conducted in the United States, 84% of the caries experience for 5- to 17-year olds involved surfaces with pits and fissures. For permanent first molars, the prevalence of occlusal caries is 20% by age 8 and 70% by age 17 (Swango and Brunelle, 1983).

The high prevalence and rapid onset of occlusal caries in children is most likely related to several factors, including the bacterial and nutrient harboring ca-

pacity of the deep pits and fissures, the close proximity of its base to the dentinoenamel junction, and the total inaccessibility of this area to any mechanical means of debridement (Fig 8-1). Susceptibility of the occlusal surface to caries is related to the steepness of the cuspal inclines or, conversely, the depth of the occlusal fissure. Deeper fissures tend to be more susceptible to caries. As the steepness of the cuspal inclines increases, so does the prevalence of dental caries (Bossert 1937). It has been shown that it takes approximately 3 years for occlusal caries to reach its peak incidence in newly erupted molars (Berman and Slack, 1973).

Historic development of preventive techniques for the occlusal surface

Because of the predominant nature of occlusal caries in children, several methods of prevention have been attempted in the past to reduce its prevalence. As stated previously, mechanical cleaning of occlusal pits and fissures by use of a toothbrush is largely ineffective. In fact, Taylor and Gwinnet (1973) found that debris remained in fissure sites regardless of the means of prophylaxis. In 1923, Hyatt reported a technique termed *prophylactic odontotomy* in which noncarious fissures were prepared and restored with a shallow sil-

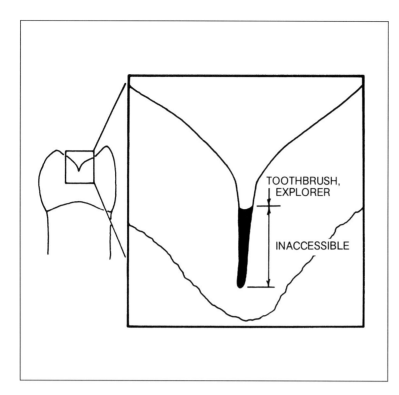

Fig 8-1 The inability of a toothbrush bristle to penetrate the depths of a fissure and the proximity of some deep fissures to the dentinoenamel junction explain a probable mechanism for the accelerated caries progression reported on occlusal surfaces

Table 8-1 Prevalence of caries in the nonfluoridated community of Culemborg, Holland, compared with 15 years of optimal fluoride exposure in Tiel, Holland*

	Mean No. of Carious Surfaces per Child			Reduction %
Type of caries	Culemborg†	Tiel‡	Difference	
Pit and fissure caries	12.9	8.2	4.7	36
Smooth proximal caries	10.1	2.5	7.6	75
Smooth gingival caries	3.6	0.5	3.1	86
Total caries	26.6	11.2	15.4	58

*Adapted from Becker-Dirks (1974).
†Water fluoride level of 0.1 ppm.
‡Water fluoride level of 1.0 ppm.

ver alloy as a prophylactic measure. However, this technique along with the technique of fissure eradication (Bodecker, 1929), where the fissures were removed and smoothed but not restored, was not widely practiced and soon was abandoned. In the 1950s, the development of topical and systemic fluorides greatly affected the prevalence of dental caries in children, but they were found to be least effective on the occlusal surface. Not until 1955, when Buonocore introduced a method of adhering resin to an acid-etched enamel surface, was there potential for a truly effective preventive measure that could be applied directly to the occlusal surface. In 1967, the first clinical trail was reported by Cueto and Buonocore, who used cyanoacrylate as the sealant material placed over an etched occlusal surface. Later, a bisphenol A-glycidyl methacrylate (bis-GMA) ultraviolet light-activated resin was substituted (Buonocore, 1971) and investigated for approximately 10 years. The recent development of new systems employing either autopolymerization or visible light polymerization have evolved the technique to its current status.

Ineffectiveness of fluoride

Systemic fluoride ingestion has been found to be more selective in its caries-reducing benefits on the smooth surfaces than on the pit and fissure surfaces. For example, after 15 years of systemic fluoride ingestion in Tiel, Holland, caries reduction for pit and fissure lesions was only 36% compared with smooth-surface caries reduction of approximately 80% (Backer-Dirks, 1974) (Table 8-1).

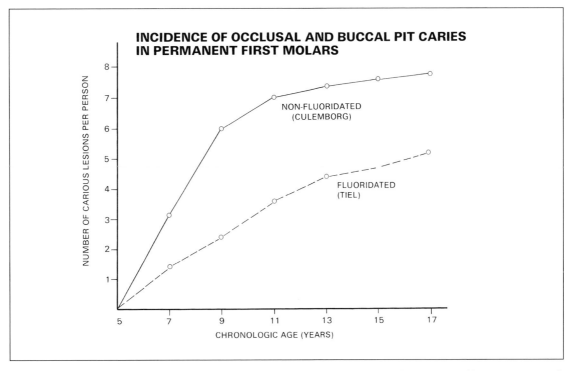

Fig 8-2 When permanent first molars were analyzed 3 years after eruption, the caries prevalence for pit and fissure sites was much greater for the nonfluoridated community of Culemborg (70%) than for the fluoridated community of Tiel (30%).

The rapid nature of occlusal caries is supported by its high prevalence in a nonfluoridated community only 3 years after eruption. Although the prevalence is much less for those molars from a fluoridated community, the difference between the two curves declines after 3 years as the prevalence of caries in Tiel approaches that of Culemborg, Holland (Fig 8-2). In a recent survey conducted by the National Preventive Dentistry Demonstration Program, there was no difference found in the occlusal caries experience of children (Bohannan, 1983) from fluoridated and nonfluoridated communities.

Therefore, in a fluoridated community, because of the selective protection afforded the smooth enamel surface, the relative incidence of occlusal caries will actually rise. The ingestion of systemic fluoride during the preeruptive development of a tooth contributes to the reduced caries susceptibility of its occlusal surface, most probably by enhancing the coalescence of occlusal pits and fissures. The enhanced coalescence of occlusal pits and fissures reduces the steepness of the cuspal inclines, thereby reducing the susceptibility to caries.

In conclusion, even with optional fluoride therapy, pit and fissure caries may be delayed, but not prevented, on the same scale as smooth-surface lesions. Therefore, it is felt that the use of occlusal sealants could be an important adjunct in any caries control program because it is intended for those caries-susceptible areas least benefited by fluoride.

Effectiveness of sealants

Occlusal sealants are defined as the application and mechanical bonding of a resin material to an acid-etched enamel surface, thereby sealing existing pits and fissures from the oral environment. This mechanism prevents bacteria from colonizing in the pits and fissures and nutrients from reaching the bacteria already present.

Several long-term studies evaluating the effectiveness of a single application of sealant are available. These studies evaluated either an ultraviolet light–polymerized agent, such as Nuva-Seal (L.D. Caulk Co.) (Leake and Martinello, 1976: Going et al, 1977; Horowitz et al, 1977; Meurman et al, 1978; Richardson et al, 1981) or autopolymerized agents, such as Kerr Pit and Fissure Sealant (Kerr Manufacturing Co) (Charbeneau and Dennison, 1979), Concise White Sealant (3M Co) (Simonsen, 1981), and Delton (Johnson and Johnson) (Houpt and Shey, 1983a, 1983b; Mertz-Fairhurst et al, 1984). Many of these studies were designed to use a half-mouth technique where eligible pairs of contralateral caries-free teeth are randomly selected (one to receive sealant, the other to remain as an untreated control). The studies evaluated the percentage of surfaces retaining the singularly applied sealant and the percentage of caries reduction afforded by it when compared with the controls. In a recent review, Ripa (1985) calculated the mean percent retention and caries reduction of singularly applied

Table 8-2 Mean retention and caries reduction from a single application of sealant on permanent teeth*†

Duration (y)	Sealant retention (%)	Caries reduction (%)
1	80	82
2	71	68
3	58	65
4	51	43
5	43	36
6	54	40
7	49	34

*Adapted from Ripa (1985).
†Calculated from 70 reports of 48 clinical trials using different means of sealant polymerization.

sealants to permanent teeth from 70 reports of 48 clinical trials (Table 8-2).

Therefore, it can be shown that a single application of occlusal sealant is an effective caries-reducing agent provided that it is meticulously applied. Single application is not, however, the recommended regimen for placement. On the contrary, reapplication every 6 months, if needed, is recommended (ADA, 1987). The recommended sequence of treatment is prophylaxis first, followed by sealant placement, and then topical fluoride application, repeated every 6 months if needed. One study has demonstrated the effectiveness of sealants when the recommended regimen is used (Bagramian et al, 1979). They found that when sealants were used in a fluoridated community as part of a comprehensive preventive program that included semiannual dental health education, prophylaxis, and topical fluoride applications, caries reduction was 87.5% over a 3-year period. These encouraging results were obtained even in the absence of rubber dam use for isolation. Sealants were replaced on suspicion of loss, which resulted in 47% to 81% of teeth requiring reapplication over the 3-year period, depending on tooth type and age of the patient. The mean number of reapplications per tooth was 1.8 times. Other investigators have been more successful in reducing the incidence of retreatment or reapplication of lost sealant over a 3- to 5-year period—15% (Doyle and Brose, 1978) and 31% (Straffon et al, 1985). A large percentage of the failures recorded were due to the placement of occlusoproximal restorations because of the development of proximal, not occlusal, caries. In nonfluoridated areas, loss of a single application of sealant over a 5-year period due to proximal restoration placement was calculated to be 19% (Horowitz et al, 1977) and 32% (Meurman et al, 1978). Therefore, there is little doubt that occlusal sealant placement is effective as a caries-reducing agent. As stated by the Council on Dental Materials and Devices (ADA, 1987): "The Council recognizes that pit and fissure sealants, properly applied, form an acceptable part of proven effective preventive measures."

Although sealants have been shown conclusively to be an effective preventive measure, they have been challenged about their time and cost effectiveness. This challenge is the most severe test currently applied to sealant use. Despite the proved safety and effectiveness of sealants, acceptance and use are low among general practitioners because of its perceived cost ineffectiveness (Hunt et al, 1984). However, the adoption rate is improving, especially among pediatric dentists (Hunt et al, 1984; Jerrell and Bennett, 1984).

Calculation of cost effectiveness in terms of cost benefit ratios are conflicting, and not yet conclusive. Initial placement of sealant to prevent occlusal caries is reported to cost more than conventional restoration with amalgam after a lesion develops (Leake and Martinello, 1976; Messer and Nustad, 1979). These findings were the result of a single application over a 4-year period by inexperienced operators whose percentage of caries reduction of 22% to 24% is considerably less than the 41% to 43% obtained by other investigators (Going et al, 1977; Horowitz et al, 1977). Nevertheless, initial placement of a sealant and possible replacement on a noncarious tooth appear more costly than amalgam placement when indicated. In a 3-year study, Leske et al (1977) reported that nine sites must be sealed to prevent one site from developing caries. However, better results were obtained by Leverett et al (1983) in a fluoridated community over a 4-year period. They demonstrated that five sealants would have to placed and maintained to prevent one carious lesion from developing in a sound tooth. They suggested that delaying placement of a sealant until an incipient lesion is evident would greatly improve its cost-benefit ratio. In another fluoridated community, Simonsen (1989) was able to demonstrate even better cost effectiveness over a 10-year period. He reported that a single application of sealant, and one reapplication if necessary, was approximately two thrids the cost of treating the caries that developed in an unsealed control group.

It is generally inappropriate to compare sealant placement and amalgam restoration as alternative treatments (Smith, 1984). However, Dennison et al (1980a) compared these alternatives in the occlusal surface of newly erupted molars in terms of cost effectiveness. Contralateral pairs of permanent first and second molars were selected so that one surface was sealed while the paired surface was restored with amalgam. Both treatments were evaluated independently by two examiners at baseline and 6, 12, and 18 months after placement. The re-treatment rate for sealants was highest (17.3%) after 6 months and declined to 7.8% after 18 months. There was evidence of a generalized marginal deterioration in more than 50% of the amalgam restorations, whereas 55% of the sealant margins remained undetectable clinically. After 7 years, 50% of the sealed surfaces were maintained without reapplication, 30% received one reapplication, 10% received two reapplications, and 10% received three applications (Straffon and Dennison, 1988). Likewise, time effectiveness appeared not to be a major concern (Dennison et al, 1980b). They showed that the cumulative mean time required to place and maintain the amalgam restorations was 13 minutes, 58 seconds, whereas the cumulative times invested in the sealant treatment was 8 minutes, 45 seconds.

Although several studies have addressed cost effectiveness, it should not be the sole factor to determine whether or not sealants are used for a particular patient (Houpt and Shey, 1983b). The use of sealants must be related more to preventive philosophy and conservation of tooth structure than to absolute cost-benefit ratios (Ripa, 1985). Cost of placement can be minimized by (1) delegating treatment to auxiliary personnel where legally permitted, (2) selecting commercial products that have the highest proved success rates and are approved by the American Dental Association (ADA), (3) following meticulous application protocol, and (4) applying sealants in conjunction with optimal fluoride therapy. Thus, improvements on the cost effectiveness of sealant placement can be obtained by use of stricter guidelines in patient selection and development of more retentive sealants in the future. Because the future status and ultimate acceptance of occlusal sealant usage lie in future improvements of its retentive abilities, the morphologic characteristics of the etched enamel to which it adheres will be examined next.

Retentive characteristics of etched enamel: The bonding phenomenon

It is essential to understand basic concepts of enamel morphology to comprehend the bonding mechanism of sealants. Normal enamel is composed of hydroxyapatite crystals arranged in hexagonal prisms forming rods oriented at right angles to the surface (Fig 8-3). The

enamel surface is usually in a low-energy weakly reactive, hydrophobic state. However, when exposed to acid, it becomes a high-energy, strongly reactive, hydrophilic surface. This high-energy state provides for the rapid attraction of the sealant to the enamel surface.

The acid also etches the enamel surface, producing increased surface area and porosity (Fig 8-4). The increased surface area and porosity are the result of selective demineralization of the hexagonal prisms. Three different surface patterns are possible (Silverstone, 1975): (1) preferential removal of the prism core (type 1), (2) preferential removal of the prism periphery (type II), and (3) random pattern of both types (type III).

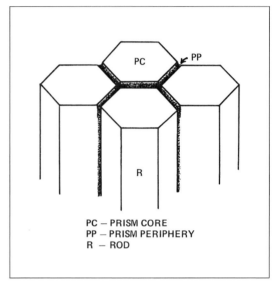

Fig 8-3 A transverse section of enamel showing the characteristic honeycomb appearance (normal density equals 30,000 to 40,000 prisms/mm²).

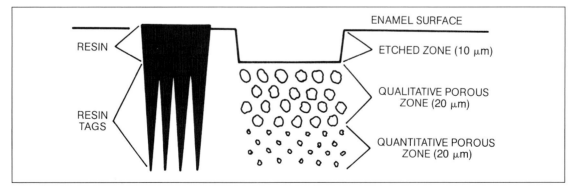

Fig 8-4 The amount of enamel surface lost to acid etching is approximately 8 to 10 μm. This loss is minimal because normal enamel depth averages about 1,500 μm. Beyond the zone of surface enamel loss, the demineralization of the rods penetrates 40 um. Mechanical retention of sealants is the direct result of resin penetration into this porous etched enamel, forming tags 40 um deep (Silverstone, 1975).

Clinically, acid-etched enamel has a chalky, dull, opaque appearance.

Research has investigated the effect of various acid concentrations on enamel etching (Silverstone, 1974). The results indicate that there exists an inverse relationship between acid concentration and changes in surface topography. Furthermore, ideal acid concentration combines the least loss in surface contour with the greatest depth of histologic change. Therefore, the most effective acid concentration appears to be between 30% and 40%

Silverstone (1975) found that phosphoric acid solutions in concentrations between 20% and 50%, when applied to enamel for 60 seconds, create the most retentive conditions and that a 30% unbuffered solution produces the most consistent and evenly distributed etch pattern. However, he did not study shorter etching periods. Laboratory testing suggested that a shorter etching time (10 to 15 seconds) may be as acceptable (Nordenvall et al, 1980; Brännström et al, 1982; Main et al, 1983). Fuks at al (1984) demonstrated that reducing etching time to 20 seconds does not increase marginal leakage as determined by dye penetration. Clinical studies have verified that a 20-second etching time produces retention rates comparably with the conventional 60-second etching time (Stephen et al, 1982; Eidelman et al, 1984; Tandon et al, 1989). Although further clinical study is required to determine optimal etching time, reduced etching time is likely to improve success rates by reducing time required to maintain a dry field. A reduction in moisture contamination would lead to fewer sealant failures and improved cost effectiveness.

Retention rates for sealants placed on permanent teeth were initially reported to be higher than those for primary teeth (Buonocore, 1971; Doyle and Brose, 1978; Richardson et al, 1981). Many theories have been proposed to explain these differences in retention rates (Silverstone, 1976). Much attention has been given to the occurrence of prismless enamel in primary teeth to account for the lower retention rates (Ripa et al, 1966). Prismless enamel is the product of reduced functional activity during the terminal stages of amelogenesis, which results in the lack of enamel rod formation during the last 25 μm of enamel formation. Therefore, no prisms (essential for sealant retention) are formed. Acid etching of this homogenous layer of enamel results in microporosities rather than the surface patterns previously described. However, on closer evaluation it was found that only 17% of primary molars studied showed areas of prismless enamel and that these areas occurred most frequently on the cervical surfaces (surfaces that are not usually sealed) (Silverstone, 1970). Thus, the occurrence of prismless enamel is not the sole factor responsible for lower sealant retention rates in primary teeth. Although the crystallite orientation within the rods is similar to that of permanent enamel (Horsted et al, 1976), the presence of more exogenous organic material within the rods of primary enamel, due to the lower mineral content and higher internal prism volume, may contribute to the poorer sealant retention rates (Silverstone, 1976).

To improve the retention rates of sealants on primary teeth, it has been shown that increasing the acid-etching exposure time on the enamel from 60 to 120 seconds produces etching patterns similar to those found with permanent teeth (Silverstone and Dogon, 1976). However, Simonsen (1978a) found no difference in retention rates for primary teeth when comparing 60- to 120-second etching times. After reviewing the literature, Ripa (1979) agreed that there was little justification for increasing the etching time for primary teeth. He concluded that more recent studies on primary teeth have demonstrated retention rates more comparable with those in permanent teeth and that it is likely that the incidence of prismless enamel on the occlusal surface of primary molars is not as high as originally assumed because of natural attrition. Recently, retention rates for sealants on primary molars were shown to be comparable to those found for permanent molars (Hardison, 1987).

Clinical problems associated with sealant use

Lack of universal usage

Not every patient should receive sealant therapy. The American Academy of Pedodontics (1983) and the National Institute of Health (1984) have developed guidelines for use by the practitioner. All guidelines agree that to achieve the greatest possible caries reduction, a comprehensive caries-preventive program must use sealants in conjunction with other caries-preventive methods, such as systemic and topical fluorides, sound dietary habits, and proper oral hygiene (ADA, 1987). Thus, patients selected for sealant placement must *(1)* be dependable on recall appointments, *(2)* be motivated and proficient in caries control, *(3)* have a low caries activity, and *(4)* receive systemic and topical fluorides.

A patient-oriented selection system relies on exercising prudent clinical judgment. Simonsen (1984) believes that both caries-free and caries-rampant patients should be left unsealed. This philosophy can be supported by research that indicated that patients with both low and high caries prevalence demonstrated the poorest sealant effectiveness (Raadal et al, 1984). But since the purpose of the sealant placement is to prevent caries formation, the risk of carious development on a particular surface should be the most important factor in determining selection factors. An extreme but highly cost-effective method would be to delay sealant placement until the first evidence of caries and then seal all susceptible surfaces (Leverett et al, 1983). This selection criterion, however, results in sealant place-

Table 8-3   Tooth-oriented indications and contraindications for the use of pit and fissure sealants*

Surface diagnosis	Clinical considerations	Do seal	Do not seal
Carious	Occlusal anatomy	If pits or fissures are separated by transverse ridge, a sound pit or fissure may be sealed	Carious pits or fissures
Questionable	Status of proximal surface(s)	Sound	Carious
	General caries activity	Many occlusal lesions; few proximal lesions	Many proximal lesions
Sound	Occlusal morphology	Deep, narrow pits and fissures	Broad, well-coalesced pits and fissures
	Tooth age	Recently erupted teeth	Teeth caries free for 4 years or longer
	Status of proximal surface(s)	Sound	Carious
	General caries activity	Many occlusal lesions; few proximal lesions	Many proximal lesions

*Adapted from Ripa (1985).

ment over incipient or early carious lesions and is, therefore, not a true preventive measure.

Another alternative would be that all children should be considered potential candidates for sealants (Ripa, 1985). This philosophy of treatment removes the decision-making process away from patient selection to the level of appropriate tooth selection. A tooth-oriented criteria system allows for the use of a clinicians's diagnostic skills. Under this system, a questionable tooth surface would be an ideal candidate for sealants. Although the decision to seal a known carious surface should be the responsibility of the practitioner to exercise prudent judgment, surfaces clearly diagnosed as carious would not be sealed under this criterion system. Table 8-3 summarized the tooth-oriented system as outlined by Ripa (1985).

In addition, the clinician must be aware that effectiveness is greatly affected by the tooth type selected (Table 8-4). For example, examination of caries prevalence by tooth type indicates that occlusal caries on permanent molars occurs at a rate four times that of premolars (Swango and Brunelle, 1983); therefore, sealant placement on premolars may not be as cost effective even though they are more retentive. Differences in caries distribution pattern has dictated that newly erupted permanent first and second molars should receive priority over premolars and primary molars even in high-risk groups (NIH, 1984).

Technique sensitivity

Strict and meticulous adherence to the manufacturer's recommendation for placement is critical. The quality

Table 8-4   Success of sealant retention based on tooth selection*†

Factor	Counterpart
Older (10–14 years)	>Younger (5–8 years)
Permanent	>Primary
Mandibular	>Maxillary
Premolars	>Molars
Occlusal	>Buccal or lingual

*Adapted from Going et al (1973) and Meurman et al (1978).
†Factors on the left have shown better retentive qualities than their counterparts on the right.

of the etch and sealant coverage and polymerization are greatly influenced by the quality of the isolation. Difficulty in maintaining a dry field during placement is compounded by the fact that teeth to be sealed are recently and often not completely erupted. In fact, teeth that were in an early stage of eruption and had a tissue operculum over the distal marginal ridge had twice the sealant loss of completely erupted molars (Dennison et al, 1990).

Caries susceptibility of etched enamel

Nonsealed, etched enamel is not more susceptible to caries formation. The carious process on the occlusal surface is initiated within the fissure and not on the cuspal inclines. Since it has been shown that only the cuspal inclines are etched and not the fissures (Taylor and Gwinnett, 1973), it seems unlikely that a carious lesion would develop in a nonsealed, etched site. In addition, it has been shown that etched enamel remineralizes completely within 48 hours because of the deposition of salivary calcium and phosphate salts (Albert and Grenoble, 1971; Arana, 1974; Kastendieck and Silverstone, 1979).

Furthermore, those occlusal sites that have lost sealant coverage are not more susceptible to future caries development because of the etching (Charbeneau and Dennison, 1979). In fact, the converse may be true. There appear to be initial cariostatic benefits to the occlusal surface following sealant loss (Hinding, 1974), but these effects do not last beyond 3 years (Cline and Messer, 1978). These initial cariostatic benefits have been related to the presence of resin tags remaining in the enamel surface following sealant loss. Other long-term studies confirm the lack of prolonged, enhanced cariostasis to the occlusal surface following sealant loss (Horowitz et al, 1977; Going et al, 1977).

Detection of lost sealant

Several commercial products are available whose opaque color is more visually detectable. The clinical effectiveness of one such sealant has been shown to be comparable to other products in its retentive abilities (Simonsen, 1979).

The chief criticism of opaque sealants in the inability to visually detect progression of caries underneath. Partial loss of sealant to occlusal wear could potentially expose the terminal ends of fissures, thereby inducing microleakage and enhancing cariogenesis (Charbeneau and Dennison, 1979). Therefore, the early detection of stain penetration underneath sealants would indicate marginal failure and need for replacement. It has been demonstrated that 26% of the sealants placed after 4 years illustrated marginal discoloration and stain penetration (Charbeneau and Dennison, 1979).

Inadvertent placement over active carious sites

Although it is not recommended to place sealant over a detectable carious lesion, recent research has indicated that if the sealant's marginal integrity is maintained, the carious site may become inactive. In a 5-year study, Going et al (1978) reported that 89% of the active carious test sites that were sealed became sterile. Other investigations have reported marked reductions in viable organisms cultured from sealed fissures (Handelman et al, 1973; Mertz-Fairhurst et al, 1979a; Jensen and Handelman, 1980). The reduction in cultivable bacteria appears to be progressive over time (Handelman et al, 1976; Jensen and Handelman, 1980). The inactivity of sealed carious lesions was confirmed by lack of radiographic progression observed over time (Handelman et al, 1976; Mertz-Fairhurst et al, 1979b; Handelman et al, 1981).

Thus, the previous concern over inadvertent sealing of undetected carious lesions does not appear to be warranted based on current findings. The sealing of active caries can be supported because the widely accepted practice of indirect pulp treatment sets the precedent (Fairbourn et al, 1980). The progressive reduction in viable bacterial counts recorded from sealed carious fissures results from the initial acid pretreatment and the effective elimination of the nutritional source by the impenetrable marginal seal (Jensen and Handelman, 1980; Handelman, 1982). Although bacteria sealed in fissures are greatly reduced with time, some bacteria undoubtedly remain viable and presumably retain their potential for pathogenicity. Nevertheless, improvements in sealant retention and the decreased viability of bacteria under it may actually provide therapeutic as well as prophylactic value to the inhibition of occlusal caries in the future (Going et al, 1978).

Occlusal sealant technique

Recommendation for use

It is apparent that occlusal sealants are a clinically proved caries-inhibiting agent when properly applied. Placement of sealants is a noninvasive technique that maintains tooth integrity while it provides an acceptable resolution of the carious process. Because sealants may be inadvertently used to reverse the progression of questionably carious fissures, Meiers and Jensen (1984) have described sealant therapy as interceptive rather than preventive. The term interceptive may be a more accurate description when questionable fissure lesions are sealed, as supported by the finding that 71% of 380 teeth with questionable fissures progressed to clinically evident carious lesions over a 41-month period (Miller and Hobson, 1956).

Occlusal sealants are useful in the maintenance of selected patients through the caries-active period (ages 6 to 15 years) and will at least delay the need for an occlusal restoration until a proximal lesion develops. This factor is an important consideration, since 82% of the occlusoproximal restorations in 12-year-old children from a nonfluoridated community had previously placed occlusal restorations (Roder, 1975). It is recommended that those patients selected to receive sealants meet the following requirements:

1. Be dependable on recall appointments
2. Be aged 6 to 15 years
3. Be motivated and effective in caries control
4. Have low caries activity
5. Have eligible teeth, namely, recently erupted (within 3 years), caries-free permanent teeth with steep cuspal inclines

Material selection

Several commercially available sealants are currently approved by the ADA (ADA, 1987). These products vary as to their acid concentration, means of polymerization, composition, and setting times. Acid concentration of the tooth conditioner varies between 35% and 50% depending on the manufacturer. Although it has been demonstrated that varying the acid concentration influences the quality of the etched pattern (Silverstone, 1975), there is no indication that varying the acid concentration within the 35% to 50% range has any affect on the clinical performance of the sealant (Hardison, 1983; Ripa, 1985). Likewise, the composition (unfilled or filled resin) and the color (clear, tinted, or opaque) of the different manufactured sealants vary considerably. It is not known, however, if these variables affect clinical effectiveness (Ripa, 1985). Measuring volumetric loss between unfilled and filled sealants, Jensen et al (1985) reported no significant difference between the two; 50% of the applied sealant volume was lost within the first month, and 75% was lost after 2 years.

On the other hand, the method of polymerization does have an effect on the clinical performance of the sealant. In general, autopolymerizaton is better than ultraviolet light polymerization. In a 7-year study, Mertz-Fairhurst et al (1984) reported that an autopolymerized sealant was superior to an ultraviolet light–activated sealant in sealant retention and caries protection. These results have been supported by other investigators (Ferguson and Ripa, 1980; Li et al, 1981). No difference in retention between an autopolymerized sealant and a visible light–activated sealant was shown after 5 years of evaluation (Shapira et al, 1990).

Any difference between autopolymerized and light-polymerized sealants can be accounted for by marginal microleakage at the enamel-sealant interface. The slower speed of polymerization and reduced viscosity during setting of the autopolymerization method do not allow the depth of penetration into the etched surface (Hicks and Silverstone, 1982). Polymerization by light allows time for flow under normal viscosity, thereby increasing the number and length of tags and decreasing the risk of microleakage. However, the tag length is not that important in regard to tensile strength (Retief and Mallory, 1981). It appears that resin penetration is dependent more on the etch pattern than the sealant's penetration coefficient.

Placement Technique

1. *Isolation (Fig 8-5)*. A dry surface is paramount to the successful retention of occlusal sealants. Saliva contamination must be avoided to prevent remineralization of the etched enamel surface; moisture contamination during sealant placement and polymerization must likewise be avoided. Ferguson and Ripa (1980) indicated that rubber dam isolation provides better retention rates for an ultraviolet light–activated sealant, but not for an autopolymerized sealant, placed without the aid of an assistant. This finding would support the use of autopolymerized sealants when using cotton roll isolation and operating unassisted.

In addition, other reports confirm that the retention rates of autopolymerized sealants were not significantly affected by the method of isolation (Eidelman et al, 1983; Straffon et al, 1985). Since rubber dam isolation does not significantly improve the retention of autopolymerized sealants, routine use of rubber dam during application of sealants is not indicated (Ripa, 1985). Rubber dam placement, however, is required when sealant placement is part of a quadrant approach to operative dentistry (Ferguson and Ripa, 1980: Eidelman et al, 1983). Otherwise, cotton roll isolation is adequate, but in a young child, under certain conditions, may be less comfortable to the patient and require more effort by the operator to maintain.

2. *Cleaning (Fig 8-6)*. The manufacturer recommends the use of a rubber cup prophylaxis with a slurry of pumice to thoroughly clean the enamel surface before etching. The primary objective should be to remove plaque and debris from the surface. As an alternative means to achieve the same purpose, Houpt and Shey (1983a) used a toothbrush with dentifrice. Using this method, they achieved sealant retention rates comparable to those in other reports where a pumice prophylaxis was used.

It has even been suggested that a preliminary prophylaxis (by any means) need not be performed. Previous investigation has demonstrated that the phosphoric acid etch removes surface plaque, acquired pellicle, and up to 10 μm of the enamel surface (Silverstone, 1983). Main et al (1983) reported that elimination of the prophylaxis step produced surface etch patterns and tensile bond strengths of the applied sealant comparable to those demonstrated when a pumice prophylaxis was completed. Although these results are provocative, suggesting that the clinician be concerned only with the removal of gross debris, there is still insufficient evidence to recommend a change from the manufacturer's instructions. Air polishing the surface with pumice, however, has been shown to produce similar sealant retention rates as found with traditional pumice prophylaxis (Scott, et al, 1988). In addition, sealant retention can be improved if the occlusal fissures are widened with a small round bur to increase the bonding surface area (Shapira et al, 1986).

3. *Etching (Fig 8-7)*. Investigation into the appropriate technique for applying the etching solution to the enamel surface has recently been reported. A continuous but gentle dabbing or agitation of the solution on the enamel surface, in contrast to rubbing, had been recommended because it preserves the maximal length of the delicate enamel prism sheaths (Speiser

and Segat, 1980; Silverstone, 1983). Although dabbing the etching solution has been shown to improve the microscopic quality of the fragile surface topography, further investigation has failed to demonstrate a difference in either tensile (Bates et al, 1982) or shear (Hormati et al, 1980) bond strengths for the applied sealants, regardless of the application method tested. It is doubtful, therefore, that the specific technique employed to apply the etching solution will have any impact on the clinical effectiveness of the sealant.

4. Washing and drying (Fig 8-8). The enamel surface should be rinsed with water for 10 to 20 seconds and dried for an additional 10 seconds, with care being taken not to use an oil-contaminated air syringe. If the surface is not dull, frosty, and opaque, the surface must be re-etched using the same procedure described previously.

The bond between the etched enamel surface and the applied sealant is sensitive to prior surface contamination. Recent investigations of etched enamel exposed to saliva for periods of 1 to 60 seconds showed sufficient contamination of the surface to warrant re-etching (Evans and Silverstone, 1981; Silverstone et al, 1985). However, minimal salivary exposure for less than 10 seconds after acid etching may not be adverse provided that immediate washing is performed. A 5- to 10-second wash is sufficient to maintain tensile bond strength after a short period of salivary surface contamination (Bates et al, 1982). The critical period for preventing saliva contamination is immediately before sealant placement and during its polymerization.

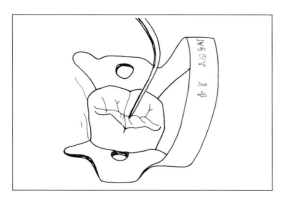

Fig 8-5 The maintenance of a dry field is critical to sealant retention. Cotton rolls may be used for isolation, but a rubber dam is preferred. After adequate isolation is obtained, the surface is dried and reexamined for the presence of any carious lesions. If caries is suspected, placement of a preventive resin restoration would be the treatment option of choice.

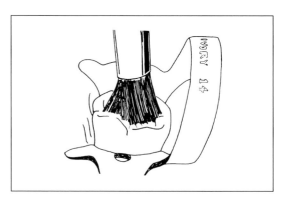

Fig 8-6 A prophylaxis is performed with a nonfluoride oil-free paste, and the tooth is rinsed with water very thoroughly. Regardless of the means of prophylaxis, only the inclined cuspal planes are cleaned. Little, if any debris is removed from the fissure sites (Taylor and Gwinnett, 1973). An effective alternative would be to eradicate the pits and fissures with a dental bur (Shapira et al, 1986).

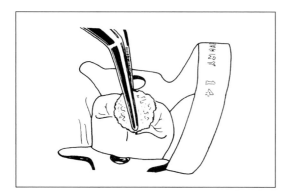

Fig 8-7 The pellet is applied to the enamel surface for 20 to 60 seconds using a continuous application of fresh acid. It is essential that a wet surface be maintained by applying additional conditioner, not allowing the solution to dry on the surface. (Caution: Etching liquid contains 35% phosphoric acid. Avoid contact with soft tissue.) A safe and effective alternative would be to use a gel instead of a solution.

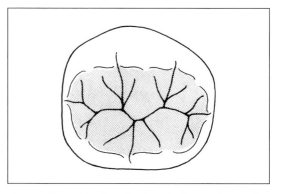

Fig 8-8 The etching liquid is placed only over the area that is to receive the sealant, generally the entire occlusal surface up to the cusp tips. The surface is rinsed with water for 10 seconds and then dried for an additional 10 seconds, being careful not to use an oil-contaminated air syringe. If the surface is not dull, frosty, and opaque, it is re-etched using the same procedure.

Moisture contamination is the most common reason for bond failure (NIH, 1984). Recently, Feigal et al (1993) reported that a dentin bonding agent placed as an intervening layer and air thinned before sealant application allowed successful sealant retention on enamel wet with saliva. This finding may result in the recommendation that a dentin bonding agent be used in difficult-to-isolate surfaces, such as those found on newly erupted teeth. Other, less significant, causes of sealant bond failure include occlusal trauma and dimensional change caused by differences in the coefficient of thermal expansion between the tooth and sealant or from polymer shrinkage during polymerization.

5. Application (Fig 8-9). A disposable tube is inserted in the applicator provided. This applicator is a unique improvement over the brush-on technique in the delivery of the sealant to the surface. The desired physical properties of a good sealant are its low viscosity and high wetting ability. The operator can quickly disperse the sealant up the grooves of the tooth with an explor-

er, and excessive sealant may be removed with a cotton tip applicator prior to polymerization.

6. Evaluation (Fig 8-10). The surface is wiped off with a wet cotton roll or pellet to remove the surface film (unpolymerized resin) that accumulates after setting. Removal of the surface film results in a more pleasant aftertaste and will also provide for a clearer inspection of the surface. The surface is checked with an explorer for any voids or incomplete coverage. Extra sealant is reapplied if required (Figs 8-11a and b).

7. Adjustment. Slight occlusal interference should be of no concern with unfilled sealants, because any interference will be quickly worn away. However, filled sealants should be adjusted with a green stone. Fluoride treatment should follow, not precede, sealant application (NIH, 1984).

8. Reevaluation (recall). Sealants should be examined for loss every 6 months. Bitewing radiographs are important in the diagnosis of caries progression under the

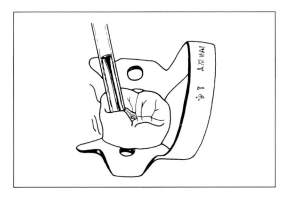

Fig 8-9 The sealant is carried to the surface and applied smoothly by slowly depressing the lever. The sealant is allowed to flow ahead into the crevices as the tip is advanced from one end of the tooth to the other. This method minimized entrapment of air bubbles better than a brush-on technique.

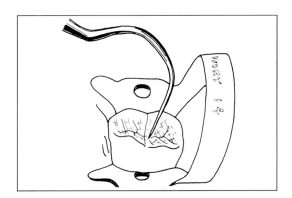

Fig 8-10 Evaluation of the sealant should include an attempt to remove the sealant with an explorer to determine if adequate bond strength is established. The use of this immediate test of retention has resulted in excellent future retention rates because potential failures are identified and rectified early (Houpt and Shey, 1983a).

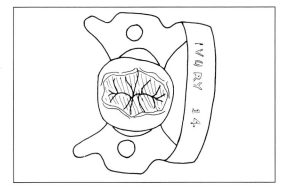

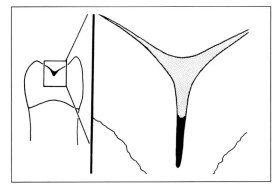

Figs 8-11a and b The sealant should completely cover the occlusal surface.

sealant if microleakage has occurred since placement. If sealant is completely lost, the entire procedure is repeated. If it is partially lost, the attachment is tested with a sharp instrument. If it is firm, the sealant surface is freshened with a fine stone or medium pumice, the exposed area is reetched, and the procedure repeated as previously described.

Preventive resin restorations

The preventive resin restoration is a natural extension of the use of occlusal sealants. It integrates the preventive approach of the sealant therapy for caries-susceptible pits and fissures with the therapeutic restoration of incipient caries with composite resin that occur on the same occlusal surface. The development of the preventive resin technique provides the most conservative approach toward confined, incipient occlusal caries in young permanent teeth whereby restoration occurs with a minimum of tooth preparation while ensuring the prevention of future caries formation through sealant placement (Meiers and Jensen, 1984).

The preventive resin restoration is the conservative answer to the conventional "extension for prevention" philosophy of Class I amalgam cavity preparation. Extension for prevention dictates that the outline form of the cavity preparation be extended beyond the margins of the carious lesion to incorporate all susceptible pits and fissures. This extension prevents future caries formation but does so at the expense of losing substantial healthy tooth structure. Even a conservative amalgam preparation significantly weakens the tooth (Larson et al, 1981). The preventive resin restoration preserves sound tooth structure by incorporating a conservative composite resin restoration with sealant application.

There are three types of preventive resin restorations based on the extent and depth of the carious lesion as determined by exploratory preparation. These types have been classified as types A, B, and C (Simonsen, 1978b, 1978c). Type A comprises suspicious pits and fissures where caries removal is limited to enamel. A slow-speed round bur is used to remove any decalcified enamel, and local anesthesia is not required. Type B is defined as the incipient lesion in dentin that is small and confined. Type C is characterized by the need for greater exploratory preparation in dentin. The Type C restoration would require the administration of local anesthesia and liner placement over the exposed dentin. Most clinical situations cannot be classified according to type until the operator has completed the required exploratory preparation to determine the extent of the carious lesion. Classification according to type is necessary only as a basis to determine the restorative material that is to be selected for placement.

Initially Simonsen (1978b, 1978c) advocated an unfilled sealant for type A, a diluted composite resin for type B, and a filled composite resin for type C. The concept of a diluted composite resin was adopted from Ul-

vestad (1976), who demonstrated superior retention for a mixture of filled composite resin and an unfilled bonding agent over an unfilled sealant after a 3-year period. The superior retention was attributed to the greater wear resistance of the filled resin particles, whereas the dilution with the unfilled resin provided the necessary viscosity for flow.

This pioneer investigation did not use the mechanical preparation of the pits and fissures, nor did it attempt placement of an intermediate layer of an unfilled resin bonding agent before the diluted composite application. Simonsen (1978b) defended the use of an intermediate unfilled resin layer because it would provide enhanced retentive tag formation in the etched enamel surface, thereby reducing microleakage around the margins of the restoration. However, in vitro investigation failed to demonstrate marginal microleakage around preventive resin restorations when such a layer was absent (Raadal, 1978a; Hicks, 1984).

As with the placement of an intermediate resin layer, the beneficial influence of fissure enlargement on the retentiveness of the composite resin is also uncertain. When an unfilled sealant was applied to mechanically enlarged fissures, no improvement in retention was found (LeBell and Forsten, 1980). On the other hand, Shapira and Eidelman (1984), using the same procedure, reported higher retention rates and attributed their finding to the fact that fissure enlargement resulted in increased surface layer for etching, elimination of the organic material surface layer, and a thicker sealant. In addition, they were able to demonstrate that a 20-second etching time provided a better retentive surface than a 60-second etching time following the mechanical preparation advocated for type A preventive resin restorations (Shapira and Eidelman, 1985).

The use of diluted composite resin in preventive resin restorations has provided comparable retention rates with unfilled sealants (Raadal, 1978b; Simonsen, 1980). The early clinical success of these restorations and the development of improved composite resin systems have encouraged recent investigators to use new materials and techniques. For example, Houpt et al (1984) reported the results of 273 type B restorations evaluated after 3 years. They demonstrated that an autopolymerized filled resin inserted into the preparation with a syringe and followed by complete coverage of all pits and fissures on the surface with an unfilled sealant is as successful in retention and caries reduction as previously reported techniques. After 4 years, the study reported that 76% of the placed restorations were completely retained and only 6% demonstrated recurrent carious lesions (Houpt et al, 1985).

With the development of wear-resistant (filled), light-activated, radiopaque composite resin systems for posterior teeth, a new generation of materials will enhance the success of preventive resin restorations (Simonsen, 1985). The following technique uses the advantages of these materials.

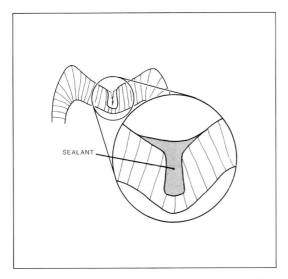

Fig 8-12 Type A preventive resin restoration. Enamel fissure caries are removed with slow-speed round bur. Enamel surface is etched and covered completely with sealant.

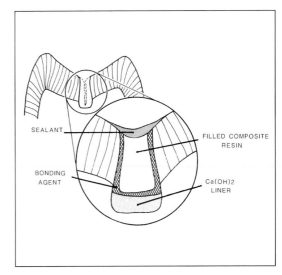

Fig 8-13 Type B preventive resin restoration. Following preparation, the material layers are placed in order: liner, bonding agent, filled composite resin, and sealant. All resin layers are polymerized simultaneously by a visible light source. An alternative would be to use a glass-ionomer cement liner instead of a bonding agent (Ripa and Wolff, 1992).

Placement technique

Armamentarium

Local anesthesia (optional)
Rubber dam or cotton rolls
Cotton pellets
Burs: slow-speed No. $\frac{1}{4}$, $\frac{1}{2}$ round, white finishing stone; high-speed No. 330, carbide fluted finishing
Etching gel (tooth conditioner)
Sealant
Applicator
Bonding agent
Calcium hydroxide liner
Polymerization unit (visible light)
Composite resin (filled)
Plastic (Teflon) instrument or condensor
Marking paper

Type A restoration (Fig 8-12)

1. Clean the surface.
2. Isolate with cotton rolls or, preferably, a rubber dam.
3. Remove decalcified pits and fissures with a slow-speed No. $\frac{1}{4}$ or $\frac{1}{2}$ round bur. (The caries must be limited to the enamel to be classified type A; do not attempt to place retentive area in the preparation.)

4. Place acid-etching gel over the entire occlusal surface for 20 to 60 seconds.
5. Wash (20 seconds) and dry (10 seconds) the surface.
6. Apply the sealant carefully, avoiding air entrapment (voids) in the preparation site.
7. Polymerize with the visible light for 20 seconds.
8. Adjust the occlusion, if needed, with finishing burs.

Type B restoration (Fig 8-13)

Type B preventive resin restorations are indicated where exploratory removal of caries has included dentin to a slight extent. After prophylaxis of the surface and placement of a rubber dam (local anesthesia is optional), follow the procedural steps illustrated in Figs 8-14 to 8-21 for completion of the restoration.

Type C restoration

Repeat all steps listed for the type B restoration. Since the type C restoration is, by definition, larger and deeper, add additional polymerization time (30 seconds). In most cases, local anesthesia will also be required.

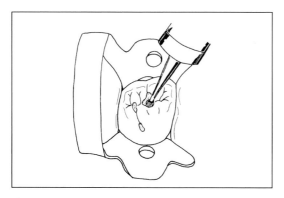

Fig 8-14 Removal of caries with a high-speed No. 330 bur, followed by a slow-speed No. $^1/_2$ round bur, is accomplished in an exploratory manner. After caries removal, calcium hydroxide liner is placed over exposed dentin.

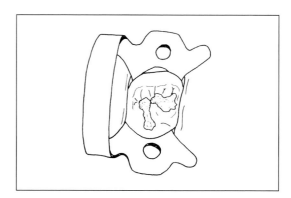

Fig 8-15 Acid-etching gel is applied over the entire occlusal surface for 20 to 60 seconds, then washed (20 seconds) and dried (10 seconds).

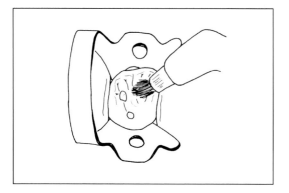

Fig 8-16 The walls of the preparation are coated with bonding agent, which acts as an intermediate resin layer. This step may be optional with small preparations.

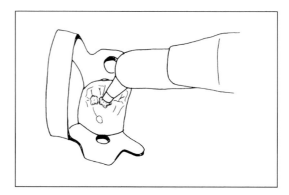

Fig 8-17 Filled composite resin is injected into the preparation from prepackaged ampules placed in the syringe provided by the manufacturer.

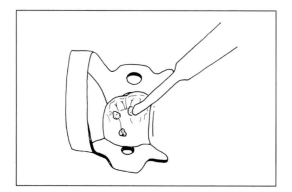

Fig 8-18 The composite resin is condensed and smoothed with a plastic or Teflon instrument.

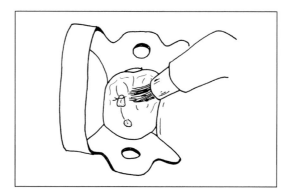

Fig 8-19 Filled sealant material is applied over the entire occlusal surface.

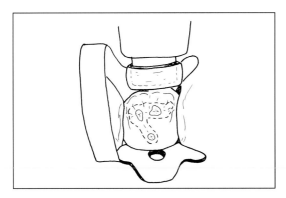

Fig 8-20 All layers are simultaneously polymerized with visible light produced by the polymerization unit.

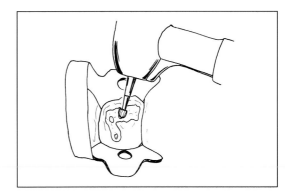

Fig 8-21 The occlusion is adjusted, where required, with finishing burs.

References

Albert, M., and Grenoble, D.E. An in vivo study of enamel remineralization after acid-etching. J. South. Calif. Dent. Assoc. 39:747, 1971.

American Academy of Pedodontics. Rationale and guidelines for pit and fissure sealants. Pediatr. Dent. 5:89, 1983.

American Dental Association (ADA), Council on Dental Materials, Instruments, and Equipment. Pit and fissure sealants. J. Am. Dent. Assoc. 114:671, 1987.

Arana, E.M. Clinical observations of enamel after acid etch procedure. J. Am. Dent. Assoc. 89:1103, 1974.

Backer-Dirks, O. The benefits of water fluoridation. Caries Res. 8(suppl. 1):2, 1974.

Bagramian, R.A., Srivastava, S., and Graves, R.C. Pattern of sealant retention in children receiving a combination of caries-preventive methods: Three-year results. J. Am. Dent. Assoc. 98:46, 1979.

Bates, D., et al, Effects of acid etch parameters on enamel topography and composite resin—enamel bond strength. Pediatr. Dent. 4:106, 1982.

Berman, D.S., and Slack, G.L. Susceptibility of tooth surfaces to carious attack. Br. Dent. J. 134:135, 1973.

Bodecker, C.F. The eradication of enamel fissures. Dent. Items Int. 51:859, 1929.

Bohannan, H.M. Caries distribution and the case for sealants. J. Public Health Dent. 43:200, 1983.

Bossert, W.A. The relation between the shape of the occlusal surfaces of molars and the prevalence of decay. J. Dent. Res. 16:63, 1937.

Brännström, M., et al. Etching of young permanent teeth with an acid gel. Am. J. Orthod. 82:379, 1982.

Brunelle, J.A., and Carlos, J.P. Changes in the prevalence of dental caries in U.S. school children, 1961-1980. J. Dent. Rest. 61:1346, 1982.

Buonocore, M.G. A simple method of increasing the adhesion of acrylic filling materials to enamel surfaces. J. Dent. Res. 34:859, 1955.

Buonocore, M.G. Caries prevention in pits and fissures sealed with an adhesive resin polymerized by ultraviolet light: A two-year study of a single adhesive application. J. Am. Dent. Assoc. 82:1090, 1971.

Charbeneau, G. T., and Dennison, J.B. Clinical success and potential failure after single application of a pit and fissure sealant: A four-year report. J. Am. Dent. Assoc. 98:559, 1979.

Cline, J.T., and Messer, L.B. Relative caries inhibition following loss of sealants. J. Dent. Res. 57:359, 1978 (IADR abstract No. 1138).

Cueto, E.I., and Buonocore, M.G. Sealing of pits and fissures with an adhesive resin: Its use in caries prevention. J. Am. Dent. Assoc. 75:121, 1967.

Dennison, D. et al. Evaluating tooth eruption on sealant efficacy J. Am. Dent. Assoc. 121:610, 1990.

Dennison, J.B., et al. A clinical comparison of sealant and amalgam in the treatment of pits and fissures. part 1. Clinical performance after 18 months. Pediatr. Dent. 2:167, 1980a.

Dennison, J.B., et al. A clinical comparison of sealant and amalgam in the treatment of pits and fissures. part 2. Clinical application and maintenance during 18-month period. Pediatr. Dent. 2:176, 1980b.

Doyle, W.A., and Brose, J.A. A five-year study of the longevity of fissure sealant. J. Dent. Child. 45:23, 1978.

Eidelman, E. et al. The retention of fissure sealants: Rubber dam or cotton rolls in private practice J. Dent. Child. 50:259, 1983.

Eidelman, E., et al. The retention of fissure sealants using twenty second etching time. J. Dent. Child. 51:422, 1984.

Evans, T., and Silverstone, L.M. The effect of salivary contamination in vitro on etched human enamel. J. Dent. Res. 60:1247, 1981.

Fairbourn, D.R., et al. Effect of improved Dycal and IRM on bacteria in deep carious lesions. J. Am. Dent. Assoc. 100:547, 1970.

Feigal, R.J. et al. Retaining sealant on salivary contaminated enamel. J. Am. Dent. Assoc. 124:88, 1993.

Ferguson, F., and Ripa, L. Evaluation of the retention of two sealants applied by dental students. J. Dent. Educ. 44:494, 1980.

Fuks, A.B., et al. In vitro assessment of marginal leakage of sealants placed in permanent molars with different etching times. J. Dent. Child. 51:425, 1984.

Going, R.E., et al. Four-year clinical evaluation of a pit and fissure sealant. J. Am. Dent. Assoc. 95:972, 1977.

Going, R.E., et al. The vitality of microorganisms in carious lesions five years after covering with a fissure sealant. J. Am Dent. Assoc. 97:455, 1978.

Handelman, S.L., Buonocore, M.G., and Schoute, P.C. Progress report on the effect of a fissure sealant on bacteria in dental caries. J. Am. Dent. Assoc. 87:1189, 1973.

Handelman, S.L., Washburn, F., and Wopperer, P. Two-year report of sealant effect on bacteria in dental caries. J. Am. Dent. Assoc. 93:967, 1976.

Handelman, S.L., et al. Use of adhesive sealants over occlusal carious lesions: Radiographic evaluation. Community Dent. Oral Epidemiol. 9:256, 1981.

Hardison, J.R. The use of pit and fissure sealants in community public health programs in Tennessee. J. Public Health Dent. 43:233, 1983.

Hardison, J.R. Retention of pit and fissure sealant on the primary molars of 3- and 4-year-old children after 1 year. J. Am. Dent. Assoc. 114:613, 1987.

Hicks, M.J. Preventive resin restorations: Etching patterns, resin tag morphology and the enamel-resin interface. J. Dent. Child. 51:116, 1984.

Hicks, M.J., and Silverstone, L.M. Fissure sealants and dental enamel. A histological study of microleakage in vitro. Caries Res. 16:353, 1982.

Hinding, J. Extended cariostasis following loss of pit and fissure sealant from human teeth. J. Dent. Child. 41:201, 1974.

Hormati, A.A., et al. Effects of contamination and mechanical disturbance on the quality of acid-etched enamel. J. Am. Dent. Assoc. 100:34, 1980.

Horowtiz, H.S. The potential of fluoride and sealants to deal with problems of decay. Pediatr. Dent. 4:286, 1982.

Horowtiz, H.S., Heifetz, S.B., and Poulsen, S. Retention and effectiveness of a single application of an adhesive sealant in preventing occlusal caries: Final report after five years of a study in Kalispell, Montana. J. Am. Dent. Assoc. 95:1133, 1977.

Horsted, M., et al. The structure of surface enamel with special reference to occlusal surfaces of primary and permanent teeth. Caries Res. 10:287, 1976.

Houpt, M., et al. Occlusal restoration using fissure sealant instead of "extension for prevention." J. Dent Child. 51:270, 1984.

Houpt, M., et al. Occlusal composite restorations: 4-year results. J. Am. Dent. Assoc. 110:351, 1985.

Houpt, M., and Shey, Z. Cost-effectiveness of fissure sealants. J. Dent. Child. 50:210, 1983a.

Houpt, M., and Shey, Z. The effectiveness of a fissure sealant after six years. Pediatr. Dent. 5:104, 1983b.

Hunt, R.J., et al. The use of pit and fissure sealants in private dental practices. J. Dent. Child. 51:29, 1984.

Hyatt, T.P. Prophylactic odontotomy. Dent. Cosmos 65:234, 1923.

Jensen, O.E., et al. Occlusal wear of four pit and fissure sealants over two years. Pediatr. Dent. 7:23, 1985.

Jensen, O.E., and Handelman, S.L. Effect of an autopolymerizing sealant on viability of microflora in occlusal dental caries. Scand. J. Dent Res. 88:382, 1980.

Jerrell, R.G., and Bennett, C.G. Utilization of sealants by practicing pedodontists. J. Pedod. 8:378, 1984.

Kastendieck, M.J., and Silverstone, L.M. Remineralization of acid etched human enamel by exposure to oral fluid in vivo and in vitro. J. Dent. Res. 58:163, 1979.

Larson, T.D., et al. Effect of prepared cavities on the strength of teeth. Oper. Dent 6:2, 1981.

Leake, J.L., and Martinello, B.P. A four year evaluation of a fissure sealant in a public health setting. J. Can. Dent. Assoc. 42:409, 1976.

LeBell, Y., and Forsten, L. Sealing of preventively enlarged fissures. Acta Odontol. Scand. 38:101, 1980.

Leske, G.S., Pollard, S., and Cons, N. Cost effectiveness considerations of a pit and fissure sealant. J. Dent. Res. 56:B71, 1977 (AADR abstract No. 77).

Leverett, D.H., et al. Use of sealants in the prevention and early treatment of carious lesions: Cost analysis. J. Am. Dent. Assoc. 106:39, 1983.

Li, S.H., et al. Evaluation of the retention of two types of pit and fissure sealants. Community Dent. Oral Epidemiol. 9:151, 1981

Main, C., et al. Surface treatment studies aimed at streamlining fissure sealant application. J. Oral Rehabil. 10:307, 1983.

Meiers, J.C., and Jensen, M.E. Management of the questionable carious fissure: Invasive vs noninvasive techniques. J. Am. Dent. Assoc. 108:64, 1984.

Mertz-Fairhurst, E.J., et al. Clinical progress of sealed and unsealed caries. part I. Depth of changes and bacterial counts. J. Prosthet. Dent. 42:521, 1979a.

Mertz-Fairhurst, E.J., et al. Clinical progress of sealed and unsealed caries part II. Standardized radiographs and clinical observations. J. Prosthet. Dent. 42:633, 1979b.

Mertz-Fairhurst, E.J., et al. A comparable clinical study of two pit and fissure sealants: 7-year results in Augusta GA. J. Am. Dent. Assoc., 109:252, 1984.

Messer L.B., and Nustad, R. Cost-effectiveness of sealants vs. amalgams on first permanent molars. J. Dent. Res. 58:331, 1979 (abstract No. 956).

Meurman, J.H., Helminen, S.K., and Louma, H. Caries reduction over 5-years from a single application of a fissure sealant. Scand. J. Dent. Res. 86:153, 1978.

Miller J., and Hobson, P. Determination of the presence of caries in fissures. Br. Dent. J. 100:15, 1956.

National Institutes of Health (NIH). Consensus development conference statement on dental sealants in the prevention of tooth decay. J. Am. Dent Assoc. 108:233, 1984.

Nordenvall, K., et al. Etching of deciduous teeth and young and old permanent teeth. A comparison between 15 and 60 seconds of etching. Am. J. Orthod. 78:99, 1980.

Raadal, M. Follow-up study of sealing and filling with composite resins in the prevention of occlusal caries. Community Dent. Oral Epidemiol. 6:176, 1978a.

Raadal M. Microleakage around preventive composite fillings in occlusal fissures. Scand. J. Dent. Res. 86:495, 1978b.

Raadal, M., et al. Fissure sealing of permanent first molars in children receiving a high standard of prophylactic care. Community Dent. Oral Epidemiol. 12:65, 1984.

Retief, D.H., and Mallory, W.P. Evaluation of two pit and fissure sealants: An in vitro study. Pediatr. Dent 3:12, 1981.

Richardson, B.A., et al. A 5-year clinical evaluation the effectiveness of fissure sealant in mentally retarded Canadian children. Community Dent. Oral Epidemiol. 9:170, 1981.

Ripa, L.W. Occlusal sealing: Rationale of the technique and historical review. J. Am. Soc. Prev. Dent. 3:32, 1973.

Ripa, L.W. Sealant retention on primary teeth: A critique of clinical and laboratory studies. J. Pedod. 3:275, 1979.

Ripa, L.W. Occlusal sealants: An overview of clinical studies. J. Public Health Dent. 43:216, 1983.

Ripa, L.W. The current status of pit and fissure sealants. A review. J. Can. Dent. Assoc. 51:367, 1985.

Ripa, L.W., Gwinnett, A I., and Buonocore, M.B. The prismless outer layer of deci. ous and permanent enamel. Arch. Oral Biol. 11:41, 1966.

Ripa, L.W., and Wolff, M.S. Preventive resin restorations: Indications, technique, and success. Quintessence Int 23: 307, 1992.

Roder, D.M. The treatment of first permanent molars in a school dental programme: Implications for fissure sealants. Aust. Dent. J. 20:94, 1975.

Scott, L. Retention of dental sealants following the use of air-polishing and traditional cleaning. Den. Hyg. 24:402, 1988.

Shapira, J., et al. Six-year evaluation of fissure sealants placed after mechanical preparation: A matched pair study. Pediatr. Dent. 8:204, 1986.

Shapira, J., et al. A comparative clinical study of autopolymerized fissure sealants: Five-year results. Pediatr. Dent. 12:168, 1990.

Shapira, J., and Eidelman, E. The influence of mechanical preparation of enamel prior to etching on the retention of sealants: Three-year follow up. J. Pedod. 8:272, 1984.

Shapira, J., and Eidelman, E. Fissure topography after combined 20- and 60-seconds etching and mechanical preparation viewed by SEM. Clin. Prev. Dent. 7:27, 1985.

Silverstone, L.M. The histopathology of early approximal caries in the enamel of primary teeth. J. Dent. Child. 37:17, 1970.

Silverstone, L.M. Fissure sealants: Laboratory studies. Caries Res. 8:2, 1974.

Silverstone, L.M. The acid etch technique: In vitro studies with special reference to the enamel surface and the enamel-resin interface. In Silverstone, L.M., and Dogon, I.L. Proceedings of an International Symposium of the Acid Etch Technique. St. Paul, Minn.: North Central Publ. Co., 1975.

Silverstone, L.M. The use of pit and fissure sealants in dentistry—Present status and future developments. Pediatr. Dent. 4:16, 1982.

Silverstone, L.M. Fissure sealants: The enamel-resin interface. J. Public Health Dent. 43:205, 1983.

Silverstone, L.M., et al. Oral fluids contamination of etched enamel surfaces: An SEM study. J. Am. Dent. Assoc. 110:329, 1985.

Silverstone, L.M. and Dogon, I.L. The effect of phosphoric acid on human deciduous enamel surface in vitro. J. Int. Assoc. Dent. Child. 7:11, 1976.

Simonsen, R.J. Fissure sealants: Deciduous molar retention of colored sealant with variable etch time. Quintessence Int. 9:71, 1978a

Simonsen, R.J. Preventive resin restorations. I. Quintessence Int. 9:69, 1978b.

Simonsen, R.J. Preventive resin restorations. II. Quintessence Int. 9:95, 1978c.

Simonsen, R.J. Preventive resin restorations: 3 year results. J. Am. Dent. Assoc. 100:535, 1980.

Simonsen, R.J. The clinical effectiveness of a colored pit and fissure sealant at 36 months. J. Am. Dent. Assoc. 102:323, 1981.

Simonsen, R.J. Pit and fissure sealants in individual patient care programs. J. Dent. Educ. (suppl.) 48:42, 1984.

Simonsen, R.J. Conservation of tooth structure in restorative dentistry. Quintessence Int. 15(1):15, 1985.

Simonsen, R.J. Cost effectiveness of pit and fissure sealant at 10 years. Quintessence Int 20:75, 1989.

Smith, D.C. The appropriateness of comparing sealants with restorations. J. Dent. Educ. 48:103, 1984.

Spieser, A.M., and Segat, T.E. The influence of technique modification on sealant leakage. J. Dent Child. 47:93, 1980.

Stanley, R.T. Preventive resin restorations: An alternative approach. Ohio Dent. J. 58:21, 1984.

Stephen, K. W., et al. Retention of a filled fissure sealant using reduced etch time. Br. Dent. J. 153:232, 1982.

Straffon, L., et al. Three-year evaluation of sealant: Effect of isolation on efficacy. J. Am. Dent. Assoc. 110:714, 1985.

Straffon, L.H., and Dennison, B. Clinical evaluation comparing sealant and amalgam after 7 years: Final report. J. Am. Dent. Assoc. 117:751, 1988.

Swango, P., and Brunelle, J. Age-and surface-specific caries attack rates from the National Dental Caries Prevalence Survey. J. Dent. Res. 62:270, 1983 (abstract No. 909).

Tandon, S., et al. The effect of etch-time on the bond strength of a sealant and on the etch-pattern in primary and permanent enamel: An evaluation. J. Dent. Child 56:186, 1989.

Taylor, C.L., and Gwinnett, A. J. A study of the penetration of sealants into pits and fissures. J. Am. Dent. Assoc. 87:1181, 1973.

Ulvestad, H. Evaluation of fissure sealing with a diluted composite sealant and an UV-light polymerized sealant after 36 months' observation. Scand. J. Dent. Res. 84:401, 1976.

Weintraub, J.A. The effectiveness of pit and fissure sealants. J. Public Health Dent. 49:317, 1989.

Questions

1. The incidence of occlusal caries in children is alarmingly high. Which of the following factors is true regarding occlusal caries formation in children?

   a. Onset is rapid, frequently occurring by the third year after eruption
   b. Susceptibility is directly proportional to the steepness of the cuspal inclines, or conversely, the depth of the fissures
   c. Susceptibility is relatively greater than on smooth surfaces
   d. Relative incidence may be higher in a fluoridated community because of the selective protection afforded the smooth surfaces by the systemic fluoride
   e. All of the above

2. Occlusal sealants are retained on the enamel surface chiefly by:

   a. Mechanical retention in deep pits and fissures
   b. Chemical bonding between the sealant and enamel
   c. Direct adhesiveness of the sealant
   d. Mechanical retention by sealant penetration into the etched enamel
   e. Chemical bonding between the sealant and etched enamel surface

3. Which of the following factors will reduce the retention of occlusal sealants?

   a. Saliva contamination of the etched surface
   b. Moisture contamination during sealant polymerization
   c. Presence of prismless enamel surface
   d. a,b
   e. All of the above

4. Before the application of pit and fissure sealant to permanent teeth, the enamel is etched with a 30% to 50% phosphoric acid for:

   a. 30 seconds
   b. 60 seconds
   c. 90 seconds
   d. 120 seconds
   e. None of the above

5. Indications for the placement of occlusal sealants in children include all of the following except:

   a. Immediately following topical fluoride application
   b. Recently erupted, caries-free tooth
   c. Low caries activity in patients proficient in caries control
   d. Dependable recall patients
   e. Steep cuspal inclines with deep fissures

Chapter 9

Behavior Management

Objectives

After studying this chapter, the student should be able to:
1. Discuss the role of systematic desensitization, modeling, and behavior modification in management of child behavior in the dental setting.
2. Discuss attitude as a modifier of child behavior in the dental setting.
3. Discuss the use of euphemisms and voice modulation in communication with the pediatric patient.
4. Describe the application of tell, show, and do in shaping behavior.
5. Discuss the concept of patient retraining.
6. Discuss the contingencies that exist with aversive conditioning.

The objective in the delivery of dental care to the child is to provide quality dental care with optimum patient cooperation. Behavior management methods may include use of the following:

1. Tell-Show-Do (TSD)
2. Voice control methods
3. Hand-over-mouth exercise (HOME)
4. Nitrous oxide-oxygen analgesia
5. Conscious sedation
6. Use of restraints
7. The combination of nitrous–oxide oxygen analgesia, and conscious sedation, with and without restraints
8. General anesthesia, on an inpatient or outpatient basis.

This chapter will present non-pharmacologic techniques for behavior management. The use of conscious sedation and general anesthesia will be discussed in Chapters 10 and 11, respectively.

Learning and conditioning

The child who has had a poor experience at the dental office and encountered a reactivation of his or her fear on returning to the dental office illustrates the phenomenon of *stimulus generalization.* The child has been preconditioned by the first visit to the dentist, and his or her return to the dental office awakened the original stimulus response, although this was a new situation. It makes little difference whether the new situation occurs in the same office with the same personnel or whether the dental office and staff are different. The reaction will be the same because of the similarity of the environment and event.

Should the child experience a more comfortable stimulus to a procedure that on prior occasion was disturbing, his or her response will likely be different. This behavior change is known as *response generalization.*

A young child accustomed to the care of a physician may feel some fear as a result of the medical visits. The child will likely exhibit this same fear when going to the dental office if the child is told he or she is "going to the doctor's office." It is a language label to which the youngster attaches a single response (Lenchner and Wright, 1975). The use of different terms might help significantly in alleviating this occurrence. The response is referred to as *mediated generalization.*

As a child's interpersonal relations and ability to reason mature, his or her differentiation becomes more specific. The generalizations that have been expansive and all inclusive shrink, becoming more localized and singular. He or she is beginning to distinguish and recognize the differences between the physician as a doctor and the dentist as a doctor. This ability is referred to as *discrimination.*

The child who experiences a particular procedure and responds with cooperative behavior is usually complimented or rewarded in some manner for his or her behavior. The compliment or reward establishes within the child a desire to continue the response. This technical procedure is referred to as *reinforcement*. The child who experiences a particular procedure and responds with undesirable behavior does not receive positive reinforcement. Responses that go unrewarded or are punished become weaker and will eventually disappear. This type of behavior change is referred to as *extinction*.

Modification of behavior

Behavior modification is defined as "the attempt to alter human behavior and emotion in a beneficial manner according to the laws of modern learning theory." This behavioral conversion technique is not confined to the areas of psychiatry and psychology. It has been applied by dentistry, medicine, education, the advertising media, governments, and many other disciplines (Beech, 1976).

The original idea of the modification of behavior came from the early studies of Pavlov and Bechterev and were reported by Pavlov in 1927. The psychologists' entry into this arena was prompted by the need for investigative substantiation and understanding of the methods wherein the behavior of organisms is altered. Theories have evolved, many of which are not dependable. Behavioral psychologists express the fact that more experimental investigation needs to be performed.

Behavior modification

The term *behavior modification* emerges from early work by Skinner (1953), Honig (1966), Reese (1966), and Grunbaum (1966). The concept is based on the establishment of competent behavioral engineering skills to bring about change in child behavior. The operational base involves the use of selected reinforcers that, being learned, it is hoped will change a child's behavior from an inappropriate to an appropriate form (Sawtell et al, 1974).

Rosenberg (1974) refers to *behavior* as that *response* by the child and the reaction of the dentist as the *consequence*. The consequence can be answered with a *reinforcer*, which strengthens behavior in a patient, or with a *punisher*, which weakens behavior.

One of the principal advantages of behavior modification is that the reinforcement process and the reinforcers are custom made and tailored to the particular child. Behavior modification is a formalized but generalized, readily adaptable tool. The freedom and flexibility of the instrument permits the dentist and dental auxiliaries to readily learn and adapt it in acceptable fashion to the child's behavior.

Reinforcers

Some reinforcers are unlearned and are related to the necessities and enjoyments of life that seemingly have always been with us, such as protection, food, and comfort. Other reinforcers concentrate more on the opportunities for personal attainment through an act of acceptable behavior. Still other reinforcements issue from the dental operator and assistant, or the dental staff, and are in the form of praise, smiling, patting, and varied signs of affection or caring.

Punishers

Punishers are those negative attitudes or actions used to extinguish inappropriate behavior and, unfortunately, on occasion appropriate behavior. A failure to reinforce may be by critique of behavior, admonitions, aversive restraints, or inadequate presentations of praise.

In recent years, pediatric dentists have been investigating various behavior modification modes in an effort to establish meaningful techniques to apply and favorably alter child behavior in the dental environment. The research has produced varying and sometimes inconclusive results, and yet a good amount of valuable information has been attested. Although the study on behavior modification procedures by Machen and Johnson (1974) revealed little difference between the modification therapies of desensitization and modeling, there was positive support of the preappointment visit for the child before the dental experience. Fields and Pinkham (1976) hypothesized that the preappointment visit of a child and parent to a reception area would be more positive than no previsit at all and that a previsit modeling session would be the most positive. The results of the study were not conclusive. However, it was observed that when the analysis incorporated maternal anxiety as a covariant with modeling of cooperative behavior, there was significant support to the modeling procedure.

Likewise, behavior management techniques vary with the individual and personnel using them. Personalities, office organization and philosophy, educational qualities of the personnel, staff concerns for patient welfare and comfort, each and all, have marked effects on and contribute to the degree of success of the procedure in changing behavior.

There are specific ways in which the behavior of a child can be modified. It is important to understand the theory behind each method and become skillful in applying it to behavior control. When the dentist has sufficient clinical experience to have developed a feeling for the child management process and has determined the merits peculiar to each method of behavior control, he or she will begin to be more proficient in selecting and applying a particular method toward a particular behavior.

Systematic desensitization

The animal studies of Masserman (1943) and Wolpe's (1952) research have carried behavior modification practices a substantial distance. Wolpe's contribution has been the systematic desensitization technique . Systematic desensitization as a behavior modification procedure used two important elements: (1) gradational exposure of the child to his or her fear and (2) induced state of incompatibility with his or her fear.

The therapist creates a list of steps arranged as a hierarchy from the least to the most stressful. The patient, while in a state of deep relaxation, is exposed one step at a time, each step presented repeatedly until there is no evidence of stress or antagonism on the patient's part. On satisfactory completion of the hierarchy procedure, the patient should be desensitized to the predominant fear.

Addleston (1959) introduced the concept *Tell-Show-Do* as a behavior modification procedure. It contains certain elements of systematic desensitization. Ingersoll (1982), however, considers Tell-Show-Do to be an information-exposure method of behavior shaping because it excludes the preparatory format contained in the original studies on systematic desensitization. McTigue (1984) describes the desensitization process Tell-Show-Do as a retraining procedure in the event a child has dental-related anxieties. He refers to the use of substitute measures as "new and more pleasant associations with the anxiety provoking stimuli."

Modeling

Bandura (1969) developed from social learning principles a behavioral modification technique called *modeling* or *imitation.* He states that learning occurs only as a result of a "direct experience which can be vicarious—witnessing the behavior and the outcome of that behavior for other people." He found earlier that children exposed to an aggressive model will imitate that type of behavior both verbally and nonverbally (Bandura, 1961).

Effective observational learning, according to Bandura (1969), is dependent on four requirements of the modeling technique:

1. Concentrated attention must be expended toward the witnessing of the model. Brief exposure to the modeling procedure is not productive.
2. There must be sufficient retention of desirable behavior in the absence of a model.
3. One must be able to reproduce effectively the behavior modeled.
4. The newly acquired behavior must be appropriately rewarded to retain it.

Authorities generally believe that modeling is the most dependable modification procedure to use with the apprehensive child introduced for the first time to the dental experience. According to Ingersoll (1982), the display of cooperative behavior accomplishes more for the dentally uneducated child than any other means. Modeling is a preparatory method of behavior modification easily adapted to the observance of older siblings receiving dental care, demonstrations by reliable actors, or presentations through prepared videotape recordings.

Attitude

A project conducted by Sawtell et al (1974) investigated the effects of certain preparational methods to establish child behavior. Four preparational methods and a control were devised for the study. There were desensitization, vicarious symbolic modeling, behavior modification, placebo, and the control group, which was not subjected to predental preparation. For the placebo group, however, preparation comprised an individual posing as a member of the dental staff, white coat and all, who led a child from the reception room to a conference area. There, the attendant, in a warm and friendly manner, conversed with the child at his or level or interest but never alluded to the dental encounter the patient would soon experience. The intent of the placebo method was to determine in some fashion whether a genial member of the dental staff could contribute in a nondentally related preparatory fashion toward cooperative behavior of the child in the dental office. The most interesting finding in the investigation was that the placebo group demonstrated the least uncooperative child behavior. The control group demonstrated the highest, but patients in the desensitization, modeling, and behavior modification groups manifested significantly more uncooperative behavior than did the placebo subjects.

As pointed out by the investigators of the study, is there a possibility that the predental preparation in the areas of desensitization, modeling, and behavior modification failed to change anxious behavior or possibly even intensified it? Did the placebo study point out the potential of positive behavior from an anxious child when introduced to a nonthreatening condition and in the company of a warm-hearted other? Perhaps the ease of the placebo preparational approach should be considered before the introduction of the new patient to the dental setting.

Communication

In all of life, an individual's association and response to another is involved with communication. It is verbal or nonverbal. An individual speaks with another or one person smiles at another. Communication is both objective and subjective.

The normal dental office can cope effectively with the average child's behavior and perform the required services. But this same dental team may be confronted by a child with whom verbal communication is not possible. If the team understands communication in the subjective as well as objective sense, management will be more effective for this potentially cooperative child.

Communication with the child patient is the prime objective to achieve behavior control (Lenchner and Wright, 1975), and it may be verbal, nonverbal, or a combination of the two.

The dentist and members of the staff should each develop his or her own individual styles of conversation. The style should be natural and comfortable for each team member because the occasion will arise when each must initiate or sustain communication with the child patient. Not only should conversation be natural, but the language choice should consist of words that express pleasantness, friendship, and concern. Initial remarks should include statements about the child's appearance or dress. He or she should be encouraged to converse by posing questions as to the child's likes. "What do you like to do best?" Do you have a pet?" " What is your cat's name?" " I bet you are a good ball player!" This approach helps establish a direct communication to which the child can relate and respond. This style of conversation also opens the mind to further thought exchange. The dental team will have prepared an avenue for the dentist to explain dental procedures to the child.

When an individual walks by another on the sidewalk and a smile is exchanged, a nonverbal communication of friendliness is expressed. When a young woman looks warmly into a young man's gaze, a powerful nonverbal communication is manifested. Nonverbal communication such as this is effective in concert with verbal expression. It can be infinitely meaningful even when used by itself. The dental team members must acquire its magic and apply it to every child to whom they have a responsibility. It is the pat on the back, the smile, and the warmth and understanding radiated from one to the other through eye contact.

Effective communication

The choice of words used by the dentist and staff or the manner in which the words are voiced can influence the emotional state of the average child. As previously mentioned, some dental students and their clinical partners, or even dentists and their staffs, give little thought to their choice of phrases and refer to the "needle" or the "shot," stating, "This will hurt a moment." For even the average child these are disturbing, often upsetting, remarks.

Lenchner and Wright (1975) indicate that the dentist must develop a "second language" by substituting "mild expressions," or euphemisms, for those that im-

ply harm in the child's mind. Pediatric dentists use many different catchy words and phrases. The family dentist should be as euphemistic. Listed below are a few examples:

Dental nomenclature	Euphemisms
Amalgam	Silver filling
Anesthetic (topical, local)	Tooth putter to sleeper
Bur	Germ chaser
Crown, stainless steel	Shiny cap
Dental caries	Tooth bugs
Liner	White filling
Matrix band	Queen's (king's) crown
Prophylaxis paste	Toothpaste
Radiograph	Tooth picture
Rubber dam	Raincoat
X-ray machine	Camera

Voice modulation controls the manner in which thoughts are expressed. Speaking quietly and in a kind voice has appeal for many children. Amplitude in the voice will cause the child to heed direction. There must be awareness between two people before communication can take place. An example might be to say in an ample voice, "Johnny! Give me your attention!"

When we use gestures in an objective way during child management procedures, their use can garner attention when purposefully overdone. "Examples of this manner of communication can be suddenly clapping the hands, staring meaningfully, or suddenly pointing with an index finger and verbalizing at the same instant "You straighten up!"

Management procedures

First dental visit preparation

To assure a successful and pleasant first dental visit, the dentist and staff must enlighten the child to the expectations of the appointment. The child needs to know the nature of the visit and must become acquainted with the dental office and its personnel. The accomplishment of these details involves:

1. *A previsit letter* from the dentist welcoming the child and explaining in brief but understandable terms the nature of the visit. An information booklet is usually included for the parent to better inform the family of subjects related to dental health. Also, the date for the get-acquainted visit is enclosed.

2. *A get-acquainted visit* is held in a conference room with certain of the dental auxiliaries present. It should be one of friendliness and warmth.

Behavior modification procedure

Modeling

Modeling of the dental experience immediately follows the get-acquainted visit. It may be a film or videotape demonstrating the dental experience. During this period the patient is in the company of an auxiliary person who, at the end, reinforces what the patient has observed by asking questions.

The first dental visit will often be subsequent to an interim period of 2 or 3 days. However, the visit may ensue the modeling session. The dental visit should include mention of policy and rules of behavior, a reinforcement of learned behavior if required, the dental examination, radiographs, oral prophylaxis, toothbrushing instruction and demonstration (including the parent), topical fluoride, and consultation with the parent and child on preventive dental measures.

To attain appropriate patient conduct, the dentist must first explain the desired behavior, possibly demonstrate it, and then guide the patient into the desired behavior. This goal may need to be accomplished by modeling the appropriate behavior. Every correct performance demands immediate reinforcement to maintain and strengthen the behavior. To eliminate behavior that is unacceptable, the dentist must consistently fail to reinforce the behavior.

Desensitization

There is some question of the effectuality of desensitization for the inexperienced, fearful child (Melamed, 1982). However, as has been previously mentioned, McTigue (1984) recommends the use of the desensitization process in retraining, referring to the effectiveness of Tell-Show-Do. Some use Tell-Show-Do for all of their behavior modification procedures. As an example of a behavior-shaping technique Tell-Show-Do is applied as follows:

1. The dentist, using language tailored to the child's understanding, tells the patient what is to be done. It is presented slowly and repetitiously to help the child comprehend the measure to be performed.
2. The dentist demonstrates to the patient, by role model or other medium, showing how the procedure is accomplished. The presentation is painstakingly developed. The operator demonstrates the procedure either on himself or herself, an assistant, or an object until the child understands. The demonstration should be performed slowly and carefully.
3. The dentist proceeds to do the dental measure exactly as described and demonstrated.

The child who is carried through a Tell-Show-Do procedure successfully should be rewarded immediately. Prompt reinforcement is necessary for strong, appropriate behavior.

Retraining

The dentist, on occasion, will encounter the child who has had a previously poor dental experience or who displays a negative behavior for other reasons. The individual will require retraining, a technique similar to behavior shaping, but it is designed to fabricate positive values to replace the negative behavior that has developed.

Before retraining devices are used, the cause or causes of the child's negative behavior should be established. With this type of knowledge in hand, the task of retraining can be augmented with a more effectively structured set of devices.

The approaches to retraining fall into three main categories: *(1)* avoidance, *(2)* deemphasis and substitution, and *(3)* distraction.

Lenchner and Wright (1975) draw on a real example of avoidance as a retraining technique. If a student is assigned a negatively behaviored child who has suffered an inept dental experience, rather than run the risk of repeating the same distracting procedure, the student provisionally restores the carious tooth. This technique is referred to as an *avoidance*, and it accomplishes two things. First, the student has moved on an entirely different treatment track, and second, he or she has performed a relatively painless service. As Lenchner and Wright state, this style of approach allows final treatment to be performed at a more appropriate time. The child patient expected the encounter to be an uncomfortable ordeal.

Once a child's particular dislike is established, one or both of the modification skills of deemphasis or substitution may be applied. The effective use of these tools will require empathetic involvement and understanding between the operator and the child. Should it be a particular instrument that produces the anxiety, the dental operator, understanding the response, should substitute another instrument if possible. If a substitution is out of the question, the operator should let the child know that the instrument will be used as little as possible and with great care. The tastes of certain materials may be objectionable to the child patient. Substitution may be the best approach toward alleviating the objection.

The dentist will discover that diversion can be an effective modification technique. The operator must learn that while accomplishing a certain dental procedure there may be a need for distraction if the child is uneasy. It may be in the form of storytelling, repetitive statements of encouragement, particular gestures, or the use of audio or visual aids. Distraction is a particularly useful technique during the administration of a local anesthetic.

Aversive conditioning

The child who displays a negative behavior and does not respond to the moderate behavior modification technique falls into a category requiring careful judgment and determination. This type of behavior would be classified on the Frankl scale as definitely negative (– –). As stated by Lenchner and Wright (1975), most authorities on pediatric dentistry subscribe to some form of restraint for the child when the gentler technique have failed. The use of restraint discipline (Lenchner and Wright, 1975) will depend on the urgency of the dental need, the rationale for the behavior in the dental office, and the nature of the behavior.

When restraint discipline is considered, the dentist's personal characteristics and judgmental ability must become a consideration.

There are some clinicians whose personality and emotional makeup will not allow them to use aversive conditioning. It is not that they do not believe in strong discipline but rather that they feel more comfortable in dealing with uncontrollable behavior in other ways. Conversely, there are those whose personal characteristics demand positive behavior from a negatively behaviored child and they use restraint discipline confidently and comfortably.

Thus far, we have related to two different types of clinician, both knowing their capabilities and their preferences of behavior control for the uncontrollable child. But we need to look at one other aspect of concern—that of the operator and his or her emotional control. In this regard, the dentist must never allow the child's behavior to upset his or her emotional and judgmental faculties. If the operator loses his or her temper when forced into a physical restraint discipline, his methods may become harsh and extend beyond the operator's primary intention of behavior modification. Such performance often becomes known to the parent and others and produces concern, embarrassment, and possible legal involvement for the dentist.

Some clinicians use only the most gentle of physical restraint methods to control adverse behavior. The operator may vigorously and tellingly remove the child's hand from a path of interference during a dental procedure. The clinician may suddenly pluck the child from the chair and forcibly reseat him or her, accompanying the action with suitable language.

Restraint discipline, as referred to by Wright and Feasby (1975), involved the hand-over-the-mouth technique. It was a behavior management procedure that had been used by many clinicians over a long period of time. McBride (1932), one of the early pediatric dentists, refers to the use of the procedure "to break down the iron will of an incorrigible patient." He instituted the use of a towel between his hand and the child's mouth saying, "It was quieter that way!" Levitas (1974) referred to the procedure as hand-over-mouth exercise (HOME) and Kramer (1974) cited it as aversive conditioning.

When restraint discipline is used, certain prerequisites must be present to assure a reasonable chance of success in modifying uncontrollable behavior:

1. The operator must control the child's behavior.
2. The operator must control his or her own behavior.
3. The dental team must be familiar with their role when the procedure is used.
4. The parent must know ahead of time of the possibility that this type of behavior shaping may be used on the child.

At special issue is the use of hand-over-mouth exercise as a control method. This method of patient management or control may no longer be acceptable to parents or other health care professionals (Bross, 1984). Negligent mishandling of the child by the treating dentist constitutes professional child abuse or neglect. This method is arguable as assault and battery, especially if the method is done without consent of the parent.

However, in a study by Barton (1993) on the effects of the hand-over-mouth exercise, two groups of children were questioned about their dental experiences. One group of children had experienced the use of the exercise, a comparative group had not. These children, all older than 10 years, were evaluated using standardized questionnaires related to their fears in general and their fears of the dental office. When the two groups were compared, there was no difference in their fears in general or their dental fears; in addition, there was no difference how the two groups felt about visiting the dental office. However, twice as many children who had the HOME experience in the dental office described negative experiences in the medical environment, either a physician's office or a hospital clinic. The study suggested the practitioner should feel comfortable using this method, if done with prior parental consent.

Parents in the operatory

Should parents stay with the child during the procedure or remain in the waiting area? In many dental offices, the parent is seen as a contributor to management or behavior problems and instructed to remain in the waiting area. Less than 8% of dentists questioned routinely allow parents to remain in the operatory with the child (Kamp, 1992). Several studies have attempted to evaluate the influence of a parent's presence on the child's behavior. One study found the mother's anxiety level had a direct effect on the negative behavior of the child (Wright et al, 1973). Yet, Pfefferle (1982) found no significant behavioral differences among children who were or were not accompanied by parents. Another study described the need for increased involvement by the parent in the informed consent and treatment decision process (Pinkham, 1991). Kamp (1992) questioned 79 parents as to their preference whether they wished to accompany the child into the operatory or remain in the waiting area and found:

1. Sixty-six percent wished to be present.
2. In general parents wished to observe the young child's dental procedures or during their child's first visit.
3. The parent's felt their presence would improve their child's acceptance of the dental procedure.

Some dentists feel the parent increases the potential management problems with the child by offering unsolicited advice, attempting to placate the unmanageable child, and disrupting the dental office routine. However, other dentists feel it is an advantage to have the parent observe the behavioral patterns of the child or how accepting the child is of dental procedures. Each dentist and dental office has to establish a policy that provides the parent with the knowledge of "what's going on!" This policy is part of the dentist's responsibility to provide quality dental care. Depending on the philosophy of the dentist and the dentist's office policy, there are several options:

1. Inform parents of the indicated care needed and the methods to be used, and routinely exclude them from the operatory area.
2. If the parent wishes, allow him or her to enter the operating area.
3. Exclude most parents, with the exception of parents of the very young child or the patient with developmental disabilities.

References

Addleston, H. Child patient training. C. D. S. Rev. 38:7, 1959.

Bandura, A. Psycho-therapy as a learning process. Psychol. Bull. 58:143, 1961

Bandura, A. Principles of Behavioral Modification. New York: Holt, Rinehart and Winston, 1969.

Barton, D. H. Dental attitudes and memories: A study of the effects of hand over mouth/restraint. Pediatr. Dent. 15:13, 1993.

Beech, H. Behavior modification. In Eysenck, H. J., and Wilson, G. D. A Textbook of Human Psychology. Baltimore: University Park Press, 1976.

Bross, D. C. Legal aspects of child abuse. In Sanger, R. G., and Bross, D. C. Clinical Management of Child Abuse and Neglect. Chicago: Quintessence, 1984.

Fields, H., and Pinkham, J. Videotape modeling of the child dental patient. J. Dent. Res. 55:958, 1976.

Grunbaum, A. Causality and the science of human behavior. pp. 3-10 In Ulrich R., Stachnik, T., and Mabry, J. Control of Human Behavior. Glenview, Ill.: Scott-Foresman, 1966.

Honig, W. K. Operant Behavior. New York: Appleton-Century-Crofts, 1966.

Ingersoll, B. D. Behavioral Aspects in Dentistry. East Norwalk, Conn.: Appleton-Century-Crofts, 1982.

Kamp, A. A. Parent-child separation during dental care: A survey of parent's preference. Pediatr. Dent. 14: 231, 1992.

Kopel, H. M. The autistic child in dental practice. J. Dent. Child. 44:302, 1977.

Kramer, W. S. Aversion—A method for modifying child behavior. J. Nebr. Dent. Assoc. 51:7, 1974.

Lampshire, E. L. Balanced medication for the child patient. Dent. Clin. North Am. Nov: 514, 1961.

Lenchner, V., and Wright, G. Z. Nonpharmaco-therapeutic approaches to behavior management. In Wright, G. Z. Behavior Management in Dentistry for Children. Philadelphia: W. B. Saunders Co., 1975.

Levitas, T. C. HOME, hand-over-mouth exercise. J. Dent Child. 41:18, 1974.

Machen, J. B., and Johnson, R. Desensitization, model learning, and the dental behavior of children. J. Dent. Res. 53:83, 1974.

Masserman, J. H. Behavior and Neuroses: An Experimental Psychoanalytic Approach to Psychologic Principles. Chicago: University of Chicago Press, 1943.

McBride, W. C. Juvenile Dentistry. Philadelphia: Lea & Febiger, 1932, p. 31.

McTigue, D. J. Behavior management of children. In Spedding, R. H. Symposium on Pedodontics. Dent. Clin. North Am. 28:1, 1984.

Melamed, B. G. Behavioral approaches to fear in dental settings. In Herson M., Eisler, R. M., and Miller, P. M. Progress in Behavior Modification. vol. 7. New York: Academic Press, 1979. In Ingersoll, B. D. Behavioral Aspects in Dentistry. East Norwalk, Conn.: Appleton-Century-Crofts, 1982.

Pfefferle, J. C., et al. Child behavior in the dental setting relative to parental presence. Pediatr. Dent. 4:311, 1982.

Pinkham, J.R. An analysis of the phenomenon of increased parental participation during the child's dental experience. J. Dent. Child. 58:458, 1991.

Reese, E. P. The Analysis of Human Operant Behavior, Dubuque, la.: Wm. C. Brown Co., 1966.

Rosenberg, H. M. Behavior modification for the child patient. J. Dent. Child. 41:111, 1974.

Sawtell, D. O., Simon J. F., and Simonsen, F. J. The effects of five preparatory methods upon child behavior during the first dental visit. J. Dent. Child. 41:367, 1974.

Skinner, B. F. Science and Human Behavior. New York: Macmillan Publ. Co., 1953.

Wolpe, J. Experimental neuroses as a learned behavior. Br. J. Psychol. 43:243, 1952.

Wright, G. Z., and Alpern, G. D., and Leake, J. L. The modificability of maternal anxiety as it relates to children's cooperative dental behavior. J. Dent, Child. 50:13, 1973.

Wright, G. Z., and Feasby, W. H. Control of anxiety. In Wright, G. Z. Behavior Management in Dentistry for Children. Philadelphia: W. B. Saunders Co., 1975.

Questions

1. A well-dressed physically attractive 12-year-old is in for a periodic dental examination. George is ushered into the dental operatory by the parent, in the company of an auxiliary and seated in the chair. The dentist, after kindly words of greeting, prepares for the recall examination. He asks the patient to "Please open." There is no verbal response, no eye contact, and no effort on the patient's part to respond affirmatively to the request. The doctor repeats the request several times. "Eventually, George opens his mouth for brief moments to permit the dental assessment. Finally, the dentist, seemingly satisfied, turns to the mother and explains that George's teeth and soft tissues appear in acceptable condition. You can attribute George's behavior to:

   a. Negativism
   b. Passive resistance
   c. Emotional development
   d. Developmental impairment

2. This is Carlos' third appointment, and the treatment planned is to complete the restorative measure on the primary mandibular left first molar. Last week he became very unhappy and unruly, and treatment did not go well, ending in a provisionalized procedure. A modification of behavior to a more appropriate and beneficial state will be necessary and involves:

   a. Applying progressive stimuli until anxiety responses disappear
   b. Explaining step-by-step what the patient is to do
   c. Telling him what he should know in language he understands
   d. Showing him exactly what the procedure will be
   e. Doing for him exactly what was explained and shown
   f. c,d,e
   g. All of the above

3. Jane, aged 3, will be in for her predental visit. Preappointment information indicates an family unit possessing a respectably high dental IQ. The predental visit will consist of:

   a. A get-acquainted visit, dental examination, radiographs, oral prophylaxis, and topical fluoride
   b. A get-acquainted visit followed by a video tape session on modeling
   c. A desensitization period to condition the child for the dental experience
   d. A get-acquainted visit and a behavior-shaping session on Tell-Show-Do

Chapter 10

Conscious Sedation

Objectives

After studying this chapter, the student should be able to:
1. Understand the objectives of conscious sedation.
2. Identify drugs commonly used.
3. Identify methods of drug administration.
4. Identify the monitoring devices and personnel needed to monitor patients who are candidates for conscious sedation.
5. Evaluate the patient's need for behavior modification, selecting the appropriate drug or combination of drugs to accomplish this goal.
6. Explain the adverse side effects that may occur when drugs are used.
7. Reverse any complications that might occur.

Conscious sedation has been defined by the American Academy of Pediatric Dentistry as "a minimally depressed level of consciousness that retains the patient's ability to maintain a patient airway independently and continuously, and respond appropriately to physical stimulation and/or verbal command" (AAPD, 1993).

Philosophy of conscious sedation

As a dentist, you must decide for yourself what represents acceptable behavior from your young patients. This decision will depend on your own personality, experience, and philosophy. Having defined acceptable behavior for yourself, you can then determine how you plan to modify unacceptable behavior patterns. The judicious use of conscious sedation has its place in dentistry for children, but needless to say, it use can be abused.

Conscious sedation is often useful if long procedures are indicated for nervous and apprehensive children. To a limited degree, conscious sedation may be indicated for uncooperative and defiant children. Conscious sedation does not, however, approach the problem of teaching the uncooperative child to accept the dental situation as an experience that he or she must

meet several times a year for the rest of his or her life. The dentist must establish the frequency of use of premedication for a child patient with the realization that there is no one drug that will solve all of the dentist's child management problems.

Objectives of conscious sedation

Bennett (1978) listed the understanding of the objectives as the most important factor for success. Conscious sedation has several objectives:

1. The patient's mood should be altered. This is the prime objective. The use of a pharmacologic agent will reduce the child's apprehension and reaction to painful stimuli. The use of a mood-altering drug will render the child more receptive to dental procedures. With this result, future dosages of drugs may be reduced.
2. The child should remain conscious. Although the child's responses to verbal stimuli may be sluggish, the patient should be responsive.
3. The child should be cooperative. With an increased level of cooperation, the dental care needed is completed more quickly and productively, to the advantage of both the dentist and the patient.

4. All protective reflexes should be intact and active. The normal physiologic reflexes are in a functioning state. The airway is active, the respiratory mechanism is reflexive, and the cardiovascular system is well within normal functioning limits.

5. All vital signs must remain stable and normal. If the patient is conscious with all protective reflexes intact, all vital signs should be normal.

6. The child's pain threshold should be elevated. Even though local anesthesia is used as an adjunct to conscious sedation, an additional drug can be added to reduce pain at the level of the central nervous system.

7. Amnesia should occur. Amnesia is not a major objective, but certain drugs will eliminate the awareness of the procedure, that is, the administration of local anesthesia.

Influencing factors in the use of conscious sedation

Patient classification

Many variables influence the criteria followed in the use of drugs for mood alteration, analgesia, or patient cooperation, and all are interrelated. The first variable is the kind of patient available. Kopel (1959) has classified patients in a preoperative screening situation: (1) the very young patient; (2) the emotionally disturbed, which include (a) the child from a broken home or from a poor family, (b) the pampered or spoiled child, (c) the neurotic child, (d) the excessively fearful child, and (e) the hyperactive child; (3) the physically handicapped; (4) the mentally handicapped; and (5) the child with a previous untoward medical or dental experience. The classification developed by Frankl et al (1962) is related to an intended response to dental care. Briefly, rating No. 1 is the definitely negative child, rating No. 2 is the negative child, rating No. 3 is the positive child, and rating No. 4 is the definitely positive child.

Musselman and McLure (1975) placed children in two groups: children needing preventive conscious sedation and children needing management medication. Preventive conscious sedation is defined as conscious sedation for children who are under abnormal stress from the dental situation and whose demeanor is responsive but strained. An example is the young child whose behavior degenerates from being strained but cooperative to becoming unmanageable. A second example of children needing conscious sedation is those who are unable to cooperate. These children lack the ability to communicate with the dentist and understand the dental environment. These are children who are developmentally handicapped, emotionally disturbed, or very young.

Age

The second variable is the age of the child, and this encompasses two factors. First is the anatomic or physiologic level of maturity. The second factor is the psychologic or emotional level of maturity. You must judge if the anatomic (chronologic) age of the child correlates with the emotional age of the child. If not, then careful use of conscious sedation can help the emotionally immature child to approach limits of acceptable behavior for his or her age.

Dental history

The next variable that influences criteria for drug choice is previous dental history. Is this the first dental office visit for the child? Second, have there been previous experiences related to physical or psychologic trauma? And third, the quantity and degree of dental caries must be considered. The latter includes rampant caries, such as in the child with "baby bottle mouth" or "nursing bottle syndrome." Other factors to consider are economic; for example, would it be more economically feasible to use conscious sedation versus general anesthesia on a cost-time comparison? The other economic variable is the cost of travel for dental care.

Determinative factors for use of conscious sedation

The following list of determinative factors is suggested. First, does the child already have acceptable behavior according to Frankl's ratings No. 3 and 4? Fortunately, these ratings includes about 90% of the children of all ages seen in the dental operatory. If the child does not have acceptable behavior, the second step would be to try psychologic or behavior modification. This would be Tell-Show-Do; voice control; and restraints without sedation. This small percentage of uncooperative young patients can often be dealt with by psychologic or behavior modification. If steps one and two fail, the third would be the use of some form of conscious sedation.

The priority of use should be:

1. Nitrous oxide analgesia (see Chapter 13).
2. Conscious sedation.
3. Conscious sedation plus nitrous oxide analgesia.
4. The use of any of the above with some form of restraints.

The last resort for control of unacceptable behavior is use of a general anesthetic agent in a hospital (see Chapter 11).

Methods of drug administration

This variable is related to the age of the child, type of care indicated, and behavior.

The four common methods of drug administration are parenteral (intravenous [IV], intramuscular [IM], or subcutaneous [SQ]), oral (po), rectal, and inhalation. All are acceptable and have relative merits. The individual needs of each patient should indicate the method to be used. Generally IV and rectal routes are used with hospitalized children, and inhalation, IM, and oral methods are used for dental office patients.

Oral medications (elixirs, pills, and capsules) are well accepted by most children and are easy to administer. Some elixirs are very bitter and should be given in orange juice or soda. Best results are obtained when the patient has had nothing to eat or drink for 3 to 4 hours before the appointment. When such variables as dosage, patient needs, and digestion are controlled, and adequate time is allowed for the medication to take effect, the results are usually excellent.

Rules for drug administration

Because of the concerns related to the overuse of conscious sedation, the American Academy of Pediatric Dentistry and American Academy of Pediatrics have published guidelines outlining the use of conscious sedation (AAPD, 1993). Following is a summary of these guidelines.

Before treatment

Chart documentation

1. Verbal and written instructions should be given to the parents about preoperative and postoperative care.
2. Dietary precautions should be emphasized.
   a. No milk or solid foods should be eaten after midnight before procedure.
   b. Only clear liquids should be ingested up to 4 to 8 hours before appointment, depending on age.
3. Vital statistics should be recorded (weight and height).
4. Preoperative health evaluation:
   a. Risk assessment should be made using the American Society of Anesthesiologists' classification (see Chapter 11).
   b. Health history should be completed.
   c. Status of airway should be confirmed.
   d. Vital signs, including pulse and blood pressure, should be recorded.

During treatment

Personnel

1. The practitioner should be trained in the use of conscious sedation methods.
2. Two members of the dental team should be present—the dentist and an assistant trained in life-support methods.

Monitoring procedures

1. Blood pressure, heart, and respiratory rates should be continuously monitored by trained personnel and intermittently recorded.
2. Child's color should be visually checked, especially oral mucosa and nailbeds for cyanosis.
3. Restraints, if used, should be checked for maintenance of a patent airway.
4. Head position should be evaluated constantly (Moore et al, 1984).
5. Patient should be monitored, always, by at least one trained person.

Postoperative care

Monitoring procedures

1. Vital signs should be recorded at intervals after the procedure.
2. Discharge of the patient should occur only when:
   a. Vital signs are stable.
   b. Patient is alert, can talk, and can sit up unaided.
   c. Patient can walk with minimal assistance.

Additional monitoring aides— Use of the pulse oximeter

Hypoxemia, a low partial pressure of oxygen, can be a serious problem in the sedated child (Mueller, 1985). The pulse oximeter is a method to monitor arterial oxygen saturation and developing hypoxemia. The pulse oximeter monitor is applied to a finger or toe by a Velcro-type strip (Fig 10-1). A light passes through the vascular bed of the digit, measuring the patient's percent of oxygen saturation as an estimate of arterial oxygen saturation. Since small changes in the arterial oxygen saturation are more critical in children because of their decreased oxygen reserve, oxygen desaturation is faster than in adults, resulting in hypoxemia (Anderson and Van, 1988; Anderson et al, 1988). A pulse oximeter should be used for the consciously sedated child in addition to monitoring of blood pressure, pulse and respiratory rates, and color. In a recent survey of pediatric dentists, pulse oximeters were used by 69% of the respondents (Houpt, 1993).

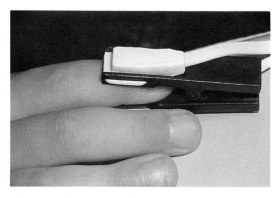

Fig 10-1 The monitoring device of the pulse oximeter attached to a finger.

Drug indications, dosage forms, and contraindications

Specific drug usage is influenced by the variables discussed earlier, that is, age of the child, defined by Kopel's or Frankl's classifications, quantity of dental care needed, and method of administration.

The calculation of the dosage to use for conscious sedation is not a simple task (Malamed, 1989). Young's rule and Clark's rule based on either age or weight have proved inconsistent in the area of conscious sedation for children (Wright et al, 1983; Brandt and Bugg, 1984). The desired effect for conscious sedation in pediatric dentistry is much different than the pediatrician's need for the child to have a good night's sleep or to reduce the child's hyperactivity in the classroom. Unfortunately, children are not constant when age and weight are compared. Wright et al (1983) described the use of a dosage chart that plotted dosages of a drug (chloral hydrate) against age. Data from three sources were used to determine dosages for conscious sedation for children. The results from this method seemed to be more consistent. The best method seems to be previous experiences—the dentist's clinical usage and the patient's past response to a specific drug—and they are the most reliable determinants for safe and effective drug usage (Malamed, 1989).

Hydroxyzine

Effect

A drug of choice is hydroxyzine, a minor tranquilizer, and an antihistaminic, antispasmodic, antiemetic, and somewhat anticholinergic drug. When used as a comedication with meperidine or chloral hydrate, it allows for a lower dosage of these otherwise high dosage–strength drugs. Hydroxyzine is readily absorbed into the gastrointestinal tract and takes effect in about 30 minutes. The oral administration reaches peak effect in about 2 hours. The influence of the medication resolves itself in about 6 hours. It will suppress of modify patient responses to physical stimuli without tempering the patient's mental perspective.

Contraindications, toxic effects, and side effects

Hydroxyzine may heighten the action of meperidine and the barbiturates. When it is used in combination with these central nervous system depressants, the dosage should be reduced. The parent should be cautioned that the child may be drowsy and should not be left alone.

Dosage forms

Hydroxyzine HCI (Atarax) is available in the following oral dosage forms:

Tablets
10 mg (orange)
25 mg (green)
50 mg (yellow)
100 mg (red)
Syrup
10 mg/5-mL tsp in 473-mL (1 pt)
    bottles

Hydroxyzine pamoate (Vistaril) is available in the following oral dosage forms:

Capsules
25 mg (two-tone green)
50 mg (green and white)
100 mg (green and gray)
Oral suspension
25 mg/5-mL tsp in 473-mL (1 pt)
    bottles
Injectable (hydroxyzine HCI)
25 mg/mL in 10-mL vials
50 mg/mL in 2- and 10-mL vials

Precautions

This drug is especially effective in reducing anxiety and tension in younger children. In some instances, as the child gains confidence in his or her ability to cope with the dental appointments, the dosage can be reduced. The child is thus weaned from its use so that by the end of the series of appointments, the child can manage the situation with his or her own inner strength and newfound self-confidence.

Chloral hydrate

Effect

Chloral hydrate is a hypnotic that stimulates sleep at the cortical level, with no loss of reflexes, no after-effects, and a wide margin of safety.

Blood pressure and respiration are not affected if it is used within recommended limits. Chloral hydrate is an emetic, which is a disadvantage. Several authors discourage its use without combining it with another drug to counter this disadvantage (Brandt and Bugg, 1984; Barr et al, 1977).

Contraindications, toxic effects, and side effects

Chloral hydrate is contraindicated in patients with marked hepatic or renal impairment, patients receiving anticoagulants, and patients with previous hypersensitivity or idiosyncrasies. It should not be used for patients with severe cardiac disease. It has a tendency to produce nausea and vomiting.

Dosage forms

Syrup
500 mg/5mL in 473-mL (1-pt)
    or 3.8-L (1-g) container
Capsules
250 and 500 mg

Precautions

Nausea and vomiting are factors with chloral hydrate, but there is no antidote to reverse the effects.

Meperidine (Demerol)

Effect

Meperidine reduces pain and acts as an analgesic and sedative. When used within normal limits, it has little effect on the cardiovascular system.

Contraindications, toxic effects, and side effects

Its use is contraindicated in patients with severe liver dysfunction. In addition, it may cause respiratory depression in patients with increased intracranial pressure and intracranial lesions. Side effects include vertigo, dysphorea, nausea and vomiting, flushing of the face, syncope, and blurred vision.

Dosage forms

Syrup
50 mg/5mL
Tablets
50 mg
100 mg
Injectable
50, 75, and 100 mg/1 mL

Precautions

Local anesthesia usage should be minimized because of the relationship among local anesthesia, meperidine, and the increased tendency for convulsions (Brandt and Bugg, 1984).

Emergency care

Narcotic antagonists are administered IV, IM, or SQ:

1. Naloxone (Narcan, 0.4 mg/mL, does not depress respiration
2. Nalorphine (Nalline, 5 mg/1 mL
3. Levallorphan tartrate (Lorfan), 1 mg/1 mL, used only for severe respiratory depression

Drug combinations

Comedication is when one or more drugs, when combined, complement each other. However, these combinations do not provide a panacea for those dentists looking for a "magic potion."

A number of combinations of various drugs have been reported to be effective, Houpt (1993) surveyed the pediatric dentistry training programs in the United States to determine which drugs are used. He found 14 individual drugs and/or combinations of drugs. Among the popular combinations used, with or without nitrous oxide are:

1. Chloral hydrate and hydroxyzine
2. Chloral hydrate and hydroxyzine plus meperidine
3. Chloral hydrate and promethazine
4. Chloral hydrate and diazepan
5. Hydroxyzine and meperidine

When the drugs are combined, the side effects of one drug may offset the ill effects of another.

Management of complications

Procedures for handling airway obstruction, vomiting respiratory depression, bradycardia, and hypotension are given in Table 10-1. The dentist who elects to use conscious sedation must have the proper facilities, per-

Table 10-1 Management of complications

Airway obstruction
1. Extend the neck of the child.
2. Clear the mouth with your finger and then suction.
3. Perform oral airway maintenance.
4. Give oxygen by mask using a nitrous oxide analgesia machine. Use oxygen only.

Vomiting
1. Place the head down and turn to one side.
2. Suction the pharynx and oral cavity thoroughly.
3. Establish a clear airway.
4. If the child is nauseated after the treatment, give room-temperature carbonated soft drink.
5. If vomiting persists, consider the use of rectal trimethobenzamide (Tigan) as an antiemetic.

Respiratory depression
1. Be certain the airway is clear.
2. Reverse narcotic with a narcotic antagonist either SQ, IM, or IV.
3. Ventilate with positive-pressure oxygen.

Bradycardia
1. Give 0.5 mg of atropine IV, IM, or SQ.
2. Give positive-pressure oxygen.

Hypotension
1. Give positive-pressure oxygen.
2. Put patient in supine position.

sonnel training, and emergency equipment to manage the child in the dental operatory. Both the dentist and the staff should not only have the training to initiate a procedure using conscious sedation but also be able to reverse any undesirable reaction.

Postoperative instruction for parents

The last important act of the dentist before administering drugs to a child is to give the parent or guardian postoperative instruction. The following is a typical set of instructions that should be discussed in detail with the parent by the student or the dentist. (Note: This discussion should be recorded in the patient's chart.)

It is necessary to use sedative drugs to achieve dental care for your child. Please note the following:

1. It is most important that you tell the dentist of any drug reaction, unusual medical history, illness, or hospitalization your child has experienced.
2. The child must be accompanied by a parent for all appointments.
3. The first appointment may be necessary for adjustment of the proper drug dosage; therefore, little dental work may be accomplished.
4. The child may remain sleepy for a time after the appointment. Do not be alarmed as the drugs are wearing off. Your child can be irritable as this occurs.

5. Do not allow the child to bite his or her lip, tongue, or cheek if a local anesthetic is used.
6. After dental care, your child should be under adult supervision and not allowed to play near streets, stairways, or other areas where he or she may be injured by falling.
7. Cold drinks such as ginger ale or a cola will help reduce any nausea and help stimulate the patient to be more alert.
8. Should any unusual situation arise, please call the dentist as soon as possible.

Restraints

Restraints are used for infants, medicated children, and children with developmental disabilities. As with other methods of behavior control in the area of dentistry for children, the use of restraints has its followers and detractors. Kelly (1976) lists indications for the use of restraints:

1. The very young child, usually less than 3 years of age, with whom communication is a problem
2. The medicated child
3. The handicapped child, who, despite all good intentions, cannot control his or her involuntary movements
4. The potentially cooperative patient who misbehaves but has the potential to become a cooperative patient

Before any form of restraint is used, the patient and parent should have an explanation of its use, with the intent not to allow the child to harm himself or herself. As he or she learns to cooperate, the restraining device can be altered.

Two types of mouth props are in use (Fig 10-2). The bite block, with a piece of dental floss added, is used to hold the mouth open. The molt prop is adjustable and can be used at different degrees to open the child's mouth. The metal portion should be taped or covered with tubing to protect the child's teeth and tissue.

To control unwanted leg and arm movements, assist children with neurologic disabilities, or assist children with undue stress or stimulation, one commercial device available is a Pedi-Wrap (Fig 10-3). This device is a nylon sheet that encircles the child and is secured with Velcro straps. The Pedi-Wrap is for small children who are medicated for long, extensive restorative appointments.

A similar device is a Papoose Board, which is like the Pedi-Wrap but has a firm board (Fig 10-4). The Pedi-Wrap and Papoose Board are available in three sizes. The Papoose Board is excellent for larger children who have a developmental disability.

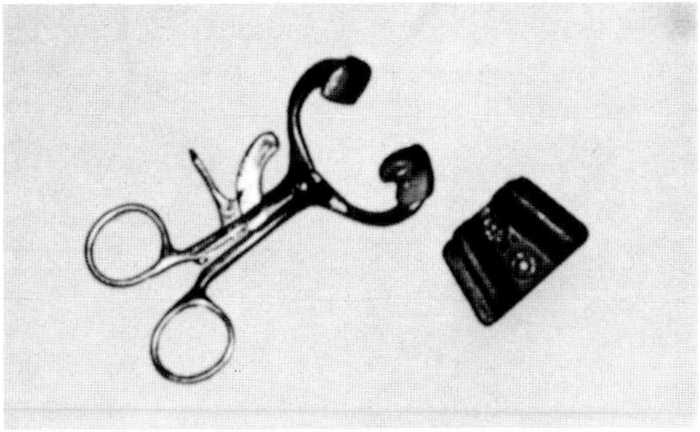

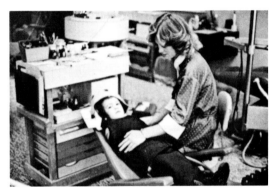

Fig 10-2 Several types of mouth props are available as aids to management.

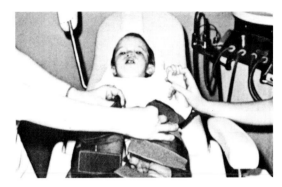

Fig 10-3 The Pedi-Wrap, using a mesh material and self-adhering straps, is one type of restraining device.

Parental attitudes and restraints

Assessments of parental attitudes on the use of restraining methods such as the Papoose Board have produced mixed results. Several studies report the use of such devices as least acceptable to parents (Murphy et al, 1984). However, Frankel (1991) evaluated 74 mothers whose children were uncooperative. With the use of nitrous oxide, local anesthesia, and a Papoose Board, dental care was completed. Fifty mothers gave the following responses to a questionnaire:

1. Ninety percent realized the restraint protected the child.
2. Seventy percent felt the child was comfortable during the procedure.
3. Sixty percent did not feel the child was more afraid.
4. Sixty-eight percent did not report a residual negative effect.
5. Eighty-six percent would elect to allow the same procedure again.

Again, the use of restraints depends on parental consent and the dentist's comfortableness with the procedure.

Sources

The Papoose Board is available from Olympic Medical Corporation, Seattle, Washington. The PediWrap is available from Clark Associates, Worcester, Massachusetts.

Documentation

The patient's chart should contain several items: *(1)* a copy of the signed consent form; *(2)* type of restraints used; *(3)* vital signs, including pulse, respiratory rate, blood pressure, and percent oxygen-hemoglobin satu-

Fig 10-4 The Papoose Board is similar to the Pedi-Wrap, but has the additional advantage of having a board attached to the back.

ration before, during, and at termination of treatment, and at discharge of the patient (Lout and Mathewson, 1988); *(4)* any unfavorable responses to the procedure; *(5)* medications given—route, site, type of drug, and dose; *(6)* copies of any prescriptions written; and *(7)* patient's status on discharge to the parent.

Success or failure of conscious sedation

Success or failure in the use of drugs to alter behavior may be affected by numerous factors:

1. Time of day of the appointment. An old debate has been whether the child should be seen in the morning when the child and the dentist are at their peaks or, with younger children, at naptime.
2. Parental anxiety and how the parents react to dentistry and their interrelationship with the dentist and the child.
3. Dentist's expectation. Does the dentist expect the drug or drugs used to completely immobilize the

child? Are the drugs used to relieve the anxiety of the dentist instead of the child? If these answers are "yes," the dentist may want to refer the child to someone who has the confidence to manage the situation.

4. Office environment. Is the dental office conducive to relaxation during the conscious sedation, or is it a stimulating atmosphere?

5. Children's much higher rate of metabolism, especially under stress, such as a dental appointment. The most frequent lack of success with conscious sedation is insufficient dose of the drug or drug combination.

6. Parental anxiety about the use of conscious sedation; they inadvertently give the wrong dosage.

7. Regurgitation of the medication, causing failure.

Finally, the management of children, with or without conscious sedation depends on the individual dentist's identification with the child, his or her philosophy of dental care, and the dentist's own sense of well being in the daily practice environment.

Note

This chapter provides the dental practitioner with general recommendations about prescription and administration of different drugs commonly used in pediataric dentistry. For more specific information concerning these medications, product package inserts, pharamacology textbooks, and pediatric dental literature are the best sources. The authors do not accept responsibility for the administration of these drugs in the private dental operatory.

References

American Academy of Pediatric Dentistry (AAPD). Guidelines for the elective use of pharmacologic conscious sedation and deep sedation in pediatric dental patients. Pediatr Dent 15:297, 1993.

Anderson, J. A., et al. Pulse oximetry: Evaluation of accuracy during out patient general anesthesia for oral surgery. Anesth. Prog. 35:53, 1988.

Anderson, J. A., and Van, W. F. Jr. Respiratory monitoring during pediatric sedation: Pulse oximetry and capnography. Pediatr. Dent. 10:94, 1988.

Barr, E. S., Wynn, R. L., and Spedding, R. H. Oral premedication of the problem child: Placebo and chloral hydrate. J. Pedod. 1:272, 1977.

Bennett, R. C. Sedation in Dental Practice. 2nd ed. St. Louis: The C. V. Mosby Co., 1978.

Brandt, S.K. and Bugg, J. L. Problems of medication with the pediatric patient. Dent. Clin. North Am. 28:563, 1984

Frankel, R. J. The Papoose board and mother's attitudes following its use. Pediatr. Dent. 13:285, l991.

Frankl, S. N. Shiere, F. R., and Fogels, H. R. Should the parent remain with the child in the dental operatory? J. Dent Child. 29:150, 1962.

Houpt, M. Project USAP the use of sedative agents in pediatric dentistry: 1991 update. Pediatr. Dent 15:36, 1993.

Kelly, J. R., The use of restraints in pedodontics. J. Pedod. 1:57, 1976.

Kopel, H. M. The use of ataractics in dentistry for children. J. Dent Child. 25:14, 1959.

Lout, R. K. and Mathewson, R. J. Effectiveness and safety of chloral hydrate hydroxyzine sedations in an undergraduate pediatric dental clinic. J. Dent. Res. 67:1988 (IADR abstract No. 385).

Malamed, S. F. Sedation: A Guide to Patient Management 2nd ed. St. Louis: The C. V. Mosby Co., 1989.

Moore, P. A. Therapeutic assessment of chloral hydrate premedication for pediatric dentistry Anesth. Prog. 31:191, 1984

Mueller, W. A., et al. Pulse oximetry monitoring of sedated pediatric dental patients. Anesth. Prog. 32:237, 1985.

Murphy, M. G., Fields, H. W. Jr. and J. B. Machen. Parental acceptance of pediatric dentistry behavior management techniques. Pediatr. Dent. 6:193, 1984.

Musselman, R. J. and McClure, D. B. Pharmoatherapeutic approaches to behavior management. In Wright G. Behavior Management in Dentistry for Children. Philadelphia: W. B. Saunders Co., 1975, p. 172.

Wright, G. Z. Starkey, P. E., and Gardner, D. E. Managing Children's Behavior in the Dental Office. Philadelphia: W. B. Saunders Co., 1983.

Additional readings

Aubuchon, R. W. Sedation liabilities in pedodontics. Pediatr. Dent. 4(1):171, 1982.

Badalaty, M. M., et al. A comparison of chloral hydrate and diazepam sedation in young children. Pediatr. Dent. 12:33, 1990.

Hasty, M. F., et al. Conscious sedation of pediatric dental patients: An investigation of chloral hydrate, hydroxyzine-pamoate, and meperidine vs. chloral hydrate and hydroxyzinepamoate. Pediatr. Dent. 13:10, 1991.

Houpt, M. I., et al. Comparison of chloral hydrate with and without promethazine in the sedation of young children. Pediatr. Dent. 7:41, 1985.

Moore, P. A., et al. Sedation in pediatric dentistry: A practical assessment procedure. J. Am. Dent. Assoc. 109:564, 1984.

Poorman, T. L. Farrington, F. H., and Mourino, A. P. Comparison of a chloral hydrate/hydroxize conbination with and without meperidine in the sedation of pediatric dental patients. Pediatra. Dent. 12:289, 1990.

Tobias, M. Lipshultz, D. H., and Album, M. M. A study of three preoperative sedative combinations J. Dent. Child 42:453, 1975.

Verwest, T. M., Primosch, R. E., and Courts, F. J. Variables influencing hemoglobin oxygen desaturation in children during routine restorative dentistry. Pediatr. Dent. 15:25, 1993.

White, T. R., and Dalzell, D. P. Drug Syllabus for Pediatric Dentistry. Oklahoma City: Oklahoma University Press, 1993.

Wilson, S. Chloral hydrate and its effects on multiple physiological parameters in young children: A dose-response study. Pediatr. Dent. 14:171, 1992.

Questions

1. A small patient, aged 3, is referred to your office as a "behavior problem." What is the most accurate statement?

   a. Arrangements should be made to medicate the patient so that the initial visit will be pleasant

   b. The child should be seen initially without medication

   c. Nitrous oxide will likely be needed to examine the child

   d. This problem is not unusual; all small children present behavior problems

2. A 4-year-old child needs some assistance for acceptable behavior in the dental office. Conscious sedation is desired. What factors will aid in predicting and controlling desired results of orally administered medication?

   a. Emotional age of the patient

   b. Weight, height, and chronologic age of the child

   c. Stomach contents

   d. Emotional maturity of the parents

   e. All of the above

3. A 4-year-old patient visits your office for her initial dental examination. You evaluate her as a timid, shy patient. Which medication would be the best for this patient?

   a. Hydroxyzine (Atarax) and hydroxyzine pamoate (Vistaril) in divided doses

   b. Diazepam (Valium) alone

   c. Promethazine (Phenergan) alone

   d. Meperidine (Demerol) alone

   e. Naloxone (Narcan)

4. A 6-year old boy is medicated with meperidine HCl. He has a negative medical history, however, and he experiences respiratory depression. Which antagonist can be given this patient without the risk of further respiratory depression?

   a. Naloxone (Narcan)

   b. Nalorphine (Nalline)

   c. Levallorphan tartrate (Lorfan)

   d. Epinephrine

   e. Alphaprodine (Nisentil)

5. A 2-year-old patient visits for treatment of "nursing bottle syndrome." He has to have four anterior crowns completed in one visit. The rest of the primary teeth are free of dental caries. The patient is difficult to treat, and you decide to use conscious sedation. The medication of choice is:

   a. Nitrous oxide analgesia

   b. Meperidine (Demerol)

   c. Naloxone (Narcan)

   d. Promethazine (Phenergan)

   e. Chloral hydrate plus either hydroxyzine HCl (Atarax) or hydroxyzine pamoate (Vistaril)

Chapter 11

Hospital Dentistry

Objectives

After studying this chapter, the student should be familiar with:
1. The indications for hospital treatment of a patient.
2. The record systems necessary for hospital treatment of a patient.
3. The sequence of procedures used in the practice of hospital dental care.
4. Alternative to inpatient care, that is, outpatient or ambulatory general anesthesia.

Philosophy

As a dentist, you must decide what represents acceptable behavior from dental patients. If the behavior is unacceptable following behavior modification and conscious sedation, you should consider hospitalizing the patient to provide treatment.

Educational background

Dentists electing to treat children in the hospital should have formal training as a general practice resident where a hospital rotation is part of the experience or as a graduate student in pediatric dentistry with a hospital rotation that may include hands-on training in general anesthesia.

Hospital selection

Musselman and Roy (1974) suggested several criteria for selection of a hospital for the general practitioner:

1. An established dental service or clinic
2. Acceptance by the hospital's physicians and administrators of the need to use general anesthesia to complete dental care for young children and the handicapped
3. Hospital staff experiences in using anesthesia for dental procedures

4. Availability of operating room time and patient beds
5. Outpatient general anesthesia service
6. Pediatric department with personnel who understand the needs of children during the hospital stay
7. Availability of mobile, portable, or modified dental equipment for providing dental care
8. Close proximity to the dentist's private office

Staff membership

The dentist who would like hospital staff privileges must make application for a staff appointment and privileges. This application is usually handled by the hospital administration. The application will state what kind of privileges are available and will allow the dentist to select which privileges he or she would like. The application is reviewed by the appropriate committee, and privileges are extended commensurate with training and experience.

Patient selection and evaluation

The selection and evaluation of patients to be admitted to the hospital for dental surgery under general anesthesia usually are discussed according to patient eligibility and patient classification of physical status. The following categories illustrate patients whose dental care can most appropriately be accomplished in the hospital:

1. Patients with serious medical problems who may be compromised in an outpatient, nonhospitalized environment
2. Patients who pose a serious medical or anesthesia risk in an outpatient, nonhospitalized environment
3. Patients with a need for complex or extensive (or both) dental care that can be accomplished more safely and conveniently with a multidisciplinary team of health care professionals
4. Patients with handicapping medical conditions or disorders, whether they be physical, emotional, or mental, that may not be appropriately treated in an outpatient, nonhospitalized environment
5. Patients in very young age categories who require special medical or anesthesia considerations
6. Patients with emergency dental needs isolated from or in conjunction with emergency medical needs where a multidisciplinary health care team approach is desirable
7. Patients with oral disease who require special preoperative diagnostic and consulting services where a multidisciplinary health care team approach is desirable

Physical status classification system

In 1962 the American Society of Anesthesiologists adopted what is now commonly referred to as the ASA physical status classification system. It represents a method of estimating the medical risk factor presented by a patient about to undergo a surgical procedure in a hospital setting. The system was designed primarily for patients about to receive a general anesthetic, but, since its introduction, the classification system has been used for all surgical patients, regardless of the anesthetic technique employed (eg, general anesthesia, regional anesthesia, or sedation).

Physical status 1: patient without systemic disease; a normal, healthy patient
Physical status 2: patient with mild systemic disease
Physical status 3: patient with severe systemic disease that limits activity but is not incapacitating
Physical status 4: patient with incapacitating systemic disease that is a constant threat to life
Physical status 5: moribund patient not expected to survive 24 hours with or without operation
Physical status E: emergency operation of any variety that precedes the number (eg, E-3)

Hospital procedures

What are the steps needed to hospitalize a child and complete dental care?

Step 1: Initial examination

At the time of the initial dental appointment, perform a complete examination: *(1)* obtain a health history, including any medication or other abnormal medical findings; *(2)* determine the family and social background; and *(3)* identify the chief complaint. If at all possible, complete an oral, clinical, and radiographic examination. Follow-up radiographs and a more in-depth oral diagnosis with a resulting treatment plan may have to be postponed until the child has been given a general anesthetic. If possible, from the above information, establish a sequence of dental care. At this time decide if further consultations are needed.

Step 2: Parental consultation

Discussion with the parent the need for hospital admission. For example, in a certain case you might explain:

1. A large quantity of active dental caries requires restoration
2. The age of the child results in his or her failure to understand and cooperate
3. Because of these two factors, the best method would be to admit the child for a general anesthetic in a hospital

Describe the risks involved with general anesthesia. If possible, give the parent an estimate of the expense of hospitalization, medical costs, anesthesia costs, and cost of the restorative procedures. Because the child is unmanageable, an estimate of cost may have to be postponed because of the lack of oral and clinical data. Outline to the parents the sequence for any necessary consultation, physical examination, dental insurance procedures, and admission to the hospital.

It is appropriate to discuss the various preventive measures with the parent to avoid further oral health problems.

Emphasize that if there are any problems or questions, the parent is to call you for any information.

Steps 3: Consultations

Discuss with the child's physician the nature of the dental care and medical clearance for both the dentistry and the anesthesia. If no special medical or surgical clearance is indicated, proceed to arrange the time for the operating room. If there is any contraindication to dentistry or to anesthesia, schedule the patient with the appropriate physician and await his or her consultation before scheduling the surgery. If the patient is free of any known contraindication, as determined by the physician, proceed with the scheduling. The child's physician will see the patient before admission or during admission (or both) for an updated medical survey and physical examination.

Step 4: Preadmission

If the parent has hospitalization insurance coverage, including anesthesia benefits, prior authorization may be needed before hospital admission and surgery. Many times a physician's statement of patient health care needs is required by an insurance carrier before coverage is granted for hospitalization and anesthesia for dental care. If so, the patient must be scheduled to see an attending staff physician for consultation. If the patient has insurance coverage for dental care, prior authorization must obtained before the performance of dental surgery. This authorization usually requires submission of clinical and, where feasible, radiographic examinations to determine and approve the prescribed treatment plan.

Call the surgical scheduling office at the hospital to arrange for a tentative time for the procedure and reservation of the operation room suite. Call the patient admitting office at the hospital to arrange for a bed the day of surgery as well as the day before surgery. Both the surgical scheduling office and the patient admitting office will usually require the following information:

1. Date of desired admission
2. Name and service of dentist and physician
3. Name, age, and sex of patient
4. Diagnosis and approximate days of hospital stay
5. Accommodations required (private room, intensive care unit)
6. Parent's name, address, telephone number
7. Insurance company group number

Step 5: One week before appointment

Check on any insurance authorization that was pending approval for hospitalization, anesthesia, or dental care. If this approval has not been obtained, verbal authorization of impending written authorization is necessary before proceeding on any scheduled hospitalization. If authorization has been denied for hospitalization, anesthesia, or dental care, the parent must be notified. The parent then will incur the full expenses of the procedures.

Check with the attending staff physician concerning the confirmation of the admitting date and your coadmission of the patient. The attending staff physician in many hospitals is responsible for the medical survey and the management of any concurrent or arising medical problems. Many times the attending staff physician will want to do a medical survey within 48 hours before the admission if he or she is unable to do the medical survey at the time of admission.

Check with the patient admitting office and the surgical scheduling office to ensure specific dates on admission day, operating day, time duration, and tentative discharge day. Check with the supervisor of the operating room regarding operating room personnel and the equipment needed for the dental surgery. Inform the parents of the impending hospital admission date. Answer any questions that they might have. Confirm arrangement for the admission procedures as to:

1. When (date and time).
2. Where (place in hospital).
3. What to bring (personal hygiene equipment, insurance forms, etc).
4. Legal consent; because the patient is a minor, a legal guardian must accompany patient to sign necessary consent form and to give pertinent information. If legal guardian(s) cannot be in attendance, signed surgical consent must be forwarded to the hospital before admission of the patient.

Step 6: Patient admittance

The patient should report to patient admitting office per your directions according to date and time, with the prescribed articles, insurance documents, signed consent, etc. The patient will get a hospital card, hospital chart, and identification bracelet. A financial screening will usually be accomplished at this time. A consent form for anesthesia and surgery will be completed if it has not already been done. Completion of this form is very important.

The patient will be visited in the ward, room and/or bed by:

1. Nursing service for nursing notes
2. Patient representative for social notes
3. Physician for medical survey
4. Dentist for preoperative orders
5. Anesthesiology for preanesthesia orders
6. Laboratory technician for blood, urine, etc
7. Radiology technician for chest radiograph

Step 7: Preoperative procedures

Visit with the patient on the ward as soon as possible after patient admission. By this time the patient will have been visited by nursing services and should have a medical chart on the ward. Check the medical chart for accuracy in the patient's background data and consent.

Review admission nursing notes in the progress notes section of the chart. Write admission notes in the progress notes section, the purpose of which is to communicate to all ward personnel the purpose of the admission and general status of the patient. Included is the following information:

1. Number of previous admissions
2. Patient resume: *(a)* patient background, *(b)* social family history, *(c)* health history, *(d)* chief complaint, *(e)* current medications, *(f)* previous hospitalization or surgeries (dates, types, complications), and *(g)* allergies and which types
3. A general dental diagnosis (problem oriented, priorities, reason for admission, patient category)
4. Date and time of prospective operation and nature of operation (treatment plans)
5. Any medical alerts

Check to ensure the patient's medical history and physical examination has been performed by the child's physician and review this survey. Many times it is advantageous to do this review in conjunction with the physician. In some hospitals the anesthesiologist will be the attending coadmitting staff physician assigned to the patient. Write preoperative orders in the physician's orders section.

These preoperative orders should include:

1. Diet description and restrictions
2. Activities description and restrictions
3. Laboratory studies needed for anesthesia and surgical clearance
4. Medication continuance and special medications needed
5. Consultation requests as needed
6. On call for operating room

Check to ensure the preanesthesia evaluation is scheduled for anesthesiology. Preanesthesia orders must be written by the anesthesiologist in the physician's orders section of the medical chart and progress notes.

Visit the patient on the ward the evening before surgery. The purpose of this late visit is to ensure the patient's readiness for the surgery to follow. A preoperative visit note should be written in the progress notes section of the medical chart. It should include specific comments on:

1. Patient's comfort
2. Patient's adjustment to hospital environment
3. Patient's vital signs and appearance
4. Laboratory results
5. Consultation reports
6. Anesthesia preoperative orders

The responsible physician or dentist should record and authenticate the preoperative diagnosis. This diagnosis should include a written summary of clinical and laboratory findings.

Step 8: Equipment preparation

During the week before the dental operation, make a list of all necessary equipment that must be in the operating room at the hospital. Call the hospital operating room supervisor and inquire as to the status of the equipment that is usually furnished by most hospitals. Equipment and supplies that are not supplied by the hospital are the responsibility of the dentist and his or her staff. These supplies should be prepared well in advance of the impending dental operation to ensure their availability. All equipment that can be sterilized should be. All other equipment and supplies should be as disinfected as possible. The dentist and staff should bring all necessary equipment and supplies to the hospital the day of the operation. In some hospitals, the operating room staff will scrub and sterilize the instruments before the dental appointment.

During the week before the dental operation, review your dental assistant utilization program for the dental operation. Many hospitals will furnish you with a nurse in the operating room, but his or her skills may be limited in areas of dentistry. It is advisable for the dentist to bring one or two dental assistants from the dental office who are well trained in hospital operating room procedures and dental assisting.

The day of the dental operation arrive at the hospital at least 1 hour before the scheduled dental operation. Proceed to the surgical area where you will change from your street clothes to your surgical clothes, normally including shirt, trousers, shoe covers, head or face cover, and surgical mask. All jewelry should be kept in your locker. Inform the supervising nurse that you are available so that the patient's floor can be notified for transport to the operating room suite.

Step 9: Anesthesia induction

Arrange to meet your patient in the surgical holding area. The patient will be premedicated and may or may not be able to converse with you. Review the medical chart to ensure that all necessary data is in order for general anesthesia.

Proceed to the assigned operating room. If no one is operating in the room, place your mask on your face and enter the room. Check all equipment you intend to use for the dental operation. Have your dental assistant, who is similarly gowned, prearrange your dental instruments and supplies so as not to interfere with the transferring of the patient and his or her anesthesia induction. The instruments are usually placed on Mayo stands.

The patient will be brought into the operating room and transferred to the operating table from the mobile cart. The anesthesiologist and staff will attend to the patient, usually as shown in Fig 11-1.

After the anesthesiologist has the established monitoring devices and intravenous (IV) route, induction begins. In younger children, induction may begin with a low percentage of anesthetic gases. In older children, a barbiturate may be used. Intravenous succinylcholine or a similar drug is now administered to assist in the induction of the patient.

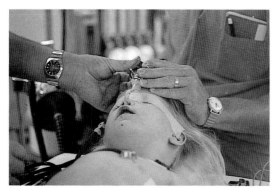

Fig 11-1 A precordial stethoscope and a pulse monitor are taped to the patient's chest. A rectal or axillary temperature monitor is placed on the patient. Cardiac monitoring equipment may also be placed on the patient.

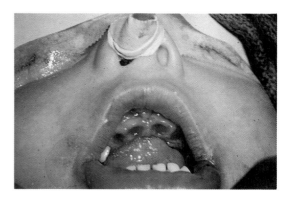

Fig 11-2 The nasal endotracheal tube taped in place.

The dentist should request nasal intubation versus oral intubation for maintenance of the anesthetic state. When the anesthesiologist has completed the placement of the nasal tube, the tube should be taped in place on the child's face and nose. Some anesthesiologists will place in ophthalmic ointment in the eyes and then tape them shut to prevent conjunctivitis and foreign bodies in the eyes (Fig 11-2).

Step 10: Restorative procedure

The patient should now be draped for the dental procedure. The dental surgery equipment is brought into place using instrument setups.

Follow the specific hospital operating room protocol as to further clothing procedures and scrubbing procedures that are necessary. In general, a presurgical scrub for you and your staff is necessary. For soft tissue surgical procedures, gloves as well as sterilized secondary clothing are usually mandatory.

A throat pack is now placed carefully by the dentist, using tied sponge material or sutured 5-cm (2-in.) gauze. Petroleum jelly or other suitable lubricant should be placed on the patient's lips.

If intraoral radiographs are to be taken, they should be accomplished as rapidly as possible. Lead aprons and gloves should be available and used for attending personnel.

While the radiographs are being processed, the patient should have a routine prophylaxis with necessary scaling and polishing. With processed radiographs, a definitive diagnosis and treatment plan can be established and recorded. Proceed with the necessary dental care. Use rubber dam wherever possible.

Several rules of thumb are considered standard operating procedures. Remember that this patient is a management problem and the restorative procedures should be done with the intent to function for a long time:

1. Any two or more surfaces of caries should be restored with a stainless steel crown.
2. Any incipient interproximal or developmental precarious lesions should be restored.
3. There should be no heroic pulp therapy with the intent to use the procedure with the highest percentage of predicted success. In other words, indirect pulp capping and direct pulp capping procedures should not be done as pulp procedures in the primary dentition. If there is doubt as to pulpal success, remove the tooth.
4. Where possible in normal younger children, direct space maintainers should be fabricated.

All tissues removed during the procedure should be forwarded to the hospital pathologist for diagnosis and his or her signed report.

Always keep the anesthesiologist informed as to the anticipated finishing time because the time will influence anesthetic choice on the patient and the postoperative recovery time. If oral surgery is anticipated, do not leave these procedures to the last, because the patient will recover without a proper period of time for you to evaluate postoperative hemorrhage. The use of sutures should definitely be considered whenever possible.

About 15 minutes before the procedure is to be completed, tell the anesthesiologist that you are about finished with the procedure. The amount of gaseous anesthesia can be reduced, and the patient will receive a high percentage of oxygen.

Rinse and thoroughly aspirate the mouth. Gently remove the throat pack and inspect the area for any debris. The anesthesiologist will use an aspirating tube to clear the nasal area, pharynx, and throat of debris and accumulated fluids.

Step 11: Postoperative procedures

Do not leave the operating room until the patient is extubated and reacting. Remain in the operating room and organize your operative summary, postoperative orders, and dictated operative report. Accompany the patient to the recovery room and do an immediate follow-up oral examination. Many times, the patient will have an oral airway tube in place. Reassurance to the patient during this period is often very helpful for recovery.

Complete the operative summary and postoperative order forms in the patient's medical chart while the patient and chart are still in the recovery room. The operative summary, or the record of operation, is a brief form used in hospitals for the purpose of detailing the parameters of the operation itself. It is primarily used for legal and accounting purposes. The dictated operative report will explain in greater detail the dental procedures. The operative summary should include:

1. Names of surgeons and assistants
2. Preoperative diagnosis
3. Anesthesia type and duration
4. Postoperative diagnosis
5. Surgical procedure description or charting
6. Amount and type of intravenous fluids
7. Tubes and drains placed
8. Closures and sutures
9. Pathology specimens submitted
10. Complications
11. Risks
12. Postoperative condition of patient

The postoperative orders are very important because these instruct other professionals in the hospital on the manner and way in which you wish the patient to be cared for until discharge from the hospital. These orders are completed in the physician's orders section of the patient's chart and must be signed. Postoperative orders should include:

1. Vital signs recording
2. Position of patient
3. Lip and nostril medications
4. Removal of packs, etc
5. Intravenous fluids continuance
6. Diet restriction
7. Activities restriction
8. Medication continuance and commencement
9. Special orders
10. Patient discharge orders
11. On call information for dentist

After you have finished the operative report and postoperative orders and visited the patient in the recovery room, go immediately to the patient's ward or bed where you can discuss the anesthesia and surgery with the parents or guardians.

Return to the surgical suite area and dictate the operative report. This report is usually done on a telephone or dictating machine following a prescribed format for each hospital. Check the patient once again before leaving. When a report is dictated, the format usually is:

1. Dictating physician
2. Patient's name
3. Hospital number
4. Date of operation
5. Surgeon
6. Assistants
7. Preoperative diagnosis
8. Postoperative diagnosis
9. Name of operation
10. Indication for surgery
11. Gross findings*
12. Procedure†
    a. Preparation
    b. Procedure
    c. Tissues removed
    d. Closure
    e. Drains
    f. Sponge and needle counts
    g. Condition of patient

Go back to the surgeon's lounge and change from your surgical clothes. You may wish to leave the hospital to return to your office. It is advisable to be available during this time to direct any postoperative orders that might become necessary to overcome a complication.

Return to the hospital and see the patient for a postoperative visit and write a postoperative visit note in the progress notes in the patient's chart. This note is simply an assessment of the patient's postanesthesia course and a comment on any postoperative sequelae. Any time a patient is visited on the ward by the dentist, a progress note should made on the chart. If the patient is to stay the night, so state in the progress notes. Routine postoperative visit notes should include the following information:

1. General status of the patient (eg, awake, asleep, agitated, crying).
2. Vital signs: temperature, respiration, blood pressure, pulse.
3. Fluid balance: IV infusing, infiltrated, or discontinued? If IV is not in place, is the patient taking fluids postoperatively? On the output side, has the patient voided or is he or she vomiting?
4. Patient comfort: Does the patient seem to be experiencing pain or discomfort (is he or she restless, unable to sleep, or feeling nauseous)?

---

*Describe all pathologic findings and all organs explored, normal and abnormal.
†Describe technique of all operations performed.

5. Bleeding: Does the patient seem to be clotting normally in sites of extraction or incision?
6. Restorations: Are there any obvious restorations in disrepair (crowns that have dislodged or amalgam restorations that have fractured)?

Also note any palliative treatment rendered for problems associated with Nos. 1 to 6. Note your name and a telephone number where you can be reached should emergency or postoperative complications develop.

Step 12: Discharge and follow-up care

Review the patient's progress and determine if the patient is ready for discharge. Discharge orders should not be written until the nurse's notes have been reviewed to clear any problems in voiding, bleeding, eating, vital signs, etc, and the patient has been evaluated by the attending anesthesiologist and attending physician. If these steps have been taken, you may write the discharge orders in the physician's orders section of the patient's chart and in the progress notes.

After you write the discharge order, you now must write the discharge note in the progress notes. The purpose of the discharge note is to summarize the hospital course and discharge status of the patient. The discharge note temporarily functions in lieu of the more complete discharge summary (which is dictated and is therefore not returned to the chart for several weeks). The discharge note should include:

1. Date of admission
2. Diagnosis
3. Procedure performed
4. Complications
5. Discharge status
6. Date of discharge
7. Disposition (to parents at ____ am/pm)
8. Follow-up
9. Dentist's signature

Dictate a discharge summary for the patient's chart. The discharge summary is a condensation of all information bearing on the present admission. For legal and accounting purposes it is important that all details that substantiate the whole period of hospital stay be included in the discharge summary. It should include:

1. Date admitted
2. Date discharged
3. Brief summary statement describing this admission and the patient's background
4. Social family history: indicate marital status, family situation, etc
5. Health history: indicate medical and dental findings of significance
6. Chief complaint

7. Previous hospitalizations: type, dates, complications
8. Previous surgeries: type, date, complications
9. Present medication
10. Allergies
11. Physical examination
12. Discharge diagnosis: the problem for which the patient was originally admitted, followed by the treatment status of that problem at the time of discharge (example: rampant dental caries; status after dental oral rehabilitation)
13. Discharge medications
14. Recommendations
15. Disability
16. Dentist's signature

The patient who has had restorative procedures in the hospital should have an immediate follow-up appointment as indicated by the type of surgery. In general dental cases, the normal follow-up is 1 week later in the dental office. In other surgical cases involving periodontal or oral surgery, the follow-up should be sooner.

At the follow-up visit, the following items should be discussed with the parent or patient:

1. Review of the radiographs, plus the diagnosis and treatment plan that was completed in the operating room
2. Nature of the restorative procedure that was accomplished
3. Continuation of postoperative instruction and commencement of new instructions for preventive maintenance
4. Any medications that should be continued or commenced
5. The preventive dental program for the patient, including nutritional counseling
6. A recall program for the patient
7. Any insurance forms that were not yet discussed or completed
8. Any follow-up visits deemed necessary for anesthesia or medical consultations

All dictated reports accomplished at the hospital must be completed.

At the time of signing out all dictated reports in the chart, review the chart for completeness and designate that you have done so in the progress notes section of the chart. This chart should include:

1. Patient identification
2. Complaints
3. Personal history, family history, and history of present illness
4. Physical examination
5. Special report, consultation, and clinical laboratory reports
6. Radiographs
7. Provisional diagnosis

8. Medical and dental treatment
9. Operative reports
10. Pathologic findings
11. Progress notes, final diagnosis, and condition on discharge
12. Discharge summary and follow-up

This step-by-step procedure follows the procedures used in most hospitals. The dentist, with careful planning in consultation with the hospital support staff, will find care for dental patients in the hospital a rewarding and enjoyable experience.

Ambulatory or outpatient anesthesia

With higher cost of hospitalization for inpatient dental care, use of outpatient anesthesia for selected patients has increased (Davis and Bierenbaum, 1982). Insurance programs, both private and governmental have expressed interest in this mode of care. Costs have been reduced by this type of service. Patient selection uses the same ASA guidelines but selection is limited to those in the ASA physical status categories 1 and 2. Ferretti (1984) lists several additional factors in the patient-selection process, including *(1)* the ability of the parents or guardians to provide reliable preoperative and postoperative care for the child and *(2)* the parents' financial status. Steps 1 through 12 as previously described for inpatient treatment are similar in the ambulatory method, but the patient is admitted and discharged the same day. Only postoperative and discharge procedures are abbreviated. Some authors believe the discharge decision is one of common sense (Brown, 1978; Stark, 1985). A follow-up telephone call in the evening will allow you to assess the quality of care and determine if any complications are present. Ferretti (1984) lists the advantages of this approach to anesthesia:

1. Tremendous monetary savings
2. Reduction in the volume of records needed
3. Effective and efficient use of medical personnel time
4. Reduction of the psychologic trauma caused when the child is separated from parents

References

Brown, B. R., Jr., ed. Outpatient Anesthesia. Philadelphia: R. A. Davis Co., 1978.

Davis, M. J., and Bierenbaum, H. J. Hospital care in pedodontics: A survey of current practices. Pediatr. Dent. 4:245, 1982.

Ferretti, G. A. Guidelines for outpatient general anesthesia to provide comprehensive dental treatment. Dent. Clin. North Am. 28:107, 1984.

Musselman, R. J., and Roy, E. K. Hospital management of the handicapped patient. Dent. Clin. North Am. 18:699, 1974.

Stark, D. C., ed. Practical Points in Anesthesiology. 3rd ed. New Hyde Park, N. Y.: Medical Examination Publ. Co., Inc. 1985.

Questions

1. Which of the following patients should be considered candidates for hospitalization for completion of dental care?

   a. An 11-year-old boy with type A hemophilia requiring several retained primary molar extractions

   b. A 3-year-old girl with rampant caries needing seven pulpotomies, eight stainless steel crowns, and four extractions

   c. An 18-year-old woman with cerebral palsy, who is also mentally retarded, with 21 surfaces of active caries

   d. A 4-year-old boy with a history of chronic heart disease needing a minimum of seven stainless steel crowns, where oral examination is difficult due to his immaturity

   e. A 3-year-old girl needing 16 primary teeth restored but living 250 miles from the nearest dentist

   f. b,c,d

   g. c,d,e

   h. a,d,e

   i. a,e

   j. All of the above

2. A 3-year-old child has complete restorative care using general anesthesia. The radiographs reveal small incipient interproximal caries on the first and second maxillary right primary molars. The teeth should be treatment planned for:

   a. Back-to-back silver amalgam restoration

   b. Pulpotomies plus stainless steel crowns

   c. Stainless steel crowns

   d. None of the above

3. For the dentist doing the restorative procedure in the hospital operating room, the first step after the patient has been intubated, had the eyes taped shut, been draped and prepped, is to:

   a. Take any needed radiographs

   b. Do an oral examination

   c. Place a throat pack

   d. Do a thorough prophylaxis before doing an oral examination

   e. Complete the treatment plan

4. A 5.5 year old child is having complete dental care done using general anesthesia. The radiographs reveal that the four primary maxillary incisors have pulpal exposures. These incisors should be treatment planned for:

   a. Extractions

   b. Pulpotomies plus anterior crowns

   c. Pulpotomies only

   d. Pulpotomies plus anterior crowns

   e. Extractions plus a removable space maintainer

5. The anesthesiologist has been informed that the restorative procedures will be done in 15 minutes. The last crowns have been cemented and cleaned, the rubber dam removed, occlusion checked, and the mouth rinsed with all remaining debris removed. The next step is to:

   a. Remove any dental instruments from the area

   b. Fill out the operating room report

   c. Complete the treatment plan

   d. Remove the throat pack

   e. Write the postoperative orders

Chapter 12

Local Anesthesia

Objectives

After studying this chapter, the student should be able to:
1. Describe the psychologic preparation of the child for the local anesthesia procedure.
2. Describe the rationale for choosing a local anesthetic agent suitable for the child patient.
3. Describe the philosophy of the local anesthetic syringe exchange process.
4. Identify the penetration site landmarks used in the local anesthesia procedures.
5. Describe the techniques for anesthetizing pertinent areas of the oral cavity.
6. Describe the maximum safe dose of a local anesthetic agent permissible for a given pediatric patient.

The control of pain while performing dental procedures for the child is one of the most fundamental and important components supporting sound principles of behavior management.

Pain control for the child is provided in most instances by means of a skilled and sensible local anesthetic delivery technique. The successful administration of the anesthetic agent is based on the concept of psychologic preparation and a skillful administration of the agent.

Agent types

Duration of action and potency

The duration of action of local anesthetics is directly proportional to protein-binding characteristics (Covino, 1981). Agents that are highly protein bound (for example, etidocaine and bupivacaine) have the longest duration of action, whereas those with lower protein-binding capacities (for example, lidocaine and mepivicaine) have shorter durations of action. The relationship between protein-binding of local anesthetic agents and their duration of action is consistent with the basic structure of the nerve membrane. Proteins account for approximately 10% of the nerve membrane. Agents that penetrate proteins,

therefore, will tend to possess a prolonged duration of anesthetic activity.

Local anesthetics such as mepivicaine, lidocaine, and prilocaine are most commonly employed in the dentistry, but recently etidocaine and bupivicaine, which have a higher potency and longer duration of action, have become popular to control postsurgical pain. These latter agents can produce conduction anesthesia for up to 20 hours; however, the average duration is 4 to 8 hours. Their greatest advantage is that they can produce prolonged relief of pain, thereby eliminating or significantly reducing the need for systemic analgesics.

Local anesthetics may also be classified according to their potency. Potency is usually described in terms of the minimal anesthetic concentration that blocks impulse conduction within a specified period of time. Local anesthetic potency is related to a number of physicochemical properties, including intrinsic vasodilator activity, tissue diffusion characteristics, and lipid solubility. Lipid solubility is the single most important determinant of local anesthetic potency. Highly lipid-soluble anesthetics are very potent, whereas those with low lipid solubility have low potency. Etidocaine, with a relatively high potency, has a lipid-solubility coefficient of 141. Lidocaine, with a lipid-solubility coefficient of 2.9, is one fourth as potent as etidocaine (Milam and Giovannitti, 1984).

Difficulty in obtaining profound regional anesthesia

may be a consequence of the pH of the tissue into which the solution is injected, the pKa of the local anesthetic drug, or the pH of anesthetic solution itself. The free base, or un-ionized, form of the local anesthetic molecule is responsible for diffusion across the membrane to the receptor site. The charged, or ionized, form of the local anesthetic molecule is believed to be responsible for binding at the receptor and producing conduction blockade. The relative proportion between the base form and the ionized form depends on the pH of the tissues and the pKa of the specific local anesthetic agent. The pKa is defined as the pH at which 50% of a drug is ionized. In general, among local anesthetics at the same concentration, the lower the pK value, the more rapid the onset of anesthesia and vice versa. The most effective local anesthetics in a tissue environment with low pH (for example, an area of inflammation) are those with the lowest pKa values (etidocaine) (Covino, 1981).

Duration of action may also be related to the volume of anesthetic solution administered, but the evidence is conflicting. Aberg and Sydnes (1978) achieved a significant difference in duration of anesthesia in permanent teeth by increasing volume from 0.9 to 1.8 mL, but found no difference between 0.45 and 0.9 mL. They also demonstrated that duration increases with increasing concentration of solution. In a pulp test study evaluating local anesthetics, Vreeland et al (1989), however, found that increasing neither the volume nor the concentration of lidocaine increases the success of pulpal anesthesia. The current recommendation for the initial volume of solution administered in children is not clearly defined. Malamed (1990a) recommended using 1.5 mL of 2% lidocaine for achieving mandibular anesthesia in adults, while the manufacturer (Astra Pharmaceuticals, 1987) suggests 0.9 to l.0 mL is sufficient in children younger than 10 years old.

Mechanism of action

Because local anesthetic agents are weak bases, they are commonly combined with a strong acid (for example, hydrochloric acid) to improve water solubility, tissue diffusibility, and stability in solution. When the acid is injected into the tissue, it is presumed to interact with tissue buffers, forming free base, or un-ionized form. This un-ionized form permits diffusion of the local anesthetic across the nerve membrane, where it then dissociates into a charged or ionized form. The charged form of the local anesthetic molecule is believed responsible for the resulting nerve blockade.

Several mechanisms of action have been proposed for nerve conduction blockade by local anesthetics, although the exact mechanism is not clear. Local anesthetics are suggested to interfere with the conduction of action potentials along peripheral nerve fibers by impairing the functions of sodium ion channels. Nerve impulses cannot be proprogated when inadequate numbers of sodium channels are available (Courtney, 1988). Propagation of impulses along a nerve fiber will be blocked when a sufficiently large length of nerve membrane is impaired. That length has been determined to be three consecutive nodes of Ranvier (Blair and Erlanger, 1939) which is approximately a 1.8-mm length of the inferior alveolar nerve (Brown, 1981). Recovery from nerve blockade is dependent on redistribution and metabolism of the local anesthetic solution.

Metabolism and excretion

The amino-ester local anesthetics are hydrolized by plasma cholinesterase. Any factor that would contribute to a decrease in plasma cholinesterase activity could allow serum concentrations of an ester-linked local anesthetic to rise and thus increase the likelihood of systemic toxicity. The use of amino-ester local anesthetics should be avoided when possible if decreased cholinesterase activity is suspected.

Amino-amide local anesthetics are metabolized mainly in the liver by microsomal enzymes. The most rapidly metabolized of this group is prilocaine, which in part accounts for its relatively low systemic toxicity. Hepatic metabolism of amide-linked local anesthetics can be affected by any factor that alters liver function, such as hepatic disease and drugs (Yagiela, 1985). The renal clearance of amide agents is inversely related to their protein-binding capacity. Renal clearance also is inversely proportional to the pH of urine, suggesting urinary excretion by nonionic diffusion. (Covino, 1981).

Innervation to the primary and permanent teeth

Effective local anesthesia for the maxillary and mandibular teeth and their related structures first requires familiarity with the manner in which these areas are innervated. Only then will the operator understand the fundamentals for the prescribed techniques.

There are variances in the anatomic arrangements of nerve systems, or the way in which systems commingle. Any variance can create a less than adequate anesthetic response. A particular nerve branch may be congenitally absent (Mink and Spedding, 1966). What may seem the logical anesthetic procedure may fail to provide the desired anesthetic effect. A complete pulpal anesthesia may require the deposition of an agent around an accessory nerve branch. Knowing where anomalies exist and how to adjust makes pain control more effective.

Superior alveolar branches
of the maxillary nerve

The maxillary division of the trigeminal nerve gives rise to the sphenopalatine ganglion in the pterygopalatine fossa and to the zygomatic and posterior superior alveolar branches while traversing forward through the infratemporal fossa. The main trunk then enters the infraorbital fissure at the posterolateral surface of the tuberosity of the maxilla, becoming the infraorbital nerve coursing the floor of the orbit, cradled in the infraorbital groove. The infraorbital nerve fosters the middle and anterior branches of the superior alveolar complex.

The posterior superior alveolar nerve branch, at its origin, usually divides into two branches that pass down to the distal surface of the maxilla. One branch will remain external to the maxillary bone and supply the buccal mucosa and the mucous membrane of the cheek. The other enters the posterior wall by way of the posterior superior alveolar canal and innervates the posterolateral wall of the maxillary sinus and the supporting structures of the three permanent molars and their root ends with the exception of the mesiobuccal root of the permanent first molar.

The middle superior alveolar nerve, when present, arises from the infraorbital nerve, its site varying (Malamed, 1980). It appears as a differentiated entity about 30% of the time. The nerve descends along the lateral wall of the maxillary sinus, innervating the epithelial surface of the sinus and the root ends and supporting structures of the primary first and second molars or permanent first and second premolars and the mesiobuccal root of the permanent first molar (Romanes, 1981).

The anterior superior alveolar branch arises a short distance posterior to the external orifice of the infraorbital canal. It courses within the anterior wall of the maxillary sinus and provides sensory fibers to the maxillary incisor and canine root ends and periodontal structures. Its branches commingle 70% to 80% of the time, with those of the posterior superior alveolar nerve to form the superior dental plexus (Malamed, 1980). Otherwise, its fibers decussate with those of the middle superior alveolar branch.

Effect of accessory nerve innervations

Because of the anomalous factors that exist within the framework of the superior alveolar nerve system, specific techniques have been developed to accommodate them. As examples, the maxillary permanent first molar and primary second molar require adjusted techniques.

In that the permanent first molar's mesiobuccal root is innervated by fibers from the anterior (or middle) superior alveolar branch, it becomes necessary to anesthetize not only the posterior superior alveolar aspect but also the anterior (or middle) superior alveolar network to accomplish adequate pulpal anesthesia. Too, the primary maxillary second molar has a different pattern of innervation. Because of the comingling of the posterior superior alveolar branch with the anterior (or middle) alveolar nerve ends, it is sound procedure to routinely anesthetize both the posterior and anterior (or middle) superior alveolar branches. This technique will more completely block the sensory response of the primary second molar.

There is some clinical evidence of accessory innervation by the anterior and nasopalatine nerves, and on occasion the palatal areas require the deposition of an anesthetic agent to reduce sensory response (Spiro, 1981).

Anterior palatine and nasopalatine branches
of the maxillary nerve

The anterior (greater) palatine nerve emerges from the pterygopalatine canal by way of the greater palatine foramen, followed by the middle and posterior branches of the palatine nerve that pass posteriorly to innervate the tissues of the soft palate and tonsillar area. The anterior palatine nerve courses anteriorly midway between the midline of the palate and the palatal gingivae. The nerve terminates just distal to the maxillary canine tooth, its fibers overlapping those of the nasopalatine nerve. The nerve supplies sensory fibers to the tissues of the hard palate. Spiro (1981) suggested that there is some clinical evidence that accessory fibers perhaps innervate, to some extent the palatal roots of the primary and permanent molar teeth.

In the course of a maxillary posterior operative procedure, the operator is alerted to a child's discomfort. The source of the distress may be the rubber dam clamp impinging on sensitive palatal tissue. If not that, the discomfort may result from less-than-adequate pulpal anesthesia. In either instance, this situation invariably occurs when the operator, for one reason or another, fails to perform a routine anterior palatine nerve infiltration.

The nasopalatine branch of the maxillary nerve directs itself anteriorly along the vomer, exiting from the nasal cavity by way of the incisive canal at the midline of the vault at its most anterior point. Its location is evidenced by the nasopalatine papilla. The nerve fibers innervate the soft and hard tissues of the anterior quadrant from the midline laterally to the maxillary canine tooth.

Again, Spiro (1981) stated that clinical observation suggests that the nasopalatine nerve may be accessory to innervation of the incisor teeth, the same as the anterior palatine nerve branch. Again, the policy of using a palatal infiltrative procedure of the nasopalatine nerve in concert with anterior superior alveolar anesthesia could ensure a more secure pulpal anesthesia and a more comfortable rubber dam clamp application.

Inferior alveolar (mandibular) nerve

The inferior alveolar nerve is the largest branch of the mandibular division of the trigeminal nerve. It arises at the level of the external pterygoid muscle and descends between the sphenomandibular ligament and the medial surface of the ramus of the mandible entering the mandibular canal by way of the mandibular foramen. It courses the canal anteriorly and divides into two terminal branches, the mental and incisive nerves.

The only means to accomplish adequate pulpal anesthesia for all the mandibular teeth is through the use of the nerve block procedure. The supraperiosteal infiltrative technique, for the most part, is unsatisfactory. The cortical plate of bone is heavier over the primary and permanent molars and presents a barrier to constantly effective pulpal anesthesia. On the other hand, acceptable pulpal anesthesia can be achieved through supraperiosteal injections for primary and permanent incisors.

The nerve block can offer problems of anesthetic effectiveness. With young children the procedure is 90% effective, but effectiveness decreases to approximately 80% in older individuals (Malamed, 1981). Anatomic variability, below-average technical performance, and accessory innervations are attributable causes.

Anatomic change is elicited through normal growth and development processes. As an example, the location of the mandibular foramen in the child is inferior to its site in an older individual. Too, the mandibular ramus is narrower anteroposteriorly in the child than in an adult. The factors cited require adjustments in the steps of the block procedure. The line of delivery of the syringe will be in a slightly downward direction to accommodate the more inferior location of the foramen. The needle's depth of penetration will not be as great.

Erroneous technique can result from an anesthetic syringe's misdirection, too-shallow deposition of an anesthetic agent, or the volume of drug deposited. Corrections for poor anesthetic procedure require a careful review of the subject, noting and understanding how the mistake may be remedied.

Mental and incisive nerves

The mental and incisive nerve branches emerge from the inferior alveolar nerve as its terminal branches. The mental nerve exists from the mental foramen and innervates the skin and mucosa of the lower lip and chin as well as the gingival tissues labial to the mandibular incisors. The incisive nerve furnishes sensory fibers to the first premolar, the canine, and the mandibular incisor teeth. The innervations are through a plexus of nerve branches that also decussate with like branches of the opposite side of the midline. Roberts and Sowray (1970) pointed out that mental injection is a greatly misused, erroneous term, because in reality the procedure involves the incisive nerve.

Long buccal nerve

The long buccal nerve is the first branch from the inferior alveolar nerve. It runs downward and forward along the masseter muscle, progressing onto the medial surface of the ascending ramus. The nerve passes over the anterior border of the ramus, level with the mandibular occlusal plane, and to the lateral surface of the body of the mandible. Sensory fibers are distributed to the buccinator muscle, the buccal mucosa, and the buccal gingivae over the mandibular molars and second premolar.

Lingual nerve

The lingual nerve is the second branch from the inferior alveolar nerve. It courses downward, lying lateral to the internal pterygoid muscle, medial to the ascending ramus, and within the pterygomandibular space. The nerve courses forward in the lateral lingual sulcus, supplying anterior two thirds of the tongue and the inferior surface of the sublingual salivary gland. There is sensory innervation to the floor of the mouth and the gingiva of the lingual surface of the body of the mandible.

Mylohyoid nerve

The mylohyoid nerve has both sensory and motor functions. It is a branch of the inferior alveolar nerve, arising from it as the parent enters the mandibular foramen. The nerve is directed along the medial surface of the ramus, anteriorly along the mylohyoid groove of the body of the mandible toward its motor destination in the mylohyoid muscle. Sensory fibers supply the skin about the mental protuberance.

Occasionally accessory innervation will exist in the mandibular region, and although an inferior alveolar nerve block has been implemented, certain teeth reflect poor pulpal anesthesia. The mylohyoid nerve is usually the branch that is implicated. Its fibers may innervate the mandibular molars and incisors. Pulpal response usually arises from the mesial aspect of the tooth being operated. After it has been determined that there is no fault with the inferior alveolar block, and that pulpal response persists, a submucosal deposition of an anesthetic agent at the medial surface of the mandible at its juncture with the floor of the mouth will usually block accessory sensory innervation by the mylohyoid nerve.

Traditional techniques

Anatomic structures in children are naturally smaller than those in an adult. Therefore, there is good reason to reduce the depth of penetration of the needle during injection procedures. There are three specific anatomic differences to be conscious of in children: (1) the proximity of vascular structures in the maxillary tuberosity area, where penetrating too deeply with the needle can result in injury to the pterygoid venous plexus or posterior superior alveolar artery and resultant hematoma; (2) the mandibular ramus is shorter and is narrower anteroposteriorly; therefore, for an inferior alveolar nerve block, the depth of penetration of the needle must be reduced; and (3) the bone is less calcified, permitting expetiated diffusion of the local anesthetic agent (Malamed, 1990b).

There are also variations in the origin and degree of innervation between mature permanent teeth of adults to primary and immature permanent teeth of children. Primary teeth have fewer myelinated nerve fibers and lose them early during their resorptive process (Johnsen and Johns, 1978). Immature permanent teeth have an increased threshold to electrometric pulp testing that has been attributed to the immature integration of the nerve fibers with the odontoblastic processes (Fulling and Andreasen, 1976). Innervation for the primary maxillary first and second molars is usually from the middle superior alveolar nerve branches. The primary maxillary second molar in some instances, however, may not have a complete block of sensation following middle superior alveolar injection because fibers from the posterior superior alveolar branch are still capable of being stimulated and the middle superior alveolar nerve is frequently congenitally missing (Mink and Spedding, 1966). Therefore, it is sound practice to infiltrate both branches when establishing anesthesia for primary maxillary molars. The permanent maxillary first molar receives innervation from the posterior superior alveolar nerve for the most part, but many times will have nerves from the middle superior alveolar branch that supply the mesiobuccal root. Thus both branches should also routinely be anesthetized for permanent maxillary first molars.

There is no perfect technique that guarantees complete success in anesthetizing children, but there are a few errors that can guarantee failure. Four common mistakes are made by dentists attempting to anesthetize a child: (1) waving the needle in front of the patient, (2) not getting supportive control of the patient's head and hands, (3) using long needles, and (4) using inappropriate doses (Wei, 1988). In addition, to ensure the child's comfort and safety, injection of local anesthetics should always be made slowly (approximately 1 mL/min), preceded by application of topical anesthesia and aspiration to avoid intravascular injection, which may result in systemic reactions to the local anesthetic ingredients. Traditionally, local anesthesia is achieved by either infiltration or nerve block, sometimes in combination.

Local infiltration amounts to the deposition of local anesthetic solution, or flooding of the terminal nerve branches, for achieving anesthesia. The area to be treated, or the procedure to be accomplished, will dictate whether local infiltration will be sufficient. Most soft tissue surgeries, and many restorations can be achieved by buccal infiltration (O'Sullivan et al, 1986).

Palatal infiltration may be accomplished for procedures invasive enough to stimulate palatal nerve supply, such as a stainless steel crown restoration, but not invasive enough to require palatal nerve block. Palatal infiltration might be easily approached via the buccogingival papilla (intrapapillary injection). There are also instances where infiltration might provide adequate anesthesia for accomplishing minor restorations on primary mandibular molars as well, but the actual effectiveness of this approach has not been reported (Malamed, 1990b).

Nerve blocks are accomplished by depositing the local anesthetic close to a distal nerve trunk, thus giving a larger region of anesthesia. The inferior alveolar nerve block can prove to be one of the most frustrating of all nerve block techniques; it has a 15% to 20% failure rate in achieving adequate anesthesia (Malamed, 1990c). When an anesthetic solution is administered for an inferior alveolar nerve block, the attempt is made to place the solution near the mandibular foramen. Because the mandible grows anteroposteriorly, the foramen moves posteriorly in approximately the same way. With age there is a progressive increase in distance of the mandibular foramen above the occlusal plane as a result of greater posterior maxillary basal and alveolar bone growth. In children, the mandibular foramen is near the height of the occlusal plane; the mandibular foramen moves posteriorly and slightly occlusally with age, averaging approximately 7 mm above the occlusal plane in adults (Benham, 1976). If the first attempt at an inferior alveolar nerve block is unsuccessful, a second attempt may be made using a higher landmark for needle insertion.

One of the most difficult tasks for the dentist is to test for adequate anesthesia following an inferior alveolar nerve block. Most commonly the dentist uses lip numbness as a subjective sign to indicate a sufficient block of the ipsilateral inferior alveolar nerve. A study performed by Ellis and coworkers (1990) indicated that the loss of gingival response to stimulation (positive gingival test) is a more rapid sign of anesthesia onset and a more reliable predictor of success than are tongue and lip signs. Thermal response does not provide any information regarding the onset of anesthesia. The most reliable indication of an efficacious inferior alveolar nerve block is a combination of three signs (tongue, lip, and gingiva).

Armamentarium

Aspirating syringe

To prevent, or at least minimize, the intravascular expression of an anesthetic agent during an injection procedure, the use of an aspirating-type syringe is advocated. Its plunger end harbors a harpoonlike blade that engages the pistonlike stopper in the anesthetic carpule. When the 1.8-mL glass anesthetic cartridge is inserted into the syringe, the plunger is quickly and firmly pressed, engaging the harpoon into the stopper. When the plunger mechanism is withdrawn, fluids are aspirated at the injection site.

Presterilized disposable needle

Many gauges and lengths of needles are available to the dental practitioner. The needle gauges most commonly used in pediatric dentistry are 25, 27, and 30; the most common lengths are 1 in. (short) and 1.5 in. (long). A ⅝-in. (extra short) needle is recommended for intraligamental injections.

The 27-gauge needle is adequate for the aspiration measures used, although it has been advocated that the 25-gauge needle be used because of its larger diameter (McClure, 1968). Fuller and coworkers (1979), using dentists as subjects, found no significant differences in perception of pain produced by penetrations of 25-, 27-, and 30-gauge needles in the retromolar fossa. However, a study of 138 pediatric dental patients showed that the 30-gauge needle tends to have slightly lower pain scores (Brownbill et al, 1987). The authors declared, however, that the level of discomfort was insignificant, and suggested that patient comfort would not be compromised by the use of either a 25- or a 30-gauge needle. The large number of very low scores in both groups indicated that children did not think that needle penetration for inferior alveolar nerve block was very uncomfortable.

Menke and Gowgiel (1979) used cadavers to determine the depth of penetration of the needle from the oral mucous membrane to the interior alveolar nerve at the mandibular foramen. The depth of penetration at the narrowest anteroposterior width of the ramus and pterygotemporal depression was determined to be half the narrowest anteroposterior width of the ramus plus or minus 1 mm. This depth was within the limits of a short needle length. A short needle was recommended for use because it was easier to estimate the depth of penetration and was less likely to penetrate too deep and deviate from its course than was a long needle.

Anesthetic agents

There are three anilide-link anesthetic agents, suitable for the child patient. All are the amide type and rarely evoke allergic reactions. They are lidocaine HCl, mepivacaine HCl, and prilocaine HCl (Malamed, 1980).

1. Lidocaine (Xylocaine) HCl 2% with epinephrine 1:100,000
2. Mepivacaine (Carbocaine) HCl 2% with levonordefrin (Neo-Cobefrin) 1:20,000
3. Prilocaine (Citanest Forte) HCl 4% with epinephrine 1:200,000

4. Prilocaine (Citanest Plain) HCl 4%
5. Mepivacaine (Carbocaine) HCl 3%

Mepivacaine HCl has a more rapid onset and a more prolonged effect than lidocaine HCl. Both are well-suited and dependable anesthetic agents for the child.

Prilocaine HCl 4% with epinephrine 1:200,000 is a shorter-acting agent. Its use may be advantageous in the child for whom long-term anesthetic effects are undesirable. Prilocaine HCl should be used in sparing amounts. Unlike lidocaine HCl or mepivacaine HCl, it undergoes metabolic breakdown in both the liver and the kidneys. Ortho-toluidine, one of its metabolites, can excite the production of methemoglobin, and high doses of the anesthetic agent can induce the chance development of methemoglobinemia. Prilocaine HCl should be avoided in patients who are anemic, exhibit cardiac failure, or who display hypoxic sings of respiratory failure. Patients taking phenacetin or acetaminophen should not receive this agent (Malamed, 1980). Mepivacaine HCl 3% does not contain a vasoconstrictor and with its reactively low toxicity is a dependable agent to use in the child with cardiovascular disease.

Topical anesthetic agents

A dependable topical anesthetic agent applied to a dried mucous membrane for 1 minute substantially reduces the mild discomfort of the injection procedure. These agents are in gel, ointment, or liquid form. The ointment form of the product has an advantage over the liquid agents. An ointment tends to remain where placed, whereas solutions, if ineptly handled, escape and run elsewhere, producing topical effects not required and, in some instances, contributing to undesirable patient behavior.

Lidocaine (Xylocaine 5%) and 20% ethyl aminobenzoate (Topicale), benzocaine are effective agents. They have low toxicity a rapid onset, and a pleasant taste. Rarely, with repeated or overextended use, the ester agents can become locally allergenic.

Mouth props

A pediatric patient may require a prop of some type to support the jaws in an open position. The device will always be required in patients receiving dental treatment under a general anesthesia. Other children requiring a mouth prop are certain of those who are handicapped or medically compromised or those under the process of conscious sedation. Too, a prop lends jaw support for those patients who are unaware of gradual jaw closure while restorative measures are in progress.

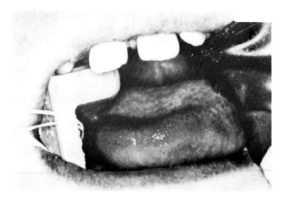

Fig 12-1 The rubber mouth prop, such as the medium-sized McKesson, affords adequate vertical accommodation but in some mouths diminishes overall space to operate without some restriction. It provides stability and requires little attention to adjustment.

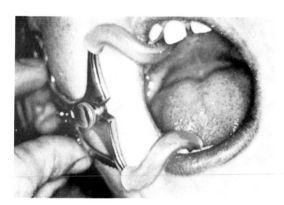

Fig 12-2 A Molt gag or mechanical mouth prop is used by many practitioners to maintain an oral opening when the patient's voluntary control is of no avail. It affords ample operating space but requires some attention to adjustment and positioning.

The most adaptable prop for pediatric use is the rubber bite block, such as the one developed by McKesson (Fig 12-1). The medium size is the most popular, but the small one may be more appropriate for smaller tots and infants. Once the prop is placed in the mouth, it remains relatively secure. The bite block tends to be bulky, however, and takes up valuable room in small mouths. Some clinicians prefer the mechanical mouth gag (Molt), which fits posteriorly and to one side. The device has a tendency to move about after placement and requires stabilization (Fig 12-2).

Patient preparation

The preparation of the pediatric patient for the local anesthesia procedure must be carefully considered. Throughout all of dental care, patient cooperation is essential, and as such, the administration of a behaviorly successful local anesthetic procedure becomes paramount. In other words, a satisfactorily accomplished anesthetic measure provides the operator with a comfortable leeway for other potentially troublesome procedures during the dental appointment.

Patient preparation in the dental environment is dependent on a well-trained team of auxiliary personnel. The auxiliaries must be attentive to the child and must, as efficiently as the dentist, explain in understandable terms why the patient is in the dental office, what is going to be done, and how it will be done.

Semantics is a fundamental component undergirding patient preparation and management. The language level used must be appropriate to the age and understanding of the child. A liberal use of euphemistic terms should be used to soften what otherwise could be disturbing phrases. The following are examples:

1. Toddler-preschooler (2 to 6 years). Explanations and descriptions of the procedures must be in simple, understandable terminology. For example:

"John do you know there are some sugar germs in your teeth? They make holes in your teeth. You don't want them in your teeth, do you? Here's what I'm going to do. First, I'll put your teeth to sleep, but you will be awake. There will be a little feeling when the sleepy medicine goes on. When your teeth are asleep, I will chase the germs from them and fill the holes they made. Do you understand?"

2. School-age child (6 to 12 years). The semantics must be adjusted to the patient's level of maturity. For example: "John, we are going to put your tooth to sleep before we work on it to get the decay out. Afterward we will fill the tooth. Do you understand?"

3. Adolescent (13 years and older). When one is communicating with adolescents, the language level must fit their more mature understanding. Explain why the procedure is necessary and indicate that with his or her understanding and cooperation, and the use of a local anesthetic, the procedure will be accomplished easily and with relative comfort. The average teenager is usually cooperative and understands adult-level communication.

Anesthesia for the maxillary tissues

The needle penetration site is determined by two anatomic landmarks, the mucobuccal fold and mucogingival junction (Sweet's line), a visible white border between the fixed gingiva and the red alveolar mucosa. The penetration site is 2 to 3 mm apical to the

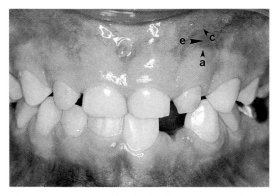

Fig 12-3 Injection site landmarks for the superior alveolar nerve branches: *(c)* the mucobuccal fold and *(e)* the penetration site, 2 to 3 mm superior to *(a)* the mucogingival junction.

mucogingival junction and into the alveolar mucosa and 2 mm from the labial or buccal surface (Fig 12-3). Syringe angulation places the needle in line with and addressed toward the apex of the root. The bevel is adjacent to the labial or buccal tissue. Needle penetration is quickly accomplished by pulling the loose alveolar tissue of the lip or cheek over the positioned needle. Penetration is rapid and relatively pain free. Aspiration is an essential step in the local anesthetic procedure. Immediately following needle penetration, the thumb ring is withdrawn slightly, producing a negative pressure in the anesthetic cartridge. If the needle is within a vessel, blood will be seen in the cartridge. In event of a positive aspiration, the needle is withdrawn slightly, directed to a new position and aspirated again. If the aspiration is negative, a slow deposition of the agent is begun. A hematoma may likely form should the needle injure a large vessel or plexus of veins and extravasation occur. Too, should there be an intravascular expression of the anesthetic agent, a systemic reaction, varying from minor to major proportions, may be evidenced. The supraperiosteal technique requires a very careful deposition of the anesthetic agent to minimize patient discomfort. After the initial aspiration, a few drops of solution are deposited at the penetration site. The needle is probably no more than 2 to 3 mm deep. The needle tip should be advanced adjacent the apex of the root of the tooth, the area aspirated, followed by the deposition of 0.60 mL (one third carpule) of the anesthetic agent.

Superior alveolar nerve branches

The superior alveolar nerve network (superior alveolar dental plexus) is anesthetized by the supraperiosteal field block. The effect produces anesthesia for multiple teeth and their related soft tissues along their labial and buccal aspects (Bennett, 1984).

The anterior superior alveolar nerve has as its general landmark the loose alveolar tissue superior to the maxillary canine tooth. The penetration site is at the mucobuccal fold apical to the canine. The range of anesthesia includes the incisors to the midline and extends posteriorly by branches supplying the superior dental plexus (Figs 12-4a and b).

The middle superior alveolar nerve has as its prevailing target the loose alveolar tissue apical to the first primary molar or first premolar. According to Jorgenson and Hayden (1980), because of the heavy cortical bone of the zygoma adjacent to the buccal roots of the permanent first and primary second molars, these teeth are not inclined to complete insatience following a middle superior alveolar anesthetic procedure. A supraperiosteal injection in the posterior superior alveolar region, blocking accessory fibers eminating from the posterior superior alveolar nerve, is also required (Figs 12-5a and b).

The posterior superior alveolar nerve has as its penetration site the red, loose alveolar tissue adjacent to the mucobuccal fold and apical to the most posterior erupted molar tooth distal to the zygomatic process. The supraperiosteal injection produces complete anesthesia of all the permanent molars with the exception of the mesiobuccal root of the permanent first molar. The molar requires a supraperiosteal deposition of solution in the middle superior alveolar region to suppress accessory innervation arising from that area and supplying the mesiobuccal root (Figs 12-6a and b).

Anesthesia for the palatal tissues

Anesthesia of the hard palate becomes necessary when a surgical procedure is required or manipulations of the free gingival tissues of the palate will take place, such as the fitting of stainless steel crowns or bands or the placement of a rubber dam clamp, any one of which may produce palatal discomfort.

This anesthetic procedure can be a painful, traumatic endeavor unless managed carefully. An unfavorable procedure can be the undoing of any effort to manage patient behavior. A favorable procedure includes adequate topical anesthesia, firm, steady control of the needle, slow deposition of the anesthetic agent, and confidence in oneself. The topical anesthetic should be in place and under pressure for at least 1 minute. An ischemic area is thus produced. A cotton applicator that contains a topical anesthetic and is maintained under pressure helps accomplish the topical numbness. The slow deposition of the agent following needle insertion is the essence of a relatively comfortable palatal procedure (Fig 12-7). A forced expression of solution can prove very uncomfortable for the patient.

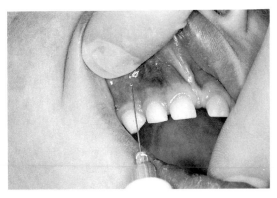
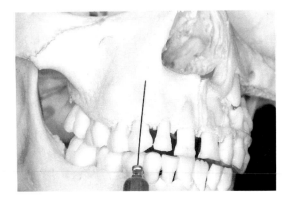

Figs 12-4a and b   The penetration site for the anterior superior alveolar nerve branch is the loose alveolar tissue at the mucobuccal fold just apical to the canine. Following the needle penetration and appropriate aspirative measures, the needle is directed toward the apex of the root, avoiding contact or penetration of the periosteum. The distance is only a few millimeters. The deposition of 0.60 mL of solution is slowly and carefully executed.

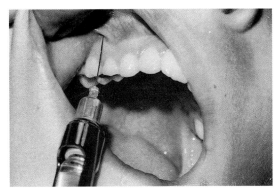
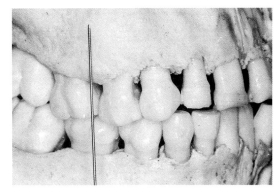

Figs 12-5a and b   The penetration site for the middle superior alveolar nerve branch is the loose tissue superior to the mucogingival junction and apical to the primary first molar. The cortical bone is thinner over this tooth, and the supraperiosteal injection usually results in complete anesthesia for the primary first molar and most of the primary second molar.

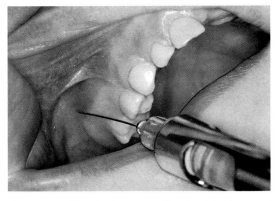
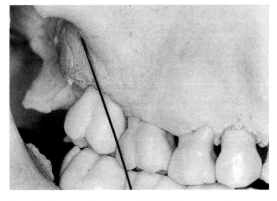

Figs 12-6a and b   The direction and landmark for the posterior superior alveolar nerve branch are distal to the zygomatic process and apical to the last erupted tooth in that region. The penetration site is the loose alveolar tissue at the mucobuccal fold. It is necessary that the middle superior alveolar area be anesthetized for pain-free procedure on the permanent first molar tooth. The mesiobuccal root receives accessory nerve supply from the middle (or anterior) superior alveolar plexus.

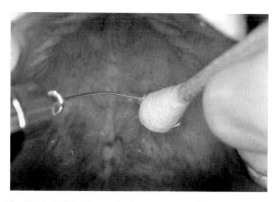

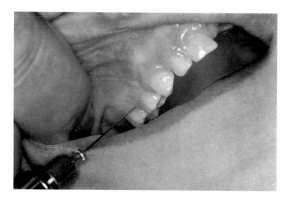

Fig 12-7 While the topical-pressure anesthetic process is maintained, the syringe needle is positioned adjacent to the applicator tip, the bevel palatally oriented. When the needle is flexed, the pressure forces the bevel firmly against the mucosa, and solution is expressed into its surface, producing additional surface anesthesia. Ischemic tissue reaction (blanching) will be observed.

Fig 12-8 The needle is directed into the interseptal area, entering the interdental papilla and passing a minimal distance of 2 to 4 mm to palatal interseptal tissue. A drop or so of solution is deposited. With accurate needle placement, immediate ischemia should be noted. The needle is withdrawn. The needle is reinserted into the ischemic interseptal tissue, the area aspirated, and the needle advanced about 2 mm along the hard surface of the palate. Following aspiration, the syringe is advanced again no more than 2 mm, and a final deposition of the agent is made.

Anterior palatine nerve

The supraperiosteal injection of the anterior (greater) palatine nerve is initiated while pressure is still maintained. The target area is any desired location posterior to the maxillary canine and anterior to the greater palatine foramen, and midway between the midline of the hard palate and the palatal surface of the posterior teeth.

With the pressure still in effect, the needle is placed with the bevel resting against, but not penetrating, the mucous membrane. A palatal pressure is applied to the needle at its bevel, and a small volume of the anesthetic agent is forced against the mucous membrane, producing some ischemia. The pressure is released and the bevel permitted to penetrate the ischemic tissue. Small amounts of solution continue to be deposited slowly and carefully, as the needle is advanced until it lightly contacts the bone. About 0.2 to 0.3 mL of solution is slowly deposited and then the needle is withdrawn.

Interdental papillary injection of palatal nerves

An alternate method of palatal anesthesia is the interdental papillary approach. If used, this step will follow the superior alveolar anesthetic procedure. The needle is inserted into the anesthetized interdental papilla at its labial or buccal aspect, and a few drops of solution are deposited as the syringe is advanced 2 to 4 mm toward the palatal free gingiva. The palatal tissue should be observed for blanching at that point. The syringe is withdrawn and inserted into the blanched palatal tissue. About 0.25 mL of solution is deposited as the needle is advanced along the palatal surface 4 mm or so.

The interdental papillary injection, carefully executed, can be fairly atraumatic and is a procedure of choice with a young child. In addition, this method of anesthetizing can be effectively concealed with the retracting hand (Fig 12-8).

Nasopalatine nerve

The penetration site for the nasopalatine nerve is the mucous membrane lateral to the incisive papilla. There are two ways of accomplishing the anesthetic procedure. One method is the interdental papillary approach at the midline between the maxillary central incisor teeth. An anterior superior alveolar anesthesia must be performed initially. After 2 minutes the anesthetic needle is introduced into the interseptal tissue. An anesthetic agent is slowly expressed, and the needle is carefully directed through the interdental papilla into the lateral surface of the incisive papilla. The second and most prescribed way of procuring nasopalatine anesthesia is using the pressure-topical anesthetic approach suggested by Malamed (1980) as indicated for the greater palatine nerve. However, the interdental papillary method may be the choice procedure for the young child (Figs 12-9a and b).

Anesthesia for the mandibular tissues

Buccal nerve

Buccal nerve anesthesia is accomplished by a field block or submucosal infiltration. The field block is

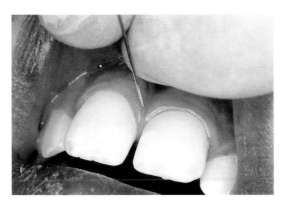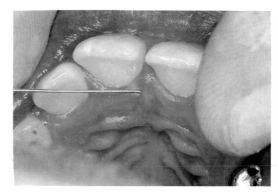

Figs 12-9a and b   The interdental papillary approach to nasopalatine nerve anesthesia requires an initial supraperiosteal injection of the anterior superior alveolar nerve branch, followed by an access to the palatal surface lateral to the incisive papilla by way of the interdental papilla at the midline. The needle slowly and carefully traverses between the maxillary central incisor teeth, through the interdental papilla, as the anesthetic agent is expressed along with way. About 0.2 to 0.3 mL of solution is deposited at the lateral surface of the incisive papilla.

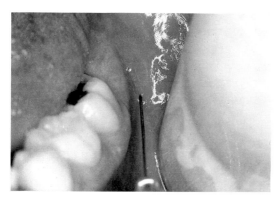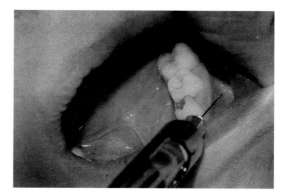

Figs 12-10a and b   The buccal nerve anesthetic procedure is accomplished in either of two ways. Using a field block procedure, the operator deposits the anesthetic agent into the buccal soft tissues distal to the most posterior tooth in the mandibular arch. The optional procedure involves the deposition of solution in the mucobuccal fold adjacent to the tooth being treated. With either method, 0.25 mL of the agent is sufficient.

achieved by depositing a small amount of solution into the buccal soft tissues of the vestibule distal to the most posterior tooth in the mandibular arch. The range of anesthesia includes the buccal tissues and alveolar gingival mucosa to the primary second molar or premolar tooth. A submucosal infiltration into the buccal tissues adjacent to the tooth being attended will also furnish required anesthesia. The deposition of 0.25 mL of solution will be adequate (Fig 12-10).

Mental nerve

Mental nerve block anesthesia may be indicated on occasion in pediatric dentistry. It is achieved after hav-ing initially established the location of the mental foramen by palpation. It is usually targeted at the mucobuccal fold area and apical to the primary first and second molars or interradicularly of the first and second premolars. Anatomically, its site will vary mesially or distally of its usual location. The needle penetration site is just anterior to the mental foramen, and the syringe is directed posteriorly to the area. With negative aspiration, 0.5 to 1.0 mL of solution is slowly expressed and then the syringe is removed. Anesthesia includes the buccal tissues distal to the permanent first molar and mesially to the midline, including the lower lip (Fig 12-11).

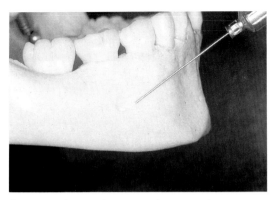

Fig 12-11 The mental nerve anesthetic procedure requires a supraperiosteal injection adjacent to the mental foramen. The needle penetration site is in the mucobuccal fold inferior to the primary first molar or over the first premolar root. The needle is directed downward and posteriorly 4.0 mm. About 0.5 mL of the agent is slowly deposited subsequent to aspiration.

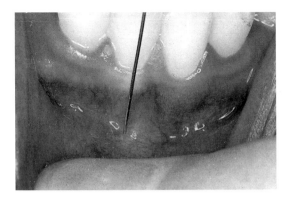

Fig 12-12 Incisive nerve anesthesia may be by block or supraperiosteal means. For the block, which is seldom used, needle penetration is distal to the mental foramen. The needle is directed downward and posteroanteriorly, enters the orifice, is aspirated, then deposits about 0.5 mL of solution. The supraperiosteal injection requires the submucosal deposition of the anesthetic solution near the apex of the mandibular incisor or canine. About 0.5 mL of the agent is required.

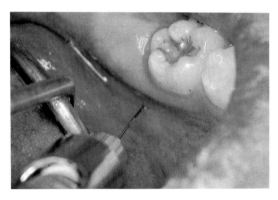

Fig 12-13 To accomplish mylohyoid nerve anesthesia, the operator directs the anesthetic syringe from the opposite side of the mouth. Needle penetration is at the juncture of the medial surface of the mandible and the floor of the mouth, one tooth posterior to the tooth being operated. The depth of penetration is 3 to 5 mm, and about 0.5 mL of solution is slowly deposited following aspiration.

Incisive nerve

Incisive nerve block anesthesia is used only minimally in pediatric dentistry. After the mental foramen is located, needle penetration is made distal to it, entering the orifice in a downward, posteroanterior direction. Anesthetic solution is expressed in small amounts with the excursion of the needle. Once in the foramen, the area is aspirated, and 0.5 to 1.0 mL of solution is deposited. This block provides the mental nerve block and, additionally, sensory suppression of the teeth anterior to the mental foramen to the midline. The supraperiosteal incisive nerve procedure is accomplished through the deposition of a small amount of the anesthetic agent apically to the incisor or canine tooth being attended (Fig 12-12).

Lingual nerve

Lingual nerve anesthesia can be achieved by three means. The usual method is the block anesthesia by way of the direct-thrust inferior alveolar nerve block procedure. Another way is the supraperiosteal injection into the juncture of the lingual surface of the mandible and the floor of the mouth adjacent to the area being attended or just lingual to the tooth being operated in which solution is deposited into the gingival mucosa of that area. The interdental papillary form of anesthetizing the lingual innervation is used in conjunction with the incisive nerve supraperiosteal process. It is a procedure of choice when a mandibular incisor or canine is anesthetized for an operative procedure.

Mylohyoid nerve

Mylohyoid nerve anesthesia is not often required. But if the mylohyoid nerve is suspected of supplying accessory sensory innervation to a mandibular tooth being operated, the measure is indicated. The procedure is best achieved initiating a submucosal deposition of the anesthetic agent at the juncture of the lingual surface of the mandible with the floor of the mouth in the vicinity of the tooth being operated (Fig 12-13).

Inferior alveolar nerve

Inferior alveolar nerve block anesthesia is the most widely accepted local anesthetic procedure employed in dentistry and is the only block required for pediatric dental pain control. The effect of the anesthetic measure includes sensory suppression of the areas sup-

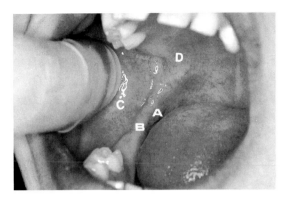

Fig 12-14 The needle penetration site for the inferior alveolar nerve block is a depression identified by an imaginary line dividing the tip of the finger (or thumb) and intersecting with an imaginary vertical line extending superiorly from the apex of the pterygomandibular triangle. The triangle is formed next to (A) the internal pterygoid ligament and includes: (B) the apex of the triangle, (C) the anterior border of the ramus of the mandible, (D) the vault of the palate.

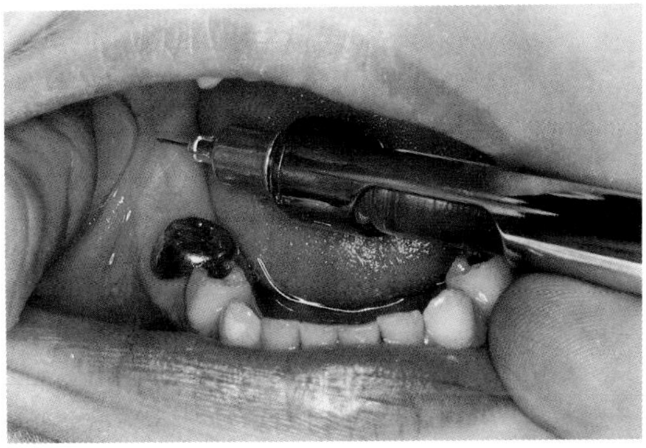

Fig 12-15 The barrel of the anesthetic syringe is positioned parallel to the line of occlusion of the posterior teeth and is directed from over the primary mandibular molar or premolar of the opposite side. After needle penetration and the needle tip encounters the medial surface of the mandibular ramus, its hub should be about 3.0 mm from the mucosa. At this point the area is aspirated, followed by a slow deposition of solution to affect the inferior alveolar nerve block.

plied by the inferior alveolar nerve itself and its mental and incisive branches. The process also provides block anesthesia to the lingual nerve.

The direct-thrust approach to this nerve block involves directing the anesthetic syringe from the primary mandibular molars of the opposite side of the arch toward a targeted area on the medial surface of the ramus of the mandible. In the child the ramus is shorter in vertical dimension and is narrower anteroposteriorly than in the adult, but the site of injection as such is relatively the same. When the anterior border of the ramus is palpated, with the finger or thumb resting in its greater curvature, it can be observed that as the internal pterygoid ligament passes inferiorly and laterally to attach at the base of the mandible, a triangle is formed by the anterior border of the ramus, the internal pterygoid muscle, and the vault of the palate. The apex of the triangle is placed inferiorly. An imaginary, longitudinal line dividing the tip of the finger or thumb as it rests in the coronoid notch passes medially over a depressed area just above the apex. The penetration site is the point of intersection (Fig 12-14).

The anesthetic syringe is introduced into the oral cavity parallel with the occlusal plane of the mandibular posterior teeth. Further, it is positioned and directed from over the primary mandibular first and second molars or premolar on the opposite side (Fig 12-15). This compensates for the anteroposterior divergence of the ramus and places the mandibular foramen in line with the contemplated needle direction. As the needle penetrates the tissue, the barrel of the syringe may need to be repositioned distally or medially or removed and reinserted should needle passage meet with tissue or bone resistance. Tissue obstruction will be medial to the penetration site and is usually the internal pterygoid muscle. Laterally, the internal oblique ridge on

the medial surface of the ramus of the mandible may offer obstruction.

The deposition of the anesthetic agent is performed in stages, slowly and carefully, expressing a prescribed amount of solution at each step.

1. Initial needle penetration is 2 to 3 mm submucosally. Sequential to negative aspiration, a small volume of solution is expressed.
2. The syringe is carried on a direct thrust to within 3 mm of the needle hub, adjusting the bearing of the syringe if obstruction dictates. Usually, the medial surface of the ramus is easily encountered. If the aspiration is negative, a slow deposition of 1.0 mL of the anesthetic agent is effected.
3. The needle is withdrawn half way, and the syringe is positioned over the primary molar and premolar teeth on the side being anesthetized. Then 0.5 mL of solution is deposited. This measure anesthetizes the lingual nerve.
4. The final step is the buccal nerve anesthetic procedure described earlier regarding anesthesia for the mandibular tissues. The deposition of 0.25 mL of solution is usually adequate.

Alternative techniques

Although the previously mentioned techniques for local anesthesia will usually produce an adequate anesthetic response, there are situations that (1) necessitate supplemental anesthetic dose; (2) dictate that the amount of local anesthetic be kept minimal, as in the cases of certain medically compromised and low-

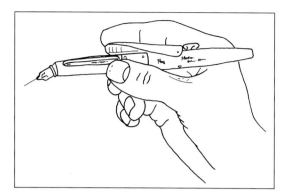

Fig 12-16a The pen-grip design (Microject, Medidenta International) is easily concealed in the hand.

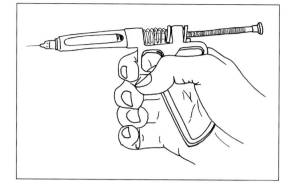

Fig 12-16b The pistol-grip (or palm-grip) design (Ligmaject, Healthco) is difficult to conceal but provides stability and control during handling.

weight patients, and (3) necessitate use of a different technique to achieve anesthesia.

Gow-Gates technique

Since its first mention in the literature, the Gow-Gates technique (Gow-Gates, 1973) for mandibular anesthesia has gained in popularity, not only as a supplemental form of anesthesia, but as a primary method (Malamed, 1981). Reports have described the effectiveness of such a technique in children (Yamada and Jasstak, 1981; Carroll, 1981). Unlike conventional techniques, the Gow-Gates relies on a target zone of the internal condylar neck while using the extraoral landmarks of the tragus of the ear and the opposite corner of the mouth for guidance and proper orientation of the injection. This technique has been claimed to have higher reliability and need fewer supplemental injections than a conventional inferior alveolar nerve block. Other advantages are that only one injection is required for total anesthesia of the third division of the trigeminal nerve (inferior alveolar, lingual, long buccal, and mylohyoid nerves) and that there is less chance of positive blood aspiration.

Intraligamentary technique

Another commonly used technique to achieve anesthesia is the intraligamentary, or periodontal ligament (PDL), injection (Primosch, 1986; Herod, 1989). The injection of a local anesthetic solution directly into the periodontal ligament space as a supplement to conventional techniques following incomplete anesthesia is not a recent development in dentistry. The intraligamentary, or periodontal ligament, injection has often been advocated during endodontic treatment where conventional anesthetic approaches have failed to achieve adequate anesthesia (Walton and Abbott, 1981). Historically, to obtain intraligamentary anesthe-

sia, operators delivered the anesthetic solution into the periodontal ligament space with a conventional aspirating syringe. This technique required the application of great pressure, which was often difficult for the operator (Malamed, 1982; Walton and Abbott, 1981). However, since the introduction in the mid-1970s of the pistol- or palm-grip syringes, which provide greater operator ease in delivering anesthetic solution under pressure, the intraligamentary technique has tended to be the primary choice for obtaining supplemental anesthesia (Primosch, 1986).

The two most significant design characteristics of pressure syringes are the lever system and cartridge housing. The lever system provides the mechanical advantage of applying sufficient pressure without discomfort or physical stress to the hand. The mechanical advantage provides a twofold to threefold increase in applied pressure over conventional syringes. A complete depression of the lever ejects an individual dose of 0.2 mL (one-eighth carpule) of anesthetic solution. There are two basic grip designs: pen and pistol (palm) (Figs 12-16a and b). The pistol grip is the most popular because it provides the best stability and control during handling. However, it is large, bulky, and difficult to conceal. The gunlike design may elicit a more negative patient reaction. On the other hand, the pen-grip design, more easily concealed in the hand, avoids a potentially menacing connotation.

The cartridge housing completely covers the glass anesthetic cartridge to protect the patient from inadvertent breakage during pressure application and is either closed or open to visual inspection. The open design, such as the transparent Teflon sleeve of the Ligmaject system, provides an important advantage to the operator by allowing visual inspection of the amount of solution delivered and signs of possible cartridge breakage.

Listed below are the sequence of steps employed in the delivery of intraligamentary anesthesia with a pressure-type syringe but which may also be followed, with certain limitations, when a standard syringe is used (ADA, 1983; Khedari, 1982; Malamed, 1982; Miller, 1983; Smith et al, 1983).

1. Assembling the syringe. Use a 30-gauge extrashort (1.25-cm [0.5-in.]) needle because it is less flexible and resists buckling and bending during insertion and injection.

2. Preparing the injection site. There is not consensus as to the necessity for preparing the injection site. Some suggestions have included plaque removal and application of topical anesthetic and disinfectant to the papillary gingiva.

3. Inserting the needle. The mesiobuccal and distobuccal proximal sites of the selected tooth are used. The needle is inserted into the gingival sulcus at a 30° angle to the long axis of the tooth with the bevel toward the bone. With the tooth surface used as a guide, the needle is penetrated approximately 2 to 3 mm into the periodontal ligament space until firm wedging of the needle between the crestal bone and root is tactually sensed (Fig 12-17).

4. Injecting the solution. If the needle is properly placed, injection should occur under positive back pressure (resistance to flow). Injection under positive back pressure is critical to maximizing success (Malamed, 1982; Smith et al, 1983; Walton and Abbott, 1981). If injection occurs without resistance, resulting in leak back of solution from the gingival sulcus, repositioning of the needle is necessary. Another sign indicating proper needle placement is the presence of gingival blanching (Grundy, 1984; Miller, 1983) when injecting under positive back pressure. After proper needle placement is confirmed, a slow rate of injection (10 to 20 seconds/deposit) is required (Fig 12-18). The recommended dose is 0.2 mL/site (one-eighth carpule), with a maximum of 0.4 mL/site (ADA, 1983).

When intraligamentary anesthesia delivered by a pressure syringe was used as the primary technique for permanent teeth, the success rates ranged from 70% to 96% (Grundy, 1984; Miller, 1983). When intraligamentary anesthesia was used as a supplemental technique following incomplete anesthesia by conventional methods, the percentage of success was 83% with a pressure syringe (Smith et al, 1983). When the effectiveness of the syringe type used was compared, there were no significant differences in success rates. For use as the primary technique, the success rates were 88% for the pressure-type syringe (Smith et al, 1983) and 92% for the standard syringe (Walton and Abbott, 1981). Therefore, there appears to be no selective advantage to pressure-type syringes solely in regard to success rate. Although the mechanical advantage of pressure syringes may not be critical to obtaining successful anesthesia, the mechanical advantage does provide an ease of administration preferred by operators (Malamed, 1982).

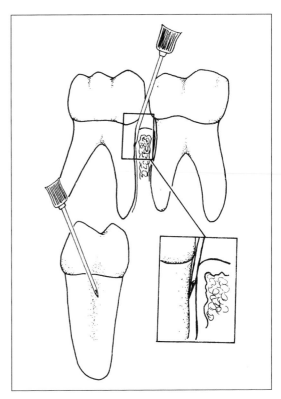

Fig 12-17 Proper needle placement is critical to achieving intraligamentary anesthesia The needle is inserted at a 30° angle to the long axis of the tooth, with the bevel toward bone. The tip is wedged approximately 2 to 3 mm between the root surface and crestal bone near the midline of the root. Both the mesiobuccal and distobuccal proximal sites are to be used.

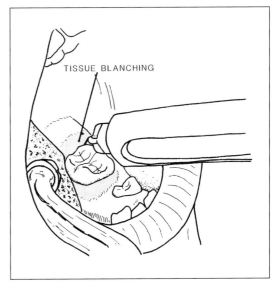

Fig 12-18 Insertion of the needle into the distobuccal site. After proper placement of the needle, injection should occur under positive back pressure to achieve success. Some gingival blanching and back flow of anesthetic solution will occur. The suction tip is placed adjacent to the site to help prevent the patient's reaction to the unpleasant taste of the solution.

Advantages

There are several advantages to the use of intraligamentary anesthesia (ADA, 1983; Khedari, 1982). The following is a list of advantages and indications for use:

1. Immediate onset within 30 seconds and an intermediate duration of action ranging from 30 to 60 minutes.
2. Patient preference. Although there is pain reported during the injection, the majority of patients interviewed preferred it to conventional block anesthesia (Malamed, 1982).
3. Supplemental injection for inadequate pulpal anesthesia without requiring rubber dam removal.
4. Alternative primary anesthesia (selective anesthesia). It is an alternative to conventional regional anesthesia that provides the opportunity to anesthetize selected teeth without obtaining unnecessary soft tissue anesthesia of the lips and tongue. Selective anesthesia is most beneficial in young patients. It also facilitates treatment of multiple, isolated teeth, such as the extraction of four first premolars. In addition, the small dosage required for anesthesia greatly reduces the potential for toxicity and adverse reactions.

Disadvantages

There are certain disadvantages to the routine administration of intraligamentary anesthesia (ADA, 1983). Among the disadvantages are the additional cost of a specialized syringe and difficulty in achieving proper needle placement. Other disadvantages are created by complications often due to the operator's unfamiliarity with the proper technique, such as injection of excessive solution volume. Even with experience in its administration, the following complications have been reported in clinical trials:

1. Glass cartridge breakage if subjected to rapid injection pressure.
2. Unpleasant, bitter taste created by back flow of anesthetic solution from the gingival crevice.
3. Postoperative gingival inflammation and pain.
4. Postoperative dental pain associated with either tooth extrusion and subsequent high occlusion or from periodontal ligament damage secondary to mechanical trauma or ischemia from vasoconstrictors. The reported incidence of postoperative dental pain ranges from 2% to 8% (Grundy, 1984; Khedari, 1982; Malamed, 1982; Miller, 1983).
5. Enamel defects produced on developing permanent teeth. When 16 primary teeth of monkeys received intraligamentary anesthesia with a pressure syringe, 15 of the succedaneous permanent teeth demonstrated enamel defects, while there were no visible defects on the contralateral control teeth (Brannstrom et al, 1984). These enamel defects were believed to result from the cytotoxic activity of the anesthetic agent. Although the enamel defects were not considered extensive, care should be exercised when intraligamentary anesthesia is considered for primary teeth during amelogenesis of the underlying permanent teeth.

In 1982, the American Dental Association Council on Dental Materials, Instruments, and Equipment evaluated intraligamentary anesthesia with pressure syringes. They concluded that it was a valuable adjunct to conventional techniques but that there was insufficient scientific evidence to support its routine use for primary anesthesia.

Local anesthetic complications

The amide-type agents rarely produce anesthetic agent complications. Most problems are caused by syncope or faulty technique (USHEW, 1979)

Syncope

Syncope is usually brought on by psychologic factors within the patient. The child becomes pale, cold, and clammy. The pulse is rapid, the pupils are dilated or constricted, and there is a drop in the blood pressure. Procedures are discontinued; the patient is placed in a reclining position with the head up 10° and the feet elevated 10°. This position provides more efficient blood circulation to the brian and encourages adequate venous return to the heart. Cold compresses should be applied to the head to arouse and comfort the patient.

Operator technique

Operator technique may produce some postanesthetic complications, such as sensory nerve damage, trismus, hematomas, and tissue trauma caused by sudden, pressured anesthetic injections.

Self-inflicted trauma

A numb feeling is produced following the local anesthetic procedure. Numbness can cause postoperative problems. Such problems may be avoided by explaining ahead of time the numb feeling. Failure to inform the young child of this out-of-the-ordinary feeling invites the possibility of an unnecessary and unwanted emotional upset on the part of the child. For example, you may say, "Johnny, we're going put your sick tooth to sleep so we can work on it and make it well. You will know the tooth is asleep because of the funny feeling. When the funny feeling leaves, then that is the sign your tooth is awake. Do you understand?"

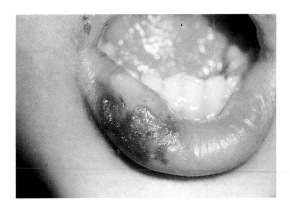

Fig 12-19 Lip laceration following the inferior alveolar nerve block procedure. Because of the large, heavy feeling of numbness, it is not unusual for the pediatric patient to squeeze the anesthetized area between his or her teeth or chew the affected region, contusing or lacerating the mucous membranes of the lip, tongue or cheek.

Lip, tongue, and cheek biting results in self-inflicted soft tissue wounds that may be prevented providing there is timely warning. Such a warning should be given immediately after the injection procedure and repeated before the young child and parent depart the operatory following dental treatment. Figure 12-19 depicts trauma inflicted by a young child while anesthetic numbness prevailed.

The warning can be in the form of an admonition such as: "Johnny, look at me! If you were asleep you would not want anyone to bite on you. It wouldn't feel good, would it? Now, Johnny, when your lip feels sleepy, and your tongue tingles on the side, and your cheek feels funny, don't bite on them! They will be sore! Leave your lip, tongue, and cheek alone and they will awaken feeling good!"

Pulling and rubbing are two other ways of producing trauma following the perception of anesthetic numbness. The dental team must be observant of and discourage the child from pulling or rubbing anesthetized soft tissues. The child may pull strongly on a numb area or vigorously rub such region and produce uncomfortably inflamed soft tissues.

Vasoconstrictor effects

Adverse effects from vasoconstrictor drugs in the amide-type anesthetic agents, used in recommended concentrations, are rare for the well child. According to Malamed (1980), the optimal concentration of epinephrine for the anesthetic agent should be 1:250,000. The strongest concentration of the drug should not exceed 1:100,000. An agent containing 1:50,000 epinephrine far exceeds recommended limits and establishes the possible risk of an overdose for a young patient. It can cause an excitement demonstrated by increased heart rate and dizziness. The patient will know something is wrong and anxieties will emerge. Reassurances that the feeling will subside momentarily may allay some of the fear (Bennett, 1984).

Local anesthetic agents used with vasoconstrictor drugs are contraindicated for certain medically compromised patients. Those with severe cardiovascular disease, hepatic or renal impairment, or hyperthyroid conditions will require medical consultation and the use of local anesthetic agents without vasoconstrictors (Allen, 1984).

Allergic reactions

Allergic reactions to local anesthetic drugs are uncommon. Bennett (1984) estimates that less than 1% of the reactions to the local anesthetic agent are allergy related. Should a reaction occur, it may be caused by the injection procedure or direct contact., The reaction may be immediate or delayed and may be minor or acute (Bennett, 1984).

Hypersensitivity that appears following the injection procedure may vary from a minor occurrence to a bronchoconstriction. Treatment may require an intravenous or intramuscular injection of 0.1 to 0.5 mL of 1:1,000 epinephrine, depending on the age and size of the child. One excellent area for injection is the base of the tongue.

Contact dermatitis exhibits as edema, eczema, or urticaria and treatment may require the use of steroids. Often no treatment is indicated other than avoidance.

Anaphylaxis can occur. It is an immediate onset and can result in cardiac arrest. The injection of 0.1 to 0.5 mL of 1:1,000 epinephrine into the base of the tongue may be necessary (Sanders et al, 1979).

Toxicity

Toxicity from the administration of local anesthesia in children is rare but its occurrence can be insidious and tragic. Severe morbidity and mortality have been reported from cases of inadvertent systemic overdose and in combination with narcotic sedative regimens

(Lalli and Amaranath, 1982; Goodson and Moore, 1983; Allen and Hayden, 1988; Hersh et al, 1991). A recent survey of 117 Florida dentists who routinely treat children demonstrated that some practitioners are unclear as to the recommended maximum dose for the local anesthetics that they are administering every day (Cheatham et al, 1992). The anatomic, metabolic, and physiologic differences of children from that of an adult population must be understood and appreciated by the clinician calculating the safe maximum pediatric dosage (Cheatham and Primosch, 1991). Adherence to safe maximum dose calculations, use of proper injection techniques, and attention to past medical history by the clinician will reduce the potential for adverse complications (Milam and Giovannitti, 1984 and Malamed, 1990d).

Prevention

Prevention is the most important phase of the management of unwanted systemic toxicity from lidocaine. Although individual susceptibility, as influenced by the drug's rate of absorption, distribution, metabolism, and excretion, plays a major role in determining toxicity potential, preventing inadvertent intravascular injection is critical to the avoidance of a toxic reaction (Malamed, 1990e). Kuster and Udin (1985) investigated the potential frequency of accidental intravascular injection of local anesthesia in children as determined by the positive aspiration of blood, The incidence of positive aspiration was reported to be 3.1% for the inferior alveolar nerve block when a 27-gauge needle is used in children. Aspiration with a 27-gauge needle appears to be adequate in preventing inadvertent intravascular injection in children, but many clinicians prefer the narrower 30-gauge needle. Selection of the 30-gauge needle as the needle of choice by 37% of the surveyed Florida dentists (Cheatham et al, 1992) seems to indicate that patient comfort is considered more important than the ability to aspirate. Several investigators concluded, however, that there is no significant difference in patient pain perception among the use of 25-, 27-, and 30-gauge needles (Fuller et al, 1979; Brownbill et al, 1987)., Most contemporary pediatric dental textbooks endorse the use of 25- and 27- gauge needles, especially when the risk of aspiration is high, because the ability to aspirate is decreased with a 30-gauge needle (Cheatham and Primosch, 1991). Multiple aspiration tests, in at least two different planes, are required to prevent a false-negative aspiration, because the negative pressure created during aspiration may draw the vessel wall against the needle bevel, preventing blood from entering the needle lumen.

The rate of the injection is another extremely important factor in preventing overdose reactions, even more so than aspiration techniques. Because the incidence of seizures increases with increasing rate of intravascular infusion of a local anesthetic agent, Mala-

med (1990e) believes that under no circumstances should the duration of injection be less than 1 minute for a 1.8-mL cartridge, and ideally the proper rate should be about 1 mL/min. Intravascular injection of the entire contents of a cartridge in less than 30 seconds creates plasma levels in excess of that required to produce an overdose reaction.

Without proper aspiration techniques, inadvertent and rapid intra-arterial injection of even a single cartridge of local anesthetic can produce seizure activity in the dental patient (Tomlin, 1974). This reaction is most commonly explained by the creation of a retrograde flow following rapid intra-arterial injection of the anesthetic agent. If pressures exceeding those of the arteries are produced rapidly in the process of injecting, the reverse flow to the common carotid artery and then to the internal carotid artery will result in an evanescent high concentration of the drug in the cerebral circulation (Aldrete et al, 1977). On the other hand, intravenous injection of the anesthetic agent is often minimized by the buffering capacity of the lung, as 90% of a bolus injection will be initially bound in the lung and then more slowly released to the systemic circulation (Yagiela, 1985). Intravenous administration of lidocaine has been demonstrated to produce seizures in monkeys at a dosage of 14.2 mg/kg (Munson et al, 1970) and in man at a dosage of 6 to 8 mg/kg (Usubiaga et al, 1966) or when the serum concentration usually exceeds 7.5 ug/mL in the cerebral circulation (Malamed, 1990e).

Although small volumes of intravascular injections have the potential to produce toxic effects, extravascular administration of excessive doses (overdosage) is the more common culprit in severe adverse reactions in children and is frequently associated with a combined narcotic sedation. The American Dental Association (1982) recommended that local anesthetic dosage be reduced when narcotic analgesics are used or with antiemetics, because they lower the convulsive threshold to lidocaine in animals (Smudski et al, 1964). A survey of pediatric dental sedations found a direct linear relationship between the number of cartridges of local anesthetic administered and the frequency of severe adverse reactions (Aubuchon, 1982). Goodson and Moore (1983) reported that the recommended maximum dosage of local anesthetic had been exceeded in 86% of the pediatric dental sedations that were reported to have resulted in severe adverse reactions.

The significant respiratory-depressant effects of a narcotic, by inducing respiratory acidosis (increased PCO_2 and decreased pH and PO_2), may play a very important role in the toxicity of local anesthetics (Moore, 1988). Respiratory acidosis decreases the central nervous system (CNS) threshold concentrations needed for local anesthetic-induced seizures and increases cerebral blood flow, thereby increasing the CNS concentration of local anesthetic solution. Respiratory acidosis also decreases the plasma protein binding of local anesthetic; with this release of previously bound drug, more local anesthetic is available for re-distribution to the CNS (McNamara et al, 1981). These mechanisms will perpetuate continuation of the seizure and further increase CNS concentration of the local anesthetic.

In 1982, the ADA recommended lowering the maximum local anesthetic dosage to 2 mg/lb (approximately one cartridge per 20 pounds) for a sedated child younger than 6 years old (ADA, 1982). During the past decade, revision of a popular textbook (Malamed, 1990e) on local anesthesia recommended a reduction in the maximum dosage to 4.4mg/kg (2 mg/lb), regardless of the vasoconstrictor concentration selected or the sedated state of the patient. Adjusting anesthetic dosage based on inclusion of a vasoconstrictor is no longer recommended. Table 12-1 demonstrates the revised recommended maximum dose for various amide anesthetic agents (Cheatham and Primosch, 1991).

Local anesthetics are potentially more toxic in small children because the margin of safety is lower. It is common practice to calculate drug dosage on the basis of body weight because body mass is related to blood volume, which correlates to the plasma concentration achieved for a given dose. Given an equal dose, a healthy child with greater blood volume will have a lower plasma level of anesthetic than will a child with lesser blood volume and body weight. Obese children are at risk for toxicity if given body weight-determined dosages because their blood volume is relatively less than their weight would indicate. Unfortunately, plasma levels of a drug are also influenced by its degree of absorption, distribution, and elimination, so that a direct relationship between body weight and plasma levels of a drug is not always reliable for a given, constant dose administered. (Scott et al, 1972).

The operator should not fail to recognize the contribution that absorption of excessively applied topical anesthesia, typically employed in greater concentration than suitable for parenteral administration, has on systemic toxicity. Only small amounts of topical agents should be applied at any one time to the oral mucous membranes because of the potential for rapid absorption into the systemic circulation. Seizures have been reported to be caused by the oral application of prescribed viscous lidocaine by overenthusiastic parents treating the symptoms of teething (Mofenson et al, 1983) and herpetic gingivostomatitis (Hess and Walson, 1988).

The typical volume and concentration of local anesthetic agents employed by dentists may possibly be greater than necessary for children (Vreeland et al, 1989; Wilson et al, 1990). Practitioners using greater volumes of anesthetic solution (more than 1.0 mL) for an initial injection may be doing so without the benefits of improved success rates and at the risk of achieving potential toxicity. Studies have demonstrated that increasing volume from 0.9 to 1.8 mL does not increase the success rate or the duration of anesthesia achieved in humans (Vreeland et al, 1989; Aberg and

Table 12-1 Maximum recommended dose of amide local anesthetics by weight of child (dosage = 2 mg/lb)

		Maximum Number of cartridges		
	mg/cartridge	40lbs	60 lbs	80 lbs
Lidocaine 2% (Xylocaine)	36	2	3	4
Mepivacaine 2% (Carbocaine)	36	2	3	4
Mepivacaine 3% (Carbocaine)	54	1.5	2	3
Prilocaine* 4% (Citanest)	72	1.5	2	3

*Maximum dosage for prilocaine is 2.7 mg/lb.

Sydnes, 1978). In children, the volume of lidocaine for initial interior alveolar nerve blocks, recommended by both the manufacturer (Astra Pharmaceutical, 1987) and a popular textbook (Malamed, 1990e), is 1.0 mL. The cumulative doses given to a small child receiving multiple-quadrant restorative dentistry must be kept to a minimum and below the maximum recommended dose based on weight. Selective employment of intraligamentary injection and mandibular infiltration may help to reduce the amount dministered.

It is therefore imperative that the clinician administer safe and effective local anesthesia slowly (less than 1 mL/min) and at reduced volume (one-half to two-thirds cartridge) following negative aspiration in at least two planes from a needle larger than 30 gauge. Excellent technique must be employed to reduce failure rate and to avoid supplemental injections of additional volume. An excellent discussion of the reasons for local anesthesia failures has been recently published and merits review (Wong and Jacobsen, 1992).

Recognition

The two organ systems most profoundly affected by the actions of local anesthetic agents are the central nervous system and the cardiovascular system. Local anesthetics readily cross the blood-brain barrier and, in the presence of high plasma levels, allow depression of the inhibitory pathways on the cerebral cortex, which permits the facilitory pathways to act unopposed, resulting in CNS stimulation (excitatory phase of toxicity). Initial CNS stimulation may cause a variety of reactions, such as restlessness, a feeling of being cold, apprehension, tachycardia, tremor, talkativeness, and nausea and vomiting, as well as the desired numbness of the lips and tongue. More pronounced CNS stimulation may result in seizures (Englesson and Matousek, 1975). The initial excitatory phase may be ex-

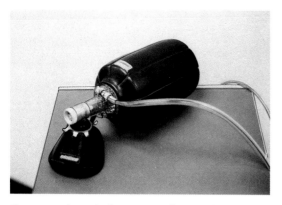

Fig 12-20 The Ambu-bag is an excellent portable device for emergency resuscitory measures. When it is adapted to an oxygen tank system, ventilation is provided through the act of manual bag compression.

tremely brief or absent depending on the level and rapidity of plasma concentrations achieved. As the drug concentration continues to rise in the brain, the facilitory pathways also become inhibited, and generalized CNS depression occurs as manifested by lethargy, drowsiness, disorientation, loss of consciousness, and respiratory depression or arrest (Wagman et al, 1968).

Depression of the central nervous system may occur without apparent stimulation and may be characterized by vasomotor depression. If the vasomotor center is affected, the resulting cerebral anemia may cause syncope, pallor, cyanosis, palpitations, and precordial discomfort. When these responses are superimposed on the direct effect of the local anesthetic agent on the cardiovascular system, an accurate diagnosis of toxicity may be difficult to make. It is likely that many patients who lose consciousness after a local anesthetic injection are reacting to central nervous system toxicity rather than a vasovagal response (syncope) attributed to apprehension and anxiety (Bartlett, 1972). Initial drug plasma levels will cause elevated blood pressure and heart and respiration rates, but increasing plasma concentrations will eventually exert a negative inotropic (contraction) and chronotropic (rate) effect on the myocardium and can produce peripheral vasodilation and severe bradycardia, resulting in hypotension and circulatory collapse. This response occurs at approximately twice the plasma levels necessary to produce CNS toxicity.

Intervention

Early recognition of the signs of toxicity and immediate intervention are key to the management of lidocaine toxicity. In most cases, the adverse reactions will be self-limiting, mild, and transitory. Rarely, are additional measures, other than patient reassurance and supplemental oxygen delivery, necessary to manage the situation (Fig 12-20). Supplemental oxygen administration is essential to counteract respiratory acidosis. Since life-threatening allergic reactions are extremely rare in patients receiving local anesthesia, adverse reactions should never be simply labeled as "allergic," because the potential for mismanagement that will complicate additional treatment is disadvantageous (Malamed, 1990e).

Severe, rapid-onset overdose reactions associated with intravascular injection are best managed by basic life support, including adequate airway and oxygenation of the patient. If seizure activity lasts beyond 3 minutes, an anticonvulsant medication, such as Valium or midazolam, should be administered intravenously, if feasible, or intramuscularly, if necessary. The assistance of medical personnel should be obtained, and the patient should be thoroughly evaluated before discharge. Postseizure reactions, especially when managed by medications, will manifest as postexcitatory depression and the patient often requires further basic life support. During the entire period, the patient's vital signs must be monitored and recorded.

Nearly all systemic toxicity from local anesthesia administration is preventable. The clinician will prevent untoward adverse reactions if:

1. A complete medical evaluation is obtained.
2. Anxiety and fear are reduced.
3. The injection is given with the patient in a supine position.
4. The weakest concentration of an agent with a vasoconstrictor is used in the minimum volume required to achieve success.
5. The injection is given slowly (< 1 mL/min) following negative aspiration in two planes.
6. The patient is continuously observed during and after the procedure for any undesirable reaction.

References

Aberg, G., Sydnes, G. Studies on the duration of local anesthesia. Int. J. Oral Surg. 7:141, 1978.

Aldrete, J. A., Narang, R., Sada, T. et al. Reverse carotid blood flow—A possible explanation for some reactions to local anesthetics. J. Am. Dent. Assoc. 94:1142, 1977.

Allen, G. D. Dental Anesthesia and Analgesia (Local and General). 3rd ed. Baltimore: The Williams & Wilkins Co., 1984.

Allen, G., and Hayden J. Complications of Sedation and Anesthesia in Dentistry. Mass. PSG Publishing Co., 1988, pp. 137-147.

American Dental Association (ADA): Accepted Dental Therapeutics. 39th ed. Chicago: ADA 1982, pp. 149-150.

American Dental Association (ADA) Council on Dental Material, Instruments, and Equipment. Status report: The periodontal ligament injection. J. Am. Dent. Assoc. 106:222, 1983.

Astra Pharmaceutical Products, Inc. Xylocaine (lidocaine hydrochloride): Injections for Local Anesthesia in Dentistry (package insert). Westborough, Mass.: revised April, 1987.

Aubuchon, R. Sedation liabilities in pedodontics. Pediatr. Dent. 4:171, 1982.

Bartlett, S. Z. Clinical observations on the effects of injections of local anesthetic preceded by aspiration. Oral Surg. 33:520, 1972.

Benham, N. R. The cephalometric position of the mandibular foramen with age. J. Dent. Child. 43:233, 1976.

Bennett, C. R. Monheim's Local Anesthesia and Pain Control in Dental Practice. 7th ed. St. Louis: The C. V. Mosby Co., 1984.

Blair, E., Erlanger J. Propagation, and extension of excitatory effects, of nerve action potential across nonresponding intermodes. Am. J. Physiol. 126:97, 1939.

Brannstrom, M., Lindskog, S., Nordenvall, K. F. Enamel hypoplasia in permanent teeth induced by periodontal ligament anesthesia of primary teeth. J. Am. Dent. Assoc. 109:735, 1984.

Brown, R. The failure of local anesthesia in acute inflammation: Some recent concept. Br. Dent. J. 151:47, 1981.

Brownbill, J. W., Walker, P. O., Bourcy, B. D., et al. Comparison of inferior dental nerve block injections in child patients using 30-gauge and 25-gauge short needles. Anesth. Prog. 34:215, 1987.

Carroll, D. P. Local anesthetic dosage in children's dentistry. J. Mich. Dent. Assoc. 63:141, 1981.

Cheatham, B. D., and Primosch, R. E. Pediatric local anesthesia—Current concerns and future challenges. Update Pediatr. Dent. 6:1, 1991

Cheatham, B. D., Primosch, R. E., and Courts F. J. A survey of local anesthetic usage in pediatric patients by Florida dentists J. Dent. Child, 59:401, 1992.

Courtney, K. R. Local anesthetics. Int. Anesth. Clin. 26:239, 1988.

Covino, B. G. Physiology and pharmacology of local anesthetic agents. Anesth. Prog. 28:98, 1981.

Ellis, R. K., Berg J. H., Raj, P. Subjective signs of efficacious inferior alveolar nerve block in children. J. Dent. Child. 57:361, 1990.

Englesson, S., and Matousek, M. Central nervous system effects of local anaesthetic agents. Br. J. Anaesth. 47:241, 1975.

Fuller, N. P., Menke, R. A., and Meyers, W. J. Perception of pain to three different intraoral penetrations of needles. J. Am. Dent. Assoc. 99:822, 1979.

Fulling, H. J., Andreasen, J. O. Influence of maturation status and tooth type of permanent teeth upon electrometric and thermal pulp testing. Scan. J. Dent. Res. 84:286, 1976.

Goodson, J. M., and Moore, P. A. Life-threatening reactions after pedodontic sedation: An assessment of narcotic, local anesthetic, and antiemetic drug interaction. J. Am. Dent. Assoc. 107:239, 1983.

Gow-Gates, G. A. E. Mandibular conduction anesthesia: A new technique using extraoral landmarks. Oral Surg. 36:321, 1973.

Grundy, J. R. Intraligamentary anesthesia. A survey of use by general practitioners and by staff and students in a dental school. Res. Dent. 1:36, 1984.

Herod, E. L. Periodontal ligament injection: Review of the literature. Quintessence Int. 20:219, 1989.

Hersh, E. V., Helpin, M. L., and Evans, O. B. Local anesthetic mortality: Report of a case. J. Dent. Child. 58:489, 1991

Hess, G. P., Walson, P. D. Seizures secondary to oral viscous lidocaine. Ann. Emerg. Med. 17:725, 1988.

Johnsen, D., Johns, S. Quantitation of nerve fibres in the primary and permanent canine and incisor teeth in man. Arch. Oral Biol. 23:825, 1978.

Jorgenson, N. B., and Hayden, J., Jr. Sedation, Local and General Anesthesia and Dentistry. 3rd ed. Philadelphia: Lea & Febiger, 1980.

Khedari, A. J. Alternative to mandibular block injections through intraligamental anesthesia. Quintessence Int. 13:231, 1982.

Kuster, C. G., and Udin, R. D. Frequency of accidental intravascular injection of local anesthetics in children. J. Dent. Child. 52:183, 1985.

Lalli, A. F., and Amaranath, L. A critique on mortality associated with local anesthetics. Anesth. Rev. 10:29, 1982.

Malamed, S. F. Handbook of Local Anesthesia. St. Louis: The C.V. Mosby Co., 1980.

Malamed, S. The Gow-Gates mandibular block. Evaluation after 4.275 cases. Oral Surg. Oral Med. Oral Pathol. 51:463, 1981.

Malamed, S. F. The periodontal ligament (PDL) injection: An alternative to inferior alveolar nerve block. Oral Surg. Oral Med. Oral Pathol. 53:117, 1982.

Malamed, S. F. Handbook of Local Anesthesia. 3rd ed. St. Louis, The C.V. Mosby Co. 1990, (a) p. 203, (b) pp. 237-238, (c) p. 199, (d) pp. 48-49, (e) pp. 258-284.

McClure, D. B. Local anesthetic for the preschool child. J. Dent. Child. 35:441, 1968.

McNamara, P., Slaughter M., and Pieper, J., et al. Factors influencing serum protein binding of lidocaine in humans. Anesth. Analg. 60:395, 1981.

Menke, R. A. Gowgiel, J. M. Short-needle block anesthesia at the mandibular foramen. J. Am. Dent Assoc. 99:27, 1979.

Milam S. B., and Giovannitti, J. A., Jr. Local anesthetics in dental practice. Dent. Clin. North Am. 28:493, 1984.

Miller, A. G. A clinical evaluation of the Ligmaject periodontal ligament injection syringe. Dent. Update 10:639, 1983.

Mink, J. R. Spedding, R. A. An injection procedure for the child dental patient. Dent. Clin. North Am. :309-325, 1966.

Mofenson, H. C., Caraccio, T. R., Miller, H., et al. Lidocaine toxicity from topical mucosal application. Clin. Pediatr. 22:190, 1983.

Moore, P. A. Local anesthesia and narcotic drug interaction in pediatric dentistry. Anesth. Prog. 35:17, 1988.

Munson, E. S., Gutnick, M. J. and Wagman, I. H. Local anesthetic drug-induced seizures in rhesus monkeys. Anesth. Analg. 6:986, 1970.

O'Sullivan, V. R., Holland, T., O'Mullane, D. M., et al, A review of current local anaesthetic techniques in dentistry for children J. Irish Dent. Assoc. 32:17, 1986.

Primosch, R. E. The role of pressure syringes in the administration of intraligamentary anesthesia. Compend. Con. Educ. Dent. 7:340-348, 1986.

Roberts, D. H., and Sowray, J. H. Local Anesthesia in Dentistry. Bristol, England: John Wright & Sons, Ltd., 1970.

Romanes, G. G. Cunningham's Textbook on Anatomy. 12th Ed. London: Oxford University Press, 1981, p. 752.

Sanders, B., Blain, S., and Carr, S. Local Anesthesia. In Sanders, B. Pediatric Oral and Maxillofacial Surgery. St. Louis: The C.V. Mosby Co., 1979.

Scott, D. B., Jebson, P. J. R., Braid, D. P., et al. Factors affecting plasma levels of lignocaine and prilocaine. Br. J. Anaesth. 44:1040, 1972.

Smith, G. N., Walton, R. E., and Abott, B. J. Clinical evaluation of periodontal ligament anesthesia using a pressure syringe. J. Am. Dent. Assoc. 107:953, 1983.

Smudski, J. W., Sprecher, R. L., and Elliott, H. W. Convulsive interactions of promethazine, meperidine and lidocaine. Arch. Oral Biol. 9:595, 1964.

Spiro, S. R. Pain and Anxiety Control in Dentistry. Englewood, N.J.: Jack Burgess, Inc., 1981.

Tomlin, P. J. Death in outpatient dental anaesthetic practice. Anaesthesia 29:551, 1974.

Usubiaga, J. E., Wikinski, J., Ferrero, R. et al. Local anesthetic-induced convulsions in man—an electroencephalographic study. Anesth. Analg. 45:611, 1966.

Vreeland, D. L. Reader, A., Beck, M., et al. An evaluation of volumes and concentrations of lidocaine in human inferior alveolar nerve block. J. Endod. 15:6, 1989.

Wagman, I. H., de Jong, R. H., and Prince, D. A. Effects of lidocaine on spontaneous cortical and subcortical electrical activity. Arch. Neurol. 18:277, 1968.

Walton, R. E., and Abbott, B. J. Periodontal ligament injection: A clinical evaluation. J. Am. Dent. Assoc. 103:571, 1981.

Wei, S. Pediatric Dentistry—Total Patient Care. Philadelphia: Lea & Febiger, 1988, pp.157-158.

Wilson T., Primsoch, R. E., Melamed, B., et al. Clinical effectiveness of 1% and 2% lidocaine in young pediatric dental patients. Pediatr. Dent. 12:353, 1990.

Wong, M. K. S., and Jacobsen, P. L. Reason for local anesthesia failures. J. Am. Dent. Assoc. 123:69, 1992.

Yagiela, J. A., Local anesthetics: A century of progress. Anesth. Prog. 32:47, 1985.

Yamada, A., Jasstak, J. T. Clinical evaluation of the Gow-Gates block in children. Anesth. Prog. 28:106, 1981.

Questions

1. Which of the following local anesthetic techniques is recommended for anesthetizing a primary mandibular second molar before its removal?

   a. Buccal and lingual infiltration adjacent to second primary molar
   b. Inferior alveolar nerve block
   c. Inferior alveolar and lingual nerve block
   d. Inferior alveolar, lingual, and buccal nerve block

2. Which of the following local anesthetic procedures is recommended for anesthetizing a primary maxillary first molar before its removal?

   a. Middle superior alveolar and anterior palatine nerve infiltrations
   b. Posterior and middle superior alveolar and anterior palatine nerve infiltration
   c. Tuberosity block
   d. All of the above

3. James Johnson, age 4, is in for his first restorative work. You are about to anesthetize. You must develop a sound patient-dentist relationship between James and yourself. This philosophy is based on the following concept(s):

   a. Patient preparation
   b. Skilled administration of the local anesthetic
   c. Armamentarium and anesthetic agents adaptable to the child patient
   d. A well-trained chairside assistant
   e. Requiring the parent to remain in the reception room
   f. c,d
   g. b,c
   h. a,e
   i. a,b

4. James, as has been stated, is 4 years old. Your approach in working with him requires explanations and descriptions of the local anesthetic procedure. As such you would explain and describe the procedure:

   a. In a mature, straightforward way
   b. In terms that are simple and understandable
   c. In semantics adjusted for his level of maturity
   d. In childlike language
   e. a,b
   f. b,c
   g. c,d
   h. All of the above

Chapter 13

Nitrous Oxide–Oxygen Inhalation

Objectives

After studying this chapter, the student should be able to discuss:

1. The indications for and the limitations of using nitrous oxide–oxygen inhalation in the dental operatory.
2. The mechanism of action of this agent on physiologic and psychological functioning.
3. The contraindications, potential abuse, and adverse side effects of its application.
4. The equipment used in its delivery.
5. The procedural guidelines for its use.

Nitrous oxide–oxygen inhalation is a commonly used aid to alleviate patient anxiety and apprehension and to augment the dentist's ability to communicate with the patient. Additionally, it may help to overcome a child's fearful behavior permanently. The outcome of this management technique is successful only when the patient no longer requires it.

Indications

The inhalation of nitrous oxide gas combined with oxygen provides the patient with a sedative-euphoric state of being. In the proper concentrations, an altered state of awareness can be created with effects that include relaxation (sedation) and alterations in memory (amnesia) and perception (analgesia). The current approach in the use of nitrous oxide is to deemphasize the amnesiac and analgesic effects obtained at higher concentrations (greater than 40%) and to emphasize the psychosedative benefits obtained at lower concentrations (less than 40%) (Simon and Vogelsberg, 1975; Bennett, 1978).

The indications for the use of nitrous oxide–oxygen inhalation include the need to *(1)* ease anxiety and apprehension associated with the dental environment, especially "needle phobia" (Sorenson and Roth, 1973), *(2)* create a hypnotic state, *(3)* increase tolerance to long appointments, *(4)* increase the pain reaction threshold, *(5)* suppress the gag reflex, and *(6)* preclude sedative premedication or enhance its effects,

thereby reducing the need for general anesthesia (Manford and Roberts, 1980). All of these indications obviously support its use for the behavior management of children in the dental setting.

Nitrous oxide–oxygen inhalation is the pharmacotherapeutic modality most used by dentists to overcome a patient's anxiety. However, its administration should be considered only as an adjunct to nonpharmacotherapeutic management techniques and not as a panacea. The psychosedation created by nitrous oxide should be used to augment, not replace, other routine methods of child behavior management. It is best applied to help children learn how to cope with stress and anxiety. Monitoring and management of the patient are still required, because sedation, by itself, does not control behavior but rather provides an avenue by which the patient can be taught to modify behavior and reduce apprehension. For behavior modification to work, the patient must be conscious and responsive to suggestions.

Unfortunately, in some situations, the ease and effectiveness of its application may result in its abuse. Failure to select appropriate circumstances for the administration of nitrous oxide may result in its becoming a crutch for both the dentist and the patient. The dentist may routinely use nitrous oxide to avoid having to deal directly with the patient's anxiety or to prevent the patient's interference with efficient operative procedures. For the patient, it may be abused by providing a means to avoid dealing realistically with his or her fear. Therefore, nitrous oxide–oxygen inhalation should not be considered as a method of eluding responsibility for managing fear and apprehension but as a means to teach the child patient to modify his or her behavior in the dental operatory (Pruhs and Williams, 1978). The dentist's responsibility to use behavioral modification techniques does not end with the passive act of placing the nasal mask on the child patient.

Mechanism of action

Nitrous oxide is a colorless, odorless, inert, nontoxic gas. However, when inhaled, it is only nontoxic if a minimum concentration of 20% oxygen is simultaneously administered (Bennett, 1978). A minimum concentration of 20% oxygen is required to prevent anoxia. Nitrous oxide is considered only a 15% potent anesthetic agent because surgical levels of anesthesia are unobtainable safely without causing asphyxia (Bennett, 1978).

When inhaled, nitrous oxide enters the pulmonary alveoli and passes through their epithelium to enter the blood stream. Passage of nitrous oxide through the pulmonary epithelium is regulated by the nitrous oxide partial pressure gradient between the pulmonary alveoli and the blood stream. Nitrous oxide is carried in the serum and thus does not compete with oxygen or carbon dioxide for hemoglobin in the red blood cells. It quickly arrives at all highly perfused organs such as the brain. There it affects the central nervous system by depressing the cerebrum, creating an altered state of awareness. At optimal level of delivery (40% nitrous oxide, 60% oxygen), an alteration in memory may occur (amnesia) (Robson et al, 1970). This amnesia may be more a reflection of not caring rather than not remembering because the ability of total recall has been demonstrated following termination of the procedure (Hogue et al, 1971).

There are also reports that optimal levels of nitrous oxide administration may impair motor function and performance (Trieger et al, 1971; Machen et al, 1977), but it appears that learning and memory are not sufficiently altered to affect methods of behavioral modification employed by the dentist. Whatever changes occur are completely reversible by an adequate period of 100% oxygenation (Machen et al, 1977).

However, there is a great deal of debate concerning the effect of nitrous oxide on perception and as to whether dental analgesia is achieved at the recommended level of administration. Although there is absolutely no effect on proprioception, some studies have indicated that nitrous oxide has the ability to elevate a patient's pain reaction threshold when used at the 40% concentration (Hogue et al, 1971; Berger, 1972; Devine et al, 1974). Other investigators believe that these results are more likely due to a placebo influence (Trieger et al, 1971; Everett and Allen, 1971; Allen, 1974; Bennett, 1978). Studies on adults have demonstrated that nitrous oxide elevates the pain threshold level to electrical pulp stimulation (Dworkin et al, 1983; Heft et al, 1984). In children, there is evidence that nitrous oxide sedation maintained at the level of relative analgesia significantly decreases the intensity of pain perceived during cavity preparation of primary molars (Hammond and Full, 1984).

The sedative effect of nitrous oxide produces relaxation of the neuromuscular system. The respiratory tract system is slightly stimulated, resulting in increased tidal volume. However, the potential for respiratory tract depression created by some premedications used to manage patient behavior may be increased by nitrous oxide. The cardiovascular system becomes slightly depressed, causing a decreased heart rate (Hogue et al, 1971) and lowered blood pressure (Aspes, 1975). These changes are likely due to the reduced demand for cardiac function created by the administration of the high oxygen level with the nitrous oxide.

Also reported are gastrointestinal disturbances mainly in the form of nausea and vomiting. The incidence of nausea and vomiting appears to be very low (Hogue et al, 1971; Houck and Ripa, 1971; Hallonsten et al, 1983). No correlation exists between the incidence of nausea and vomiting and the concentration of nitrous oxide used, length of treatment, age of patient, or health status (Hallonsten et al, 1983). Therefore, no special eating instructions before administration are routinely required (Hogue et al, 1971) unless past history indicates that the child has a propensity to vomit (Houck and Ripa, 1971). In such cases, an antiemetic may be given in addition to instructions not to eat 2 to 3 hours before the appointment.

Nitrous oxide is not metabolized by the body but is excreted mainly through the lungs. Longer administrations may cause saturation in the lungs that can alter the oxygen–carbon dioxide exchange. Therefore, for maintenance beyond a 30-minute duration, the nitrous oxide dosage should be reduced by one half (Simon and Vogelsburg, 1975). As the nitrous oxide leaves the blood to enter the alveoli, it will dilute the amount of oxygen delivered to the alveoli. When the nitrous oxide administration is terminated, the outpouring of nitrous oxide into the lungs will dilute the availability of oxygen to the patient, causing a condition termed *diffusion hypoxia* (Sheffer et al, 1972).

Although this danger is probably insignificant in healthy patients with normal alveolar ventilation (Simon and Vogelsburg, 1975), it is recommended that the patient receive 100% oxygen for 5 minutes at the termination of nitrous oxide use to prevent the possibility of diffusion hypoxia.

Contraindications

There are no absolute contraindications to administration of nitrous oxide–oxygen inhalation, only relative ones (Langa, 1968; Stuebner, 1973; Bennett, 1978; Wald, 1983; Malamed, 1985). Chronic obstructive pulmonary disease (bronchitis, emphysema), upper respiratory tract infections, otitis media, multiple sclerosis, and severe emotional disturbances are definite concerns warranting medical consultation before use. Emphysema is a real concern because the high oxygen concentrations delivered during administration actually suppress the drive to breathe in these patients.

Most commonly, the patient's inability to perform nasal respiration because of obstruction from a cold, deviated septum, or enlarged adenoids prevents its use. The presence of otitis media during the administration of nitrous oxide poses an additional warning. Any gas-filled space, such as the middle ear, will develop increased volume/pressure as nitrous oxide diffuses into the space. An increased pressure differential develops because nitrous oxide diffuses faster into the space than nitrogen leaves, because nitrous oxide is 35 times as soluble as nitrogen in the blood. In addition, interference of the venting function of the eustachian tube by upper respiratory tract infections will allow for further increase in middle ear pressure. The result of increased middle ear pressure can range from mild auditory changes to deafness (Wald, 1983; Malamed, 1985). An appropriate regimen of antihistamines or decongestants before use may be helpful. This type of pressure-volume change created by nitrous oxide may also cause gastrointestinal distention, resulting in nausea and vomiting.

Some authors warn against its use in patients with heart disease, epilepsy, asthma, and sickle cell anemia (Stuebner, 1973; Barenie, 1979). However, most feel that the sedative ability of nitrous oxide to reduce stress and the high levels of oxygenation provided may be highly beneficial from a preventive viewpoint (Langa, 1968; Bennett, 1978; Wald, 1983; Malamed, 1985). Other conditions possibly precluding its use include a history of dislike from a previous experience or defiant and hysterical behavior in a child who has lost contact with reality, nor should it be used as an analgesic or general anesthetic to avoid administering local anesthesia (Simon and Vogelsberg, 1975).

Adverse effects

Although nitrous oxide–oxygen inhalation has a remarkable record of safety, occasional, and sometimes fatal, complications have occurred that should prevent complacency toward its use. Among the many hazards reported are asphyxia resulting from equipment failure, diffusion hypoxia, malignant hyperpyrexia, bone marrow depression, pressure-volume effects, adverse psychologic reactions, and nausea or vomiting (Ducan and Moore, 1984). There is concern about the effects of long-term exposure to nitrous oxide on dental personnel (Bussard, 1976; Greenfield, 1977). In 1971, a survey of female operating room nurses and anesthetists revealed that their miscarriage rate was 29.7% compared with a prevalence of 8.8% among general duty nurses (Cohen et al, 1971). A follow-up survey confirmed the increased risk of spontaneous abortion among operating room nurses and documented an increased risk of congenital abnormalities in infants of unexposed wives of male operating room personnel (Cohen et al, 1974). Another survey of female nurse anesthetists found that the 16.4% prevalence of birth defects in children whose mothers worked during pregnancy was significantly greater than the 5.7% prevalence found in those who did not (Corbett et al, 1974). Although no direct cause and effect relationship can be proved nor any specific agent cited (nitrous oxide is used with halothane as a general anesthetic), the implications of these surveys were alarming enough to stimulate investigation of dental personnel.

In 1974, Millard and Corbett measured the levels of nitrous oxide in the dental operatory when 60% nitrous oxide was used at a flow rate of 4 L/min. Their measurements revealed that the air concentration of nitrous oxide increased with the length of the procedure. After 15 minutes of use, the concentration of nitrous oxide in the breathing zone of the dentist and assistant was recorded as 3,800 and 1,900 ppm, respectively, whereas the concentration in the corner of the room was 1,750 ppm. After 1 hour, the concentration of nitrous oxide had risen to 6,800, 5,900, and 3,100 ppm for the dentist, assistant, and room, respectively. These concentrations are much higher than recorded in the operating room of a hospital. Therefore, it was not surprising to learn that when dentists, exposed to nitrous oxide for periods greater than 3 hours a week, were compared with those with less exposure, there was a reported 156% increase in liver disease among those dentists with chronic exposure and a 78% rise in spontaneous abortion among their wives (Cohen et al, 1975).

A more extensive survey of dental personnel in 1980 defined chronic exposure to nitrous oxide as greater than 8 hours a week (Cohen, 1980). The results of this survey indicated the fold increase for the following conditions: liver disease (1.7), kidney disease (1.2), and neurologic disease (1.9) for male dentists; spontaneous abortion (1.5) for wives of dentists; and liver disease (1.6) kidney disease (1.7), neurologic disease (2.8), and spontaneous abortion (2.3) for female chairside assistants.

Recent epidemiologic evidence supports the finding of reduced fertility among female dental assistants exposed to ambient levels of unscavenged nitrous oxide for longer than 5 hours per week (Rowland et al, 1992). To date, however, neither the concentration of trace ambient nitrous oxide that is harmful to humans nor the length of exposure that produces biologic deleterious effects is known (Henry, 1992).

The hazard of chronic use of nitrous oxide in the dental operatory is related to its method of delivery.

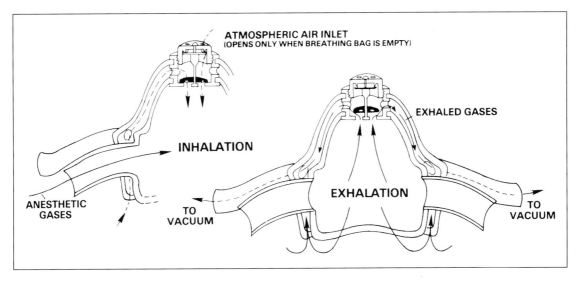

Fig 13-1 Diagram of scavenging nasal mask (Brown, Porter Instruments).

Since the system of delivery is open, allowing for waste nitrous oxide to contaminate the environment, a more stringent monitoring program must be enforced (Whitcher et al, 1978). Chronic nitrous oxide exposure should be kept at a minimum by (1) eliminating leakage in the system, (2) limiting mouth breathing or speech by the patient during use, (3) providing adequate laminar flow circulation of room air, and (4) reducing the level of nitrous oxide concentration to 50 ppm in the breathing zone of the operating personnel (Whitcher et al, 1978). The amount of waste gases is significant because one recent report indicates that inhaled concentrations by the patient are approximately only one third that delivered by the machine (Sher et al, 1984).

To achieve sufficient protection from this potential hazard, many ventilation and scavenging devices have been manufactured (Swenson, 1976; Hallonsten, 1982a), although these systems seem to vary greatly in their effectiveness (Hallonsten, 1982a; Brown and Bell, 1984; Christensen et al, 1985). In particular, a double nasal mask has been shown to reduce the amount of residual gas by 97% (Whitcher et al, 1978; Tonn and Whitcher, 1980). The scavenging mask is a mask within a mask, with two hoses supplying nitrous oxide to the inner mask and two hoses attached to the outer mask to retrieve the expired and residual gas by evacuation with a central suction system (Fig 13-1).

Even with careful technique and safe equipment, the efficiency of scavenging equipment to remove expired and waste gasses is diminished by poorly fitting masks and mouth breathing from uncooperative patients. When a scavenger mask is used on uncooperative child patients, the level of waste nitrous oxide can be five times that recommended (Badger and Robertson, 1982). Casual patient talking or the use of a rubber dam does not significantly influence the effectiveness

of scavenging systems to reduce ambient levels of nitrous oxide (Christensen et al, 1985). A local exhaust system placed near the patient using a scavenging mask has been successfully employed to overcome local air contamination in the breathing zone of dental personnel (Hallonsten, 1982b). Clearly, the modification of current breathing circuits and development of scavenging devices with improved physical properties are warranted (Brown and Bell, 1984). The modifications required should be directed toward reducing (1) gas flow resistance in the tubing, (2) carbon dioxide retention in the mask and subsequent rebreathing, and (3) influence of scavenging devices on the degree of rebreathing and the concentrations of gas administered (Hallonsten and Lofstrom, 1982).

Studies have revealed that, even in the presence of scavenging devices, ambient nitrous oxide levels routinely exceed National Institute of Safety and Health (NIOSH) recommendations of 25 ppm (Henry and Primosch, 1991). Use of scavenging devices alone, without monitoring, will not guarantee compliance with federal guidelines. Scavenger effectiveness can be reduced by patient behavior, certain dental procedures, and improper delivery and suction rates (Henry et al, 1992). Building ventilation rates and leaking equipment also influence levels of ambient nitrous oxide. A room air exchange rate of 10 changes per hour was recommended to minimize ambient levels (McGlothlin et al, 1989), and pressure leakage around loose connections and/or faulty rubber goods should be periodically monitored.

Another potential problem with using nitrous oxide is its availability for recreational use. The potential for its abuse is real, and therefore the equipment must be safely secured. Long-term exposure of 40% nitrous oxide in rats has revealed neurologic damage to the occipital cortex of the brain (Hayden et al, 1974). In humans, case reports of habitual recreational use by dentists show the development of neuropathy that includes numbness and pain in the distal extremities, loss of bladder control, and multiple sclerosis–like symptoms (Layzer et al, 1978; Paulson, 1979; Gutmann and Johnsen, 1980).

Equipment

Numerous machines are available for the administration of nitrous oxide–oxygen inhalation (Figs 13-2 to 13-6) (Allen, 1974; Malamed, 1985). These machines should have the capacity to accurately regulate gas flow and maintain the minimum level of 20% oxygen flow to prevent asphyxia. In addition, they should be of continuous flow design and have an audible or visual warning system or system shut-down if oxygen flow is interrupted. There should also be an oxygen flush lever that will deliver 100% oxygen at 30 L/min. The designs for converting this system into one using a full mask and intermittent positive pressure ventilation for emergency resuscitation are available (Nozik et al, 1975).

The gas cylinders are required to be color coded green (oxygen) and blue (nitrous oxide). The nitrous oxide cylinders should be of medical quality to assure freedom from inadvertent contamination by toxic by-products such as nitrous dioxide and nitric oxide.

There are basically two sizes of cylinders: small (for portable use) and large. The large cylinders (size G or H) contain approximately 12,000 to 16,000 L (3,200 to 4,200) ga). These are more discreet because they can be hidden from view and are more economical than the smaller-size cylinders. The large cylinders contain ten times the volume but cost only three times as much as the smaller cylinders. The small cylinders (size D or E) contain approximately 950 to 1,596 L (250 to 420 ga). The nitrous oxide is packaged by compression of the gas into its liquid form and stored at 650 to 800 psi (Bennett, 1978). Since the contents are mostly liquid, it holds a constant pressure, and its use will not register on the pressure gauge until the liquid is used up and converted to gas. When this conversion occurs, a marked decrease in pressure will be recorded; although pressure is not a direct indicator of amount, it may be used for this purpose at this time. Generally, if you were to use an E-sized cylinder of nitrous oxide that contains 1,596 L (420 ga) at a continuous flow of 3.5 L/min, you could expect it to last 7.5 hours. On the other hand, the oxygen cylinder stores oxygen gas at 2,000 psi, and its pressure will drop in proportion to its usage. An E-sized cylinder of oxygen contains 627 L (165 ga), which at a 5 L/min flow rate would be exhausted in approximately 2 hours.

The regulator is designed to maintain a constant pressure. Within the regulator is a reducing valve that steps down the high pressure of the gas to atmospheric level (50 psi) before delivery (Langa, 1968). It is normal for the external surface of the regulator to frost up during usage. The higher pressure gauge is attached to the regulator.

Routine sterilization of the nasal mask is essential because the nasal mask can cause bacterial transmission and cross-contamination of succeeding patients (Hunt and Yagiela, 1977). In addition, upstream contamination of the hoses and inhalation apparatus may occur. Therefore, it would be advisable to clean the bag and breathing tube by soaking them in soap and water, leaving them to dry in room air, once weekly.

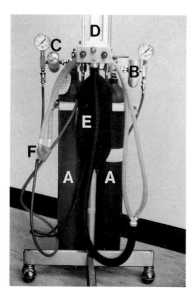

Fig 13-2 The various components of a portable unit: (*A*) cylinder, (*B*) regulator, (*C*) pressure gauge, (*D*) flowmeter, (*E*) reservoir bag, and (*F*) nasal mask.

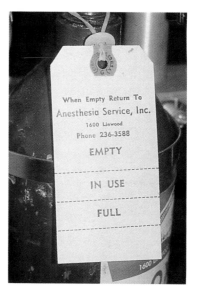

Fig 13-3 A gas cylinder should have a tag system allowing identification of the cylinder as full, in use, or empty.

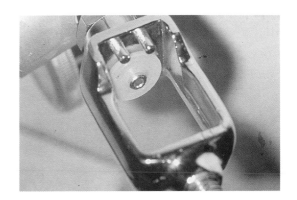

Fig 13-4 The cylinders are directly attached to the regulator gauge by means of a pin-indexed yoke system. This is a safety system to prevent attachment of the wrong gas cylinders.

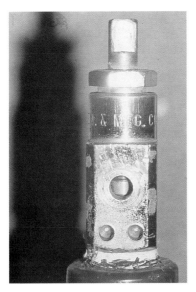

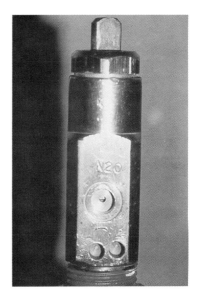

Figs 13-5a and b The different distance between pinholes among the various gas cylinder prevents inadvertent placement of the wrong cylinder on the yoke. The distance between pinholes is wider for the oxygen cylinder than for the nitrous oxide cylinder.

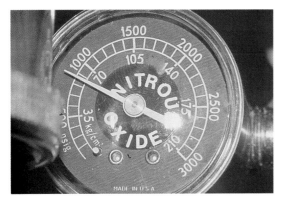

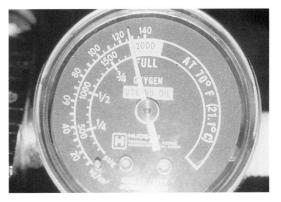

Figs 13-6a and b When the cylinders are full, the nitrous oxide gauge will read approximately 800 psi, and the oxygen gauge will register approximately 2,000 psi.

Procedure for administration

1. Select the appropriate patient through visual and verbal clues given from the manifested anxiety level expressed by the patient, parent, and siblings (Sorensen and Roth, 1973).
2. Review the medical history.
3. Obtain parental consent.
4. Introduce the patient to the equipment before the appointment to avoid anxiety over the technique and to gain patient acceptance.
5. Complete advanced preparation and organiza-

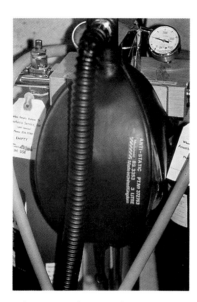

Fig 13-7   The reservoir bag provides the operator with a visual check as to the patient's depth and frequency of respiration. The flowmeter should be adjusted at a sufficient rate to prevent the bag from either collapsing on inspiration or remaining overinflated.

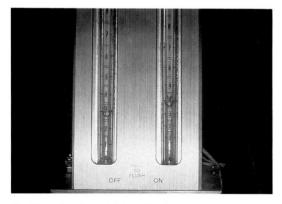

Fig 13-8   The flow (L/min) of each gas is separately controlled by the operator and displayed on the flowmeter by floating beads. The accuracy of the flowmeter is ± 5% and is directly proportional to its length. The liter flow must be converted into percent by the operator's calculations.

tion before seating the patient. This step includes:

a. Inspecting the equipment for adequate gas supply by opening the cylinder with the wrench provided and checking pressure gauge. A half turn counterclockwise is sufficient to open the cylinder.
b. Placing a sterilized, scented nasal mask of appropriate size onto the tubing and turning the suction on the scavenging system.
c. Ensuring that a trained assistant is constantly present to assist if complications should arise.
d. Sending the patient to the bathroom before beginning.

6. Introduce the child (if not done during a prior visit) to the equipment being used in terms he or she will understand (euphemisms). Tell the child that you have magic air that when breathed will make him or her feel happy and comfortable. Using the technique of tell, show, and do, place the mask over your nose so that the child can observe how it works. An analogy of the mask is one like pilots or astronauts use should be sufficient. Then tell him or her that we are going to pretend to take a space trip by placing the mask on the child's nose instead. Most children readily accept fantasy and are very receptive to the power of suggestion.
7. Fill the reservoir bag with 100% oxygen (Fig 13-7), using the flush valve, before placing the mask on the nose so not to startle the child. Do not display a hurried or forceful approach.
8. Tighten the adjustment on the breathing tubes behind the back of the chair so that the mask fits comfortably but firmly over the nose.
9. Begin the flowmeter with 100% oxygen at 5 to 8 L/min for 2 to 3 minutes (Fig 13-8). This amount will delete the nitrogen in the bloodstream and better prepare the system for nitrous oxide uptake (Bennett, 1978; Barenie, 1979).
10. Tell the patient to close or touch the lips together to encourage nasal respiration. Place your fingers over the lips if a reminder is needed.
11. Begin induction of nitrous oxide by either a slow or rapid method. Slow induction technique uses increasing increments of 0.5 to 1.0 L/min nitrous oxide while simultaneously decreasing oxygen flow in equal increments. This method allows a slow adjustment of the patient to its effects and allows the operator to monitor the patient's progress. However, the rapid induction technique delivers immediate concentration or 40% (2 to 4 L/min) nitrous oxide and 60% (3 to 5 L/min) oxygen to the patient. This method is recommended for preschool children who cannot adequately communicate their level of sedation (Simon and Vogelsberg, 1975).
12. During induction. explain the psychosedative effects to the child in a positive but not overelaborate manner to prepare him or her for the events that will transpire. Although there is a consider-

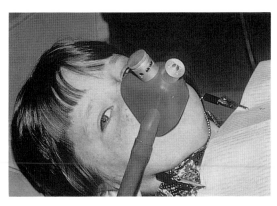
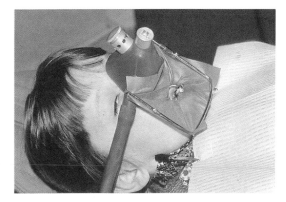

Figs 13-9a and b Note the changes produced after 5 minute induction of 40% nitrous oxide—the centrally fixed pupils, with a faraway, distant stare and the sagging eyelids are classic signs of adequate sedation.

Table 13-1 Patient symptoms obtained at various nitrous oxide levels

Nitrous oxide concentration (%)	Symptoms
10–20	Tingling feeling (paresthesia) Sensation of warmth
20–40	Numbness of the extremities Sensation of floating Auditory changes (distinct but distant humming noise)* Dissociation (inability to perceive spatial orientation)* Analgesia Euphoria
40–60	Dreaming, laughing, or giddiness Sweating Nausea and vomiting Uncoordinated movement Loss of eyelid reflex

*These changes may be unpleasant to the patient. Therefore, it is important to maintain physical contact with the patient, to give verbal reassurances, and to avoid startling movements or loud sounds.

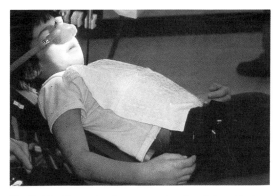

Fig 13-10 The patient's eyes may be closed, but this does not always indicate that sleep is occurring. Therefore, be aware that the patient may still hear your remarks even though he or she appears asleep. Sedation may produce deep relaxation with heavy arms, open hands, and a stationary position usually spread out over the chair. A mouth prop may be indicated in this situation.

able range in patient response, the list of symptoms in Table 13-1 can be used as a guide according to the percent concentration of nitrous oxide (Bennett, 1978).

13. Peak effect will occur within 3 to 5 minutes (Fig 13-9). Let the child's reactions to the sedation guide your judgment, not the flowmeter. You want to achieve relative analgesia (stage 1, plane 2, of anesthesia). Relative analgesia is defined by the following criteria: respiration is normal; general muscles are relaxed; pupils are normal and contracted with exposed to light; rate of blinking is reduced; eyes have a relaxed, dreamy, faraway look; mouth is maintained open without props; patient follows directions, is relaxed, euphoric, and less aware of immediate surroundings; some patients experience a tingling in fingers, toes, lips, or

tongue; some patients feel a warm wave suffuse the entire body; patients experience a humming, droning, or vibratory sensation and feeling of lethargy or drowsiness; voice becomes throaty; and thoughts wander beyond the treatment room environment (Hammond and Full, 1984).

14. The patient should now be ready for administration of the local anesthetic. The careful use of suggestion will help increase the patient's hypnotic state (Barber et al, 1979). In addition, the exposure to new equipment and the unfamiliar sensations of euphoria will act as a distraction.

15. Once the injection is completed, reduce the nitrous oxide level to 20% to 30% during the maintenance phase.

16. The patient should always be capable of rational response to verbal command (Fig 13-10). Verbal

contact is the best method of monitoring the patient, but do not encourage the patient to speak frequently. Speaking promotes mouth breathing; therefore, verbal commands such as "open or close your mouth" should be sufficient to monitor patient responsiveness.

17. Vomiting seldom occurs, but its occurrence is influenced by prior history, overdosage (more than 50% nitrous oxide), frequent fluctuations in concentration, and prolonged administration (because of the saturation effect). Young children will seldom give a verbal warning of nausea, but violent contraction of the abdomen may indicate an impending episode of vomiting. If vomiting should occur do not panic. Lower the head and turn it to the side. Suction the mouth clear. Aspiration will not occur because the laryngeal reflex is still intact (Allen et al, 1977). Terminate the nitrous oxide delivery and give 100% oxygen while bringing the dental procedure to completion as quickly as possible.

18. Following the termination of the procedure, place the patient on 100% oxygen during the withdrawal phase for 3 to 5 minutes to prevent diffusion hypoxia.

19. Have the child sit up in the chair for a few additional minutes to avoid postural hypotension. Although all changes are completely reversible by oxygenation, the child patient may still be withdrawn, sleepy, and unresponsive, similar to waking up from a nap.

20. Record all results and the concentrations used, in the patient's records for future guidance.

References

Allen, G. D. Nitrous oxide–oxygen sedation machines and devices. J. Am. Dent. Assoc. 88:611, 1974.

Allen, G. D., Ricks, C. S., and Jorgensen, N. B. The efficacy of the laryngeal reflex in conscious sedation. J. Am. Dent. Assoc. 96:901, 1977.

Aspes, T. The effect of nitrous oxide sedation on the blood pressure of pediatric dental patients. J. Dent. Child. 42:364, 1975.

Badger, G. R., and Robertson, C. W. Nitrous oxide waste gas in the pedodontic operatory. J. Am. Dent. Assoc. 104:480, 1982.

Barber, J., et al. The relationship between nitrous oxide conscious sedation and the hypnotic state. J. Am. Dent. Assoc. 99:624, 1979.

Barenie, J. Inhalation conscious sedation: Nitrous oxide analgesia. In Ripa, L. R., and Barenie, J. Management of Dental Behavior in Children. Littleton, Mass.: PSG Publ. Co., 1979.

Bennett, R. C. Inhalation sedation: Nitrous oxide and oxygen. In Bennett, R. C. Conscious-Sedation in Dental practice. 2nd ed. St. Louis: The C. V. Mosby Co., 1978.

Berger D. E. An assessment of the analgesic effects of nitrous oxide on the primary dentition. J. Dent. Child. 39:265, 1972.

Brown, J. P., and Bell, S. Efficiency of three nitrous oxide relative analgesia scavenging systems. Dent. Anaesth. Sedat. 13:5, 1984.

Bussard, D. A. Congenital anomalies and inhalation anesthetics. J. Am. Dent. Assoc. 93:606, 1976.

Christensen, J. R., et al. Measurement of scavenged nitrous oxide in the dental operatory. Pediatr. Dent. 7:192, 1985.

Cohen, E. N., et al. Occupational disease among operating room personnel. A national study. Report of an ad hoc committee on the effects of trace anesthetic agents on the health of operating room personnel. Anesthesiology 41:321, 1974.

Cohen, E. N., et al. A survey of anesthetic health hazards among dentists: Report of an ad hoc committee on the effects of trace anesthetic agents on the health of operating room personnel. J. Am. Dent. Assoc. 90:1291, 1975.

Cohen, E. N. et al. Occupational disease in dentistry and chronic exposure to trace anesthetic gases. J. Am. Dent. Assoc. 101:21, 1980.

Cohen, E. N., Belleville, J. W., and Brown, B. W. Anesthesia, pregnancy and miscarriage: A study of operating room nurses and anesthetists. Anesthesiology 35:343, 1971.

Corbett, T. H., et al. Birth defects among children of nurse anesthetists. Anesthesiology 41:341, 1974.

Devine, V., et al. Controlled test of the analgesic and relaxant properties of nitrous oxide. J. Dent. Res. 43:486, 1974.

Ducan, G. H., and Moore, P. Nitrous oxide and the dental patient: A view of adverse reactions. J. Am. Dent. Assoc. 108:213, 1984.

Dworkin, S. F., et al. Analgesic effects of nitrous oxide with controlled painful stimuli. J. Am. Dent. Assoc. 107:581, 1983.

Everett, G. B., and Allen, G. D. Simultaneous evaluation of cardiorespiratory and analgesic effects of nitrous oxide–oxygen inhalation analgesia. J. Am. Dent. Assoc. 83:129, 1971.

Greenfield, W. Trace anesthetic gases: A possible occupational hazard. J. Am. Dent. Assoc. 95:749, 1977.

Gutmann, L., and Johnsen, D. Nitrous oxide-induced myeloneuropathy: Report of cases. J. Am. Dent. Assoc. 103:239, 1981.

Hallonsten, A. L. Nitrous oxide scavenging in dental surgery. I. A comparison of the efficiency of different scavenging devices. Swed. Dent. J. 6:203, 1982a.

Hallonsten, A. L. Nitrous oxide–oxygen sedation in dentistry. Swed. Dent J. (suppl)14:5, 1982b.

Hallonsten, A. L., and Lofstrom, J. B. Physical properties of nitrous oxide–oxygen sedation equipment used in dentistry. Swed. Dent. J. 6:133, 1982.

Hallonsten, A. L., Koch, G., and Schroder, U. Nitrous oxide–oxygen sedation in dental care. Community Dent. Oral Epidemoil. 11:347, 1983.

Hammond, N. I., and Full, C. A. Nitrous oxide analgesia and children's perception of pain. Pediatr. Dent. 6:238, 1984.

Hayden, J., et al. An evaluation of prolonged nitrous oxide–oxygen sedation in rats. J. Am. Dent. Assoc. 89:1374, 1974.

Heft, M. W., Gracely, R. H., and Dubner, R. Nitrous oxide analgesia: A psychophysical evaluation using verbal descriptor sealing. J. Dent. Res. 63:129, 1984.

Henry, R. J. Assessing environmental health concerns associated with nitrous oxide. J. Am. Dent. Assoc. 123:41, 1992.

Henry, R. J., and Primosch, R. E. Influence of operatory size and nitrous oxide concentration upon scavenger effectiveness. J. Dent. Res. 70:1286, 1991.

Henry, R. J., Primosch, R. E. and Courts, F. J. The effects of various dental procedures and patient behaviors upon nitrous oxide scavenger effectiveness. Pediatr. Dent. 14:19, 1992.

Hogue, D., Ternisky, M., and Iranpur, B. The responses to nitrous oxide analgesia in children. J. Dent Child. 38:129, 1971.

Houck, W. R., and Ripa, L. W. Vomiting frequency in children administered nitrous oxide–oxygen in analgesic doses. J. Dent. Child. 38:404, 1971.

Hunt, L. M. and Yagiela, J. A. Bacterial contamination and transmission by nitrous oxide sedation apparatus. Oral Surg. 44:367, 1977.

Langa, H. Relative analgesia in dental practice—Inhalation analgesia with nitrous oxide. Philadelphia: W. B. Saunders Co., 1968.

Layzer, R. B., Fishman, R. A., and Schafer, J. A. Neuropathy following abuse of nitrous oxide. Neurology 28:504, 1978.

Machen, J. B., Ayer, W. A., and Mueller, B. H. Psychomotor effects of nitrous oxide—oxygen sedation on children. J. Dent. Child. 44:219, 1977.

Malamed, S. F. Sedation. A Guide to Patient Management. St. Louis: The C. V. Mosby Co., 1985.

Manford, M. L. M., and Roberts G. J. Dental treatment in young handicapped patients. An assessment of relative analgesia as an alterative to general anesthesia. Anaesthesia 35:1157, 1980.

McGlothlin, J. D., Jensen, P. A., Todd, W. F. et al. In depth survey report: Control of anesthetic gases in dental operatories. DDHS (NIOSH) publication No. ECTB; 166-11b, 1989.

Millard, R. I., and Corbett, T. H. Nitrous oxide concentrations in the dental operatory. J. Oral Surg. 32:593, 1974.

Nozik, D. L., et al. Modification of a nitrous oxide sedation apparatus to provide capability for intermittent positive pressure ventilation. J. Am. Dent. Assoc. 91:128, 1975.

Paulson, G. W. Recreational misuse of nitrous oxide. J. Am. Dent. Assoc. 98:410, 1979.

Pruhs, R. J., and Williams, D. L. A psychological rationale for the use of nitrous oxide psychosedation for children. J. Dent. Child. 45:56, 1978.

Robson, J. G., Burns, B. D., and Welt, P. J. The effect of inhaling dilute nitrous oxide upon recent memory and time estimation. Can. Anaesth. Soc. J. 7:399, 1970.

Rowland, A. S., Baird, D. D., Weinberg, C. R., et al. Reduced fertility among women employed as dental assistants exposed to high levels of nitrous oxide. N. Engl. J. Med. 327:993, 1992.

Sheffer, L., Steffenson, J. L., and Birch, A. A. Nitrous oxide induced diffusion hypoxia on patients breathing spontaneously. Anesthesiology 37:436, 1972.

Sher, A. M., et al. Nitrous oxide sedation in dentistry. A comparison between Rotameter settings, pharyngeal concentrations and blood levels of nitrous oxide. Anaesthesia 39:236, 1984.

Simon J. F., and Vogelsberg, G. M. Use of nitrous oxide–oxygen inhalation sedation for children. In Wright G. Z., Behavior Management in Dentistry for Children. Philadelphia: W. B. Saunders Co., 1975.

Sorenson, H. W., and Roth, G. I. A case for nitrous oxide–oxygen inhalation sedation: An aid in the elimination of the child's fear of the "needle." Dent. Clin. North Am. 17:51, 1973.

Stuebner, E. A. Nitrous oxide analgesia or anesthesia. Dent Clin. North Am. 17:235, 1973.

Swenson, R. D. Scavenging of dental anesthetic gases. J. Oral Surg. 34:207, 1976.

Tonn, E. M., and Whitcher, C. E. Scavenging of waste nitrous oxide in pediatric dental offices. J. Int. Assoc. Dent. Child. 11:41, 1980.

Trieger, N., et al. Nitrous oxide—A study of physiological and psychomotor effects. J. Am. Dent. Assoc. 82:142, 1971.

Wald, C. Nitrous oxide—Are there any real contraindications? Quintessence Int. 14:213, 1983.

Whitcher, C., Zimmerman, D. C., and Piziali, R. L. Control of occupational exposure to nitrous oxide in the oral surgery office. J. Oral Surg. 36:431, 1978.

Questions

1. Five minutes after you infuse your patient with 40% nitrous oxide, he complains of "feeling funny." You notice that his pupils have become fixated with the appearance of a "distant stare." What is your most prudent reaction?

   a. Proceed with scheduled treatment, maintaining patient at current level of nitrous oxide
   b. Proceed with injection of local anesthetic and then reduce nitrous oxide level by 10% to 20%
   c. Delay treatment until patient falls asleep
   d. Stop treatment by turning off nitrous oxide flow because patient is entering into the preexcitatory stage of anesthesia
   e. Turn off nitrous oxide flow, administer positive pressure oxygen and call for help

2. Before demonstration of the nitrous oxide equipment to your patient, which of the following must be checked before the nasal mask is placed over the child's nose?

   a. Oxygen is flushed into reservoir bag
   b. Scavenger system is turned on
   c. Adequate pressure is in both gas cylinders
   d. Nasal mask has been wiped clean and sterilized
   e. All of the above

3. Total calculated flow rate (L/min) during respiration in children is approximately:

   a. 1 to 4
   b. 5 to 9
   c. 10 to 14
   d. 15 to 19
   e. 20 to 24

4. Which of the following medical conditions is a contraindication to the administration of nitrous oxide?

   a. Asthma
   b. Epilepsy
   c. Mental retardation
   d. Sickle cell anemia
   e. None of the above

5. Nitrous oxide is carried in the blood stream by:

   a. Hemoglobin
   b. White blood cells
   c. Red blood cells
   d. Serum
   e. None of the above

Chapter 14

Morphology of the Primary Teeth

Objectives

After studying this chapter, the student should be able to:
1. Identify and distinguish morphologic differences in primary teeth.
2. Apply the knowledge of morphology in clinical procedures for children.

There are several reasons that the dentist requires a thorough understanding of primary tooth morphology. Cavity preparations must conform to the thickness of enamel and dentin plus location and size of the pulp. Restoration of natural contours and morphology of primary teeth is needed for function. Performance of pulpal procedures, recognition of atypical situations, and judgment of indicated treatment for primary and young permanent teeth are also important considerations.

General morphologic considerations in the primary dentition

Figure 14-1 illustrates the external differences between primary and permanent teeth.

Crown

1. The primary tooth has a shorter crown than the permanent tooth.
2. The occlusal table of a primary tooth is narrower proportionally than is the permanent tooth.
3. The primary tooth is much more constricted in the cervical portion of the crown than is the permanent tooth.
4. The enamel and dentin layers are thinner in the primary tooth.
5. The enamel rods in the gingival third extend in a slightly occlusal direction from the dentinoenamel junction in primary teeth but extend slightly apically in the permanent dentition.
6. The contact areas between the primary molars are very broad and flat.

7. The mineral content is nearly the same in the primary and permanent tooth.
8. The color of the primary tooth is usually lighter.

Pulp (Fig 14-2)

1. The pulp of the primary tooth is larger than that of the permanent tooth in relation to the crown size.
2. The pulp horns of the primary tooth are closer to the outer surface of the tooth than are those of the permanent tooth.
3. The mesial pulp horn extends to a closer approximation of the surface than does the distal pulp horn of the primary tooth.
4. The mandibular molar has larger pulp chambers than does the maxillary molar in the primary tooth.
5. The form of the pulp chamber of the primary tooth follows the surface of the crown.
6. Usually there is a pulp horn under each cusp.
7. Histologically, there is very little difference between the pulpal tissue of a primary tooth and that of a young permanent tooth.

Root

1. The root of the primary anterior tooth is narrower mesiodistally than is that of the permanent anterior tooth.
2. The roots of the posterior primary tooth are longer and more slender in relation to crown size than are those of the permanent tooth.
3. The roots of the primary molar flare more as they approach the apex than do the permanent molar roots (which affords the necessary room for the development of the permanent tooth buds).

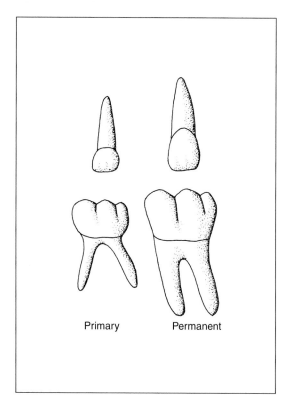

Fig 14-1 A comparison of the morphologies of primary and permanent teeth.

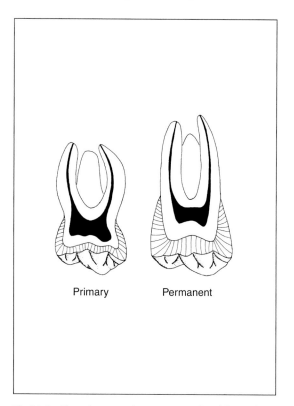

Fig 14-2 The primary and permanent pulps differ in form, size, and approximation to the occlusal surface.

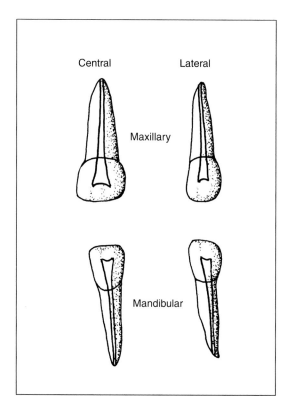

Fig 14-3 Morphology of the primary incisors.

Morphology of specific primary teeth

Mandibular incisors

Of the 20 primary teeth, the first to erupt are the mandibular central incisors (Fig 14-3), usually at age 6 to 8 months. The mandibular central incisor is almost symmetrically flat when viewed from the buccal aspect. As with all primary incisors, there are no developmental grooves or mammelons. The crown is one third the length of the root with a cingulum on the lingual surface. The root is long and cylindrical. The primary mandibular lateral incisor is distinguished from the mandibular central incisor by the distal incisal angle, which is more rounded. In overall dimensions, the primary lateral incisor is somewhat longer but narrower than the primary central incisor.

Pulpal anatomy. The pulp canal follows the outline form of the surface topography of the primary mandibular central and lateral incisors. The pulp is approximately 2.6 mm from the incisal edge in the primary central incisor. The distance to the pulp is 1.7 mm from the distal enamel surface and 1.0 mm from the mesial surface. The pulp of the mandibular lateral incisor has similar dimensions but is somewhat smaller.

Maxillary incisors

The next teeth erupting are the maxillary central and lateral incisors (Fig 14-3), usually by 10 months of age.

The primary maxillary central incisor is unique in that it is the only tooth in the human dentition that has a greater mesiodistal dimension than crown height. The contact points with adjacent teeth are broad, extending from the incisal one third to the gingival one third. Similar to the mandibular incisors, the maxillary central incisor has a flat labial surface. There is a prominent lingual cingulum. The root is conical and roughly two and a half times as long as the crown height.

Pulpal anatomy. The central incisor has two or three small projections (pulp horns) toward the incisal edge; the mesial pulp horn is most prominent. The incisal edge is 2.3 mm from the pulp horn on the mesial aspect and 2.4 mm from the distal pulp horn on the distal aspect. On both the mesial and distal aspects, the pulp horns are approximately 1.2 mm from the dentino-emanel junction (DEJ).

The maxillary lateral incisor is smaller than the maxillary central incisor. The distal incisal aspect is rounded. The tooth in general is more conical, both crown and root.

The pulp chamber is also smaller (2.6 mm from the incisal edge to the pulp). The pulp is approximately 0.9 mm from the DEJ on the mesial and distal aspects.

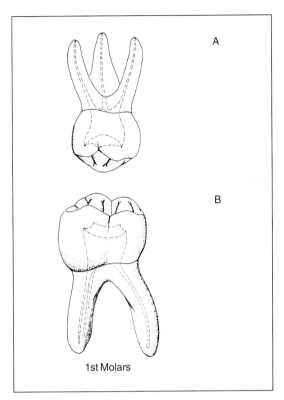

Fig 14-4 *(A)* Maxillary and *(B)* mandibular primary first molars.

Maxillary first molars

The next teeth to erupt are the primary maxillary first molars (Fig 14-4), usually by 16 months of age. The primary maxillary first molar is unique in that it looks somewhat like a molar but also like a premolar (Fig 14-4,*A*). There is no other comparable tooth in the human dentition. The occlusal surface consists of three cusps, one each on the buccal-mesiobuccal and distobuccal surfaces and one on the lingual surface. This gives the tooth a square look. There are three slender roots, one beneath each cusp tip. A characteristic of all primary molars is that the furcation of the roots begins at the cementoenamel junction. This is not apparent in permanent molars. There is a very prominent buccal cervical ridge.

Pulpal anatomy. The pulp horns correspond to each cusp; the mesiobuccal pulp horn is the most prominent. The mesiobuccal pulp horn is 1.8 mm, the distobuccal pulp horn is 2.3 mm, and the lingual pulp horn is 2.0 mm from the cusp tip.

Mandibular first molars

This primary molar erupts by the 16th month of life. It has four cusps, two buccal and two lingual (Fig 14-4,*B*). The occlusal surface is unique in that the mesiobuccal and mesiolingual cusps converge together to form a rather narrow surface. There is a very prominent ridge of enamel, the transverse ridge, that divides the occlusal surface. The enamel of this tooth is uniformly 1.2 mm thick. There are two broad but thin mesiodistal roots, one on the mesial aspect and one on the distal aspect.

Pulpal anatomy. There are four pulp horns with one pulp horn beneath each cusp. Both buccal and lingual mesial pulp horns are 2.1 mm from the DEJ while the distal pulp horns are 2.4 mm away from the DEJ.

Canines

The next teeth to erupt are primary canines (Fig 14-5), usually by the age of 20 months.

The maxillary canine is best described as being long and sharp (Fig 14-5,*A*). The crown is constricted at the cementinoenamel junction. The marginal ridges on the primary canines are usually lacking, but there is often a prominent cingulum. The long, slender root is more than twice the crown length.

Pulpal anatomy. The pulp chamber, like the other incisor, follows the general contour of the tooth with the pulp horn 3.2 mm from the DEJ at the incisal edge. On the mesial and distal surfaces the pulp is approximately 2.1 mm from the DEJ.

The mandibular canine is a long narrow tooth, much smaller than the primary maxillary canine (Fig 14-5,*B*). The distal marginal ridge is much lower than the mesial marginal ridge. The point of contact is very close to the cervical third of the tooth. The root is long and slender and is about twice the crown length.

Pulpal anatomy. The pulp chamber follows the general outline of the tooth form. The pulp is 3.0 mm from the DEJ at the incisal edge. There is 1.8 mm distance from the pulp to the mesial and distal DEJ.

Maxillary second molars

The primary second molars are the last primary teeth to erupt, completing the primary dentition by 28 months of age (Fig 14-6).

The primary maxillary second molar resembles the permanent maxillary first molar in appearance but is smaller (Fig 14-6,*A*). There are four cusps, with two on the buccal and two on the lingual aspects. Often there is a fifth cusp or prominence, the tubercle of Carabelli. The tooth is rhomboidal. A prominent transverse or

oblique ridge connects the distolingual cusp with the mesiolingual cusp. There are three roots that are curved to accommodate the developing tooth bud beneath. The enamel is usually 1.2 mm thick uniformly on the tooth.

Pulpal anatomy. There may be four or five pulp horns, which usually are most prominent beneath each cusp tip. The mesiobuccal pulp horn, as usual, is the largest and closest to the DEJ. The mesiobuccal pulp horn is usually 2.8 mm from the DEJ, while the distobuccal horn is 3.1 mm from the DEJ.

Mandibular second molars

Similar to the primary maxillary second molar, the primary mandibular second molar is a smaller permanent mandibular first molar (Fig 14-6,B). There are five cusps, three on the buccal surface and two on the lingual. The enamel is uniformly 1.2 mm thick. There are two roots which are narrow mesiodistally but very broad buccolingually. Again, the roots are somewhat curved to accommodate the developing tooth bud.

Pulpal anatomy. There are five pulp horns corresponding to the five cusp tips. The mesiobuccal pulp horn is the largest, extending 2.8 mm from the DEJ , while the

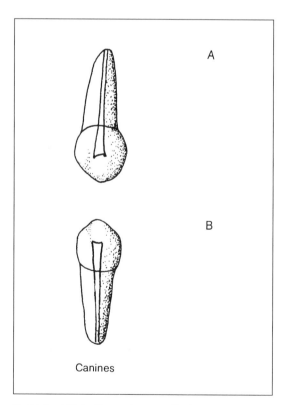

Fig 14-5   *(A)* Maxillary and *(B)* mandibular primary canines.

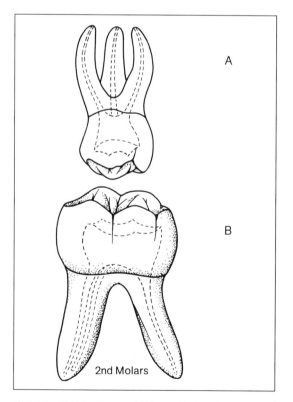

Fig 14-6   *(A)* Maxillary and *(B)* mandibular primary second molars.

distobuccal pulp horn is 3.1 mm from the dentinoenamel junction.

Influences of primary tooth morphology

Progress of caries

It is necessary to restore incipient lesions in primary teeth because of the following factors (Fig 14-7):

1. Enamel is much thinner, thus dental caries is more active in primary teeth.
2. Dentin is proportionally thinner and caries progresses to pulpal tissue faster.
3. The mesial pulp horns extend higher occlusally than on permanent teeth.

Because the enamel and dentin are much thinner, the pulp is more accessible to caries and subsequent bacterial invasion.

Tooth preparations

In general, enamel thickness as related to pulpal tissue is smaller in proportion, thus modifications are needed in cavity preparations. Because of the narrow occlusal table, cavity preparation must be altered (Fig. 14-8). The interproximal contacts of primary teeth are broad and flat compared to those of permanent teeth (Fig 14-9). The contacts of the primary teeth are restored in a "back-to-back" procedure by a firm wedge at the cervical part of the proximal box. It is important to restore the broad contacts of primary teeth to gain a bulk of amalgam to prevent restoration failure.

The specific influences of morphology and dental caries on cavity preparations are related to the individual tooth in the primary dentition.

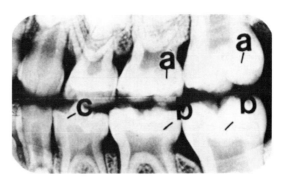

Fig 14-7 The radiographic rationale for early restoration of primary teeth: (*a*) enamel is thinner; (*b*) dentin is thinner; (*c*) the mesial pulp horns extend higher occlusally.

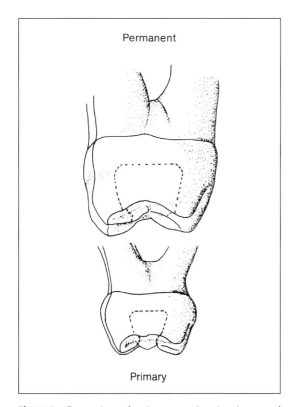

Fig 14-8 Comparison of cavity preparations in primary and permanent teeth.

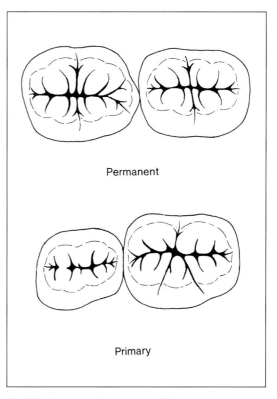

Fig 14-9 The broad, flat contacts of primary teeth versus the narrow, pointed contacts of permanent teeth.

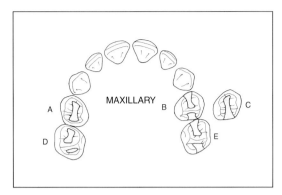

Fig 14-10 Typical outline forms of cavity preparations in primary maxillary teeth. (See the text for an explanation of the labels.)

Maxillary first molars

The primary maxillary first molar has a central groove that is usually carious. The Class I cavity outline usually includes the mesial and distal pits (Fig 14-10,*A*). It extends through the central groove and into the fissures on the mesial and distal aspects. The exception is where there is a large transverse ridge of enamel forming two distinct pits—mesial and distal. In this instance, two smaller occlusal preparations are done.

On primary first molars, the distal surface is the most caries-susceptible surface. The mesial surface is seldom carious. The preparation of all Class II cavity preparations involving the proximal surface is initiated by completing the occlusal surface of the tooth first. This allows easier access to the lesion as well as extension of the preparation for easier polishing of the restoration and prevention. The occlusal portion of the preparation is as previously described. All primary teeth have narrow occlusal tables, but the primary maxillary first molar is extreme. The widest part of the tooth is the mesiodistal contact points. The most important feature is the very large mesiobuccal pulp horn. Should the distal surface be involved, to avoid overextension into the mesiobuccal pulp horn, it is a good idea not to extend the preparation beyond the transverse ridge of enamel (Fig 14-10,*B*). Also, this is true in the rare instance when only the mesial surface is involved. Where the occlusal surface is abraded, resulting in loss of definite anatomy, a careful extension of the occlusal portion to the mesial marginal ridge is indicated (Fig 14-10,*C*). *Beware of the mesiobuccal pulp horn.* If both the mesial and distal surfaces are involved, a stainless steel crown is the restoration of choice.

Maxillary second molars

There are three occlusal pits in the primary maxillary second molar divided by a large, oblique, transverse ridge of enamel. The central pit is most often carious. When this occurs, the outline does not cross the oblique ridge. It extends to the mesial marginal ridge, including the smaller mesial pit (Fig 14-10,*D*). If the distal pit is involved, it is completed as an individual occlusal preparation. The two are combined into a single occlusal preparation if the oblique ridge is undermined with caries. If the lingual pit is involved, the preparation on the distal surface should be extended to form a two-surface restoration that includes the distal and the lingual pits.

In a Class II cavity preparation, including either the mesial or distal surfaces, the occlusal outline is completed first (Fig 14-10,*E*). The primary maxillary second molar has broad flat contacts and is larger than the primary maxillary first molar. Because this tooth is larger, the overall preparation is somewhat larger. Because the pulp does not extend as far into the dentin as the primary first molar, the proximal box preparation can be somewhat deeper than in the primary maxillary first molar. If the distal surface is involved, again, the occlusal portion is done first. The disto-occlusal cavity preparation is a difficult preparation because the contact is broad in all dimensions (Fig 14-10,*E*). The preparation should not be neglected because of its influence on the decalcification of the mesial surface of the immature permanent first molar. If the lingual pit is involved, a three-surface preparation, including the distal, occlusal, and lingual surfaces, is indicated.

Mandibular first molars

The occlusal surface of the primary mandibular first molar has three occlusal pits—mesial, distal, and central. The distal and central pits are most often cariously involved. A large transverse ridge of enamel usually connects the mesiobuccal and mesiolingual cusps. Unless the transverse ridge is undermined, it should also be kept intact. Because of the large marginal ridge, occlusal portions of cavity preparations, whether on the distal or the mesial pits, should be extended as minimally as possible (Fig 14-11,*A*).

The Class II cavity preparation on the primary mandibular first molar is influenced by the transverse ridge, which should be left intact (Fig 14-11,*B*).

If the mesial and distal surfaces are both involved, the tooth should be restored with a stainless steel crown. The occlusal portion of a mesio-occlusal cavity should include only the mesial pit. The disto-occlusal cavity preparation should include both the central and distal occlusal pits. Because of the morphology of the distal cusps, both buccal and lingual, the proximal box should be extended adequately to allow for polishing but not overdone. This causes weakening of both cusps with increased tendency to fracture. If the mesial pit is involved and a disto-occlusal preparation is indicated,

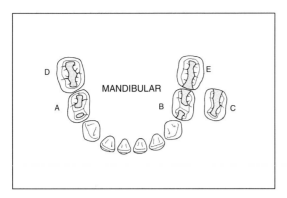

Fig 14-11 Outline forms used in cavity preparations of primary mandibular teeth. (See the text for an explanation of the labels.)

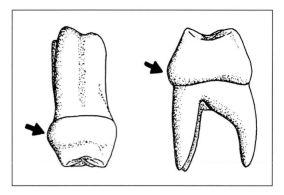

Fig 14-12 Prominent mesiobuccal cervical ridges (bulges) in primary first molars.

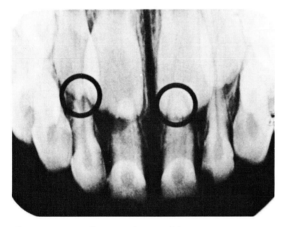

Fig 14-13 Note the conical roots of the primary anterior incisors *(circles).*

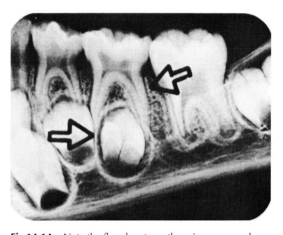

Fig 14-14 Note the flared roots on the primary second molars adjacent to the second premolar *(arrows).*

carefully extend the preparation to include the entire occlusal surface. Be aware of the mesiobuccal pulp horn (Fig 14-11,*C*).

Mandibular second molars

The occlusal cavity preparation outline is very similar to the outline for a permanent mandibular first molar (Fig 14-11,*D*). Occlusal caries usually is found in one of the three pits, primarily the central one. The cavity outline is extended through all the developmental grooves and pits on the occlusal portion. The marginal ridges on the mesial and distal portions should remain in excess of 1.5 to 2.0 mm of tooth structure. The mesial surface of the primary mandibular second molar is the surface most often involved. It contacts with the distal surface of the primary first molar in the occlusal one third of the tooth. The occlusal portion of the preparation includes all developmental grooves and pits extending to 2.0 mm from the distal marginal

ridge (Fig 14-11,*E*). The buccal and lingual grooves are extended to remove all developmental and carious defects. Remember the location of the mesiobuccal pulp horn when completing the proximal box.

Stainless steel crown preparations

The prominent mesiobuccal cervical ridge of mandibular and maxillary first molars must be accommodated in the preparation of stainless steel crowns (Fig 14-12).

Surgical procedures

Conical roots of primary anterior teeth facilitate easy removal (Fig 14-13). However, the flared roots of primary molars dictates that teeth be removed with care (Fig 14-14). The premolar tooth buds are located between the roots of the primary molars. In some instances, primary molars must be sectioned and removed in two pieces to prevent interference with the developing premolars.

Pulp therapy

Indirect pulp capping. This procedure is used to remove all the caries in a tooth except for the last small portion before the pulp tissue is exposed. Therefore, determining the "typical" location of the pulp from knowledge of morphology and from radiographs is essential. The procedure is limited to permanent teeth only.

Pulpotomy. The procedure is used in certain instances where caries has progressed into the pulp chambers. The diseased portion of the pulp is removed, the pulp is medicated, and a stainless steel crown is placed to restore the tooth. The location of the pulp, the number of pulp horns, and the location of the root canals are important.

Pulpectomy. This procedure is used when it is necessary to remove all pulpal tissue because of carious invasion. Understanding the tooth morphology, the number of root canals and location and curvature to the roots is extremely important.

Summary

Clinically, there are important differences between the primary and permanent teeth. The primary teeth are characterized by:

1. Thinner enamel and dentin layers. The occlusal enamel is of a consistent depth.

2. Pulp horns closer to the outer surface of teeth. The mesial pulp horns are closer to the surface than the distal pulp horns.

3. Pulps proportionally larger than those of the permanent teeth in relation to their crowns. The pulp chamber in primary teeth follows the outline of the occlusal crown surface; thus a pulp horn is present under each cusp. Mandibular molars usually have larger pulp chambers than maxillary molars.

4. Enamel rods in the gingival one third extending in a slightly occlusal direction from the DEJ. In permanent teeth, these rods extend slightly apically.

5. Greater constriction of the crown in the cervical region and a pronounced cervical bulge.

6. Roots that flare as they approach the apex (in molars). This is to accommodate succedaneous teeth.

7. More tortuous and irregular pulp canals.

Additional readings

Arnim, S. S., and Doyle, M. P. Dentin dimensions of primary teeth. J. Dent Child. 26:191, 1959.

Barker, B. C., et al. Anatomy of root canals. IV. Deciduous teeth. Aust. Dent. J. 20:10l, 1975.

Dental Anatomy: A self-Instructional Program. 9th ed. Norwalk, Conn.: Appleton-Century-Crofts, 1977.

Kramer, W. S., and Ireland, R. L. Measurements of the primary teeth. J. Dent. Child. 26:252, 1959.

Kraus, B. S., Jordon, R. E., and Abrams, L. Dental Anatomy and Occlusion. Baltimore: The Williams & Wilkins Co., 1969.

Puddhikarant P., and Rapp, R. Radiographic anatomy of pulpal chambers of primary molars. Pediatr. Dent. 5:25, 1983.

Russman, S. A. A study of pulp chamber anatomy in the deciduous dentition. Thesis. Ann Arbor: University of Michigan, June, 1947.

Wheeler, R. C. Dental Anatomy, Physiology, and Occlusion. 5th ed. Philadelphia: W. B. Saunders Co., 1974.

Questions

1. While planning treatment for a 4-year-old child in your office, on the x-ray you notice a pulp exposure on the maxillary second primary molar. The treatment plan should show what pulp treatment for this tooth?

   a. Indirect pulp capping, silver amalgam
   b. Direct pulp capping, silver amalgam
   c. Pulpotomy, stainless steel crown
   d. Extraction, then space maintainer

2. Clinically, you are having difficulty adapting a stainless steel crown to the primary mandibular left first molar. The anatomic feature most likely to cause this difficulty is:

   a. The occlusal transverse ridge
   b. The cervical bulge on the mesiobuccal surface
   c. The broad buccolingual contact
   d. The narrow occlusal table

3. During the next clinic period, the treatment plan indicates the need to do a disto-occlusal restoration on the primary maxillary left first molar. The caries activity is moderate but the preparation will be extended to the mesial pit. What pulp horn should be considered?

   a. Mesiobuccal
   b. Mesiolingual
   c. Distobuccal
   d. Distolingual

4. A worried parent calls your office concerned because her 4-month-old child has "no teeth yet." Your advice should be:

   a. "The child's dental development is slow."
   b. "The child is within a normal range of growth and you should not worry."
   c. "X-rays should be taken immediately to look for missing teeth."
   d. "A 'teething ring' should be used to stimulate eruption."

5. The primary pulpal tissue:

   a. In general is smaller proportionately than permanent pulps in relation to tooth crown size
   b. Is closer to the outer surface of the tooth than the permanent teeth
   c. Follows the general surface contour of the crown
   d. Has the mesial pulp horn closer to the surface than the distal pulp horn
   e. None of the above
   f. All of the above
   g. a,b,d
   h. b,c,d
   i. a,c,d

Chapter 15

Restorative Procedures for Primary Molars

Objectives

After studying this chapter, the student should be able to:

1. Understand the basic principles and imperatives of infection control and hazardous waste disposal.
2. List the advantages and indications for use of the rubber dam.
3. Use the appropriate rubber dam instrumentation and application for the child patient.
4. Visualize the specific cavity preparation indicated in primary posterior teeth, depending on the restorative material used.
5. Assess the advantages and disadvantages of specific dental materials.
6. Relate knowledge of dental materials to restorative procedures for children.
7. Elaborate on matrix systems and amalgam manipulation to restore primary teeth.
8. Develop a rationale for finishing amalgam restorations.
9. Outline a procedure for burnishing and finishing amalgam restorations.
10. Describe the indications, cavity preparation modifications needed, and instrumentation alternatives when composite resin materials are used.

Infection control

Infectious diseases can be spread in the dental operatory by *(1)* inhalation of the infective agent into the respiratory tract; *(2)* ingestion of the infectious agent into the digestive tract; and *(3)* direct contact with the infected individual's tissues (Rowe, 1991). The American Academy of Pediatric Dentistry (AAPD, 1992) has stated that measures must be taken to isolate the digestive tract, the respiratory tract, and oral mucosa of those children at risk from sources of infection. To prevent the spread of infection, the following procedures are recommended during treatment of all children:

1. A medical history must be taken to attempt to identify specific infections and current illnesses.
2. Gloves should be worn when the dental staff will be touching blood, saliva, or mucous membranes.
3. Surgical masks should be worn when the splashing or splattering of blood is possible.
4. Protective eyewear, similar to a surgical mask, should be worn when the splashing or splattering of blood is possible.
5. Surgical gowns should be worn when clothing may be soiled with blood or body fluids.
6. Rubber dam should be used wherever possible.

7. Sharp instruments and needles should considered as potentially infective and handled with extreme care.
8. Instruments, if they penetrate soft tissues, must be sterilized after use. Sterilization methods should be monitored monthly.
9. Operatory surfaces that are contaminated by blood or other fluids must be cleaned and decontaminated.
10. Impressions, appliances, etc, should be cleaned of all oral tissues and fluids before they are sent to the dental laboratory.
11. Handpieces should be sterilized between patients if possible. Burs should be changed between patients and sterilized.
12. Waste materials such as sharp items, oral tissues, and blood should be considered potentially infective and handled with extreme care. Contaminated sharp items should be placed in puncture-proof containers prior to disposal.

Extensive standards have been established by the Occupational Safety and Health Administration (OSHA) to control occupational exposure to blood-borne pathogens (US Department of Labor, 1992).

Rubber dam usage

Advantages

The rubber dam shields the child from any sensation of debris or taste of materials. Because he or she is more comfortable and thus easier to manage, the dentist has improved visibility and greater efficiency. Increased efficiency results because the dentist and an assistant can work together, and materials can be inserted in a dry field.

Indications

The use of the dam is indicated in virtually all (99.9%) cases, certainly in all operative procedures and endodontics. Its use is also imperative for reducing bacterial contamination in pulpal therapy.

With the increased emphasis on office efficiency, dentists still are hesitant to use the rubber dam. In a survey of alumni of the University of Oklahoma, College of Dentistry, less than 37% use the rubber dam routinely for children. The newer alloys which use high-copper amalgam, are influenced by moisture contamination (Yamada and Fusayama, 1981). This study found decreases in physical properties when the high-copper amalgam was exposed to moisture contamination.

Armamentarium

Rubber dam (extra heavy) 12.5 x 12.5 cm (5 x 5 in.)
Rubber dam punch
Rubber dam clamps (Fig 15-1)
    Permanent molars: Ivory 8A, 14A, 14
    Primary molars: S.S.W. Nos. 27, 26 (S.S. White Co.)
Ash Nos. 4,5, (Ash, Ltd.)
Rubber dam forceps
Rubber dam frame: Young's frame
Dental floss

Local anesthesia

Anesthetize maxillary teeth with an infiltration on the buccal surface; anesthesia is usually not necessary on the lingual surface. However, the injection may cause more discomfort than would 2 or 3 seconds of pressure from the rubber dam clamp. For the mandibular teeth, administer a mandibular block plus several drops for long buccal innervation.

Preparation of the rubber dam materials

Figure 15-2 is an illustration of the rubber dam punched for the maxillary and mandibular right quadrants. For the left side, the dam would simply be flipped over.

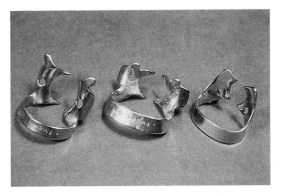

Fig 15-1 Rubber dam clamps used in pediatric dentistry.

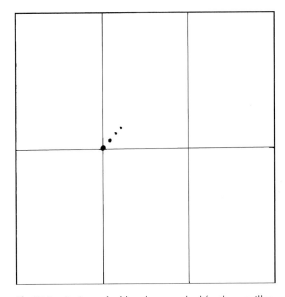

Fig 15-2 A piece of rubber dam punched for the maxillary and mandibular right quadrants.

Punch only the holes necessary for good isolation of all tooth surfaces to be restored. Treating preschool children (primary dentition) usually involves isolating the primary second molar through the canine or lateral incisor. In school-aged children (mixed dentition), the permanent first molar through the lateral incisor are usually isolated. Where it is necessary to isolate a single tooth, punch only one hole in the appropriate position, for example, for an occlusal preparation on a primary second molar or permanent first molar.

Holes for quadrant isolation should be punched approximately 3 to 4 mm apart. If they are punched too close together, the rubber dam material will not adapt itself properly around the teeth, retraction will be poor, and leakage may occur. If holes are punched too far apart, it will be difficult to pass the material through the contact area.

An aid to hole spacing is the use of a rubber stamp, which stamps both the primary and permanent denti-

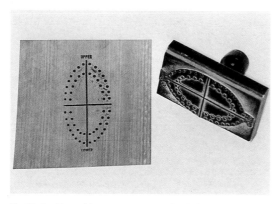

Fig 15-3 The rubber stamp as an aid to hole determination.

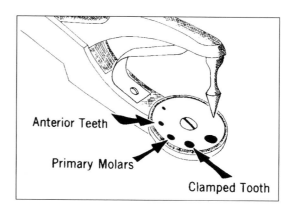

Fig 15-4 Rubber dam punch.

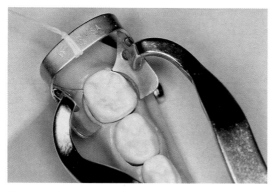

Fig 15-5 Place the rubber dam clamp with dental floss attached prior to rubber dam insertion.

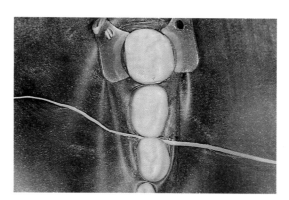

Fig 15-6 Use dental floss to push the rubber dam between the contacts.

tions (Fig 15-3). The stamp takes the guesswork out of punching and space selection.

The second largest hole on the table of the rubber dam punch is used to punch the hole that slips over the clamped tooth (Fig 15-4). The third largest hole on the table is suitable for all other posterior teeth, including the canine. The second smallest hole is suitable for all incisors. In some instances a single large hole can be used to isolate an entire quadrant.

The dark, extra-heavy rubber dam material is recommended because it affords good tissue retraction, resists tearing, is more easily placed, and provides excellent visual contrast.

Placement of the clamp

Before placing the retainer on a tooth, attach a 45-cm (18-in.) length of dental floss to the bow of the clamp as a safety measure (Fig 15-5). The floss will enable you to retrieve the clamp if it should escape control and disappear in the direction of the pharynx.

Select the clamp appropriate for the tooth, place it on the rubber dam forceps, and carry it to the mouth (Fig 15-5).

It should take only 15 to 30 seconds to apply a rubber dam clamp. If it becomes a heroic effort, check for an alternate method because *(1)* the tooth has not completely erupted and thus cannot hold the clamp, *(2)* the size of the clamp is wrong, or *(3)* the tooth has badly broken down before restorative care.

Application of the dam

Pass the dental floss through the hole receiving the clamp and carry the dam into the mouth. With the index fingers of both hands, spread the hole to be placed over the clamp.

Position the hole over the clamp, beginning on the lingual surface, and carry the dam distally over the bow of the clamp and then the buccal wing. Place the Young's frame. Isolate the other teeth. Use wax floss to carry the rubber dam material through the contacts (Fig 15-6).

In cases requiring stabilization, ligate the most anteriorly isolated tooth with length of waxed floss (Fig 15-7a). A wedge or a butterfly piece of rubber dam can be used instead of a floss ligature. The wedge is placed between the contacts of the most anteriorly isolated

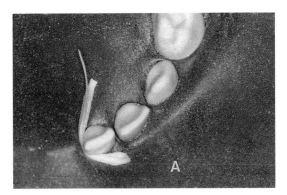

Fig 15-7a Use dental floss to stabilize the rubber dam.

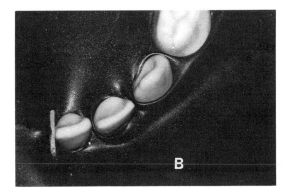

Fig 15-7b Either a wooden wedge or a piece of rubber dam can be substituted for stabilization.

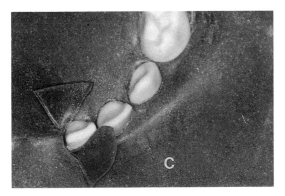

Fig 15-7c The butterfly, cut from a piece of rubber dam material, can also be used to provide stabilization.

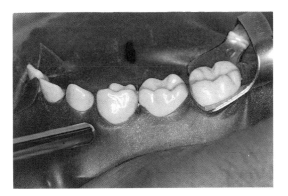

Fig 15-8 After it has been stretched, invert the rubber dam by using air.

tooth. Stretch the dam, insert the wedge, then allow the dam to snap back into position (Fig 15-7b). Cut the butterfly from a piece of rubber dam material, then stretch it and insert it between the contacts of the most anterior tooth. When released, the butterfly resumes its normal shape and maintains the dam in position (Fig 15-7c).

Invert the rubber dam material around the neck of the tooth to retract the gingiva and prevent leakage. The easiest way is to stretch the dam and have the assistant gently desiccate the entire area. When the dam is allowed to return, it will cup around the tooth (Fig 15-8).

While the dam is in place, there is no intraoral stimulation from air, water, or instruments, and no debris drops into the mouth. Salivary flow is thereby reduced and a saliva ejector is rarely needed. The saliva ejector itself acts as a stimulus and increases salivary flow, thus defeating its purpose.

Alternative application methods

There are several methods of applying a rubber dam and clamp, but none has advantages over another. The idea is to become comfortable with one method and use it routinely.

Alternative method 1. After the clamp has been placed on the tooth, place the rubber dam on the rubber dam frame. Then place the frame over the clamp.

Alternative method 2. Align the rubber dam clamp on the rubber dam. Engage the clamp in the dam material with the rubber dam faced. Place the clamp and rubber dam on the forcep. Insert it over the indicated tooth (Fig 15-9). Stretch and apply the rubber dam frame. This method is limited to winged clamps.

Alternative method 3. Punch holes indicating the most posterior tooth and the most anterior tooth to be isolated. Use a pair of scissors to connect the holes by slitting the dam material. Then place the rubber dam over the clamped tooth. Post the most anterior part of the rubber dam to the most anterior part of the tooth. This method is often used for multiple stainless steel crown procedures (Fig 15-10).

Check to be sure the rubber dam frame is not near the patient's eyes; if so, readjust the frame. If the rubber dam is uncomfortable or inhibits the child's breathing because the dam is against the nose, either fold the dam over or carefully remove some of the excess dam material with a pair of scissors.

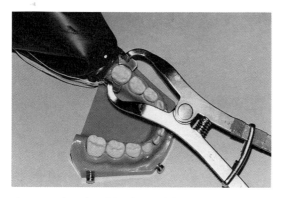

Fig 15-9 Place the rubber dam and clamp at one time.

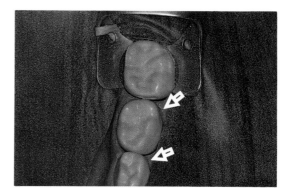

Fig 15-10 Another method is to use one large hole from the most posterior tooth to the most anterior tooth.

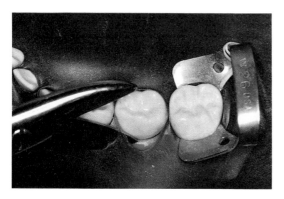

Fig 15-11 Cut the rubber dam to assist in its removal.

Removal of the dam

Remove all debris from the surface of the rubber dam. If the dam has been stabilized, with floss, cut one end of each ligature at the knot. Pull the ligature free with the other end. The knot is easily disengaged in this manner. Remove the wedges or piece of rubber dam material, if used. Stretch the dam to the buccal or lingual side, and, if necessary, cut all interproximal rubber dam material with the scissors (Fig 15-11). With forceps remove the rubber dam clamp, and then remove the rubber dam and frame as a unit. Make sure the area is thoroughly rinsed and evacuated. Inspect both the rubber dam and the teeth to make sure all fragments of the rubber dam material and floss are removed.

Amalgam restoration for primary teeth

Morphologic considerations

Primary molars have enamel rods that are inclined occlusally. In the primary dentition, the enamel and den-

tin are not as thick as in the permanent dentition. Cavity preparations in primary teeth are modified to accommodate tooth size, pulp size, and enamel or dentin thickness. Anatomically, the primary molars resemble permanent teeth with the exception of the primary mandibular first molar. In the 1950s and 1960s, studies completed at the University of Nebraska resulted in the present concept of cavity preparation for primary molars. There have been some modification because of improved dental materials and methods, but the basic principles still apply (Ireland, 1963).

Principles of cavity preparation

Occlusal

1. Outline form should be dovetailed, including all fissures, areas of caries, pits, and developmental grooves.
2. The extension of the occlusal portion of the cavity preparation depends on the primary molar involved.
   a. The occlusal portion usually is extended about one half the way across on the primary maxillary and mandibular first molars.
   b. For the primary mandibular second molar, extend the step completely across the occlusal surface.
   c. The primary maxillary second molar preparation includes only the nearest occlusal pit. The transverse ridge is not included unless undermined with carious lesions. The distal preparation is done in the same manner.
3. The walls converge slightly with the greatest width at the pulpal floor.
4. Cavosurface margins should be sharp.
5. Angles of walls and floors should be slightly rounded.
6. The axiopulpal line angle should be gently rounded.

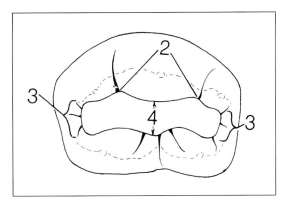

Fig 15-12 External outline form of a Class I preparation on a primary tooth. (The numbers correspond to the numbers in the technique description in the text.)

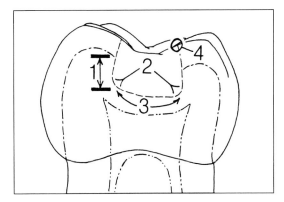

Fig 15-13 Internal outline form of a Class I preparation on a primary tooth. (The numbers correspond to the numbers in the technique description in the text.)

Proximal box

1. The buccal and lingual walls should just extend into self-cleansing areas.
2. A sharp 90° cavosurface angle is desirable.
3. The buccal and lingual walls of the proximal box should converge slightly from the gingival floor to the occlusal surface.
4. The gingival floor should be beneath the point of contact, at, or just beneath, the gingival tissue. No bevel is placed.
5. All internal line angles should be gently rounded.
6. Buccal and lingual retentive grooves are contra-indicated.
7. The axial wall should follow the contour of the tooth.

Armamentarium

Mirror
Explorer
Bin angle chisel, 17-18
Enamel hatchet, 8-9, 10-11
Spoon excavators
    No. 38-39 (American Dental Manufacturing Co.)
    No. 42-43 (American Dental Manufacturing Co.)
Burs
    No. 330 F.G.
    No. 4 or No. 6 R.A.
    No. 169L F.G.
Pliers
    No. 114 (Unitek Corp.)
    No. 110 (Unitek Corp.)
Amalgam pluggers
    No. 7 (American Dental Manufacturing Co.)
    No. 8 (American Dental Manufacturing Co.)
Cleoid-discoid carver, 4-5 DC
Matrix scissors, 1-51
Lateral condensor, 21B, PF1-21
Double-ended amalgam carrier

Double-ended T-3 carver
Amalgam
Amalgamator
Wedges, flat toothpicks
Dental floss
Pumice
Stainless steel band material (0.002-in. thickness),
    Unitek Corp
    Primary teeth, $^3/_{16}$ in. (0.47 cm)
    Permanent teeth, $^1/_4$ or $^5/_{16}$ in. (0.63 or 0.8 cm)
Curved crown and bridge scissors
T-bands, brass

Class I cavity preparation

External outline form (Fig 15-12)

1. Start preparation by penetrating the occlusal surface with the No. 330 bur. Go from distal to mesial surface.
2. Include all deep and defective grooves in the preparation. Blend the outline to form smooth-flowing arcs and curves. This blending establishes the walls of the cavity preparation.
3. Contour the outline parallel to the mesial and distal marginal ridges. Maintain a bulk of tooth structure on the marginal ridges.
4. Maintain a width approximately one third the width of the occlusal table.

Internal outline form (Fig 15-13)

1. Penetrate 0.50 to 1.0 mm into the dentin. Dentin is much softer to the touch, is not as shiny as enamel, and usually is yellow. The No. 330 bur shank is a good depth marker. It is approximately 1.5 mm from the bur tip to the shank.
2. Round line angles with the No. 330 bur. Round line angles are easier areas to condense amalgam into, and they reduce internal stress on the amalgam restoration. The walls are wider at the pulpal floor

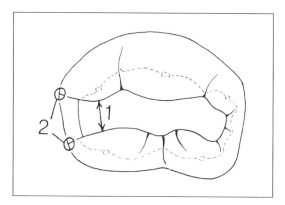

Fig 15-14 External view of a Class II amalgam preparation. (The numbers correspond to the numbers in the technique description in the text.)

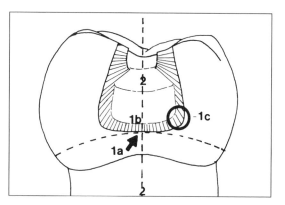

Fig 15-15 Cross-sectional view of a Class II amalgam preparation. (The numbers correspond to the numbers in the technique description in the text.)

than at the occlusal opening. This convergence aids in retention of the restorative material.

3. Slightly round the pulpal floor. All internal line angles should be rounded.

4. Establish a sharp cavosurface angle in the lateral walls with the No. 169L bur. The walls are parallel or slightly undercut to the external surfaces of the tooth. A word of caution: Watch the tip of the No. 169L bur to prevent scoring the floor of the preparation. The sharp cavosurface angle is an asset to improve carving and polishing, and reduce marginal failure (Mathewson, 1972). If the active caries has not been removed during cavity preparation, do so now. Use a No. 4 or 6 round bur in a slow-speed handpiece. A large spoon excavator works as well. Rinse the preparation with water. Inspect for caries removal, sharp cavosurface margins, and retention.

Class II cavity preparation

1. Complete a Class I cavity outline as described.

2. Use a No. 330 bur to extend the occlusal outline through the marginal ridge. If two primary molars are being done together back to back, extend the proximal box into self-cleaning areas. Attempt to leave 90° cavosurface margins. The isthmus (narrowest part of the occlusal outline near the proximal box) is approximately one half to one third the width of the occlusal surface.

3. Extend the No. 330 bur into the proximal surfaces. Keep the bur parallel to the long axis of the tooth. Move the bur in a pendulating motion from lingual to buccal.

4. Extend the proximal box gingivally beneath the contact area to the interproximal area. This area is determined by the clearance of an explorer tip.

5. The axial wall, as determined by carious lesion depth, should follow the contour of the tooth.

6. Use the enamel hatchet to remove any overhanging

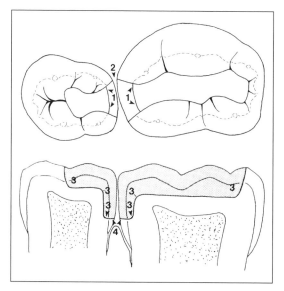

Fig 15-16 Internal and external views of two Class II primary molar restorations. (The numbers correspond to the numbers in the technique description in the text.)

enamel in the proximal box. Overuse of hand instruments is not indicated. Effective use of the bur can accomplish the same end result much faster. Rinse the debris from the cavity preparation. Check the following items:

Occlusal view (Fig 15-14)

1. Form the isthmus (most narrow portion of the occlusal outline nearest the proximal surface) so that it is one half the width of the occlusal table and connects the proximal with the occlusal dovetail.

2. Curve the proximal wall gently, creating an angle 90° to the axial surface of the tooth, if possible. The proximal extensions are governed by the adjacent tooth and determined by the clearance of an explorer tip.

Table 15-1 Comparison of effectiveness of pulpal protection materials

	Cavity varnishes	Cavity liners	
		Ca (OH)$_2$*	ZOE[†]
Sealing of margins	Yes, 48 hours	Not known	Yes
Sealing of dentinal tubules	Some	Yes	Yes
Prevention of dentin discoloration	Not known	Yes	Yes
Prevention of thermal sensitivity	No	Some	Yes
Biologic response in dentin (sclerosis)	No	Yes	Some
Hardening of surface layer	No	Yes	Yes
Visibility of material on enamel margins	Poor	Good	Good
Principle in action	Mechanical	Biologic	Biologic

*Calcium hydroxide.
[†]Zinc oxide–eugenol.

Cross-section proximal box area (Fig 15-15)

1. In establishing the gingival floor, keep in mind that *(a)* it is even with or slightly below the gingiva, as determined by the carious lesions; *(b)* it is perpendicular to the long axis of the tooth; and *(c)* it has rounded line angles.
2. Keep the proximal box in an occlusogingival direction roughly parallel to the long axis of the tooth.

Occlusal and internal views (Fig 15-16)

The proximal box area:

1. Gently curves buccolingually to follow the contour of the proximal surface.
2. Extends so an explorer tip can pass through the embrasure.
3. Has gently rounded axiopulpal line angles, as do all line angles.
4. Has no bevel at the gingival margin.

Proximal retentive grooves are not indicated. There is the possibility of a pulpal exposure. Studies have shown that, in primary teeth, retentive grooves do not reduce the incidence of marginal failure or gross fracture (Mathewson and Lu, 1975).

Failures of amalgam restorations

Marginal failure of amalgam restorations in primary posterior teeth is often blamed on the restorative material. However, amalgam has been placed in primary teeth where cavity preparations have been overextended. The amalgam is expected to perform beyond its physical limitations. A number of studies have demonstrated that if excessive tooth structure is removed, marginal failure increases (Birtcil et al, 1981; Larson et al, 1980; Mahler and Marantz, 1980; Blaser, 1985). Dawson et al (1981), reviewing 280 restorations in primary teeth, concluded that nearly 70% of the multisurface amalgam restorations needed replacement. These studies support the philosophy that amalgam should not be placed in primary teeth with more than two surfaces of dental caries.

Materials used with amalgam restorations

Reviewing the physical properties and uses of dental restorative materials here is an necessary evil. Admittedly a dry subject, it is the basis of success in restorative dentistry, and dentistry for children is no exception. The following section is a brief review of the pertinent information with the emphasis on the clinical applications (Table 15-1).

Cavity varnishes

A cavity varnish is a solution of one of several resins in an organic solvent. Copal or nitrated cellulose are dissolved in organic solvents such as alcohol, benzine acetone, or chloroform.

When carious lesions are removed from a tooth, there is a histologic response in the pulp as a result of the carious process and the trauma of cavity preparation. Dentin should be considered a vital extension of the pulpal tissue. The primary use of cavity varnishes is to minimize this insult and assist the vital pulpal tissue in the recovery process. A varnish or resin layer is formed on the dentin and tooth by evaporation of the solvent, leaving a thin, semipermeable membrane. The intent of this membrane is to seal the exposed dentinal tubules, protecting the underlying pulp from further irritation.

Cavity varnish is used to reduce marginal leakage on the cavosurface margins of amalgam restorations (Andrews and Hembree 1975; Yates et al, 1980). A thin film is placed on the margins before the insertion of the restoration. This varnish layer seems to serve as a wedge between the amalgam and cavity wall. Therefore, it is easy to leave an excess of amalgam on the margins after carving, with the amalgam sticking to the varnish material.

If a cavity liner containing calcium hydroxide, zinc oxide-eugenol, or polycarboxylate is used, a cavity varnish is placed afterward.

Placement of a cavity varnish beneath a composite resin is contraindicated unless recommended by the manufacturer's instructions. Kelsey and Panneton (1988) compared a conventional copal resin varnish (Copalite, Bosworth) with two newer resin-compatible cavity liners. The intent of these new liners was to develop a universal liner that would reduce microleakage associated with amalgam and provide a chemical barrier for composite resin materials. Unfortunately, neither of these newer products was as effective as the copal resin varnish in reducing microleakage around amalgam restorations.

Cavity liners

Cavity liners are liquid suspensions of calcium hydroxide or zinc oxide that are applied in a thin layer over exposed dentin surfaces.

In the primary dentition, after removal of deep carious lesions, a liner is used before the insertion of an amalgam restoration or cementation of a stainless steel crown to protect the exposed dentin and reduce subsequent trauma to the pulp. The cavity liners with calcium hydroxide are usually alkaline, and there may be some therapeutic effect on the pulp to form secondary dentin.

The most common type consists of two tubes. One tube is the base or active ingredient, and the other tube is the catalyst, such as Dycal (L.D. Caulk Co). In contrast to cavity varnishes, the cavity liner *should not* be left on the cavity margin. If left, increased incidence of marginal leakage occurs.

These liners are best used when thin layers are applied. If additional thickness is required, several thin layers applied in sequence are an improvement over one thick layer.

Calcium hydroxide liners (Dycal) may withstand the condensing force of amalgam. A second base is not indicated (Mitchem, 1971). McComb (1983), reporting on the properties of five calcium hydroxide liners, noted the added antibacterial function of the liners. This property is especially important in deep carious lesions and indirect pulp cap procedures. The physical evaluation of the five commercial products demonstrated that Dycal and Life (Kerr Div/Sybron Corp) had earlier strengths after 10 minutes but that Life continued to increase in strength over time. All were soluble in distilled water, but some solubility is desired to release the necessary therapeutic ions.

Cavity liners with zinc oxide–eugenol as an active ingredient should not be used beneath resin or composite resin restorations. Eugenol interferes with the final polymerization of the plastic materials.

A light-curing calcium hydroxide liner is available (Prisma VLC Dycal, L.D. Caulk Co). This material is rigid and is used as a protective base beneath cements, restorative materials, and composite resins. This type of material has several advantages:

1. It is less soluble than conventional calcium hydroxide.

2. No mixing is needed.
3. The working time is controlled by exposure to the light source.
4. If there are areas of insufficient thickness, additional material can be added before curing.

Glass-ionomer cavity liners

Glass-ionomer cavity liners are fast-setting, radiopaque versions of glass-ionomer cements. When mixed properly and applied with clinical precision, glass-ionomer liners have the following advantages (Swift, 1988; Olsen et al, 1989; Croll, 1993):

1. Glass-ionomer liners bond to dentin.
2. These liners release the fluoride ion, and may be cariostatic.
3. If the carious lesion is close to the pulp, calcium hydroxide can be used first; then the glass-ionomer liner can be applied.
4. The liners are nearly insoluble in oral fluids.
5. They have high compressive strengths.
6. Injectable liners are available.
7. A visible light-hardening glass-ionomer cement is available, simplifying application.
8. When composite resin materials are used, there is a micromechanical attachment between the composite resin and the glass-ionomer liner.

There are also disadvantages:
1. The materials are sensitive to moisture during the application and hardening process.
2. Some of the glass-ionomer liners can take 4 to 6 minutes to harden, a disadvantage when the patient is a child.

Following completion of caries removal and the cavity preparation, a debris-containing smear layer forms on the dentin surface. Polyacrylic acid should be used to remove the smear layer to increase the bond strength of the glass-ionomer liner to dentin (Swift, 1988).

Amalgam

Because of amalgam's extensive use in restorative dentistry, a brief overview of the clinical research follows.

The selection of an alloy can result in a dramatic effect on the increase of clinical success (Birtcil et al, 1981; Mahler et al, 1973; Mathewson et al, 1974; Matsson et al, 1982; Osborne et al, 1978, 1980; Osborne and Gale, 1979; Nelson and Osborne 1981; Pameijer and Benhameurlain, 1983).

Traditional dental amalgam is triturated with mercury to form a new group of alloys:

$$Ag_3Sn + Hg \rightarrow Ag_2Ag_3 + Sn_{7-8}Hg + Ag_2Sn_3$$

$$\gamma + \text{mercury} \rightarrow \gamma_1 + \gamma_2 + \gamma.$$

The gamma (γ) phase consists of particles of unreacted alloy. Gamma is a hard, strong component of the alloy system. Gamma$_1$ (γ_1) is a phase of intermediate strength. Gamma$_2$ (γ_2) is the weak link in the chain that is responsible for the defective characteristics of traditional amalgam.

In the 1960s, a new process for alloy manufacture was introduced as the spherical-shaped alloys. Amalgams made from spherical particles have some desirable characteristics. They are more plastic and have early compressive strength values, but, being more plastic may extrude beneath the matrix bands.

A later development was the dispersed-phase alloys, for which a mixture of spherical particles of 72% silver and 28% copper and regular-cut alloy was used. Now alloys that contain higher percentages of copper in the alloy system are available. The advantage of the copper-dispersed alloys is that there is a marked reduction of the gamma2. The reaction is

$$\gamma + Hg + (AgCu) \rightarrow \gamma_1 + \gamma + Cu_6 Sn_5.$$

When γ_2 is eliminated, the amalgam is referred to as the γ_2-free amalgam, resulting in an improved clinical restoration. These alloys are available in spherical-shaped, dispersed (admixed), flake-shaped, or combination alloys.

One of the more frequent causes of amalgam failure is marginal breakdown (Fig 15-17).

The alloy-mercury ratio can be reduced when the high-copper amalgams are used. Mitchem and Mahler (1968) demonstrated that the original alloy-mercury ratio influences marginal adaptation. Mahler and Adey (1979) found that if the residual mercury content of a high-copper amalgam exceeds 41%, there is a dramatic increase in creep and an increase in the γ_2.

With a lower mercury content, there is enough unreacted alloy left to combine with the Sn, thus reducing the formation of the γ_2 phase. As the residual mercury content of the amalgam increases, there is a decrease in marginal strength.

Proper mixing is needed for optimal plasticity of the amalgam mix (Mahler, 1980; Mathewson and Lu, 1975; Matsson et al, 1982). Results show that amalgams with optimum plasticity have better marginal adaptation and less marginal leakage. The high-copper spherical amalgams or those with a large percentage of spherical components have increased potential for improved plasticity.

Creep has been shown to be less with dispersed alloy than with other alloys (Osborne et al, 1974; Malhotra and Asgar, 1978). Osborne et al (1978) correlated clinical marginal failure and the physical properties of 12 commercial alloys. A high correlation (0.79) was found between creep and marginal failure. After 1 year, Dispersalloy (Johnson and Johnson) was found to be the best alloy clinically.

To test the correlation between creep and corrosion, Mahler et al (1982), compared amalgams with high γ_2

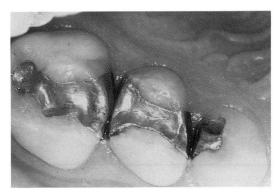

Fig 15-17 Examples of marginal failure.

content to those with no γ_2 phase. With the increase in γ_2, creep and corrosion values increased. Saraker et al, (1982) credited corrosion with the breakdown in non-γ_2 amalgams; creep plays a secondary role.

Another factor influencing the success of amalgam is condensation techniques. Influencing factors are type of condensor, force applied, and the number and size of amalgam increments used (Mahler and Marantz, 1980; Cardazzi et al, 1983). With use of an optimal method, mercury is forced to the surface, minimizing residual mercury content and reducing porosity, which contributes to the reduction of γ_2 (Clark et al, 1981).

There is an increased awareness of the potential health hazard of mercury (Avery et al, 1982; ADA, 1984). The dentist and dental assistant need to be aware of the importance of tightly closing the capsules during trituration, not handling the amalgam mix, and reducing the vaporization of mercury to a minimal level.

Fortunately, "mercury hazards to dental personnel have diminished considerably due to improved mercury hygiene and reduced caries rates" (Mandel, 1991). Further, dental amalgams do not appear to pose a risk to the health of the dental patient.

Occupational exposure to dental mercury can be minimized by adherence to these recommendations (ADA, 1991):

1. Be aware of the hazards and symptoms of mercury exposure.
2. Know the potential sources of mercury spills.
3. Provide proper ventilation in the offices.
4. Periodically monitor mercury vapor levels in the office; monitor the urine of office personnel as well.
5. Use precapsulated alloys.
6. Use amalgamators fitted with a cover.
7. Avoid skin contact with mercury.
8. Use high-volume evacuation when finishing or removing amalgams; change face masks after the procedure.
9. Store amalgam scrap under radiographic fixer solution.

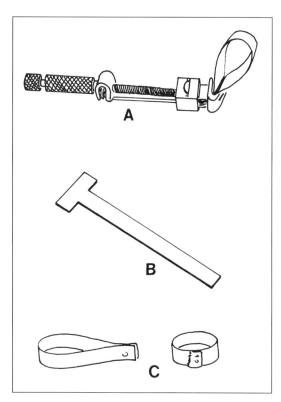

Fig 15-18 Types of matrix retainers: *(A)* Tofflemire; *(B)* T-band; *(C)* spot-welded.

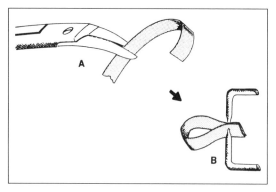

Fig 15-19 *(A)* Cut and *(B)* tack weld a piece of band material.

10. Dispose of amalgam scraps according to appropriate regulations.
11. Clean spilled mercury with commercial clean-up kits. Do not use a household vacuum cleaner.
12. Wear professional clothing only in the dental operatory.

Matrix bands and retainers

Matrix bands and retainers, properly contoured and wedged, *(1)* restore normal contact areas of primary teeth, *(2)* prevent extension of an excess of restorative

Table 15-2 Band materials available

Alloy	Thickness	Width
	T-band	
Brass	0.0015 in. (0.0038 cm)	Narrow
Steel	0.0020 in. (0.0050 cm)	Wide
	Welded	
Steel	0.0015 in. (0.0038 cm)	3/16 in. (0.47 cm) 1/4 in. (0.63 cm) 5/16 in. (0.78 cm)

material beyond the band into the gingival tissue, *(3)* are convenient and easy to use for amalgam condensation and carving, and *(4)* are easily removed.

Indications. In dentistry for children, the single Class II amalgam restoration concept is the exception rather than the rule. The use of a back-to-back matrix method is emphasized. Objections by academicians based on clinical observation are unfounded. As with all restorative procedures, if done properly, the results are optimum. Difficulties encountered in the primary dentition are due to deep cervical constriction, broad contacts, and prominent enamel buccal cervical ridges.

Three types of matrix bands or retainers are used: Tofflemire, T-band, and spot-welded. The Tofflemire matrix retainer is not suitable for use with back-to-back amalgam restorations. Its use is restricted to the rare occasion when a mesio-occlusal restoration is done on a permanent first molar. These retainers come in junior forms for pedodontics with a straight or contra-angle arm (Fig 15-18, *A*).

The T-band is available in several widths, thicknesses, and alloy construction (Fig 15-18, *B*; Table 15-2). This type of band is constructed at the time of the restoration. The disadvantage is that some difficulty may be experienced in placing this type of retainer.

The spot-welded matrix retainer lends itself to the philosophy of back-to-back amalgam restorations (Fig 15-18, *C*). It can be individually custom-made for each tooth, purchased commercially, or preformed in the dental office. It can be contoured with a suitable pliers.

Use of the T-band or spot-welded matrix bands is to be encouraged. The technique shown in Figs 15-19 to 15-25 is for multiple restorations applied to both types of matrix bands.

Custom spot-welded matrix bands

1. Cut one 5-cm (2-in.) length of band material (Fig 15-19, *A*). Weld the ends of the band together in one spot forming a closed loop Fig 15-19, *B*).
2. Place the loop around the tooth. Hold the loop firmly at the lingual surface with the index finger. With the No. 110 pliers, pinch together the buccal

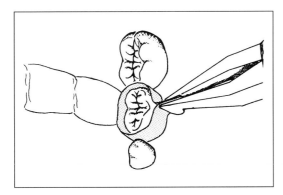

Fig 15-20   Adapt the band to the tooth.

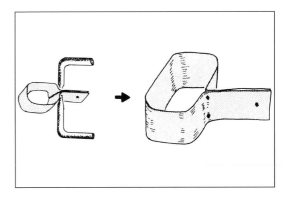

Fig 15-21   Remove the band; spot weld at the seams.

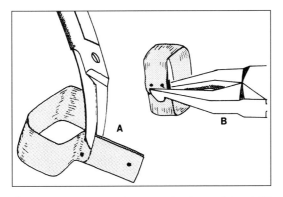

Fig 15-22   (*A*) remove the excess band material and (*B*) bend remaining excess back against the band.

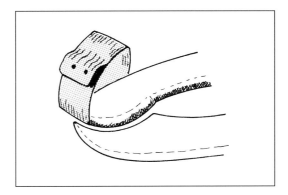

Fig 15-23   Contour the band.

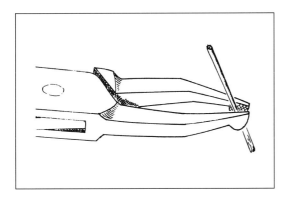

Fig 15-24   Flatten the end of the wedge.

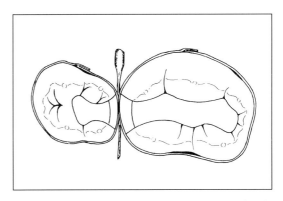

Fig 15-25   Insert the wedge carefully to stabilize the bands.

portion until the band is drawn up snugly around the tooth (Fig 15-20).

3. Remove the band and weld two spots at the seam (15-21).
4. Cut off the excess band material 1 mm beyond the welded joint (Fig 15-22, *A*). Round the cut edges of the band with the crown and bridge scissors. With the No. 110 pliers, bend the excess back against the band (Fig 15-22, *B*).
5. Contour the welded band at the cervical and con-

tact areas with the No. 114 pliers (Fig 15-23). If the tooth is isolated, burnish the band to the adjacent proximal surface.

6. Break off a toothpick about 3.8 cm (1.5 in.) long or use a preformed wedge. Use a No. 110 pliers to flatten the end (Fig 15-24).
7. Hold the bands with one finger and insert the wedge snugly at the cervical margin. The wedge can be inserted from either the buccal or lingual side with a No. 110 pliers. A slight movement of the

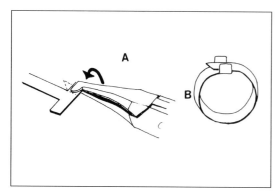

Fig 15-26 *(A)* Bend the T of the band *(B)* to form a clasp to assist in the band's formation.

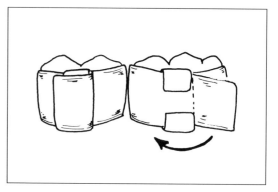

Fig 15-27   Fold the tab over to form the band.

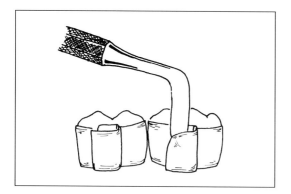

Fig 15-28   Remove the T-band by loosening the tab.

tooth is desired. With an explorer, made sure the band is snug at the gingival margins and walls of the preparation. *This is a most important step in the back-to-back method.* The purpose of the wedge is to hold the bands next to the cervical gingival margin. Remember, the broad contacts in the primary dentition should be restored (Fig 15-25).

Use of the T-band matrix

1. With the No. 110 pliers, bend the flanges of the T upward (Fig 15-26, A). Use a mirror handle or the handle of the pliers to form a circle.
2. Fold the T-wings over the circle formed. The wings should be loose enough for a sliding joint. Adjust the band so it is approximately smaller than the

tooth to be restored (Fig 15-26, B). Place the matrix on the tooth with the folded joint on the buccal side of the tooth.
3. Hold the band with one finger. Pull the tab tight with the No. 110 pliers or your finger. Fold the tab back over the joint (Fig 15-27).
4. Remove the band. Flatten the joint with a No. 110 pliers Replace the band on the tooth. Wedge tightly.
5. When the restorative procedure is finished, remove the band by raising the tab over the joint and loosening the T part of the bands (Fig 15-28). Remove the wedge. Slide the band occlusally through the contact.

Preformed spot-welded matrix bands

1. Use a copper band storage box cover. These covers are circular forms, sizes 1 to 20. Use sizes 8 to 18 for preformed matrix bands (Fig 15-29, A).
2. Cut a piece of material about 3 cm (1.25 in.) long. Give it a single weld to form a loop.
3. Place it over the form of the size needed. With a No. 110 pliers, adapt the band to the post (Fig 15-29, B).
4. Tack weld twice to form the band (Note: The weld should be just enough to hold the band together. Something greater will increase the difficulty in removing the band).

Trim off the excess band material. Repeat until a large number of the various sizes are available (Table

Table 15-3   Approximate sizes of spot-welded bands

Teeth	Maxillary	Mandibular
Primary first molars	Nos. 8 to 10	Nos. 7 to 10
Primary second molars	Nos. 12 to 14	Nos. 11 to 14
First and second premolars	Nos. 9 to 12	Nos. 8 to 11
Permanent first molars	Nos. 17 to 20	Nos. 17 to 20

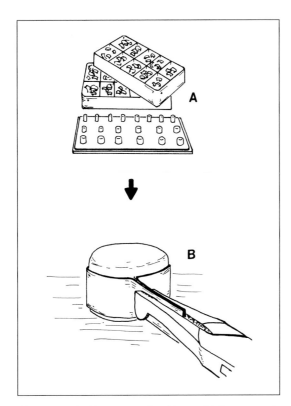

Fig 15-29 *(A)* Use a copper band box to fabricate a supply of bands; *(B)* adapt the band to the post.

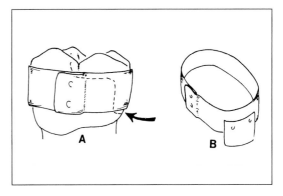

Fig 15-30 *(A)* Extend a too-short band *(B)* by spot welding a short piece of material to the original band.

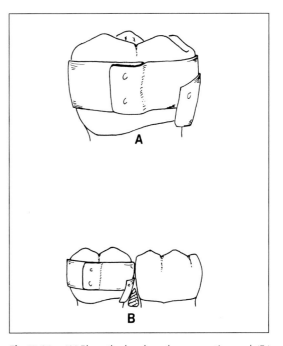

Fig 15-31 *(A)* Place the band on the preparation and *(B)* wedge it tightly.

15-3). These bands can be stored in the band box or in a durable plastic container.

Special adaptation of the matrix band. Occasions occur where the standard width of matrix material does not allow for proper wedging because the band is too short occlusogingivally. The most common site is on the distal side of a primary mandibular first molar. A method to accommodate this situation is as follows:

1. Select the proper-sized matrix band. It should fit loosely over the tooth (Fig 15-30, *A*). Cut a piece of matrix material to approximately the dimensions of the cavity preparation.
2. Tack weld a short piece to the portion of the matrix band covering the cavity preparation (Fig 15-30, *B*).
3. Place on the tooth preparation (Fig 15-31, *A*). Wedge as rightly as possible to the cervical margin (Fig 15-31, *B*).
4. Insert the amalgam, carve it, and remove the band as you would a normal matrix band.

Wooden wedge placement

Faulty wedging results in the following:

1. A concavity at the cervical portion of the proximal box can result if the rubber dam displaces the wedge or if too large a wedge is used. The purpose of the wedge in the primary dentition is to hold the matrix band at the cervical margins of the proximal box area.
2. An overextension of the restoration material (overhang) is caused if the wedge is too loose (Fig 15-32).
3. An open contact is caused by inadequate wedging pressure to separate the approximating contacts. Enough force must be exerted to orthodontically move the teeth for a short period of time. If the child has primate spacing or space between the teeth, it is not necessary to restore the contact.

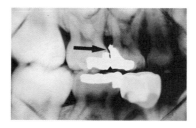

Fig 15-32 Faulty wedging results in an overhang *(arrow).*

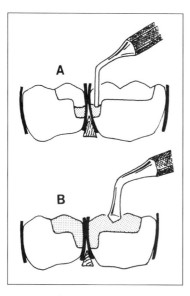

Fig 15-33 *(A)* Condense the proximal boxes at the same time, and *(B)* use the lateral condensor to burnish and carve the amalgam.

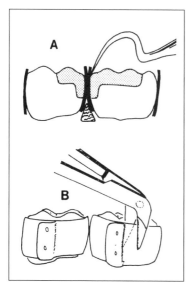

Fig 15-34 *(A)* Carve the amalgam and *(B)* remove the bands.

Condensing and carving of the amalgam

1. Mix the amalgam per the manufacturer's instructions.
2. Load a double-ended amalgam carrier. Insert one portion of amalgam into each proximal box. Fill and condense both proximal boxes at the same time (Fig 15-33, *A*).
3. With a positive finger rest, firmly condense the amalgam in the proximal boxes. If the interproximal parts of the cavity preparation are not filled and condensed equally, one of the restorations will be overcontoured at the expense of the adjacent restoration.
4. Add increments of amalgam and firmly condense both preparations until the proximal and occlusal portions are filled. Overfill the cavity preparations. Use a large condensor to condense both restorations.
5. Grossly carve the occlusal portions of both amalgams. Begin by using a lateral condensor to burnish and carve the amalgam (Fig 15-33, *B*). Because of its shape, the lateral condensor will internally carve and burnish the amalgam. If the lateral condensor is firmly pushed through the amalgam, all that needs to be done is to use carving instruments to remove the flash.
6. After the amalgam has set sufficiently, remove the excess around the marginal ridges with an explorer (Fig 15-34, *A*).
7. Use either a T-3 or cleoid-discoid carver to remove the amalgam from the margins.

Important: The amalgam carver should restore tooth structure. The inclines and angulation of the primary tooth will dictate the anatomy. If the carver stays on the tooth structure, overcarving will not occur. It is a temptation to leave a surplus of amalgam to "carve" with a finishing bur or green stone. With optimum carving, polishing is minimal. The anatomy should be shallow. Remember that primary teeth do not have a bulk of tooth structure. If overcarved, the amalgam restoration will be inherently weak.

After the amalgam is condensed and initially carved:

1. Remove the wedge.
2. Cut the band at the joint (Fig 15-34, *B*) with a matrix scissors, gold knife, or bur.
3. Carefully remove the band in a lingual or buccal direction through the contacts. The dental assistant can place a large amalgam condensor *gently* on the marginal ridge to reduce breakage as the bands are slipped occlusally.

Burnishing amalgam

After carving is completed, gently smooth the carving with a piece of moist cotton or a cupful of pumice paste. Remove any excess material from the margins of the amalgam with a suitable carver:

1. Take a small ball burnisher and smooth the occlusal surfaces. Although once thought to be detrimental, burnishing improves the adaption of amalgam, improves the surface finish, and reduces the time needed to polish (see the following section on burnishing methods).
2. Remove the rubber dam. Ask the patient to gently "tap" the teeth together. If you ask to "bite" or "close," the child may close with enough force to fracture the amalgam. Remove any occlusal prematurities with an amalgam carver.
3. Check the gingival interproximal margins for excess material.
4. Check the contact areas with dental floss by moving the floss from the buccal to lingual sides through the interproximal and gingival portions. Remove any excess material.

Figure 15-35 is the postoperative bitewing radiograph of the completed restorations. The overextension on the primary mandibular first molar resulted because either a wedge slipped or a short matrix band was used.

Finishing amalgam

Objectives

1. To have an amalgam restoration, when polished, resistant to corrosion and tarnish
2. To have a reduction in recurrent caries and marginal failure
3. To have a method that is easily used
4. To marginate the amalgam restoration

Armamentarium

Burnishing instruments
Greenstone (white stone)
Finishing burs
Abrasive points (optional)
Medium cuttle, interproximal
Fine pumice (acidulated phosphate prophylaxis paste)
Tin oxide (Amalgloss, L. D. Caulk Co)

Burnishing

Burnishing can be defined as the use of a metal instrument to smooth and shine the surface of a newly inserted amalgam restoration.

Historically, it was considered detrimental to amalgam restorations. However, current evaluations have answered some questions and suggest that burnishing may, in fact, be beneficial to amalgam restorations. Burnishing should be considered the first step in polishing.

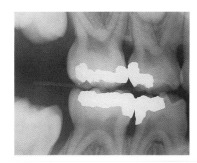

Fig 15-35 Completed Class II amalgam restorations.

Current research evaluations have concluded that burnishing is not detrimental to amalgam restorations (Birtcil et al, 1981; Boyer et al, 1980; Katora et al, 1979; Straffon et al, 1984; Yamada and Fusayama, 1981; Ulusoy et al, 1987; Lovadino et al, 1987; Woods et al, 1993).

Comparing a spherical high-copper amalgam and a conventional high-copper amalgam to a conventional fine-cut amalgam, Lovadino et al (1987) determined that burnishing during condensation improves marginal adaptation, especially in the high-copper alloys. Woods et al (1993) recommended the use of burnishing immediately before carving and as part of the condensation and finishing process.

It is suggested that burnishing is beneficial to the amalgam restoration, increasing its longevity. Burnishing reduces marginal leakage as well as the amount of mercury and the mercury-rich phase of the amalgam restoration. The timing of burnishing is important; burnishing too soon results in an uncontoured or weakened amalgam restoration. Ten minutes after the onset of trituration seems to be the best time to begin the process.

Advantages. Charbeneau (1965), evaluating various polishing methods, found that judicious burnishing to smooth a well-condensed and carved amalgam restoration improves polishing and, if done properly, is not detrimental. Kanai (1966) found burnishing to reduce residual mercury and porosity. After measuring the surface corrosion of burnished amalgam restorations, Svare and Chan (1972) suggested that burnishing might be substituted for polishing for an unpolished surface. Another advantage is the reported decrease in residual marginal mercury and decrease in the γ_2 phase (Teixera and Denehy, 1976). Boyer and Chan (1978) compared burnished amalgam restorations with mildly polished and conventionally finished amalgam restorations and found burnished restorations to be less susceptible to corrosion because of a lower porosity from the burnishing; however, too vigorous a polish can eliminate the advantage of burnishing. In a laboratory study, burnishing alone did not reduce microleakage; however, Copalite (Harry Bosworth Co), a cavity liner, did (Cothrean et al, 1978). In a clinical study, Leinfelder et al (1978) found that burnishing depends on (1) the effects of the type of alloy and the time at which amalgam restorations are burnished and that (2) regardless of the type of alloy used, unpolished amalgam restorations fail at a higher rate than those that are polished and burnished or burnished as a substitute for polishing.

Best method of burnishing. Burnishing is best accomplished by use of a round instrument. With the use of a back-and-forth movement, the surface of the amalgam is smoothed. Clinically, burnishing is done when the amalgam has begun its initial set and is resistant to deformation. Using a scanning electron microscope, Tidmarsh and Gavin (1973) found that burnishing 10 minutes after onset of trituration produces the smoothest surface. Timing of burnishing is important. Burnishing too soon results in an uncontoured and weakened amalgam restoration. Carving is important in the burnishing process!

Procedure. The following steps in the burnishing process are adopted from Tidmarsh and Gavin (1973), Schmidt et al (1975), and Teixera and Denehy (1976):

1. Overpack and overcondense the amalgam.
2. For the first, or initial, burnishing, use a lateral condensor to push the amalgam into the marginal voids (Fig 15-36).
3. Carve the amalgam, removing the excess from the cavosurface margin.
4. When the amalgam has reached sufficient hardness, burnish it, including all of the cavosurface margins (Fig 15-37).
5. After burnishing, check the cavosurface margins for excess material or flash. At this time, use a mild abrasive to complete smoothing of the amalgam (Fig 15-38).
6. If necessary, repeat step 4. The burnished amalgam should appear as in Fig 15-39.
7. If desired, polish the amalgams at the next appointment.

Because a great percentage of amalgams are not polished, burnishing at least should be done to reduce the tendency for marginal failure. Mathewson (1992) reported the results of two surveys (1976 to 1980 and 1981 to 1990) of dental graduates of the University of Oklahoma. In general, dental amalgam restorations are not polished. Only 24% of the dentists in the 1976 to 1980 sample routinely polish amalgam restorations. The results of the 1981 to 1990 survey were similar; only 18% of those surveyed routinely polish amalgam restorations. After 1980, there was an increased emphasis on the method and need for burnishing amalgam restorations. As a result, 76% of the 1981 to 1990 sample routinely burnish amalgams. If you don't polish, at least burnish!

Polishing

Objectives
1. To marginate the amalgam and enamel
2. To adjust the occlusion
3. To encourage soft tissue adaptability
4. To reduce tarnish and corrosion

Best method of polishing. Overheating of amalgam during the polishing procedure should be avoided. Christensen and Dilts (1968) found temperature increases during all polishing procedures, with a burlew disk producing the greatest rise in temperature. A hard brush with moist pumice produced the least increase. They noted a continued temperature rise even after the polishing procedure had stopped. A scanning electron microscopy study of interproximal finishing of Class II amalgam restorations showed that medium cuttle disks gave an optimum finish to interproximal amalgam margins (Swedlow et al, 1972). Tidmarsh and Gavin (1973) found that polishing could best be accomplished with finishing burs and use of a silicon paste, especially after burnishing.

Condensing and carving the amalgam, as previously described, is the first step in finishing of an amalgam restoration. Burnishing, once thought to be detrimental to the amalgam restoration, can be beneficial to amalgam restoration. The amalgam should be allowed to age for 48 hours before the polishing process is begun.

Straffon et al (1984) compared amalgam restorations that were carved and burnished with those that were carved, burnished, and then polished after 24 hours. However, after 36 months, there was little clinical difference between the amalgam restorations.

Procedure
1. Use a white stone first. The stone is used to gently remove the flash from the margins. Run from amalgam to the enamel (Fig 15-40). Always use light pressure and short strokes when polishing amalgam. The first step is to remove any marginal flash on the cavosurface margins. If the amalgam was overcarved, trim the enamel to the amalgam margin. This procedure, an *enameloplasty*, should be reserved for minor deficiencies.
2. Insert a plug finishing bur (Fig 15-41) into a slow-speed contra-angle handpiece. Accelerate the contra-angle handpiece to its maximum speed. Use a feather touch and lightly pass over the amalgam restoration. The restoration should begin to shine. Use care with the finishing bur so as not to gouge the adjacent enamel and amalgam surface. Shallow anatomy is preferred. Deep grooves in the amalgam induce stress and may serve as food traps.
3. Use a small, round finishing bur to finish the small grooves (Fig 15-42).

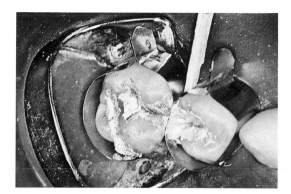

Fig 15-36 Initial burnishing of the amalgam.

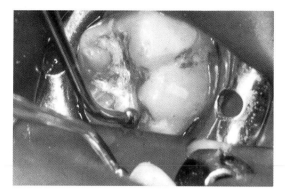

Fig 15-37 When the amalgam is hardened, it can be burnished.

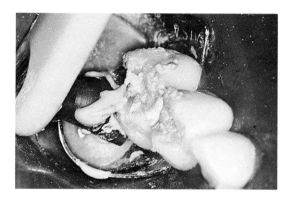

Fig 15-38 A mild abrasive finishes the initial carving.

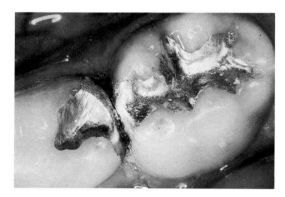

Fig 15-39 The initial step, if needed, is with a white stone.

4. Use a Wet-N-Dry medium cuttle disk (Moore Co) to polish the interproximal margins.
5. Use an acidulated phosphate prophylaxis paste with a rubber cup or a bristle brush to complete the polishing procedures (Fig 15-43). Tin oxide can be used.

Qualities of the well-polished amalgam restoration (Fig 15-44)
1. Amalgam and tooth structure of equal height—no flash and no submarginal areas
2. Anatomy and contour that resemble those of the corresponding tooth on opposite side of the arch
3. Grooves clearly defined but not deep
4. Marginal ridge height equal to that of the adjacent tooth
5. Surface free of scratches
6. Interproximal contact integrity undisturbed
7. Shiny surface finish

Factors that contribute to poor polishing results
1. Poor condensation of the amalgam, resulting in pitting of the amalgam surface

2. Inadequate carving, burnishing, and polishing methods
3. Moisture contamination during condensation
4. Unsuitable burs and polishing stones, eg, finishing burs that are too sharp or stones that are not sharpened to a point

Summary

Cavity varnishes

1. Should be used before insertion of all amalgam restorations.
2. *Should not* be used beneath composite resin restorations unless stated in the manufacturer's instructions.

Cavity liners

1. Should be used in all deep lesions in primary and permanent teeth.
2. *Should not* be placed beneath composite resin restorations if the liners contain a zinc oxide–eugenol compound.

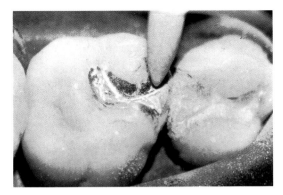

Fig 15-40 Accomplish the initial polishing, if needed, with a white stone.

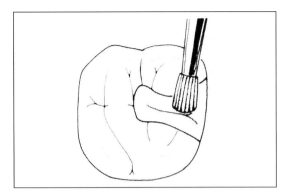

Fig 15-41 Next, use a slow-speed finishing bur.

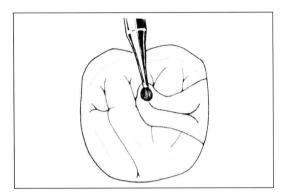

Fig 15-42 Use a small finishing bur to finish the grooves.

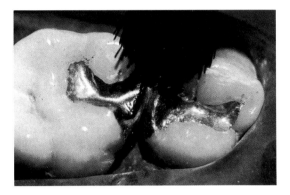

Fig 15-43 Use an acidulated phosphate prophylaxis to finish the process.

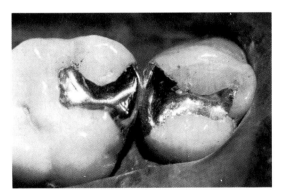

Fig 15-44 Well-finished and well-polished amalgam restorations.

Amalgam

The optimal technique includes the following:

1. Use of a rubber dam wherever possible
2. Conserve cavity preparations to counteract the weak physical properties of amalgam
3. A high-copper alloy plus the appropriate amount of mercury to achieve optimal plasticity and to reduce corrosion and creep
4. Consistent methods of trituration and condensation
5. A burnishing scheme plus a polishing method to finalize the amalgam restoration

Dental amalgam, when used as a restorative material, should meet the following criteria:

1. Have a reduced risk of marginal failure with minimal recurrent caries
2. Be resistant to corrosion and creep
3. Have characteristics for mixing, inserting, and polishing that are easily duplicated

Posterior composite resin restorations

The use of composite resins for restoration of primary posterior teeth has expanded since the 1970s, with manufacturers suggesting and advocating its substitution for dental amalgam. However, there are some peculiarities specific to composite resins that contribute to questions about their routine use for primary posterior teeth.

Advantages

1. Elimination of mercury in the dental environment
2. Improved appearance and esthetics
3. Reduced thermal stimulation to the pulp
4. Absence of expensive metals such as silver, copper, or mercury
5. Color-matching potential
6. Ability to bond to the walls of the cavity preparation
7. Longevity (with the proper technique should last 10 years)

Disadvantages

1. Increased tendency for extensive abrasion of functioning occlusal surfaces
2. Possible open interproximal contacts
3. Appearance of microscopic voids, which can cause recurrent caries, if a rigid technique is not used
4. Lack of a composite resin that is truly radiopaque, although several products demonstrate some radiopacity
5. Pulpal protection with an appropriate liner necessary
6. Shrinkage during polymerization, affecting marginal adaptation

Types and classifications

Lutz et al (1983) define and classify filled restorative resins as follows. A composite resin is composed of three phases:

1. The matrix phase, which is the organic phase common to all composite resins, is an oligomer. Other organic chemicals are added to initiate setting, either by chemicals or light, plus others to aid handling and shelf life.
2. The surface interfacial phase is an agent that serves to connect the matrix phase and the partial organic filler material.
3. The dispersed phase is the filler particle used in the composite resin system. These particles vary from system to system (Table 15-4).

Curing methods

Currently composite resins are cured either chemically or by photocuring (light curing). The chemical-curing system consists of two separate pastes that are mixed together, initiating the curing process. The single-paste method is cured by photocuring. A number of studies have described the clinical advantage of using the photocuring system (Leinfelder, 1985). There are specific advantages to the visible light system. Lutz et al (1983) lists these as:

Table 15-4 Filler characteristics of composite materials

Particle size (μm)	Examples
	Conventional
15–35	Prisma-fil (L.D. Caulk Co.), Command (Kerr Division of the Sybron Corp.)
	Hybrids
1–5	P-10, P-30 (3M Dental Products)
	Microfill
<0.04	Phase fill (Phasealloy, Inc.) Silux (3M Dental Products)

1. Less porosity with a faster, complete cure of the resin
2. Immediate finish, improving physical properties
3. A more optimum working time for larger restorations
4. Improved quality of color, translucency, and tooth morphology because of the ability to add increments
5. Higher wear resistance
6. Improved esthetics for anterior restorations

Idiosyncrasies

Several authors have described problems that are peculiar to posterior composite resin restorations (Leinfelder and Vann, 1982; Leinfelder, 1985; Reinhardt, et al 1982; Lutz et al, 1983).

1. Because composite resins are not as condensable as dental amalgam, interproximal contacts are often open. To overcome this disadvantage, the operator should prewedge the tooth before cavity preparation. Additionally, the matrix band should be burnished against the adjacent proximal surface before insertion of the composite resin material.
2. Defects, or macroscopic voids, can occur. This defect can pose a serious problem if it occurs adjacent to a cavosurface margin. Use of a condensable composite resin with a precise method of insertion can reduce this problem.
3. In permanent teeth, there have been some reports of postoperative sensitivity. It is not a factor in studies to date with primary teeth.
4. Hardison (1987) determined that the radiolucent halo noticed by clinicians is really excessive unfilled resin bonding agent. The excess bonding agent must be meticulously blown out.

Table 15-5 Summary of composite resin studies of primary teeth

Study	Length (y)	Materials	Comments
Tonn et al (1980)	2	Epoxydent (Lee Pharmaceutical Corp); Optaloy (L.D. Caulk Co)	Anatomic form better with amalgam
Nelson et al (1980)	3	Adaptic Radiopaque; Adaptic; Disperalloy; (Johnson & Johnson)	Suggested composite resins for teeth with less than 3 years longevity
Leifler and Varpio (1981)	2	Concise (Cap-C-Rynge, Radiopaque; 3M Dental Products)	Modified preparations resulted in a 34% failure rate after 2 years
Paquette et al (1983)	1	Profile (S.S. White Co); Visiofil (Den-Mat Corp)	Modified preparation not recommended
Roberts et al (1985)	2	Profile; Ease (L.D. Caulk Co)	No clinical difference between composite resin and amalgam
Oldenburg et al (1985)	2	F-70; X-55 (experimental)	Beveled cavity preparation best, irrespective of material
Tonn and Ryge (1985)	2	Prisma-Bond; F-70 (Ful-Fil) (L.D. Caulk Co)	Restorations functioned well
Leinfelder et al (1986)	3	Nine composite resin materials	Wear rates depended on method of evaluation; wear decreases with time
Donly (1987)	0	Scotchbond P-3 (3M Dental Products)	Buccolingual incremental plac ement most favorable
Oldenburg et al (1987)	2	H-120 (L.D. Caulk Co)	Compared to primary molars; permanent molar wear excessive
Wendall and Vann (1987)	2	Scotchbond Visilux (3M Dental Products)	Wear patterns similar in restorations of primary and permanent molars
Tonn and Ryge (1988)	4	Ful-Fil (L.D. Caulk/ Dentsply)	Primary molar enamel wear similar to posterior primary composite resins
Vann et al (1988)	4	Ful-Fil (L.D. Caulk Co)	Wear in primary molars is progressive
Fuks et al (1990)	1	Herculite (Kerr Co)	Incremental filling does not eliminate microleakage
Barr-Agholme et al (1991)	2	Scotchbond Visilux (3M Dental)	Clinically, composite resins more successful than amalgam

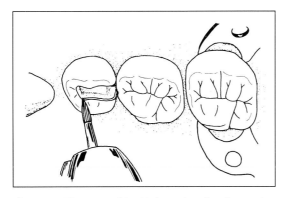

Fig 15-45 Placement of the 45-degree bevel on the margins.

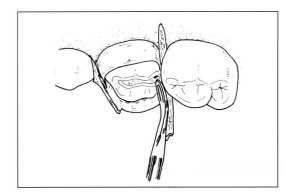

Fig 15-46 Burnish the matrix band to the adjacent tooth.

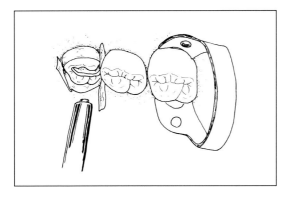

Fig 15-47 Use an air syringe to gently spread the bonding agent.

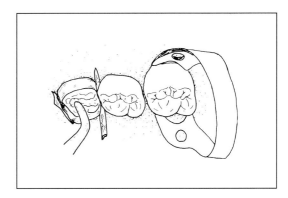

Fig 15-48 Condense the composite resin material into the cavity preparation.

Clinical studies

A summary of several clinical studies is listed in Table 15-5. The earlier studies demonstrated that dental amalgam was a better material for posterior restorations than were composite resins; excessive abrasion was the culprit. With the introduction of the intermediate or hybrid composite resins, composite resins became comparable to amalgams for posterior restorations. A modification in cavity preparation was used with a 45° bevel at the cavosurface margin (Fig 15-45).

In permanent posterior teeth, Isenberg and Leinfelder (1990) clinically demonstrated that beveling the occlusal cavosurface margin does not enhance the wear resistance properties of the composite resin material.

Armamentarium

Burs: No. 330 flamed-shaped finishing bur,
    or barrel-shaped finishing bur
Visible light source
Mylar matrix band, toothpick wedges
Articulating paper
Bonding agent
Composite material
Plastic instrument

Operative procedures

Irrespective of the system used, adhere to the manufacturer's instructions.

1. As in all restorative procedures where deep areas of caries occur, apply a calcium hydroxide material for pulpal protection.
2. With a brush, apply an acid gel to the cavity preparation.
3. Similar to an amalgam restoration, apply a matrix band. Wedge it well with a toothpick. With a suitable instrument, burnish the matrix band to the adjacent tooth (Fig 15-46). However, because of the difficulty in obtaining a tight contact, restore the cavity preparations individually.
4. Mix and spread Scotchbond (3M Dental Products) in the cavity preparation.
5. With an air syringe, gently spread the material over the cavity preparation. Do not use the visible light source at this time. Repeat the process (Fig 15-47).

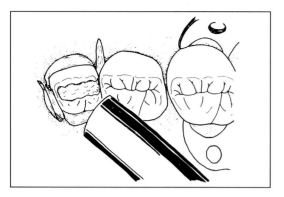

Fig 15-49 Direct the visible light source at the occlusal surface for 20 seconds after each application of composite resin.

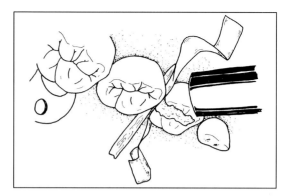

Fig 15-50 After the removal of the matrix band, cure the composite resin on the buccal side for 20 seconds and the lingual side for 20 seconds.

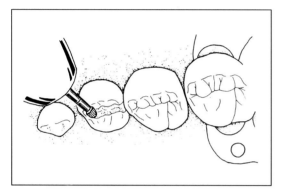

Fig 15-51 Use plug finishing burs to adjust the occlusal surface anatomy.

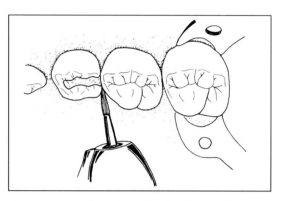

Fig 15-52 Use a flame-shaped finishing bur to polish the interproximal surfaces.

6. With the plastic instrument, tap and condense the resin material into the cavity preparation. Attempt to adapt the material to reduce the possibility of voids (Fig 15-48). By using the visible light source, you can cure the composite resin to a depth of 5 to 6 mm.
7. With the visible light source, cure the resin 20 seconds for each application of material (Fig 15-49).
8. Partially remove the matrix band. Again using the light source, cure the resin 20 seconds on the buccal surface and then 20 seconds on the lingual surface (Fig 15-50).
9. Remove the matrix band. With the flamed-shaped finishing bur, contour the interproximal areas (Fig 15-51). Remove any excess, maintaining normal proximal contour and anatomy (Fig 15-52).
10. With articulating paper, check for premature contacts. Contour and polish the occlusal surfaces (Fig 15-53).

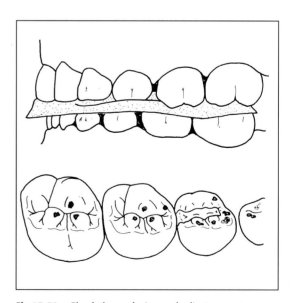

Fig 15-53 Check the occlusion and adjust premature contact spots.

Glass-ionomer cement restorative materials

Glass-ionomer cements are ion-leachable by aqueous polyacrylic acid. The cement powder is finely ground calcium aluminum fluorosilicate glass. This powder is combined with a solution of polyacrylic acid, maleic acid, and tartaric acid. The incorporation of particles of silver to cement powder creates a glass-ionomer silver "cermet" restorative material (Ketac-Silver, ESPE Premier).

The addition of silver alloy filings to the cement powder when combined with the polyacrylic acid has been referred to as the *miracle mix*.

These mixtures have several advantages:

1. The restoration is radiopaque.
2. They have a greater resistance to wear than do other glass-ionomer products.
3. They bond to dentin.
4. They can be finished soon after proper setting.
4. Fluoride can be released; thus the material may be cariostatic. Olsen et al (1989) evaluated the amount of fluoride ion released from glass-ionomer-lined amalgam restorations. The three products sampled all released the fluoride ion. However, the fluoride release varied by manufacturer and over time.
6. The mixtures do not use mercury.

The silver-glass-ionomer cements do have disadvantages (Brackett and Johnston, 1989; Smith, 1990): they have low fracture toughness and an increased potential for fracture and the silver color may be unesthetic.

Suggested indications for glass ionomer restorations (Wilson and McLean, 1988; Stratmann et al, 1989; Croll, 1993; Croll and Killian, 1993)

1. For Class I and II restorations in primary molars; for Class III restorations on the distal surface of primary canines
2. As a bonded liner under amalgam restorations in primary molars and young permanent posterior teeth
3. For repair of stainless steel crowns where the occlusal surface is abraded
4. As transitional restorations after pulp therapy in primary teeth that will exfoliate in 12 to 18 months
5. For replacement of fractured amalgam restorations

For an excellent description of the clinical use of the glass-ionomer restorative material, see Wilson and McLean. (1988, pages 221 to 227).

References

American Academy of Pediatric Dentistry (AAPD). Reference Manual. Chicago: AAPD, 1993.

American Dental Association (ADA) Council on Dental Materials, Instruments, and Equipment. Recommendations on dental mercury hygiene, 1984. J. Am. Dent. Assoc. 109:617, 1984.

American Dental Association (ADA) Council on Dental Materials, Instruments, and Equipment. Dental mercury hygiene. J. Am. Dent. Assoc. 122:112, 1991.

Andrews, J. T., and Hembree, J. H. In vitro evaluation of marginal leakage of corrosion resistant amalgam alloy. J. Dent. Child. 42:367, 1975.

Avery, K. T., Hamby, C. L., and Shapiro, S. A review of the status of mercury as utilized by the dental profession. J. Olka. State Dent. Assoc. 73:9, 1982.

Barr-Agholme, M., et al. A two-year clinical study of lightcured composite and amalgam restorations in primary molars. Dent. Mater. 7:230, 1991.

Birtcil, R. E., Pelzner, R. B., and Stark, M. M. A 30-month clinical evaluation of the influence of finishing and size of restoration on the margin performance of five amalgam alloys. J. Dent. Res. 60:1949, 1981.

Blaser, P. K. Effects of designs of Class 2 preparations on resistance of teeth to fracture. Oper. Dent. 8:6, 1985.

Boyer, D. B., and Chan, K. C. The effect of surface finish on the anodic polarization of a conventional spherical amalgam. J. Biomed. Mater. Res. 12:541, 1978.

Boyer, D. B., Edie, J. W., and Chan, K. C. Effect of clinical finishing procedures on amalgam microstructure. J. Dent. Res. 59:129, 1980.

Brackett, W. W., and Johnston, W. M. Relative microhardness of glass ionomer restorative materials as an indicator of finishing time. J. Am. Dent. Assoc. 118:599, 1989.

Caradazzi. J. L., Hadaui, F., Asgar, K. Effect on condensors on adaptability and microporosity of amalgam restorations. J. Pedod. 8:57, 1983.

Charbeneau, G. T. A suggested technique for polishing amalgam restorations. J. Mich, Dent. Assoc. 47:320, 1965.

Christensen, G. J., and Dilts, W. E. Thermal change during dental polishing. J. Dent Res. 47:690, 1968.

Clark, A. E., et al. The influence of condensing pressure on the strength of three dental amalgams. Oper. Dent. 6:6, 1981.

Cothrean, T. G., et al. Effects of burnishing on microleakage in an amalgam system. J. Prosthet. Dent. 40:163, 1978.

Croll, T. P. Light-hardened Class I glass-ionomer-resin cement restorations of a permanent molar. Quintessence Int. 24:109, 1993.

Croll, T. P., and Killian, C. M. Restoration of Class II carious lesions using light-hardening glass-ionomer-resin cement. Quintessence Int. 24:533, 1993.

Dawson, L. R., Simon, J. E., Jr., and Taylor, P. P. Use of amalgam and stainless steel restorations for primary molars. J. Dent. Child. 48:42, 1981.

Donly, K. J. Posterior composite polymerization shrinkage in primary teeth: An in vivo comparison of three restorative techniques. Pediatr. Dent. 9:22, 1987.

Fuks, A. B., Chosack, A., and Eidelman, E. Assessment of marginal leakage around Class II composite restorations in retrieved primary molars. Pediatr. Dent. 12:24, 1990.

Hardison, J. D. Radiolucent halos associated with radiopaque composite resin restorations. J. Am. Dent Assoc. 118:595, 1989.

Ireland, R. L. Operative procedures for children. J. Am. Dent. Assoc. 67:340, 1963.

Isenberg, B. P., and Leinfelder, K. F. Efficacy of bevelling posterior composite resin preparations. J. Esthet. Dent. 2:70, 1990.

Kanai, S. Structure studies of amalgam. II. Effect of burnishing on the margins of occlusal amalgam fillings. Acta Odontol. Scand. 25:47, 1966.

Katora, M. E., Moore P. A., and Jubach, T. S. Surface morphology of burnished versus non-burnished amalgam restorations. Quintessence Int. 10:93, 1979.

Kelsey, W. P., and Panneton, M. J. A comparison of amalgam microleakage between a copal varnish and two resin-compatible cavity varnishes. Quintessence Int. 19:895, 1988.

Larson, I. D., Douglas, W. H. and Geistfeld, R. E. Effect of prepared cavities on the strength of teeth. Oper. Dent. 6:2, 1980.

Leifler, E., and Varpio, M. Proximocclusal composite restorations in primary molars: A two year follow up. J. Dent. Child. 48:441, 1981.

Leinfelder, K. F. Composite resins. Dent. Clin. North Am. 29:359, 1985.

Leinfelder, K. F., et al. Burnished amalgam restorations: A two-year clinical evaluation. Oper. Dent. 3:2, 1978.

Leinfelder, K. F., and Vann, W. F. The use of composite resins in primary molars. Pediatr. Dent. 4:27, 1982.

Leinfelder, K. F., Wilder, A. D., and Teixeira, L C. Wear rates of posterior composite resins. J. Am. Dent. Assoc. 112:829, 1986.

Lovadino, J. R., Ruhnke, L. A., and Consoni, S. Influence of burnishing on amalgam adaptation to cavity walls. J. Prosthet. Dent. 58:284, 1987.

Lutz, F., et al. Dental restorative resins. Dent. Clin. North Am. 27:697, 1983.

Mahler, D. B., and Adey, J. D, The influence of final mercury content on the characteristics of a high copper amalgam. J. Biomed. Mater. Res. 13:467, 1979.

Mahler, D. B., and Marantz, R. L. Clinical assessment of dental amalgam restorations. Int. Dent. J. 30:327, 1980.

Mahler, D. B., Adey, J. D. and Marek, M. Creep and corrosion of amalgam. J. Dent. Res. 61:33, 1982.

Mahler, D. B., Terkla, L. G., and Van Eysden, J. Marginal failure of amalgam restorations. J. Dent. Res. 52:823, 1973.

Marhotra, M. L., and Asgar, K. Physical properties of dental silver-tin amalgams with high and low copper contents. J. Am. Dent. Assoc. 96:444, 1978.

Mandel, I. D. Amalgam hazards. An assessment of research. J. Am. Dent. Assoc. 122:64, 1991.

Mathewson, R. J. Determination of cavosurface angles in primary molar cavity preparations. J. Calif. Dent. Assoc. 40:1065, 1972.

Mathewson, R. J. A model for department self assessment. In Proceedings, American Academy of Pediatric Dentistry, Seattle, 1992.

Mathewson, R. J., and Lu, K. H. Influences of clinical factors on marginal adaptation and residual mercury content on amalgam. J. Dent. Res. 54:104, 1975.

Mathewson, R. J., Retzlaff, A. E., and Porter, D. F. Marginal failure of amalgam in deciduous teeth: A two-year report. J. Am. Dent. Assoc. 88:134, 1974.

Matsson, L., et al. Marginal adaptation of dispersion and traditional amalgams with reference to plasticity: A clinical comparison. J. Dent. Res. 61:1172, 1982.

McComb. D. Comparisons of physical properties of commercial calcium hydroxide lining cements. J. Am. Dent. Assoc. 107:610, 1983.

Mitchem, J. C. Resin restorations: Factors affecting clinical performance. Dent. Clin. North Am. 27:713, 1983.

Mitchem, J. C., and Mahler, D. B. The adaptation of amalgam, J. Am. Dent. Assoc. 76:787, 1968.

Nelson, G. V., et al. A three-year clinical evaluation of composite resin and a high copper amalgam in posterior primary teeth. J. Dent. Child. 47:414, 1980.

Nelson, G. V., and Osborne, J. W. A three-year clinical study of high copper amalgams in primary teeth. Pediatr. Dent. 3:186, 1981.

Oldenburg, T. R., Vann, W. F., and Dilley, D. C. Composite restorations for primary molars: Two year results Pediatr. Dent. 7:96, 1985.

Oldenburg, T. R., Vann, W. F., Jr., and Dilley, D. C. Comparison and composite and amalgam in posterior teeth of children. Dent. Mater. 3:182, 1987.

Olsen, B. T., et al. Fluoride release from glass ionomer-lined amalgam restoration. Am. J. Dent. 2:89, 1989.

Osborne, J. W., and Gale, E. N. Failure rate of amalgams with a high content of copper. Oper Dent. 4.2, 1979.

Osborne, J. W., Binion, P. P., and Gale, E. N. Dental amalgam: Clinical behavior up to eight years. Oper. Dent. 5:24, 1980.

Osborne, J. W., et al Static creep of certain commercial amalgam alloys. J. Am. Dent. Assoc. 89:620, 1974.

Osborne, J. W., et al. Clinical performance and physical properties of twelve amalgam alloys. J. Dent Res. 47:983, 1978.

Pameijer, C. H., and Benhameurlain, M. A long-term clinical comparison between a lathe-cut alloy and dispersalloy. Quintessence Int. 5:565, 1983.

Paquette, D. E. et al. Modified cavity preparations for composite resins in primary molars, Pediatr. Dent. 5:246, 1983.

Reinhardt, J. W., et al. Porosity in composite resin restorations. Oper. Dent. 7:82, 1982.

Roberts, M. W., Moffa, J. P., and Broring, C. L. A two-year clinical evaluation of a proprietary composite resin for restoration of primary posterior teeth. Pediatr. Dent. 7:14, 1985.

Rowe, N. H. Control of infection in dental practice. J. Mich. Dent. Assoc. 73:22, 1991.

Sarkar, N. K., Osborne, J. W., and Leinfelder, L. F. In vitro corrosion and in vivo marginal fracture of dental amalgams. J. Dent. Res. 61:1262, 1982.

Schmidt, J. R., et al. Burnishing (surfacing) the amalgam restoration. III. Dent. J. 44:282, 1975.

Smith, D. C. Composition and characteristic of glass-ionomer cements. J. Am. Dent. Assoc. 120:20, 1990.

Straffon, L. H., et al. A clinical evaluation of polished and unpolished amalgams: 36-month results. Pediatr. Dent. 6:220, 1984.

Statmann, R. G., Berg, J. H., and Donly, K. J. Class II glass ionomer-silver restorations in primary molars. Quintessence Int. 20:43, 1989.

Swedlow, D. B., et al. Dental amalgam polishing with discs as observed by scanning electron microscopy. J. Prosthet. Dent., 27:536, 1972.

Swift, E. J. An update on glass ionomer cements. Quintessence Inc. 19:125, 1988.

Svare, C. W., and Chan, K. C. Effect of surface treatment on the corrodibility of dental amalgam. J. Dent. Res. 51:44, 1972.

Teixeira, L. C., and Denehy, G. E. Burnishing a technique for improving the amalgam restorations. J. Ind. Dent. Assoc. 55:14, 1976.

Tidmarsh, B. G., and Gavin, J. B. Finishing amalgam restorations: A scanning electron microscope study. N. Z. Dent. J. 69:175, 1973.

Tonn, E. M., and Ryge, G. Two-year clinical evaluation of lightcured composite resin restorations in primary molars. J. Am. Dent. Assoc. 111:44, 1985.

Tonn, E. M. and Ryge G. Clinical evaluations of composite resin restorations in primary molars: A 4-year follow-up study. J. Am. Dent. Assoc. 117:(.5)603, 1988.

Tonn, E. M., Ryge, G., and Chambers, D. W. A two-year clinical study of a carviable composite resin used as a Class II restoration in primary molars. J. Dent. Child. 47:405, 1980.

Ulusoy, N., Aydin, A. K., and Ulusoy, M. Evaluation of finishing techniques of assessing surface roughness of amalgam restorations. J. Prosthet. Dent. 57:286, 1987.

U. S. Department of Labor. Controlling Occupational Exposure to Blood-borne Pathogens in Dentistry. OSHA publication No. 3129, 1992.

Vann, W. F., Barkmeier, W. W., and Mahler, D. B. Assessing composite resin wear in primary molars: Four-year findings. J. Dent. Res. 67:876, 1988.

Wendall, J. J. and Vann, W. F. Wear of composite resin restorations in primary versus permanent molar teeth. J. Dent. Res. 67:71, 1987.

Wilson, A. D., and McLean, J. W. Glass-Ionomer Cement. Chicago: Quintessence, 1988.

Woods, P. W., et al. Determining amalgam marginal quality: effect of occlusal surface condition. J. Am. Dent Assoc. 124:60, 1993.

Yamada, T., and Fusayama, T. Effect of moisture contamination on high-copper amalgam. J. Dent. Res. 60:716, 1981.

Yates, J. L., Murray, G. A., and Hembree, J. H., Jr. Cavity varnishes applied over insulating bases: Effect on microleakage. Oper Dent. 5:43, 1980.

Additional readings

Farbod, F., Hadavi, F., and Asgar, K. Marginal leakage of dental amalgam. Oper. Dent. 8:11, 1983.

Jordan, R. E., Suzuki, M., and Boksman, L. The new generation amalgam alloys: Clinical considerations. Dent. Clin. North Am. 29:341, 1985.

Leinfelder K. F. Microfilled composite resins. Gen. Dent. 30:473, 1982.

Lloyd, C. H., and Mitchell, L. The fracture toughness of tooth coloured restorative materials. J. Oral Rehabil. 11:257, 1984.

Lui, J. L. Margin quality and microleakage of Class II composite resin restorations. J. Am. Dent. Assoc. 114:49, 1987.

Mathewson, R. J. Restoration of primary teeth with amalgam. Dent. Clin. North Am. 28:137, 1984.

Mitchem, J. C. The potential of amalgam condensation causing the intrusion of capping materials into the pulp. J. Prosthet. Dent. 26:506, 1971.

Rupp, N. W., Pattenbarger, G. C., and Patel, P. R. Effect of residual mercury content on creep in dental amalgams. J. Am. Dent. Assoc. 100:52, 1980.

Rydinge, E., et al. Clinical evaluation of high copper amalgam restorations. J. Oral Rehabil. 8:465, 1981.

Wilder, A. D., May, K. N., and Leinfelder, K. L. Three-year clinical study of u.v. polymerized composites in posterior teeth. J. Dent. Child. 47:414, 1980.

Williams, V. D. Factors that effect the adhesion of composites to enamel. Gen. Dent. 30:477, 1982.

Questions

1. On recall examination, several of your "ideal" amalgams exhibit severe corrosion, a fractured margin, and loss of anatomy. A probable cause(s) is (are):

   a. Undertrituration of the amalgam
   b. Poor condensation methods
   c. Saliva contamination on insertion (despite what we said!)
   d. Excessive residual mercury content
   e. All of the above

2. Which of the following should not be used to polish or finish amalgams?

   a. A ball burnisher
   b. A rubber (burlew) disk
   c. A finishing bur
   d. A white stone
   e. A lateral condensor

3. Contrary to previous beliefs, burnishing is:

   a. Contraindicated
   b. Beneficial in permanent teeth only
   c. Beneficial on all amalgam restorations
   d. Used only when time permits
   e. Used on primary teeth only

4. Figure 15-54 is a postoperative bitewing radiograph of one of your restorations. Note the overhang on the primary maxillary primary first molar. What most likely was the cause?

   a. Improper wedging
   b. Overcondensation of the amalgam
   c. Deep carious lesions
   d. Improper cavity preparation
   e. A difficult child patient

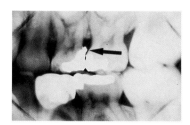

Fig 15-54

5. What would you do for the overhang in question 4?

   a. Replace the restoration
   b. Try to remove the overhang (what with?)

Chapter 16

Stainless Steel Crown Procedures for Primary Molars

Objectives

After studying this chapter, the student should be able to:
1. Describe the indications for stainless steel crowns.
2. Understand the principles of preparation, adaptation, and cementation of a successful stainless steel crown.

Stainless steel crowns were often referred to as *chrome steel crowns.* The material used was an alloy containing 18% chromium and 8% nickel (called 18-8 alloy), with a carbon content of 0.8% to 20%. The crowns exhibit the following properties:

1. Heating does not increase their strength.
2. They work-harden; strength increases from manipulation with pliers, for example.
3. Their high chromium content reduces corrosion.
4. Soldering with flux reduces their corrosion resistance.

An alternative crown material is a *nickel-chrome crown* (Ion, 3M Dental Products). The material in this crown is an alloy of 77% nickel, 15% chromium, and 7% iron. This type of crown is prefestooned and precontoured. Reportedly a minimum amount of adaptation is needed. However, the minimal adaptation can prove to be a clinical liability.

Sources of stainless steel crowns

Stainless steel crowns are available in six sizes for each primary tooth and permanent first molars (Fig 16-1). Sizes 4 and 5 are the most often used. A size 7 is available for extra-large teeth. These sizes are supplied in kit form, with the user needing to reorder only those sizes frequently used.

Indications

1. Primary or permanent teeth with extensive carious lesions; primary teeth with three carious surfaces

2. Primary or permanent teeth with enamel or dentin defects, such as hypoplastic enamel, amelogenesis imperfecta, or dentinogenesis imperfecta
3. Teeth that have been fractured
4. Teeth used as abutments for space maintainers

Braff (1975) reviewed 74 patients to compare success rates of Class II amalgam restorations and stainless steel crowns. Of the primary teeth restored with amalgam, 88.7% required replacement treatment. By comparison, only 30.03% of the stainless steel crowns required remedial care. He concluded that economics of time and cost favor stainless steel crowns. This philosophy was supported by Dawson et al (1981), who concluded that nearly 70% of the multisurface amalgam restorations in their study needed replacement with a stainless steel crown.

Armamentarium

Burs and stones
    No. 169L or No. 69L F.G.
    No. 6 or No. 8 R.A.
    No. 330 F.G.
    Tapered diamond F.G.
Green stone or heatless stone
Wire wheel
Pliers and instruments
    No. 114 Johnson pliers
    No. 800-417 crown pliers (Unitek Corp)
    No. 112 ball and socket pliers (optional)
    Sharp scaler or instrument, America No. 7
    Crown and bridge scissors
    No. 110 Howe pliers
    No. 137 Gordon pliers

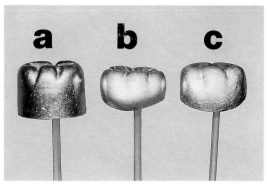

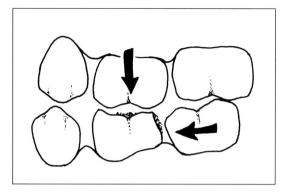

Fig 16-1 *(a)* Uncontoured or Untrimmed crowns were the initial crowns available. These are still used in special instances where extra length is needed, especially in the deep areas of interproximal carious lesions. *(b)* Precrimped crowns are made to fit primary teeth with little alteration. However, these are difficult to alter when necessary. *(c)* Pretrimmed crowns, manufactured to the approximate length of normal teeth. Trimming minimal, but contouring and crimping are needed.

Fig 16-2 Mesial drift caused by caries.

Cement medium
   Glass slab
   Spatula
   Zinc phosphate cement, liquid and powder
Rough or whiting polishing wheels
Dental floss
Rubber dam armamentarium

Clinical procedures

The stainless steel crown is different from the cast gold or fabricated crown in that the stainless steel crown is not a precision fit. With the use of pliers and good clinical judgment, the stainless steel crown is adapted to naturally occurring undercuts. Because the stainless steel crown is somewhat flexible, it will snap into and out of the undercuts.

Be wary of such statements as, "The retention of a stainless steel crown depends primarily on the retention created by adapting and contouring." Studies show that the cementing medium is the main influence on the retention of stainless steel crowns (Mathewson et al, 1974, 1975). Local anesthesia should be used routinely. If a pulpotomy or pulpectomy is to be done, do it at this time. Where there is doubt about whether to perform a pulpotomy of pulpectomy, answer the question by first removing all deep carious lesions. After assessment, complete the stainless steel crown preparation. Myers (1975) found a close association between errors in crown adaptation and gingivitis around the defective crown. Stainless steel crowns should be meticulously adapted.

1. Before placing a rubber dam, check the child's occlusion. Observe for the following situations:
   a. The opposing tooth has extruded because of longstanding carious lesions.

   b. Mesial drift has resulted because carious lesions have changed the occlusion of the adjacent tooth (Fig 16-2).
   c. Tooth reduction is needed so that the restored tooth can be returned to normal function.
2. Use a rubber dam in preparing a tooth for a stainless steel crown:
   a. To protect surrounding tissue.
   b. To improve visibility and efficiency.
   c. To better manage behavior.
   d. To prevent ingestion of the stainless steel crown during preparation.
3. You can alter the rubber dam by cutting the interproximal rubber to avoid cutting the dam with rotating instruments. Wedges can also be used to protect the dam and tissue. An alternate method is to punch a large hole and slip it over the most posterior tooth to the tooth receiving the stainless steel crown. Then stretch the dam forward to the canine area.

Tooth preparation

1. Slice the mesial and distal surfaces with a No. 169L bur. Avoid bur damage or marks on adjacent teeth. The contacts must be completely opened (Fig 16-3). The contacts of the primary tooth are broad and flat as opposed to a point contact in the permanent dentition. Hold the bur slightly at an angle to the long axis of the tooth. Extend the slice to the buccal and lingual line angles. Depth is just through the contact and beyond any interproximal caries.
2. Complete occlusal reduction with the No. 330 or tapered diamond bur. Reduce the occlusion by about 1.0 to 1.5 mm (Fig 16-4). Since the criterion for using a stainless steel crown is a gross loss of tooth structure, this step involves removing 1.0 to 1.5 mm from one or two cusp tips. The 1.0- to 1.5-

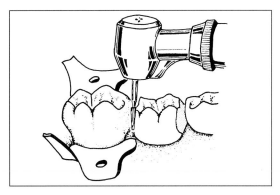

Fig 16-3   Slice the mesial and distal surfaces minimally, just breaking the contact.

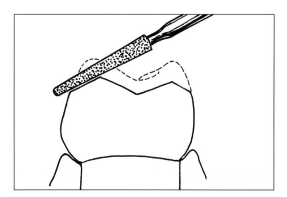

Fig 16-4   Complete occlusal reduction with a No. 330 or a tapered diamond bur.

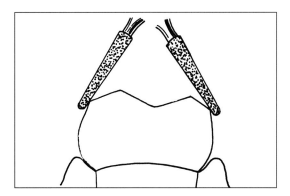

Fig 16-5   Round the sharp line angles and sharp corners.

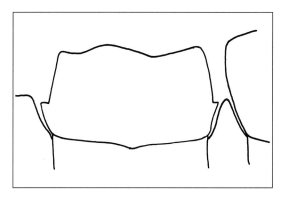

Fig 16-6   Ledges caused by overextension of the slice.

mm reduction is determined by comparing the marginal ridges of adjacent teeth.

3. Reduce and round all line angles and sharp corners of the preparation (Fig 16-5). Do not reduce the buccal and lingual aspects excessively except where there is a large buccal bulge, for example, in the primary first molar. When reduction is needed, start by taking the bur mesiodistally across the surface of the tooth, ending gingivally in a feather edge. Buccal and lingual reduction must be done to allow for the proper size crown, but too little reduction will result in the use of too large a crown.

The stainless steel crown margin must go beyond the knife-edge finish margin of the proximal surface preparation. No ledges should be apparent on the mesial and distal or the buccal and lingual sides because this would prevent crown placement (Fig 16-6).

The following is adapted from Myers (1976), summarizing the stainless steel crown preparation:

1. The dotted lines of Fig 16-7, *A* point out the correct angulation of the intended slices. The slice on Fig 16-7, *B* is correct, but the taper is extreme. Crown adaptation would be difficult. Fig 16-8 illustrates the optimum interproximal slices for the maxillary and mandibular primary molars.

2. Fig 16-9 shows the most common errors. Fig 16-9, *A* shows an excessive taper, which would reduce retention. In Fig 16-9, *B*, a shoulder has been created. It would increase the difficulty of seating the crown and adaptation.

3. Minimal but adequate reduction is needed on the buccal and lingual surfaces. The mesial and distal slices are just beneath the contacts, leaving adequate areas for retention. After the line angles are rounded, the outline of the tooth should be apparent. The contour should conform to the internal contour of the stainless steel crown. Here the old axiom prevails, "You cannot fit a square peg [the crown preparation] into a round hole [the internal structure of the crown]."

It is important to remember that the tooth preparation influences the retentive properties of the crown. Mathewson et al (1974) demonstrated that the crown preparation is a significant part of the crown's retentive potential. Others have evaluated the same principle, supporting the premise (Savide et al, 1979).

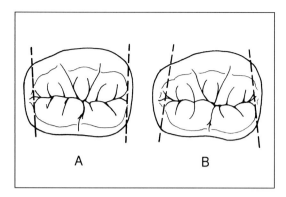

Fig 16-7 Angulation of slices: *(A)* proper slice; *(B)* improper slice.

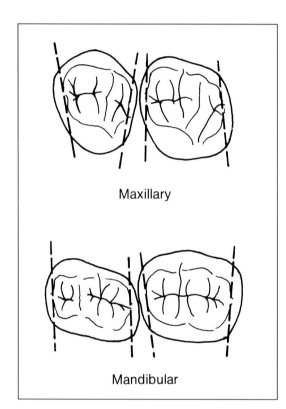

Maxillary

Mandibular

Fig 16-8 Optimum slices on the four primary molars.

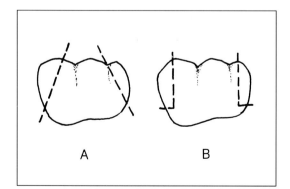

Fig 16-9 Common errors in crown slices: *(A)* excessive taper; *(B)* creation of a shoulder.

Crown selection

1. Three main considerations in selecting the proper stainless steel crown are adequate mesiodistal diameter, light resistance to seating, and proper occlusal height.
2. A crown should be somewhat larger than the tooth to which it is being adapted, especially when the gingival part of the crown is trimmed and crimped.
3. Too large a crown will rotate on the tooth preparation. Excessive time will be wasted attempting to adapt the crown.

Crown adaptation

It may be necessary to remove the rubber dam at this stage.

1. Using thumb forceps, select a crown from the supply (Fig 16-10). Use of the forceps will keep contamination to a minimum. Again, size Nos. 4 and 5 are the most frequently used. Crowns placed in a patient's mouth but not used must be sterilized again.
2. Try the crown on the tooth. Place the crown on the lingual side and rotate it toward the buccal side. The crown should fit loosely, with 2 to 3 mm excess gingivally. Crowns are prefestooned and contoured, so little trimming is needed. With a scaler, scratch around the gingival margin on the crown (Fig 16-11). This scratch line indicates the gingival line and the gingival contour, as well as the portion of the crown to be removed. In some instances, for example, where there have been gross carious lesions, preliminary cutting of the crown may be necessary to assist in seating the crown. If the crown is not trimmed, there will be excessive trauma to the gingival tissue.
3. Remove the crown from the prepared tooth, exposing the scratch line. With crown and bridge scissors, cut the crown 1 mm below the scratch line (Fig 16-12). The crown should now extend 1 mm beneath the gingiva.
4. Retry the crown on the tooth. If there is blanching of the gingiva, it may be necessary to rescribe the crown and retrim it. If the crown still does not completely seat, it may be necessary to return to step 2 of tooth preparation and reduce the occlusal surface another 0.5 to 1.0 mm.
5. The next step in adaptation is to contour the crown with pliers. Adaptation is very important to the gingival health of the supporting tissue. A poorly adapted crown will serve as a collection point for bacteria, contributing to recurrent caries or incipient periodontal disease.

Use the No. 114 pliers to recontour the gingival

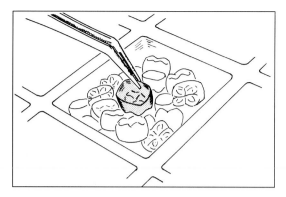

Fig 16-10   Select the crown with a thumb forcep.

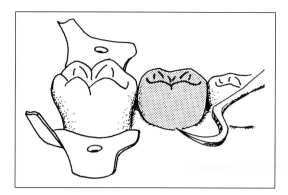

Fig 16-11   Mark the gingival margin with a scaler.

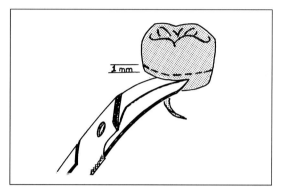

Fig 16-12   Trim the crown 1 mm beneath the scratch.

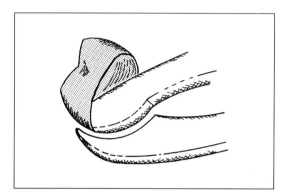

Fig 16-13   Contour the crown with a No. 114 pliers.

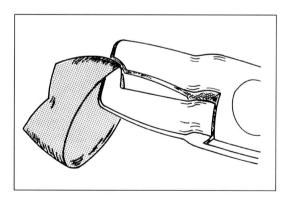

Fig 16-14   With the crown-crimping plier, crimp the margins.

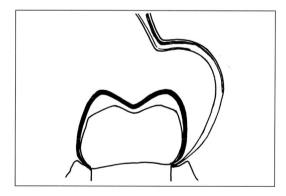

Fig 16-15   Check the margins for adaptation.

third of the crown (Fig 16-13). However, there are several other types of pliers that will suffice. It takes some practice to learn how to judge how much contouring is needed.

6. With the No. 800-417 crown-crimping pliers, crimp the margins only. This pliers is used to bend the margins gently, so as to fit into the undercut of the crown preparation (Fig 16-14). Retry the crown. Seat the crown in a lingual-to-buccal direction. It should snap into position under firm finger pressure.

7. With an explorer, check all the margins for adaptation (Fig 16-15). Where the margins are open, re-crimp with the No. 800-417 pliers. At this stage, it is easy to overcontour the crown so that it no longer snaps into place. Gently try to bend the margins out. If this results in a distorted crown, it is best to start over with a new crown.

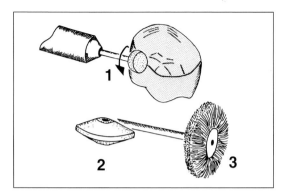

Fig 16-16 Armamentarium for finishing the crown: *(1)* large green stone; *(2)* rubber wheel; *(3)* wire brush.

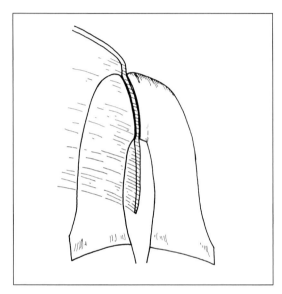

Fig 16-17 Use a No. 112 pliers to expand the contacts.

Crown finishing

1. Use a large green stone to make a knife-edge finish at the cervical margin. Operate the handpiece in such a manner that the burs and shavings are spun to the inside of the stainless steel crown. This technique should aid in retention (Fig 16-16).
2. Smooth and polish the margins with a rubber wheel.
3. Polish the entire crown with a wire brush. Rouge, whiting, or a fine polishing material can be used to give the crown a fine luster.
4. Remove the rubber dam if the crown is to be cemented with the dam off.
5. Try on the crown and check occlusion. Evaluate the opposite arch for proper cuspal and occlusal interdigitation.
6. Check the mesial and distal contacts. If they need expansion, use a No. 112 pliers (Fig 16-17). It may

be necessary to add silver solder to the contacts if the pliers do not work.

Crown cementation

You have several options when choosing a cementing media. Several factors can influence the decision, the most important of which is the status of the pulp. The following cements are currently available. However, a cavity varnish must be routinely applied before a stainless steel crown is cemented on a vital tooth (Myers et al, 1983).

Zinc phosphate cement

Zinc phosphate cement is formed by mixing zinc oxide with phosphoric acid.

Zinc phosphate cement is used mainly for luting or mechanically locking a restoration by filling in voids and defects. It is used primarily with stainless steel crowns. A second use is for cementing stainless steel bands for space maintainers. Zinc phosphate cements are easily handled and manipulated and have many years of clinical use.

If the manufacturer's instructions are followed, low film thickness and high compressive strengths can be obtained (Eames, 1977). To achieve maximum strength, low solubility, proper film thickness, and less free acid in the final mix of cement, use a high powder-liquid ratio (Savignac et al, 1965). Shepard et al (1978) found that a longer working time, a shorter setting time in the mouth, and increased retention of orthodontic bands could be achieved when refrigerated cement-mixing slabs were used to mix zinc phosphate cement.

In several studies (Mathewson, 1974, 1975), zinc phosphate cement was found to be the best choice among five different types of cements used for final cementation of stainless steel crowns.

One disadvantage of zinc phosphate is its low pH, which can cause pulpal irritation. When first mixed, zinc phosphate cement has a very low pH that can remain below 7.0 for as long as 48 hours (Norman, 1966). Wilson et al (1974) found the zinc phosphate cements to be soluble in distilled water and organic acids. Additional disadvantages include lack of antibacterial properties, solubility in oral fluids and lack of adhesion.

Zinc oxide–eugenol cements

Zinc oxide–eugenol cements consist of a mixture of zinc oxide and eugenol.

The zinc oxide–eugenol cements are used primarily for cavity base in deep lesions such as those that require indirect pulp capping.

Because it is extremely compatible with pulpal tissue, it may stimulate healing with secondary dentin formation. Unfortunately, it possesses low strength values and is very soluble in oral fluids (Phillips et al, 1968). It is used as the sub-base for pulpotomies, with or without formocresol added.

Reinforced zinc oxide–eugenol cements

The reinforced zinc oxide–eugenol cements contain additives to the liquid (eugenol) or powder (zinc oxide). These additives can be resins, accelerators, or minerals.

The improved zinc oxide–eugenol cements can be used for cementation of stainless steel crowns on vital teeth, as cavity liners in deep lesions (as in indirect pulp capping procedures), and for provisional restoration in prevention programs in children with rampant caries.

The reinforced zinc oxide–eugenol cements are somewhat less soluble in oral fluids than are zinc oxide cements. The reinforced zinc oxide–eugenol cements have greater strength than zinc oxide–eugenol but less strength than zinc phosphate cement (Phillips et al, 1968). These cements are used for final cementation of cast gold restorations.

The main advantages of these cements are their minimal pulpal irritation, easy manipulation, and optimal margin-sealing properties. They have adequate strength and can be used to cement stainless steel crowns in vital primary teeth. Unfortunately, these materials are soluble in oral fluids, cause gingival inflammation, and have minimal mechanical luting properties.

Polycarboxylate cements

Polycarboxylate cements consist of a mixture of zinc oxide powder and a polyacrylic acid liquid.

Polycarboxylate cements have a minimally irritating effect on the pulp, the same as zinc oxide–eugenol (Jendresen and Trowbridge, 1972). These cements have been used to directly bond stainless steel orthodontic brackets to enamel. The assumption was that there was a direct bonding among the stainless steel, carboxylate cement, and enamel (Mizrahi and Smith, 1968). Polycarboxylate cements have higher bond strength than either zinc phosphate or improved zinc oxide–eugenol cement (Arfali and Asgar, 1978). However, this strength is not related to increased physical properties such as tensile strength, compressive strength, or film thickness.

The main advantage of polycarboxylate cements is the low irritant factor to oral tissue. There is some adhesion to tooth substance and stainless steel alloys. Other physical properties are similar to those of zinc phosphate cement. The disadvantages are the requirements for precise proportioning and optimal manipulation, plus the need for a clean, uncontaminated tooth surface.

Glass-ionomer cements

See Chapter 15 for a description of glass-ionomer cements.

Clinical procedure

1. Apply lidocaine (Xylocaine) ointment or petroleum jelly to contact areas before cementation to assist in cement removal after cementation.
2. Use cotton rolls to isolate the quadrant containing the tooth to be restored. Every effort should be made to prevent postoperative sensitivity. If the tooth is vital, place a liner such as Dycal (L.D. Caulk Co) in the deep portions of the crown preparation, followed by Copalite (L.D. Caulk Co).
3. Zinc phosphate is still commonly used for cementation of stainless steel crowns. Cool the glass slab thoroughly under cold water and dry it with a clean towel. Place powder on one end of the slab. In the middle of the slab measure out 5 drops of liquid for each unit to be cemented. Use the spatula to divide the powder into small increments that are approximately 3 mm on a side. Move one increment across the slab and incorporate it into the liquid, mixing it for 20 seconds across a wide area. Allow this first portion to set for approximately 1 minute before continuing. This setting time will aid in neutralizing the acid. Continue to add small increments of powder, mixing each for 10 to 20 seconds, using a circular motion and covering a wide area of the slab. Check the consistency by picking up the cement on the spatula and holding it over the slab. If the cement is the right consistency, it will string out slightly between the spatula and slab before it runs back onto the slab. If it runs quickly off the spatula, it is too thin; if it must be nudged off the spatula, it is too thick.
4. Fill the crown with cement (Fig 16-18).
5. Seat the crown, usually first on the lingual side and then the buccal side. Make sure it is firmly seated. Support the child's mandible with one hand as you seat the crown with the other (Fig 16-19).
6. If the tooth is isolated with cotton rolls, place a strip of Burlew dryfoil over the crown (Fig 16-20) to help to keep the tooth free from moisture until the cement sets.
7. Remove excess cement with a scaler or explorer (Fig 16-21). Polish the crown with acidulated phosphate fluoride prophylaxis paste. Gently but firmly check all the areas of the gingival sulcus for retained cement. Excess cement can produce gingival inflammation and discomfort. Causes of stainless steel crown failures are:
   a. Poor tooth preparation.
   b. Poor crown adaptation and subsequent poor retention.
   c. Improper cementation methods with lost crowns or open margins.

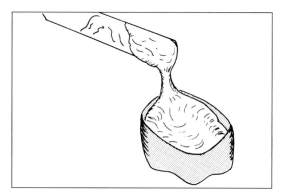

Fig 16-18   Fill the crown with cement.

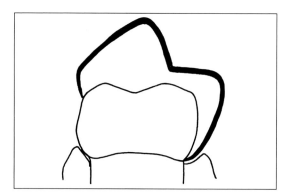

Fig 16-19   Seat the crown from the lingual side to the buccal side.

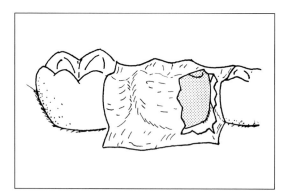

Fig 16-20   Keep the cemented crown dry.

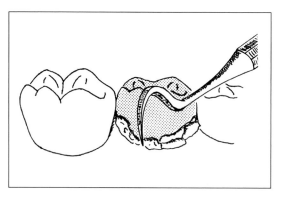

Fig 16-21   Remove excess cement with a scaler.

d. Failure of pulp treatment.
e. Induced ectopic eruption of the permanent first molar.
f. Recurrent caries, especially in the interproximal areas.
g. Crown abrasion through the occlusal surface.

Clinical modifications

The method just described is for the optimal clinical situation. Alterations and modifications need to be made for atypical situations.

Adjacent stainless steel crowns

1. When more than one stainless steel crown needs to be done in a quadrant, the two or more crowns should be:
    a. Prepared at the same time. Pulp treatment, crown reduction, and adaptation are more efficient. It also makes restoration of normal occlusion and morphology easier.

    b. Cemented at the same time. An increase in the amount of cement may be needed. The increased volume should be accompanied by a proportionate increase in mixing time.
    c. Checked for proper broad contacts. A Howe No. 110 pliers (Fig 16-22) is suitable for this procedure when the contacts need to be flattened.
2. When a stainless steel crown and a Class II amalgam restoration are to be done at one appointment, the question often is, "What is done first, cementation of the crown or completion of the Class II amalgam restoration?" The answer is to do the stainless steel crown preparation and any needed pulp treatment first, then adapt and cement the crown. However, the Class II cavity preparation is also done at the same time to allow for proper contour of the stainless steel crown's marginal ridge with the indicated amalgam restoration. After the crown is cemented, clean the excess cement from around the crown. Replace the rubber dam, and adapt and wedge a matrix band. Insert an amalgam restoration. The stainless steel crown is used as a guide in reproducing the anatomy and morphology of the silver amalgam restoration.

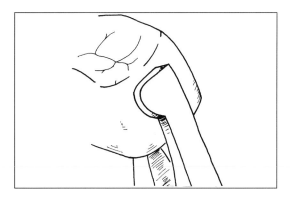

Fig 16-22 Use a Howe pliers to flatten the contacts.

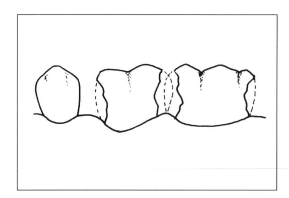

Fig 16-23 Loss of space to dental caries.

Adjacent stainless steel crowns with arch length loss (McEvoy, 1977)

1. Extensive and long-standing carious lesions can cause a shift of primary teeth into the interproximal contact areas (Fig 16-23). With this mesiodistal dimension loss, it is very difficult to restore the lost arch length. The mesial shift of the permanent first molar that may occur will influence the child's permanent occlusal relationship.
2. As previously mentioned, the manufactured stainless steel crowns come in six sizes. The tooth preparation must compensate for the need to use a smaller crown. Prepare the crown as described earlier—no proximal ledges, all line angles rounded, and prominent anatomy removed.
3. Select the crowns. Usually crowns will adjust to the tooth preparation individually but cannot be placed at the same time because of the mesial drift of the adjacent teeth.
4. The crown preparations must be reduced further. If a pulpotomy has been completed, pulpal exposure is not a problem. With a vital pulp, carefully remove tooth structure from the buccal and lingual surfaces. The crown preparation will then accommodate a smaller crown size.
5. By experimentation you can select the optimum combination of crowns. Often only one smaller crown is needed. A primary maxillary first molar from the opposite side will fit a primary mandibular first molar of the opposite side. Anatomically there is a similarity, the advantage being that the primary maxillary first molar crown is narrower mesiodistally.
6. Flatten the contacts of the crowns as described using a No. 110 pliers.
7. When the crowns are cemented, the marginal edges should be aligned. Before cement setting, use a Howe No. 110 pliers to obtain optimum alignment if necessary (Fig 16-24). With the crowns properly aligned, have the patient bite on a tongue blade until the cement is completely set.

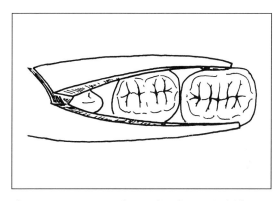

Fig 16-24 Use a Howe pliers to align the marginal ridges

Modification of the stainless steel crown size

The following is another method used to adjust crowns that are either too large or too short (Mink and Hill, 1971).

Oversized crown

1. If possible, try the crown on the tooth (Fig 16-25).
2. Use a pair of scissors to cut the crown from the gingival to the occlusal surface, either buccally or lingually, as needed (Fig 16-26).
3. Pinch the crown together, in effect reducing the crown size (Fig 16-27).
4. Again, try the crown on the tooth. The gingival margins of the crown should approximate the gingival margins of the tooth (Fig 16-28).
5. Mink and Hill recommend scratching a line along the overlapped edges. If the crown separates on removal, the cut edges can then be repositioned before soldering. If the cut edges are not repositioned, the resultant crown will again be too large or too small.
6. Spot weld the overlapped edged together. Use solder and flux to flow solder over the crown (Fig 16-29).

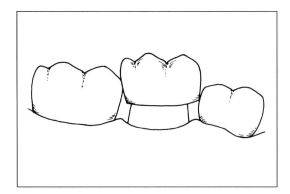

Fig 16-25   Try on an oversized crown

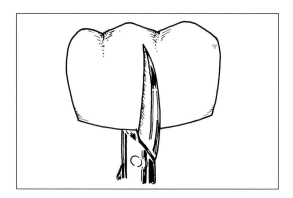

Fig 16-26   Cut the crown on the buccal or lingual surface.

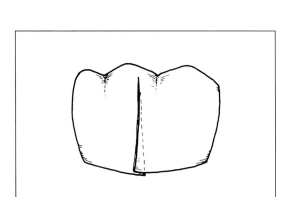

Fig 16-27   Pinch the crown together.

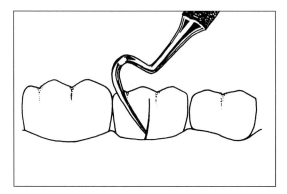

Fig 16-28   Retry the crown on the tooth.

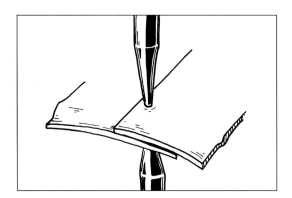

Fig 16-29   Spot weld the overlapped edges.

7. Electropolish (if available) the soldered crown. Use appropriate wheels and polishing materials to smooth the soldered part of the crown.
8. Check the crown for marginal adaptation. If no adjustments are needed, contour, crimp, and cement the crown as usual.

Undersized crown

1. Check the crown on the tooth (Fig 16-30).
2. Cut a V in the crown on the buccal or lingual side

(or both), as needed. Try the crown on the tooth (Fig 16-31).
3. Use a strip of orthodontic band material to spot weld over the V cut in the crown. Do this on one surface to allow for adjustment of the crown in the mouth (Fig 16-32).
4. Use a No. 114 pliers to adapt the band material to the crown contour. Cut off the excess, approximating the gingival contour of the crown.
5. Retry the crown on the tooth. Again, scratch the band material where it adapts to the crown (Fig 16-33).
6. Reposition the scratch and the band material. Spot weld, solder, and finish.
7. Adapt, contour, and crimp the crown.
8. Polish the soldered area and the gingival margins. Cement the crown.

Crown extension for deep proximal lesions

Often interproximal caries extend beyond the length of the manufactured crowns (Fig 16-34).

One approach is to complete whatever pulpal treatment is indicated and then restore the cavity preparation with silver amalgam. The silver amalgam is now considered as a substitute for the tooth structure. The

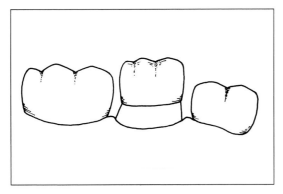

Fig 16-30 Try the crown on the tooth.

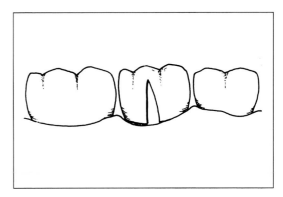

Fig 16-31 Cut a V in the crown.

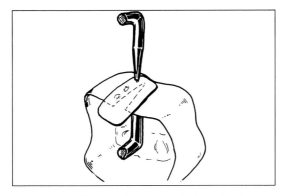

Fig 16-32 Weld a strip of material on the buccal surface.

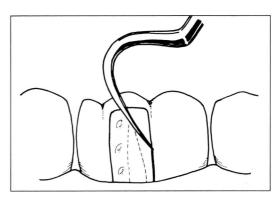

Fig 16-33 Scratch where the crown is tried on the tooth.

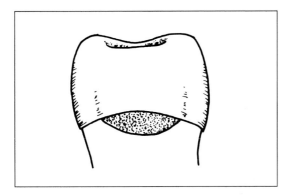

Fig 16-34 Dental caries that extend beyond the crown.

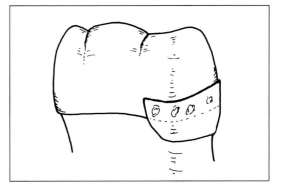

Fig 16-35 An extension soldered on the crown.

proximal areas are sliced as in a routine crown preparation. Adapt, contour, and crimp a stainless steel crown, with the amalgam substituting for tooth structure at the interproximal finishing line.

Another method is to solder an extension on the interproximal area of the crown (Fig 16-35):

1. In the area where the crown is deficient, spot weld a piece of orthodontic band material.
2. Use a pair of scissors to trim the excess material.
3. With a pair of No. 114 pliers, contour the crown as needed.
4. Polish with wheels, check the contour, and cement as described.

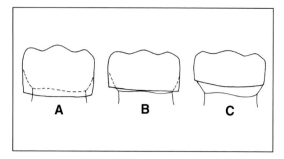

Fig 16-36 The results of three types of crowns: *(A)* overextended and poorly adapted, *(B)* correct length but poorly adapted, and *(C)* proper length and adaptation.

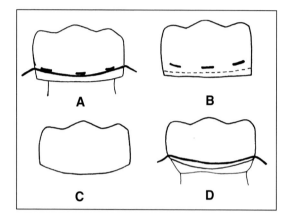

Fig 16-37 The four steps used to properly adapt a stainless steel crown: *(A)* Place the untrimmed crown on the prepared tooth; *(B)* use a No. $^1/_2$ round bur to mark the height of the gingival crest; *(C)* remove the crown and trim it in a straight line, about 1 mm below the middle mark; and *(D)* remove the remaining metal to obtain the desired shape and contour.

Methods for determining adequate crown fit

Spedding (1984) observed that most stainless steel crowns seemed acceptable when observed clinically. Unfortunately, radiographs of the same crowns revealed many to be overextended, with ragged margins. To amend these discrepancies, he proposed two principles based on the morphology of primary teeth and gingival contour.

Principle 1

When primary molars are viewed from either proximal surface, the buccal and lingual surfaces converge occlusally from the gingival crests. According to Spedding,

> Thus, any point on the tooth occlusal to the greatest diameter is on the visible clinical crown, and any point on the tooth apical to the greatest diameter is

on an undercut surface of the tooth and is not visible in the mouth.

The stainless steel crown that does not adhere to the morphologic features of the primary molar will be overextended and ill adapted (Fig 16-36, *A*, and *B*). Further, Spedding states,

> When the finished crown is correctly seated on the prepared tooth with its occlusal surface in the occlusal plane and its margin placed just apical to the marginal gingival crests, the crown is of correct length and its margins can be adapted closely to the tooth.

As seen on the buccal and proximal surfaces, when the crown is shortened and is the proper length, the crown is easily adapted to the crown (Fig 16-36, *C*).

Principle 2

According to Spedding (1984),

> If a dentist carefully examines the contours of the buccal and lingual marginal gingivae before a tooth is prepared for a stainless steel crown and produces steel crown margins of similar shapes, when these margins are adapted circumferentially against the tooth surfaces just apical to the greatest diameter of the tooth they will be located at the correct anatomic positions at all points on the tooth.

The use of principle 2 is seen in Fig 16-37. The untrimmed crown is placed on the prepared tooth (Fig 16-37, *A*). A No. $^1/_2$ round bur is used to mark the height of the gingival crest (Fig 16-37, *B*) (similar to using a scaler, as in Fig 16-11). The crown is removed and the metal is removed in a straight line, about 1 mm below the middle mark (Fig 16-37, *C*). Then the remaining metal is removed, and the desired shape and contour are obtained (Fig 16-37, *D*). The margins are contoured so that the crown is 1 mm below and approximates the gingival crest.

Considerations for successful use of stainless steel crowns

1. Removal of caries, and where needed, appropriate pulpal therapy
2. Optimum reduction of tooth structure for adequate crown retention
3. Lack of damage to adjacent teeth after opening interproximal contacts
4. Selection of appropriately sized crown to maintain arch length
5. Accurate marginal adaptation and gingival health
6. Good functional occlusion
7. Optimum cementation procedure

References

Arfali, A. H., and Asgar, K. Bond strength of three cements determined by centrifugal testing. J. Prosthet. Dent 40:294, 1978.

Braff, M. H. A comparison between stainless steel crowns and multisurface amalgams in primary molars. J. Dent Child. 42:474, 1975.

Dawson, L. R., Simon, J. E., Jr., and Taylor, P.P. Use of amalgam and stainless steel restorations for primary molars, J. Dent. Child. 48:42, 1981.

Eames, W. B., et al. Proportioning and mixing of cements: A comparison of working times. Oper. Dent 2:97, 1977.

Jendresen, M. D., and Trowbridge, H. O. Biologic and physical properties of a zinc polycarboxylate cement. J. Prosthet. Dent. 8:264, 1972.

Mathewson, R. J., Lu, K. H., and Duncanson, M. G. Effectiveness of phosphoric acid prior to stainless steel crown cementation. IADR abstract No. 332, April 12, 1975.

Mathewson, R. J., Lu, K. H., and Talebi, R. Dental cement retentive force comparison on stainless steel crown. J. Calif. Dent. Assoc. 2(8):42, 1974.

McEvoy, S. A. Approximating stainless steel crowns in space loss quadrants. J. Dent Child. 44:105, 1977.

Mink, J. R., and Hill, C. J. Modification of the stainless steel crown for primary teeth. J. Dent Child. 38:197, 1971.

Mizrahi, E., and Smith, D. C. Studies of the adhesion of orthodontic brackets to enamel using a polyacrylic cement J. Dent. Res. 47:999, 1968.

Myers, D. R. A clinical study of the response of the gingival tissue surrounding stainless steel crowns. J. Dent Child. 42:281, 1975.

Myers, D. R. The restoration of primary molars with stainless steel crowns. J. Dent. Child. 43:406, 1976.

Myers, M. L., et al. Marginal leakage of contemporary cementing agents. J. Prosthet. Dent. 50:513, 1983.

Norman, R. D. Direct pH determination of setting cements. II. The effects of prolonged storage time, powder: Liquid ratio, temperature and dentin. J. Dent. Res. 45:1214, 1966.

Phillips, R. W., et al Zinc oxide and eugenol cements for permanent cementation. J. Prosthet. Dent. 19:144, 1968.

Savide, N. L., Caputo, A. A., and Luke, L. S. The effect of tooth preparation on the retention of stainless steel crowns. J. Dent Child. 46:385, 1979.

Savignac, J. R., Fairhurst, C. W., and Ryge, G. Strength solubility and disintegration of zinc phosphate cement with clinically determined powder-liquid ratio. Angle Orthod. 35:126, 1965.

Shepard, W. B., et al. The effect of mixing method, slab temperature, and humidity on the properties of zinc phosphate and zinc siliconophosphate cement. Angle Orthod. 48:219, 1978.

Spedding, R. H. Two principles for improving the adaptation of stainless steel crowns to primary molars. Dent. Clin. North Am. 28:157, 1984.

Wilson, A. D., Abel, G., and Lewis, B. G. The solubility and disintegration test for zinc phosphate dental cements. Br. Dent. J. 137:313, 1974.

Additional readings

Adair, S. T., and Byrd, R. L. Evaluation of practitioner-developed criteria for assessing the quality of stainless steel crown. J. Pedod. 7:291, 1983.

Durr, D. P., Ashrafi, M. H., and Duncan, W. R. A study of plaque accumulation and gingival health surrounding stainless steel crowns. J. Dent Child. 49:343, 1982.

Kopel, H. M., and Batterman, S. C. The retentive ability of various cementing agents for polycarbonate crowns. J. Dent Child. 43:333, 1976.

Meyers, G. E., et al. Do's and dont's for three dental luting cements. Council on Dental Materials and Devices. J. Am. Dent. Assoc. 97:502, 1978.

More, F. G., and Pink, T. C. The stainless steel crown: A clinical guide. J. Mich. Dent. Assoc. 55:237, 1973.

Myers, D. R. Barenie, J. T., and Bell, R. A. Influence of preparation and cement on stainless steel crown retention. J. Dent Res. 252:373, 1981.

Mount, G. J., and Makinson, O. F. Glass-ionomer restorative cements: Clinical implications of the setting reaction. Oper. Dent. 7:134, 1982.

Noffsinger, D. P., Jedrychowski, J. R., and Caputo, A. A. Effects of polycarboxylate and glass ionomer cements on stainless steel crown. Pediatr. Dent. 5:68, 1983.

Phillips, R. W., Swartz, M. L., and Rhodes, B. An evaluation of a carboxylate adhesive cement J. Am. Dent. Assoc. 81:1353, 1970.

Questions

1. You have a crown for the maxillary second primary molar fairly well adapted and are ready for final cementation. However, you notice blanching of the gingival tissue on the lingual side of the molar. This blanching means you need to:

   a. Change the crown size because it is too large
   b. Recrimp the crown because it is not adapted to the tooth preparation
   c. Re-mark the crown and retrim the crown because it is still overextended
   d. Recontour the crown preparation itself because it is too conservative
   e. Do nothing, because it will go away

2. The crown preparation, in your judgment, seems to be completed. However, the stainless steel crown you have selected rotates freely on the crown preparation. Your next action should be:

   a. To yell "Help"
   b. To adapt the crown and use a thick mix of cement
   c. To trim the crown to make it smaller
   d. To select and try the next smaller stainless steel crown

3. A child 4 years of age comes to your office. The primary mandibular first molar clinically has no caries. Radiographs reveal mesial and distal carious lesions with no pulpal involvement. Outlining the treatment plan, you should:

   a. Plan on a mesio-occlusal and a disto-occlusal silver amalgam restoration
   b. Plan on a stainless steel crown
   c. Plan on a mesio-occlusodistal amalgam restoration
   d. Plan on a mesio-occlusal and disto-occlusolingual amalgam restoration

4. The crown is almost ready for cementation. However, your explorer detects a small open margin on the buccal of the primary maxillary first molar. Your next move should be:

   a. To swear (*!!.?*)
   b. To crimp the gingival margin with a No. 114 pliers
   c. To crimp the gingival margin with a No. 112 pliers
   d. To select a new crown and start over
   e. To crimp the gingival margin with a No. 800-417 pliers

5. A stainless steel crown has been adapted for the primary mandibular left second molar. The crown is well polished, extends 1 to 2 mm beneath the gingiva, and is well adapted. After the crown has been cemented, the margin on the buccal side is supragingival and has a visible open margin. The probably causes are:

   a. A poor mix of cement with improper film thickness
   b. A failure to use enough force to seat the crown
   c. Too much force; the crown has "sprung"
   d. Improper path of insertion; the crown was seated too far lingually
   e. a,b
   f. c,d
   g. b,d
   h. a,d
   i. a,c,d

Chapter 17

Restorative Procedures for Primary Incisors

Objectives

After studying this chapter, the student should be able to:
1. Restore an anterior primary tooth with a composite resin restorative material.
2. Choose one of several primary anterior crown restorative methods available.

Sequela to carious lesions

Carious lesions on the proximal and labial surfaces of primary teeth are not uncommon. Large carious areas may be found in the teeth of a few children. The cause may be poor oral hygiene or dietary habits. Fass (1967) described the syndrome called *nursing bottle mouth*, or *baby bottle syndrome*. The condition is attributed to prolonged ingestion of carbohydrates past age 1, the usual age of weaning, accompanied with decreased salivary flow during sleep. The conditions are characterized by rampant carious lesions in the primary maxillary incisors and first molars.

Restorative options

For small or incipient lesions, the typical Class III preparation is used (Fig 17-1). Composite resins are best inserted with a Centrix syringe (Centrix, Inc.) and adapted with a Teflon-coated plastic instrument (Temple, Premier Dental Products). Before the improvement in the physical characteristics of composite resins, silver amalgam was the restoration of choice. Its major drawback was its unesthetic appearance. For large carious areas, fractures, or teeth with pulpal involvement, composite resins are unsatisfactory because they lack strength. In days past, extensive carious lesions were restored with a stainless steel crown or orthodontic band. Although these restorations were adequate physically, their cosmetic potential was not likely to satisfy either child or parent. The development of preformed acrylic resin crowns (polycarbonate crowns) made it possible to restore grossly carious teeth with cosmetically pleasing results. Unfortunately,

polycarbonate crowns are very brittle and a high percentage of the crowns split, resulting in failure.

Another alternative is the use of a strip crown form as a matrix for acid-etched composite resin in a complete-coverage restoration. This type of crown gives an esthetic choice while supplying a crown that can be retained better than a polycarbonate one.

A third alternative is an open-faced stainless steel crown. This crown is the best compromise between crown esthetics and retention. It is usually used in patients with gross carious lesions. Irrespective of the type of crown used, if multiple crowns are used, they should be adapted and cemented at the same time to maintain normal spacing, appearance, and occlusion.

An improvement over the open-faced stainless steel crown is the anterior stainless steel crown with a bonded acrylic or composite resin facing. Depending on the supplier, the esthetic material is bonded or vacuum cured to the anterior surface of the stainless steel crown. Because this type of crown involves greater laboratory expense, the crowns are more expensive. The suppliers of these crowns (Cheng Crowns, Kinder Krowns, Nu-Smile, and White Bite) each claims superiority of their individual crown; minimal facing breakage; stability of the facing color; excellent tissue compatibility; and ease of adaptation.

Unfortunately, some primary teeth have carious pulpal exposures with resultant pulpal degeneration and periapical involvement. Such teeth may have to be extracted. If they are not, hypoplastic defects may develop on the permanent successors. These defects very from large opacities to irregular pits on the enamel surface. When surgical removal is indicated, a simple prosthetic appliance may be indicated to improve appearance.

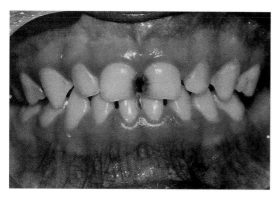

Fig 17-1 An example of caries in anterior primary teeth where Class III preparations are indicated.

For all of the restorative procedures for anterior primary teeth the initial steps are:

1. Administration of local anesthesia.
2. Selection of crown if a crown is used.
3. Use of rubber dam, if possible.
4. Removal of carious lesions.
5. Appraisal of pulpal involvement.
6. Placement of pulp-protecting materials or use of a pulp procedure, if indicated.

Composite resin is the restorative material of choice for primary anterior teeth. Esthetics is as important to children as it is to adults. Before insertion of the composite resin material, the enamel margins should be etched (Bozalis and Marshall, 1977). Studies indicate that there is an increase in retention of composite resins after primary teeth are etched (Smutka et al, 1978). The outer surface of primary teeth is different morphologically than the enamel of permanent teeth. The outer layer of primary enamel is essentially prismless. Unfortunately, the prismless layer does not respond well to acid etching. Coniff and Hamby (1976) found retentive strength increases significantly if a diamond stone is used to remove at least the prismless layer of enamel and then an acid-etch media is used. Mueller and Tinanoff (1977) found that a small, round bur is the optimum instrument to mechanically remove prismless enamel. It improves tag formation when the primary enamel is acid etched.

Evaluating primary enamel pretreatments and their effect on composite resin retention, Smutka et al (1978) examined three variables. The results showed *(1)* that pretreatment of primary enamel with 50% phosphoric acid increases the force needed to dislodge a composite resin, *(2)* that mechanical efforts to remove the prismless layer do not affect the force needed to remove the resins, and *(3)* that the use of a bonding or coupling agent before resin placement increases the force needed to remove resin.

Armamentarium

Burs
    No. 169L or No. 69L
    No. 130
    No. 4 round
    No. 35 I.V.C.
    Small diamond wheel (optional), tapered diamond
Materials
    Calcium hydroxide
    Strip crown forms: Pedo-form (Unitek Corp), four sizes for primary central and lateral incisors
    Anterior stainless steel crowns (3M and Unitek Corp)
    Composite resin restorative material
    Heavy rubber dam
Instruments
    Spoon excavator
    Scaler
    Crown and bridge scissors
    Crown pliers, Nos. 114 and 800-417 (Unitek Corp)
    Zinc phosphate cement, slab, and spatula
    Plastic instrument (Temple, Premier Dental Products)
    Matrix material, wedge
    Centrix syringe
    Finishing and polishing materials
        Heatless stone
        Rubber wheels
        Wire brush
        Prophylaxis paste, nonfluoridated

Class III cavity preparation for primary incisors

1. Where the carious process is minimal or does not extend to the incisal angle, a Class III composite resin preparation is indicated. The easiest access is from the labial side. Use an inverted cone bur (Fig 17-2).
2. Place a calcium hydroxide liner (Dycal, L.D. Caulk Co) in the deep wall of the cavity preparation. Check the manufacturer's instructions to see if cavity varnish can be used. Clean the cavity liner and Dycal from all the enamel margins (Fig 17-3). Glass ionomer liner can be used as an alternative.
3. Apply 37% phosphoric acid for 2 minutes to enamel margins.
4. After gentle rinsing and drying of the margins, a frosted look should appear.
5. The composite resin should be at room temperature. As with all dental products, it is to the user's advantage to read the manufacturer's instructions before use. Prepare the Centrix syringe by removing the Teflon plunger and disposable plastic tip. Load the resin into the Centrix syringe.
6. Hold the mylar matrix in place with a wooden wedge and inject the composite resin into the cavi-

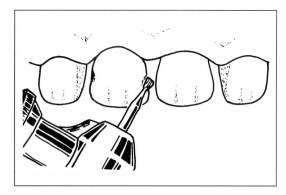

Fig 17-2   Begin cavity preparation from the labial surface.

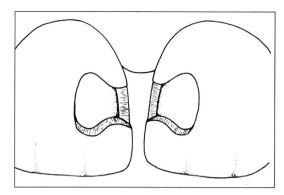

Fig 17-3   Completed Class III preparations.

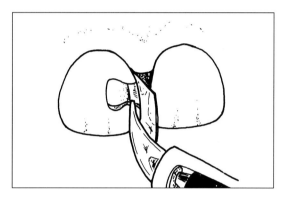

Fig 17-4   Inject the composite resin material into the cavity preparation.

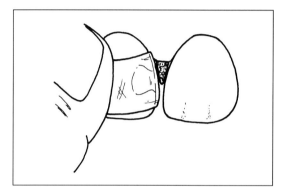

Fig 17-5   Hold the mylar strip until the composite resin sets.

ty preparation. Insert the syringe tip into the cavity portion and inject the material into the cavity (Fig 17-4). If a syringe is not used, use a plastic instrument (Temple) to insert the composite resin material. Insert the bulk of the material into the cavity preparation. Avoid trapping air in the mass. The plastic instrument can be used to shape and contour the restoration.

7. Hold the mylar matrix on the lingual surface with one hand, pull the strip tightly, and fold it over on the labial surface. Hold the strip until the composite resin sets (Fig 17-5). If autocured resins are used, hold the strip until the material polymerizes. When light-curing systems are used, polymerize 20 seconds on the labial surface and 20 seconds on the lingual surface.

8. After carefully removing the matrix, check for voids and overextensions. A sharp instrument can be used to remove any flash. Again, follow the manufacturer's recommendations for finishing. Recommendations may include:
   a. Silicone disks.
   b. Fine tapered diamonds.
   c. White stones.
   d. Carbide finishing bur.

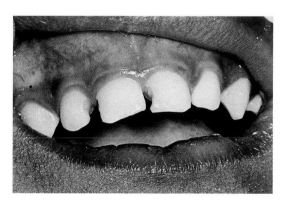

Fig 17-6   A carious lesion involving the incisal angle of a primary anterior tooth.

Finishing should be kept to a minimum because the matrix-completed surface cannot be improved.

If the carious lesion is large, involving the incisal edge, a modified preparation is used (Fig 17-6). The undermined incisal edge is removed and a labial dovetail is cut (Fig 17-7). The tooth is restored as described for incipient lesions.

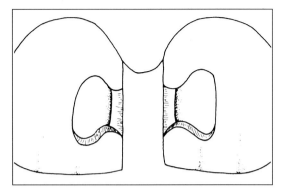

Fig 17-7   Removal of the undermined incisal edge.

Class III cavity preparation for primary canines

Maxillary primary canines:
Lingual outline form (Fig 17-8,a)

1. Use a No. 330 bur to place the mesial wall along a line of the tooth parallel to its long axis.
2. Contour the pulpal wall so that it corresponds to the external lingual surface of the tooth.
3. Leave adequate tooth structure incisal to the dovetail.
4. Maintain the gingival wall parallel to, and 1 to 2 mm above the dentinoenamel junction.

Proximal outline form

1. Maintain the labial wall parallel to the external labial surface, governing the extension by the adjacent tooth, with adequate clearance for carving with an explorer.
2. Extend the preparation incisally to remove the contact point, being careful to leave adequate tooth structure.
3. Place the gingival wall below the gingival crest, following the contour of the dentinoenamel junction.

4. Slightly round all internal line angles; make sharp cavosurface angles and smooth them with a No. 169L bur.

Mandibular primary canines (17-8,b)

The procedure is the same as for the maxillary primary canine except that the dovetail is on the labial surface.

Matrix and wedge for
Class III cavity preparation (Fig 17-9)

1. Cut a piece of matrix material 2.5 cm (1 in.) long.
2. Adapt it to the contour of the tooth.
3. Wedge it tightly at the cervical floor.

Modified Class III cavity preparation

The modified Class III preparation (Fig 17-10) is indicated in the presence of an incipient lesion with no proximal contact and excellent access:

1. Use a No. 330 bur to form a triangular preparation with gently rounded curves.

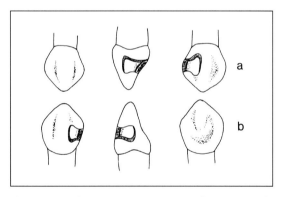

Fig 17-8   *(a)* Class III preparations in maxillary canines; *(b)* Class III preparations in mandibular canines.

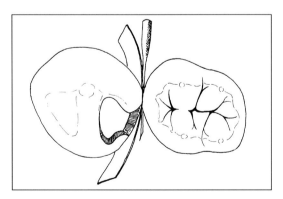

Fig 17-9   Matrix and wedge for a Class III preparation.

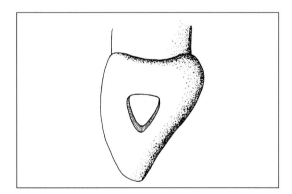

Fig 17-10   Modified Class III preparation on primary canines.

2. Penetrate about 0.5 to 1.0 mm beyond the dentino-enamel junction.
3. Retention is optional with the half-round bur at pulpal and incisal line angles.
4. Restore with a composite restorative material.

Complete-coverage composite resin restoration with strip crown forms

Crown form selection and preparation (Fig 17-11)

1. Select the appropriate crown form size from the mesiodistal measurement (in millimeters) of the tooth's incisal edge or by visually comparing the length of its incisal edge to that of an inverted crown form placed adjacent to the incisal edge of the tooth.
2. Trim off the excess form material (cervical collar and tab) with curved festooning scissors (Fig 17-12).
3. Punch holes in the incisal edge of the crown. These holes will allow a vent for the composite resin to flow through during crown placement (Fig 17-13).

Tooth preparation

1. Reduce the interproximal surfaces with a tapered diamond bur, producing a knife-edge cervical margin identical to that of a stainless steel crown preparation (Fig 17-14).
2. Remove the incisal edge approximately 1 mm (Fig 17-15).
3. Round over all the line angles slightly. Only minimal labial and lingual enamel should be removed. Minimal removal will negate the need to clean the enamel surface with a nonfluoridated prophylaxis paste while it simultaneously roughens the enamel surface and removes any areas of prismless enamel formation (thus increasing the retentive ability of the acid etching).
4. Place a small cervical undercut at the gingival margin of the labial surface with an inverted cone. This undercut area will serve as a mechanical lock to aid in retention (Fig 17-16).
5. Further reduction is accomplished only to allow placement of the selected crown form over the tooth if the previous reduction was inadequate. Minimal enamel reduction is desired because retention of the restoration is based on the quality as well as the quantity of enamel surface area exposed to the acid-etching procedure.
6. Remove existing carious lesions with a spoon excavator or round bur. Excavation of carious lesions will leave additional undercuts that will aid in the retention of the restoration. Medicate the pulp as necessary (place a calcium hydroxide liner over all areas of exposed dentin).

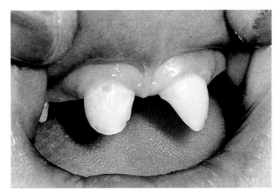

Fig 17-11 Anterior primary teeth suitable for use of strip crown forms.

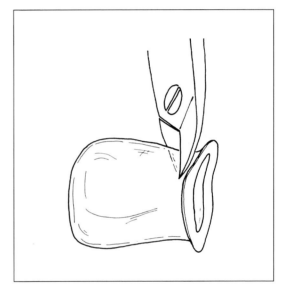

Fig 17-12 Trim excess material from the strip crown.

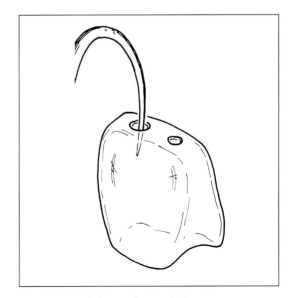

Fig 17-13 Cut holes into the incisal edge.

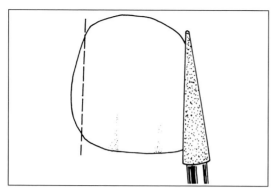

Fig 17-14 Reduce the mesial and distal surfaces with a diamond stone.

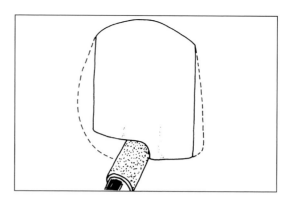

Fig 17-15 Reduce the incisal edge approximately 1 mm.

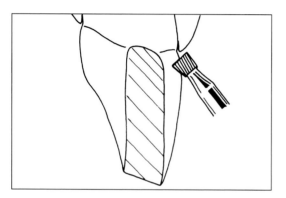

Fig 17-16 Place a cervical undercut at the gingival margin on the labial surface.

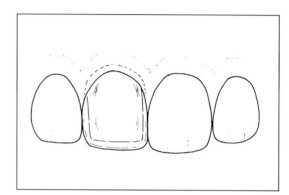

Fig 17-17 Try in the strip crown for fit.

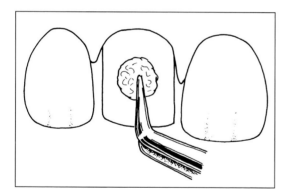

Fig 17-18 Etch the exposed enamel surfaces with phosphoric acid.

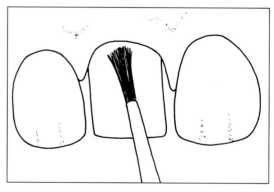

Fig 17-19 Apply the bonding agent.

Crown placement

1. Trial fitting of the crown form should be accomplished to ensure that its gingival margin extends approximately 1 mm into the gingival sulcus (Fig 17-17).

2. Coat all exposed enamel surfaces with a phosphoric acid tooth conditioner. After application, thoroughly wash the area with water and then air dry. A well-etched enamel surface will appear dull and chalky white. It is essential that the surface remain dry and free of moisture contamination from this step on (Fig 17-18).

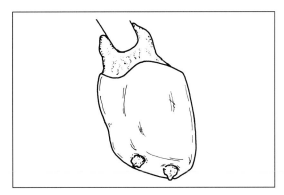

Fig 17-20 Add the composite resin material to the crown form.

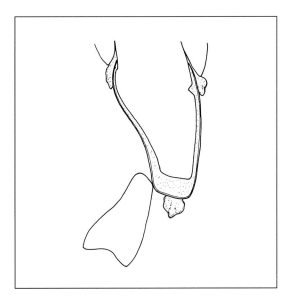

Fig 17-21 Position the crown form on the tooth.

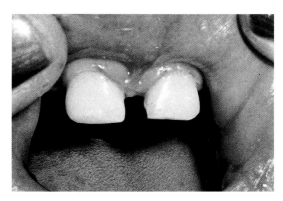

Fig 17-22 Completed strip crowns.

3. Paint the entire etched enamel surface with bonding agent (Fig 17-19).
4. Carefully pack the crown form with resin to avoid entrapment of air bubbles. Excess material should flow through the vent made in the incisal surface (Fig 17-20).
5. Position the filled crown form over the prepared tooth so that it extends 1 mm below the gingival margin and is in proper occlusion with the opposing dentition. Remove the excess composite resin from the gingival margin and incisal vent area with an explorer or scaler before it completely polymerizes (Fig 17-21).
6. After polymerization is completed, remove the crown form by slicing it on the lingual surface with a sharp scaler. Peel it away from the composite resin crown. Small adjustments with a finishing bur may be required to adjust the occlusion.
7. *Do not* finish the labial surface because the polymerization of the resin against the plastic form provides the smoothest and most stain-resistant surface finish possible (Fig 17-22).

Open-faced stainless steel crown

In children with rampant carious lesions, open-faced stainless steel crowns are used (Hartmann, 1983; Helpin, 1983). Although some esthetics is sacrificed, increased functional stability is added to these restorations (Fig 17-23).

Procedure

1. Use a thumb forceps or similar instrument to select the crown size needed (Fig 17-24). The size needed is determined by the width of the incisal edge.
2. The preparation is begun by slicing the mesial surface, slicing the distal surface, and removing about 1.0 to 1.5 mm from the incisal edge (Fig 17-25). Little reduction is needed on the lingual surface.
3. Very carefully seat the crown to see if the size is correct (Fig 17-26). If blanching occurs, the crown is overextended.
4. Scribe a line around the gingival margin. The crown should extend about 0.5 to 1.0 mm beneath the gingival crest (Fig 17-27). Use a pair of scissors to cut a V on the mesial and distal surfaces. This V should correspond to the interproximal gingival margin (Fig 17-28). At the same time, cut a hole in the labial side of the crown with a No. 58 bur to make cutting out the facing easier.
5. Use the No. 114 pliers to adapt the lingual portion of the stock crown to the lingual portion of the tooth (Fig 17-29).
6. Polish the gingival margins with a heatless stone as described for posterior stainless steel crowns (Fig 17-30). The crown in Fig 17-30 has the window cut before cementation—another alternative.

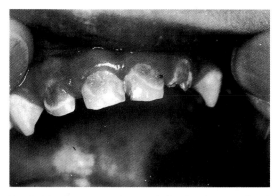

Fig 17-23 Rampant caries: an indication for open-faced stainless steel crowns.

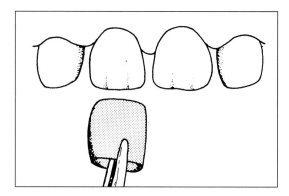

Fig 17-24 Determine the crown size.

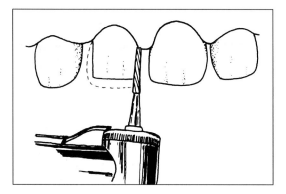

Fig 17-25 Slice the mesial, distal, and incisal surfaces.

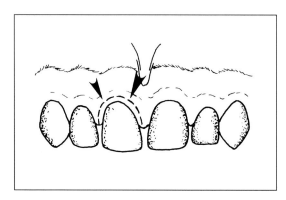

Fig 17-26 Check for appropriate crown size.

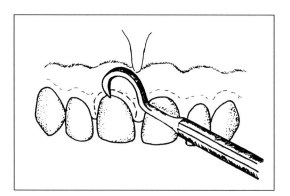

Fig 17-27 Scribe a line around the gingival margin.

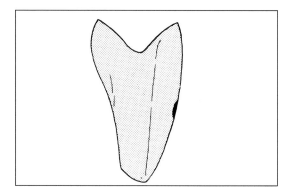

Fig 17-28 Trim the crown and cut a hold in the labial surface.

7. Try the crown on again for marginal adaptation. Apply Dycal in the deep areas if needed. Cement the crown with zinc phosphate or glass ionomer cement.
8. After the cement has set, use a No. 58 bur to cut out a window. With a small rubber wheel, smooth the rough edges. Use a No. 35 inverted cone. bur to cut an undercut around the crown window. This undercut is for retention of the composite resin (Fig 17-31).

9. A composite resin is used to restore the facing of the primary incisor. Again, this material can be injected with a syringe, or a plastic instrument can be used.
10. After the composite resin has been polymerized with a visible light source, finish with appropriate disks and diamond stones. A surface glaze can be used to complete the restoration (Fig 17-32).

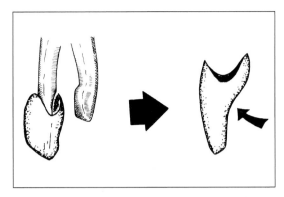

Fig 17-29 Adapt the lingual surface with a No. 114 pliers.

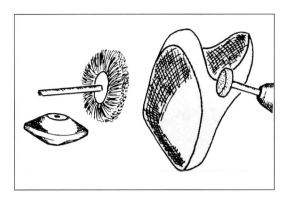

Fig 17-30 Polish the crown prior to cementation.

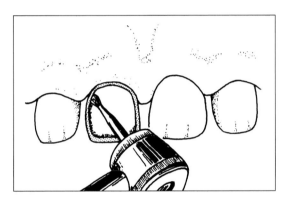

Fig 17-31 Cut a window in the crown.

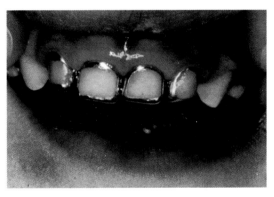

Fig 17-32 Completed open-faced crowns.

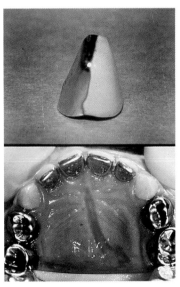

Fig 17-33 *(top)* Anterior stainless steel crown with a laboratory-cured composite resin facing. *(bottom)* Finished crowns as seen from the lingual aspect.

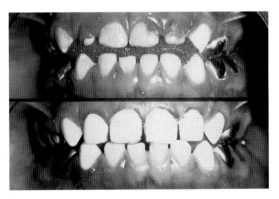

Fig 17-34 *(top)* Child with severe dental caries. *(bottom)* The four primary maxillary incisors have been restored with stainless steel crowns and laboratory-fabricated facings.

Stainless steel crowns with laboratory-added facings

Fig 17-34 illustrates a typical candidate for this type of restorative procedure.

1. Similar to the open-faced stainless steel crown method, determine the appropriate crown size (see Fig 17-24).
2. Prepare the teeth as described in Fig 17-25.
3. Use gentle finger pressure to place the crowns over the tooth preparations.
4. Depending on the dental supplier, the crown may or may not be crimped. Review the instructions that are supplied with the crown kit.
5. Check the occlusion. If more than one crown is to be cemented, cement them at the same time. The cement of choice is a glass-ionomer cement; its advantages are ease of use, strength, and fluoride release.
6. After the cement has set, round the distal corners of the crowns. The crowns are not supplied as either "right" or "left." To improve appearance, use a sandpaper disk or a fine diamond wheel (slow speed) to round these corners. Figs 17-33 and 17-34 illustrate the use of this type of crown.

References

Bozalis, W. G., and Marshall, G. W. Acid etching patterns of primary enamel. J. Dent. Res. 56:85, 1977.

Conniff, J. N., and Hamby, S. R. Preparation of primary tooth enamel for acid conditioning. J. Dent Child. 43:41, 1976.

Fass, E. N. Is bottle feeding of milk a factor in dental caries? J. Dent. Child. 29:245, 1967.

Hartmann, C. R. The open-faced stainless steel crown: An esthetic technique. J. Dent. Child. 50:31, 1983.

Helpin, M. L. The open-faced stainless steel crown restoration in children. J. Dent. Child. 50:34, 1983.

Mueller, B., and Tinanoff, N. Enhancing retention of acid-etch resin restorations in primary teeth. J. Pedod. 1:263, 1977.

Smutka, S., Jedrychowski, J., and Caputo, A. An evaluation of primary enamel pretreatments and their effects on resin retention J. Dent. Res. 57:796, 1978.

Questions

1. The use of 37% phosphoric acid as an acid-etching material has been found to:
   a. Increase the retention of composite resin materials in permanent teeth
   b. Decrease marginal leakage in permanent teeth
   c. Be of questionable value in primary teeth
   d. Be influenced by surface preparation before its use
   e. a,d,
   f. b,c,
   g. b,d
   h. All of the above

2. A 3-year-old visits the office has a primary central incisor with mesial, distal, and buccal caries. You decide to use open-faced stainless steel crowns.
   a. The crown is selected and adapted after all carious lesions have been removed
   b. The crown is selected as a preliminary step before tooth preparation or carious lesion removal
   c. It does not matter when the crown size is selected
   d. The crown is selected and adapted after the preparation has been done

3. A 3-year-old has incipient carious lesions involving the primary central incisors. These lesions do not include the incisal angle. What type of restoration is indicated?
   a. Open-faced stainless steel crown
   b. Class III amalgam restoration
   c. Polycarbonate crown
   d. Class III composite resin restoration with labial access
   e. Class III composite resin restoration with lingual access

4. An open-faced stainless steel crown is placed on the maxillary central incisor of a child 2.5 years old. His parents should be told:
   a. The life expectancy of the crown is unknown
   b. This treatment can be considered "permanent" for the primary dentition
   c. The crown will most likely need be replaced before the tooth exfoliates

Chapter 18

Pulp Treatment

Objectives

After studying this chapter, the student should be able to:
1. Use the different clinical and radiographic criteria to diagnose the etiology and to determine the indicated pulp treatment.
2. Use the several clinical procedures available for pulp care.
3. Explain the rationale for the particular pulp treatment.

The goals of pulp therapy in the primary and mixed dentitions are:

1. Successful treatment of the cariously involved pulp, allowing the tooth to remain in the mouth in a non-pathologic state.
2. Maintenance of arch length and tooth space.
3. Restoration of comfort with the ability to chew.
4. Prevention of speech abnormalities and abnormal habits.

Factors influencing success of pulp therapy are:

1. Type and amount of pulpal hemorrhage.
2. Depth of penetration of bacteria from the carious process into the pulpal tissue.
3. Speed of carious attack on the pulp.

Diagnosis

Several diagnostic considerations should be evaluated before the clinical and radiographic findings are reviewed:

1. The length of time the tooth or teeth in question are to be retained
2. The health of the patient
3. The status of the remaining dentition
4. The restorability of the tooth or teeth in question
5. Patient and parent cooperation in accepting the prevention program, including periodic evaluation

Radiographic assessment

With children, the most important aids are radiographs of the teeth in question. Current radiographs should be evaluated before treatment planning. In reviewing the radiograph, conscientiously check the following:

1. The depth of carious process related to pulpal tissue. It is important to remember that the clinical progress of dental caries is somewhat more extensive than is visible on the radiograph. A tooth demonstrating carious lesions near the pulp requires some type of pulp treatment. The photomicrograph shows acute inflammation extending into the coronal portion of the pulp (Fig 18-1).
2. The presence of calcified bodies in the pulpal tissue indicates chronic inflammation. These calcified bodies are the pulp's attempt to respond to chronic inflammation. Radiographically they appear as radiopaque bodies in the pulp chamber. The calcific bodies are seen in the pulp chamber of this photomicrograph (Fig 18-2).
3. Involvement of the bifurcation and trifurcation regions of the primary molars. It has been demonstrated that the pulpal floors of primary teeth are porous; the degenerative breakdown of the pulp causes bifurcation or trifurcation bone breakdown (Moss et al, 1965) (Fig 18-3).
4. Pathologic external root and bone resorption. As previously mentioned, resorption usually is evident in the bifurcation and trifurcation areas. With a necrotic or chronically inflamed pulp, there is often severe root resorption that is not normal (Fig 18-4). Myers et al (1987) observed that these radiolucent

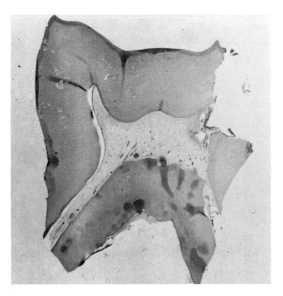

Fig 18-1   Histologic evidence of acute inflammation.

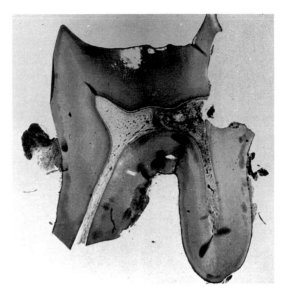

Fig 18-2   Chronic inflammation represented by calcific degeneration.

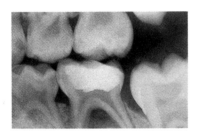

Fig 18-3   Bifurcation involvement of the primary second molar.

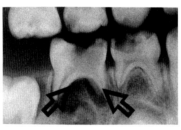

Fig 18-4   Root resorption from necrotic inflamed pulp tissue *(arrows).*

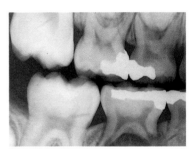

Fig 18-5   Internal resorption caused by calcium hydroxide.

bifurcation and trifurcation lesions, caused by pulpal degeneration, can produce histologic variations, ie, several forms of granulomas or lesions with cystic potential.

5. The presence of internal root resorption in the coronal or apical portion of the involved tooth. Evidence of internal root resorption is often seen on recall where a microscopic or undetected pulpal exposure has been treated with a calcium hydroxide preparation. At this time, prognosis for further pulp treatment is guarded (Fig 18-5).

Clinical assessment

Children are not good historians. Their symptoms are often misleading because of their youth, apprehension, and parental involvement. It is not uncommon for a child with large carious lesions in primary teeth to have no complaints. Questions to be asked are: Do you have any discomfort when you eat an ice cream cone or chew ice? When you eat something warm such as soup? What happens when you eat something sweet, such as a candy bar or a snow cone? Does your tooth bother you at night when you go to sleep? Is it uncomfortable for a long time? Does it jump when you hit it with a toothbrush or a fork or spoon?

These questions are an attempt to see if the tooth is influenced by thermal or chemical stimuli or percussion. Spontaneous discomfort at night indicates trouble. These questions might provide a clue as to whether the tooth is mildly inflamed, chronically inflamed, or necrotic. It is important to note that vitalometer tests with children are very unreliable. Their use is questionable (Johnson et al, 1979).

Is the tooth excessively mobile? The patient's age may influence mobility; the older child may be undergoing normal exfoliation. If there is abnormal root resorption, there will be an increase in mobility. Mobility should be used to substantiate radiographic findings.

Are soft tissue swelling or a fistulous tract present? Any swelling, with or without a fistulous tract, is indicative of a necrotic pulp. A pulpotomy is contraindicated. Removal of the involved tooth or pulpectomy is the treatment of choice.

Indications and types of pulp treatment for primary and young permanent teeth

Direct pulp capping is the placement of a calcium hydroxide preparation on a small (pinpoint) pulpal exposure. Its use should be limited to permanent teeth.

Indirect pulp therapy is indicated when a deep carious lesion is encroaching on, but not actually into, the pulp. This procedure should be reserved for permanent teeth only. A zinc oxide–eugenol (ZOE) or a calcium hydroxide [Ca(OH)$_2$] preparation is used over the carious dentin. The intent is to stimulate the tooth to assist in its own recovery from the near pulpal exposure.

Pulpotomy is indicated for carious or mechanical exposures in primary teeth and to induce root closures in the young permanent dentition. The inflamed coronal portion of the pulp is removed, and a medicament is placed over the excised pulpal tissue. The medicaments of choice are formocresol in the primary dentition and calcium hydroxide in the permanent dentition.

Pulpectomy is the treatment of choice for primary second molars and primary incisors with nonvital pulps. This treatment involves extirpation of the pulpal tissue and filling of the canals with zinc oxide–eugenol. In the permanent dentition, the pulp is removed and the pulp canals are filled with gutta-percha.

Direct pulp capping

As previously mentioned, direct pulp capping is accomplished by using calcium hydroxide on a small, mechanically induced pulpal exposure in primary and permanent teeth. Based on clinical experience, however, as a direct pulp-capping agent in primary teeth, calcium hydroxide has a higher rate of failure. An example is seen in Fig 18-6: A direct pulp cap was done using a rubber dam and all other precautions, but failure was seen on 6 months' recall.

In two relatively short-term clinical trials, the success rate was 75% (Hargraves, 1959; Jepperson, 1971). Recent histologic evidence indicates that calcium hydroxide will stimulate a healing response in mechanically exposed, noninflamed pulpal tissue of primary teeth (Jerrell et al, 1984).

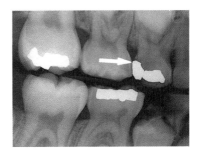

Fig 18-6   A failed direct pulp cap *(arrow)*.

A study using radioactive calcium hydroxide (^{45}Ca) over exposed pulps substantiates the hypothesis that calcium in the calcium hydroxide enters into the formation of reparative dentin. The calcium ion probably initiates secondary dentin formation (Stark et al, 1964). Schroder (1978) found that calcium hydroxide seriously impeded the healing process. She is of the opinion that the hydroxyl ion is decisive in causing the initial tissue change.

There is an indication that primary teeth respond to caries and resultant pulpal inflammation much faster. This faster response also contraindicates the use of indirect pulp capping in the primary dentition. In permanent teeth, when the bacterial carious process is 0.6 mm from the pulp, there is resultant pulpal inflammation (Rayner and Southerns, 1979). Yet primary teeth and permanent teeth have similar pulpal responses when the carious process is 1.8 mm from the outer layer of pulpal tissue. It is very tempting to do a pulp-capping procedure when confronted with a child who is a management problem or when it is late in the operating day. "The direct pulp cap is the least desirable course of treatment," with a poor prognosis, and it should rarely be used (Frank et al, 1978). Thus direct pulp capping on primary teeth, whether for a mechanical or a carious exposure, is contraindicated.

Studying carious primary incisors with possible pulpal exposures, Eidelman et al (1992) found that two-thirds of those teeth with pulpal exposures had histologic changes typical of pulpal degeneration. This degeneration was limited to the coronal portion of the pulp. Thirty percent of the primary incisors without pulpal exposures had similar histologic changes. These primary incisors from both groups were candidates for some form of pulpotomy therapy.

Even though at the time it may seem more radical, a formocresol pulpotomy is a more conservative treatment when success rates are compared—75% for direct pulp capping (Jepperson, 1971) versus 98% for formocresol pulpotomies (Morawa et al, 1975).

Calcium hydroxide is used successfully, however, as a cavity liner for deep cavity preparations in both the primary and permanent dentitions.

Table 18-1   Comparison of results in direct and indirect pulp therapy studies

Author(s)	No. of teeth	Procedure	Material*	Success (%)
Hawes et al (1963) (clinical)	475	Indirect	ZOE	97
	484	Direct	Ca(OH)$_2$	93
Dimaggio and Hawes (1963) (histologic)	84	Indirect	ZOE	88
	33	Direct	Ca(OH)$_2$	67
King et al (1965)	21	Indirect	Ca(OH)$_2$	61.4[†]
	22	Indirect	ZOE	81.8[†]
Aponte et al (1966)	30	Indirect	Ca(OH)$_2$	93
Kerhove et al (1967)	35	Indirect	ZOE	92
	41	Indirect	Ca(OH)$_2$	92
Hutchins and Parker (1972)	35	Indirect	ZOE (IRM)	94
Nordstrom et al (1974)	32	Indirect	Ca(OH)$_2$	84
	32	Indirect	SnF– ZOE	91
Nirschi and Avery (1983)	15	Indirect	Ca(OH)$_2$	93
	18	Indirect	Ca(OH)$_2$	94

*ZOE = zinc oxide–eugenol; Ca(OH)$_2$ = calcium hydroxide; IRM = interim restorative materials; SnF = tin fluoride.
[†]Sterile dentin.

Indirect pulp therapy for immature permanent teeth

Indirect pulp therapy is sometimes called the *rest treatment*. It is the procedure of choice whenever pulpal exposure seems possible during removal of deep carious lesions in a tooth that radiographically and clinically appears to have a healthy pulp.

Besic, in 1943, studied the fate of bacteria sealed in dental cavities. His method involved what has become known as the indirect pulp cap. When teeth were recultured, it was found that lactobacilli had died out in all cases within 2 to 10 months. Streptococci persisted in 30% of the cases after 1 year. He concluded that *(1)* the carious process in dentin abruptly or gradually ceases as the lesion is closed from the oral environment, even when the organisms remain alive; and *(2)* the bacteria have a tendency to die out.

Cavity preparations should be routinely lined with a calcium hydroxide or zinc oxide–eugenol protective base where there is even a remote possibility of a microscopic mechanical exposure. Direct pulp capping should be limited to mechanical exposures, such as accidental pulpal exposure in an area remote from an extensive carious lesion or in a case of minute pulpal exposure in a fractured tooth. The use of indirect pulp therapy has been questioned. Some clinicians believe all caries should be removed; others believe indirect pulp therapy should be limited to permanent teeth. However, it is our opinion that it should be limited to young permanent teeth.

Hawes et al (1963) presented convincing proof that indirect pulp therapy is successful. They left the deeper layers of carious lesions intact, sealed in a capping material of zinc oxide–eugenol or calcium hydroxide, and placed a semipermanent restoration, usually of amalgam. The success rates of direct and indirect pulp therapy procedures are shown in Table 18-1. All the teeth in the study by Hawes et al were initially diagnosed as having normal pulps. (Calcium hydroxide was used in both capping and covering the pulps of a third group of teeth treated by pulpotomy. The success rate of this group was even lower than that for teeth treated by direct capping.)

In another study, Dimaggio et al (1963) made a histologic study of 117 teeth, which had been extracted for various reasons. Their study revealed that direct capping failed more than twice as often as indirect therapy. They further included that 75% of the pulps treated by indirect therapy would have been exposed if all carious lesions had been removed initially.

King et al (1965) evaluated three capping agents. Their findings were that residual carious dentin was initially contaminated, but calcium hydroxide and zinc oxide–eugenol greatly reduced the bacteria present.

Using calcium hydroxide, Aponte et al (1966) treated 30 primary molars for 6 to 46 months. When the dentin was cultured on reentry, 93% of the teeth were free of bacteria after treatment. Clinical and radiographic evidence indicated success.

Kerhove et al (1967), using clinical and television criteria, evaluated indirect pulp therapy with a calcium hydroxide preparation and zinc oxide–eugenol. There were three failures each with zinc oxide–eugenol and calcium hydroxide in the 56 primary molars. There were no reported failures in the 20 permanent first molars. Using television densitometric evaluation, they found little increase in radiopacity when comparing the permanent dentition with the primary dentition. The same was true when the two capping materials were compared. On reentry, all 70 teeth had sound dentin and no pulpal exposures.

A total of 35 permanent teeth were evaluated by Hutchins and Parker (1972) for successful indirect pulp therapy procedures. An improved zinc oxide–eugenol cement was used. After 18 months, 33 restorations were judged radiographically and clinically successful. The durability of the IRM was considered to be functional.

Nordstrom et al (1974) compared a 5-minute application of 10% stannous fluoride solution with use of a calcium hydroxide preparation. Clinical and radiographic criteria were those described for the best prognosis. Twenty-five primary molars and 39 permanent molars were used. Bacterial cultures of the lesions before and after indirect pulp therapy procedures demonstrated a 50% increase in negative cultures for all teeth in the study. Failure rates were about equal for each material. Increased hardness of the dentin was seen with the stannous fluoride and was accompanied by an increased radiodensity of the demineralized dentin. The authors proposed that stannous fluoride may produce remineralization in vivo.

In a short-term study by Nirshci and Avery (1983) indirect pulp therapy procedures were done on permanent and primary teeth. After 6 months, success rates were judged to be in the 94% range. The author suggested further long-term studies.

Is indirect pulp therapy indicated? To simplify the decision process, Fig 18-7 assists in assessing the patient's oral health, radiographs, and clinical status. This decision-support system aims the dentist in the "correct" direction to arrive at the appropriate diagnosis and, if needed, the indicated pulp therapy.

Indications

Pain history

1. No extremes
2. May be associated with eating, especially carbohydrates
3. Sometimes dull

Clinical examination

1. No gingival pathologic condition
2. No mobility
3. Large carious lesion

Radiographic examination

1. Probable carious exposure
2. Normal periapical tissues

Justification

1. Reduction of hyperemia in pulp
2. Remineralization of carious or precarious dentin
3. Reduction of anaerobic bacteria
4. Formation of reparative dentin
5. Vital pulp maintenance
6. Continued normal root closure

Objectives

1. Reversal of bacterial invasion
2. Treatment of carious dentin
3. Maintenance of normal healthy pulp

Armamentarium—Pulp Therapy

Mirror
Explorer
Cotton forceps
Spoon excavators
Burs
    No. 330 F.G.
    No. 6 or No. 8 R.A.
Cement spatula
Plastic instruments
Irrigating syringe
Amalgam plugger
Sterile towel
Cotton pellets, paper points
Formocresol, 20% strength (Buckley, Crosby Laboratories)
Zinc oxide–eugenol (B&T, L.D. Caulk Co).
Paper mixing pad
Calcium hydroxide (Dycal, L.D. Caulk Co)
Oxidizing/irrigating agent, sodium hypochlorite
Root canal pressure syringe (Pulp dent, optional)

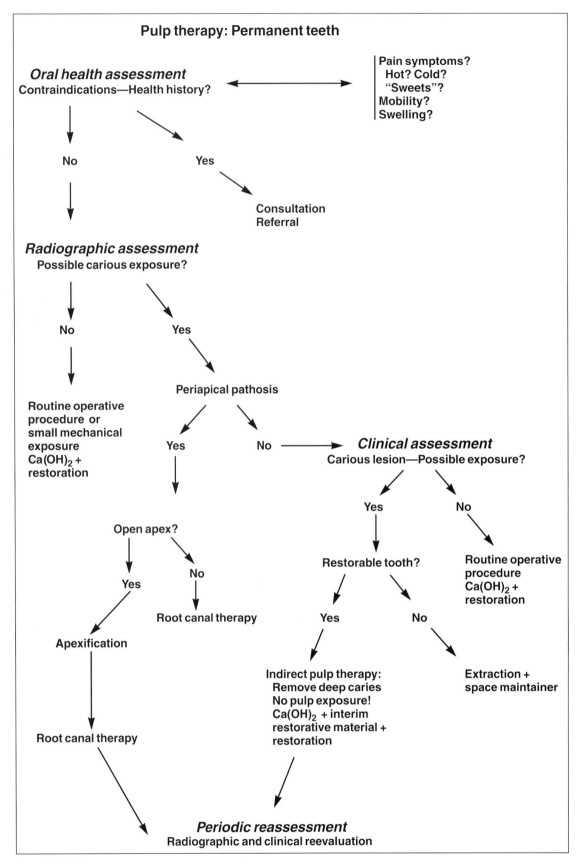

Fig 18-7 A decision-support system to determine pulp therapy for permanent teeth.

Procedure

The radiograph in Fig 18-8 demonstrates an ideal candidate for an indirect pulp therapy procedure. Complete removal of all carious dentin would result in certain pulpal exposure of the distal pulp horn, the periapical tissues are normal, and there is no evidence of coronal or apical pulpal degeneration.

1. Administer local anesthesia. This step is essential for the patient's comfort.
2. Isolate the area with a rubber dam (Fig 18-9). The use of a rubber dam in this procedure is essential. Only the permanent first molar needs to be isolated if it is only an occlusal carious lesion.
3. Use an F.G. No. 330 bur to open the carious area. Remove all unsupported enamel (Fig 18-10). The preparation is extended as dictated by the carious process.
4. Use a No. 4, 6, or 8 carbide bur at slow speed to remove carious dentin to *within 1 mm of the pulp chamber* (Fig 18-11). *Do not expose the pulp. Knowledge of pulpal morphology is important.* If hand instruments are used, a large spoon excavator is the instrument of choice.
5. Keep in mind as you progress toward the pulp chambers that:
   a. The outermost layer of dentin will be mushy, necrotic tissue (Fig 18-12,*A*).
   b. The next layer will be leathery but firmer (Fig 18-12,*B*).
   c. The last 1 mm of dentin is left—the indirect pulp cap portion of the carious dentin (Fig 18-12,*C*).
6. Apply a calcium hydroxide base over the last 1 mm of carious dentin. You will need Dycal (base and catalyst), mixing spatula and pad, and applicator.
7. With an application instrument, apply calcium hydroxide paste over the carious dentin remaining (Fig 18-13). Apply to the rest of the deeper portions of the cavity preparations.
8. Using an amalgam plugger or a plastic instrument, place a base of reinforced zinc oxide–eugenol (IRM) over the calcium hydroxide liner (Fig 18-14). Adapt the material when in a plastic state to represent as typical a cavity preparation as possible.
9. Remove excessive Dycal or zinc oxide–eugenol from the margins of the cavity preparation. Use a No. 169L bur or a hand instrument, or marginal voids will occur in the amalgam (Fig 18-15). Coat with Copalite (Harry Bosworth Co).
10. Restore with silver amalgam. If the tooth is beyond the physical limitations of silver amalgam, use a stainless steel crown.
11. Establish a recall time or appointment. The radiograph in Fig 18-16 represents the final indirect pulp therapy procedure: near pulpal exposure, a

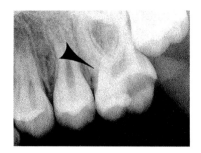

Fig 18-8 A candidate for indirect pulp therapy.

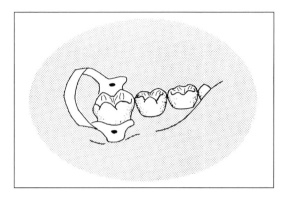

Fig 18-9 Isolate the tooth with a rubber dam.

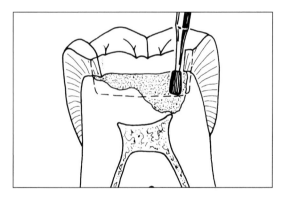

Fig 18-10 Extend the preparation with a No. 330 bur.

layer of Dycal and IRM, and final restoration with a stainless steel crown.

The reentry restorative procedure is still questionable. Research has shown that carious dentin will remineralize with the restoration. If "all systems are go" on recall, the restoration *should not* be redone. Thus, if the recall radiograph shows a layer of secondary dentin, reentry is not necessary.

If reentry is decided on:

1. Use anesthesia and a rubber dam.
2. Remove the amalgam or provisional restoration.

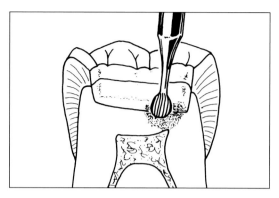

Fig 18-11 Remove the carious dentin with a slow-speed bur.

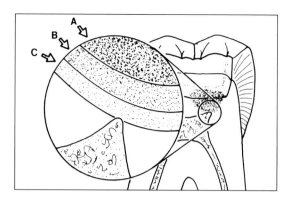

Fig 18-12 The three layers of carious dentin *(A)* necrotic tissue, *(B)* leathery, and *(C)* the 1 mm to remain.

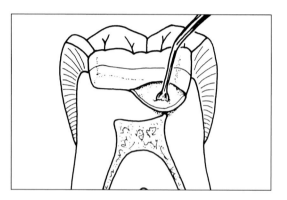

Fig 18-13 Place calcium hydroxide over the carious dentin.

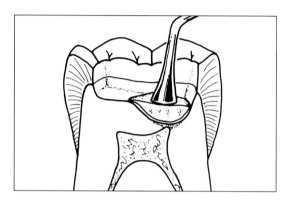

Fig 18-14 Place an improved ZOE material over the Ca(OH)$_2$.

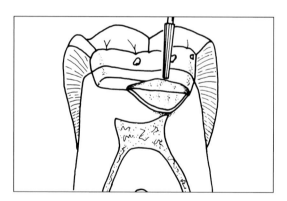

Fig 18-15 Remove excess Ca(OH)$_2$ and zinc oxide–eugenol from the margins.

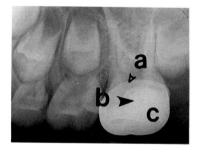

Fig 18-16 Completed indirect pulp cap and restoration: *(a)* near pulpal exposure; *(b)* layer of Dycal and IRM; *(c)* stainless steel crown.

3. Remove zinc oxide–eugenol and calcium hydroxide base with a round bur.
4. Remove flaky and fluffy material.
5. Remove any carious lesions left. Take care not to expose the pulpal tissue after all this time and effort.

6. Replace liner with Dycal.
7. Restore the tooth with silver amalgam or a stainless steel crown.

Pulpotomy

A pulpotomy is the procedure of removing the coronal part of the pulp that has been involved by dental caries. As previously mentioned, the objective of a pulpotomy is to remove the inflamed coronal portion of the pulp, allow the pulpal tissue in the root canal to remain vital, and maintain the tooth in the dental arch.

Pulpotomy with calcium hydroxide is contraindicated in primary teeth; research reveals little success with the procedure. As mentioned earlier, internal resorption is most common with failure (Via, 1955; Scröder, 1978). Evaluation of 130 primary molars treated with a calcium hydroxide pulpotomy showed that internal root resorption was present in two thirds of the roots radiographically (Magnusson, 1970).

Seventeen teeth were evaluated for success rates after pulpotomy procedures where a calcium hydroxide preparation (Life, Kerr Div/Sybron Corp) was used (Heilig et al, 1984). After 9 months, 15 teeth were radiographically successful, but the author suggested that a long-term study with a histologic evaluation was needed.

Use of formocresol

The medicament of choice, particularly for the primary dentition, has been formocresol. This drug is composed of 35% tricresol and 19% formaldehyde in a 15% water and glycerin solution. It is a very caustic drug, fixing bacteria and tissue in the upper one third of the involved pulp. Introduced by Buckley in the early 1900s, the mixture often is referred to as *Buckley's formocresol*. The formocresol pulpotomy was clinically emphasized by Sweet in the 1930s. It was not until the early 1960s that any clinical, histologic, or radiographic information was available. Unfortunately, there are still confusion and conflicting opinions on how formocresol influences the pulp and surrounding tissues.

In recent years, formocresol has been extensively evaluated using animal models. Table 18-2 is a brief representative sample of these studies. The conclusions from these studies, dependent on histologic method, animal model, and concentration of formocresol, have produced varying results. The clinical applications seem to be as follows:

1. Twenty percent dilution causes the least histologic damage.
2. A 1-minute application of formocresol is adequate to produce the desired results.
3. Teeth with a formocresol pulpotomy seem to resorb faster than those without a pulpotomy.
4. Further evaluation of the physiologic, histologic, and pathologic effects of formocresol is needed.

In 1962, Doyle et al compared use of calcium hydroxide and a two-visit, or 7-day, pulpotomy technique using formocresol. The primary canines were removed at various times. Histologic sections revealed vital tissue in the apical one third of the teeth. There was loss of cell identity in the middle third, and there was a dark-stained tissue layer beneath the amputated pulp. They found debris and dentinal chips in this layer.

Berger (1963) was the first to evaluate the formocresol technique commonly used in clinical practice. He used a one-appointment method with a 5-minute application of formocresol. This application was followed by a zinc oxide–eugenol base with formocresol added to the eugenol. The primary molars were sacrificed at intervals of 3 to 39 weeks. He reported a gradual replacement of apical tissue by granulation tissue. The replacement tissue progressed coronally, replacing tissue affected by the formocresol. This tissue was theorized to derive from the periodontal ligament.

The difference between using zinc oxide–eugenol with or without formocresol was evaluated by Beaver et al (1966). Histologic changes were noted on 60 extracted primary molars. They found that the pulp did not histologically divide into three definite zones. There were six varied tissue responses ranging from normal, or "drug fixed," to internal resorption and necrosis. The granulation tissue was not seen invading the apical one third of the tooth. The addition of formocresol to the zinc oxide–eugenol did not contribute to or detract from the success rate.

There are two methods for using formocresol. The 5-minute method, or one-stage pulpotomy, is reserved for primary teeth in which the pulp is considered vital. The 7-day method is used for teeth in which hemorrhage control is a problem. "Five-minute" and "7-day" denote the length of time a pledget of cotton moistened with formocresol is in contact with the pulp. Redig (1968) compared the two methods in 20 children. He found little clinical and radiographic difference in the teeth after 18 months.

Calcium hydroxide was reevaluated by two studies (Magnusson, 1970; Schroder, 1978). Both studies reported it to have a higher rate of failure than formocresol. The culprit was internal root resorption.

Rolling and Thystrup (1975) evaluated 98 primary molars using formocresol as the pulpotomy agent. They found a decrease in the success rate from 91% to 70% in 3 years.

Morawa et al (1975) evaluated clinically the use of a 20% dilution of formocresol. This clinical evaluation was based on a series of animal experiments at the University of Michigan (Loos et al, 1973). Loos et al found that a 20% dilution of formocresol in animals was as effective a cytostatic agent as full strength. The 20% dilution did allow some recovery of connective tissue cells. They found that the 20% dilution created similar metabolic cell changes as the full-strength formocresol. However, there was a greater and earlier cellular recovery. They also suggested that some of the

Table 18-2   Summary of experimental studies with formocresol

Author(s)	Animal subject	Results and comments
Mejare et al (1976)	Human	Used formocresol-containing formaldehyde, found routine histologic methods not appropriate for evaluation of frozen sections; histochemical demonstrations of lactate dehydrogenase best
Ranly and Fulton (1976)	Rat	Did pulpotomies using formocresol, formaldehyde, cresol, and glycerol; cresol hindered healing, formocresol slowed but did not prevent healing, and formaldehyde did not stop healing
Block et al (1977)	Dog	Found that formocresol rendered pulpal tissue antigenetically active, producing a specific cell-mediated immune response
Lazzari et al (1978)	Cow	Found that various concentrations of formocresol produced increases in tissue enzyme activity, with decreases in formocresol concentrations producing less activity
Fulton and Ranly (1979)	Rat	Used ^{3}H formaldehyde; autoradiographs of pulpotomies initially produced a random distribution; 1 week, labeling occurred in nuclei of odontoblasts; 2 weeks, pulp cells plus osteoclasts, in adjacent bone marrow and periodontal spaces were labeled
Pashley et al (1980)	Dog	Found that formocresol is absorbed rapidly into body, tissue binding was responsible for most of systemic absorption
Dilley and Courts (1981)	Rabbit	Compared four agents; found that formalin and glutaraldehyde each produced mild immunologic responses
Garcia-Godoy (1981)	Baboon	Used 20% and full-strength formocresol alone and in a zinc oxide–eugenol base; histologic responses were similar; autoradiographs demonstrated coronal uptake only
Garcia-Godoy (1982)	Dog	Compared formocresol, zinc oxide–eugenol, and polycarboxylate; severe inflammation with zinc oxide–eugenol, less with formocresol, and mild with polycarboxylate
Garcia-Godoy et al (1982)	Dog	Found that 1-minute application of full concentration formocresol produced less inflammation than 3- or 5-minute application
Chiniwalla and Rapp (1982)	Monkey	Found necrotic tissue and clotted blood adjacent to formocresol pulpotomy site, vascular architecture of pulp intact
Fuks et al (1983)	Monkey	Used diluted and full-concentration formocresol; caused primary teeth to resorb faster than antimeres
Block et al (1983)	Dog	Used ^{14}C-labeled formocresol; tissue samples revealed its presence in blood system, lymph nodes, kidney, and liver
Ranly and Fulton (1983)	Rat	Autoradiographs of formocresol demonstrated a reversible influence of pulp cells beyond zone of necrosis
Ruemping et al (1983)	Monkey	Compared formocresol pulpotomies with electrosurgical pulpotomies with similar histologic results
Myers et al (1983)	Dog	Used full-strength formocresol on 16 teeth of one dog; produced histologic changes in kidney and liver
Shulman et al (1987)	Monkey	Compared electrosurgery with formocresol; electrosurgery not effective

histopathology and subsequent clinical failures could be reduced by use of the 20% concentration. The recommended way of diluting formocresol using Buckley formocresol (Crosby Laboratories) to make a 20% 1:5 concentration is as follows (Loos et al, 1973):

1. Dilute 3 parts glycerine with 1 part distilled sterile water; *mix well*
2. Add 1 part formocresol to 4 parts diluent:

> 90 mL glycerin
> 30 mL water
> 120 mL diluent

Add 30 mL formocresol to 120 mL diluent to obtain 150 mL of dilute formocresol (20% strength).

Rolling and Lambjerg-Hanson (1978) extracted 19 teeth with formocresol pulpotomies considered to be radiographically and clinically successful 3 to 24 months after treatment. They could not find a typical histologic pattern of the pulp's reaction to formocresol. The pulpal reactions varied from vital apical tissue to chronic inflammation and necrosis. They concluded that "complete repair of devitalized pulp tissue may occur, but it is not a characteristic reaction after formocresol treatment." They believed that formocresol pulpotomies should be considered only a limited treatment.

Magnusson (1978) reviewed 84 primary molars. Radiographs showed 31 teeth with internal resorption; of the 56 teeth reviewed histologically, 15% showed some form of necrosis, 81% showed internal resorption, and 12% showed inflammation. Only 20% were considered histologically successful. According to Magnusson (1978), "Whether clinicians should accept a chronic 'silent' inflammation in residual pulp tissue is debatable."

In a retrospective study of 184 primary molars, an 80% success rate was demonstrated (Wright and Widmer, 1979). The factors contributing to success (or failure) were the time from pulpotomy to final restoration, the type of restoration placed, and the age of the child. The opinion was that pulpotomized molars exfoliated earlier than their antimeres. There was no increase of enamel defects on the succedaneous teeth.

Mejare (1979) compared pulpotomy methods using full-strength formocresol in primary teeth. The teeth were divided into two groups, those with clinical symptoms of coronal or chronic pulpitis. Zinc oxide–eugenol or a total plaster noneugenol cement was used as the vehicle for the formocresol. Initially the success rate for either method and diagnostic group was 90%. However, after 30 months, success rates in both groups and methods degenerated to 55%. The most common cause of radiographic failure was intraradicular root resorption or interradicular resorptive osteitis.

Duplicating Morawa's earlier study, Fuks and Bimstein (1981) found similar success rates of 94% and 65% for clinical and radiographic studies, respectively. They noted increased resorption rates of the roots of those teeth where a pulpotomy was completed. Garcia-Godoy (1984) advocated the use of 20% dilution of formocresol for direct pulp caps and partial pulpotomies for children who are management problems. This procedure is for emergency treatment only. When the child matures, a typical pulpotomy can be done if the tooth has not exfoliated. Results of these studies on primary dentition are summarized in Table 18-3.

Several other studies have evaluated the calcification of root canals in primary dentition after completion of formocresol pulpotomy (Willard, 1976; Fuks and Bimstein, 1981; Garcia-Godoy, 1983). They suggested that the calcific metamorphosis is the result of a vital odontoblastic response to the application of formocresol.

Using full-strength formocresol, van Amerongen et al (1986) evaluated the life span of primary molars. Primary molars judged to have vital pulps were treated with full-strength formocresol for 5 minutes; nonvital pulps were treated for 7 days. The researchers concluded that *(1)* the was no significant difference in the life span of the primary tooth with or without a pulpotomy. And *(2)* there was no difference in the life span between vital or nonvital pulpotomies. However, Fuks and Bimstein (1981) and Hicks et al (1986) disagreed. Formocresol pulpotomies on primary molars resulted in accelerated rate of resorption for 45% to 56% of the primary molars when compared to their antimeres. The cause of early resorption was speculated to be the chronic inflammatory reaction caused by formocresol seeping into surrounding periodontal tissues (Fuks and Bimstein, 1981).

There has been concern about the effects of a formocresol pulpotomy on the succedaneous teeth. The conflicting results are seen in Table 18-4.

Trask (1972), one of the first to advocate the use of formocresol on permanent teeth, reported on 43 permanent teeth treated with a 7-day or two-step, formocresol pulpotomy. In these cases endodontic therapy was not economically feasible for the parents. The procedure is suggested as an alternative to extraction. Although considered a temporary treatment, it can prevent malocclusion and periodontal disease until root canal therapy is possible.

Using similar criteria, Fiskio (1974), over a 5-year period, had a clinical success rate of 94% in the permanent dentition. Using a two-step pulpotomy procedure, Rothman (1977) reported that after 2 years 71% of 165 permanent teeth remained clinically and radiographically sound.

Reporting a retrospective study, Teplitsky (1984) determined the clinical success of formocresol pulpotomies on 76 permanent teeth. The success rates were above 90%, with some pulpotomies performed 55 months before the evaluation. Root canal calcification was evident in many of the radiographs.

Table 18-3 Results of clinical pulpotomy studies on primary teeth

Author(s)	Procedure	No. of Teeth	Success rate (%)		
			Histologic	Radiographic	Clinical
Doyle et al (1962)	Calcium hydroxide	18	50	64	71
	Zinc oxide–eugenol	14	92	93	100
Berger (1963)	Zinc oxide–eugenol	17	0	58	100
	Formocresol	30	82	97	100
Beaver et al (1966)	Formocresol	60	Varied	97	100
Redig (1968)	Formocresol, 5 min	20		85	85
	Formocresol, 7 d	20		90	90
Magnusson (1970)	Calcium hydroxide	130		20	
		119	12		
Rolling and Thylstrup (1975)	Formocresol	98			
	3 mo			91	91
	12 mo			83	83
	24 mo			78	78
	36 mo			70	70
Morawa et al (1975)	Formocresol, 20% dilution	125		98	98
Schröder (1978)	Calcium hydroxide	33			
	1 y				67
	2 y				38–59
Magnusson (1978)	Formocresol	84		62	100
		56	20		
Rolling and Lambjerg-Hansen (1978)	Formocresol	19		100	100
Wright and Widmer (1979)	Formocresol	184			80
Mejare (1979)	Formocresol				
	Coronal pulpitis	29			
	12 mo			93	
	18 mo			82	
	24 mo			68	
	30 mo			59	
	Total pulpitis	45			
	12 mo			91	
	18 mo			82	
	24 mo			61	
	30 mo			52	
Fuks and Bimstein (1981)	Formocresol, 20% dilution	70		65	94
Garcia-Gordoy (1983)	Formocresol, 20% dilution	45		96	96
van Amerongen et al (1986)	Vital, 5 min Nonvital, 7 days Formocresol IRM + formocresol	131		67	
Hicks et al (1986)	Formocresol in IRM paste	164		94	

Table 18-4 Results of research into whether formocresol affects succedaneous teeth

Author(s)	Effect
Pruhs et al (1977)	Yes
Rolling and Paulsen (1978)	None
Wright and Widmer (1979)	None
Messer et al. (1980)	Yes
Fuks and Bimstein (1981)	None
Mulder et al (1987)	None

Table 18-5 Results of formocresol pulpotomy studies on permanent teeth

Author(s)	No. of teeth	Success rate (%)	
		Radiographic	Clinical
Trask (1972)	43	98	100
Fiskio (1974)	135		91
Rothman (1977)	165	71	71
Teplitsky (1984)	76	94	96

Table 18-6   Summary of experimental studies with glutaraldehyde (GA)

Author(s)	Model	Results and comments
Ramos et al (1980)	Rats	Used 5% GA; increased cell respiratory rate
Davis et al (1982)	Rats	Used 5% GA; less inflammation and apex diffusion
Ranly and Lazzari (1983)	Bovine	Found 2% alkaline GA best
Ranly (1984)	Laboratory	Buffered; cold 2% GA most stable
Lekka et al (1984)	Human third molars	Used 2% GA; little apical diffusion
Tagger and Sarnat (1984)	Monkeys	Zone of fixed tissue than normal apical tissue
Myers et al (1986)	Dogs	3% to 5% GA pulpotomy is distributed systemically
Seow and Thong (1986)	PMNs	GA less necrotic than formocresol, eugenol, and Ca(OH)$_2$
Fuks et al (1986b)	Baboons	GA pulpotomies produced mild response
Jeng et al (1987)	Pulpal fibroblasts	2.5% GA less toxic then formocresol
Karp (1987)	Rats	GA metabolized systemically
Ranly et al (1987)	Collagen gel	Buffered GA best: 4% for 4 min 8% for 2 min
Ranly et al (1989)	Rats	25% GA distributed systemically; non toxic
Rusmah and Rahim (1992)	Human primary molars	2% buffered GA; no diffusion

Using monkeys as models, Armstrong (1979) and Fuks et al (1983) studied the effects of formocresol pulpotomies on permanent primate teeth. On these immature permanent teeth, root development continued, with subsequent apical closure.

Schwartz (1980) reported on the use of formocresol as a vital pulpotomy method either taught or used in Canada. No department of pediatric dentistry taught the method for permanent teeth. Yet, 18% of the general practitioners and 55% of the pediatric dentists surveyed used the method on permanent teeth.

Conclusions from these studies on permanent teeth are:

1. Vital pulpotomies on permanent teeth are successful.
2. In children and adolescents in whom endodontic therapy is not available, formocresol pulpotomy is a preventive alterative.
3. Root apex completion is possible, but root canal calcification can be a factor (Table 18-5).

Summary of formocresol pulpotomy studies

1. Clinical and radiographic studies of formocresol pulpotomies report a high rate of success compared with other conventional pulpotomy methods.
2. Length of application of formocresol does not increase or decrease success.
3. A 20% dilution of formocresol is optimum. A greater concentration may be a cause of adverse pulpal responses.
4. When evaluated histologically the formocresol pulpotomy causes various degrees of chronic inflammatory tissue.
5. The current trend is to reduce the overall toxicity of current drugs or find improved biocompatible substitutes (Ranly and Garcia-Godoy, 1991).

Use of formaldehyde

As Lewis and Chester (1981) state, "There is a need to evaluate the rationale underlying the use of formaldehyde in dentistry, particularly in light of its deleterious effects."

Use of ferric sulfate

Ferric sulfate has been suggested as a substitute for formocresol (Fei et al, 1991). The 1-year success rate for 25% formocresol pulpotomies was 78%, while the success rate for those primary molars treated with ferric sulfate was 96%. Additional evaluation was suggested.

Use of glutaraldehyde

Because laboratory studies have demonstrated some problems with formocresol, glutaraldehyde (GA), a bactericidal agent, has been suggested as a possible substitute. The laboratory studies are outlined in Table 18-6. Generalities from these studies are as follows:

1. There is limited diffusion from tooth structure into adjacent tissue.
2. Binding with protein tissue is irreversible.
3. There is less pupal irritation because of less apical diffusion.
4. Cold, buffered, 2% GA is most stable.

Ranly and Garcia-Godoy (1991), comparing formaldehyde to GA, concluded that *(1)* GA is a better fixative than formaldehyde and can be used in a lesser concentration; *(2)* GA is less antigenic; *(3)* extensive

Table 18-7 Clinical studies with glutaraldehyde (GA)

Author(s)	Procedure	No. in sample	Success rate (%)		
			Histologic	Radiologic	Clinical
Kopel et al (1980)	2% GA, 1 y	30	100		98
Garcia-Godoy (1983)	2% GA, 0.5–1.5 y	55		96	96
Fuks (1986)	2% GA, 0.5 y	50		94	94
	2% GA, 1 y	47		90	90
Garcia-Godoy (1986)	2% GA, 3.5 y	48		98	98
Fuks (1986)	2% GA, 0.5 y	53		94	94
	2% GA, 1 y	52		90	90
	2% GA, 2 y	50		82	82
Hernandez Pereyra et al (1987)*	2% GA, 0.5 y	10		80	
	2% GA, 2 y	10		90	
	Formocresol, 0.5 y	10		20	
	Formocresol, 2 y	10		40	

*Sample of permanent first molars.

toxicity testing has shown that GA is easily metabolized or excreted; and *(4)* GA is limited to shallow, well-demarcated fixed zone with vital tissue distal to these areas.

Clinical studies done in countries other than the United States have demonstrated that GA is as effective as formocresol (Kopel et al, 1980; Garcia-Godoy, 1983; Fuks et al, 1986; Fuks, 1991). Because of the review requirements of the Federal Drug Administration, GA has not been available for clinical use in the United States. The results of the clinical studies are in Table 18-7.

Twenty permanent molars were used to compare their reaction to 2% GA and formocresol (Hernandez Pereyra et al, 1987). Divided into equal groups of 10 permanent molars, each molar had a carious exposure, radiographic indications of slight periapical change, and closed apices. After 6 months, 80% of the GA group had normal trabecular bone pattern (NTBP); after 2 years 90% had NTBP. Among the formocresol group, after 6 months, 20% had NTBP and, after 2 years, 40% had NTBP.

Use Fig 18-17 as a guide to reach the correct diagnosis and, if needed, the appropriate pulp therapy for primary teeth.

Indications

Teeth
1. Primary teeth
2. Permanent molars where economics is a factor

Pain history
1. No extremes

Clinical examination

1. No gingival pathologic condition or evidence of a chronic fistulous tract
2. No extreme mobility of the tooth
3. Carious lesion

Radiographic examination

1. Probable carious exposure
2. Normal interradicular periapical tissues
3. Normal root development
4. No internal or external root resorption

General treatment procedures

1. Removal of the coronal portion of a vital pulp
2. Control of the resultant hemorrhage
3. Medication of the pulpal tissue
4. Placement of a pulpal dressing
5. Final restoration

Failure

Indications
1. Increased mobility, fistulous tract
2. Premature exfoliation
3. Radiographic evidence of interradicular or periapical radiolucency
4. Internal or external root resorption

Cause
1. Poor diagnosis and treatment selection

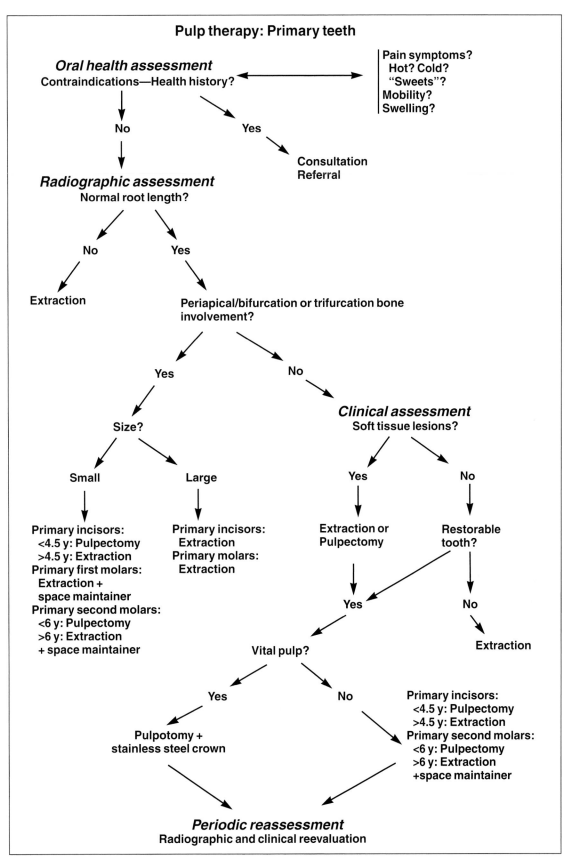

Fig 18-17 The determination of the need for pulp therapy using a decision-support system.

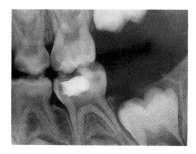

Fig 18-18   Primary molars that are candidates for pulpotomy procedures.

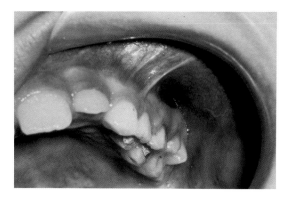

Fig 18-19   A formocresol burn.

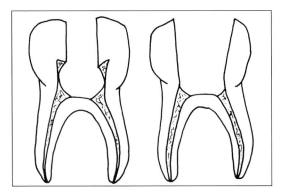

Fig 18-20   Occlusal openings in primary molars.

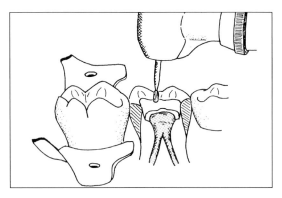

Fig 18-21   Using the same bur, remove all overhanging enamel.

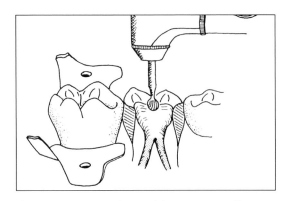

Fig 18-22   Use a sterile round bur to remove all carious dentin.

Procedure

1. Use local anesthesia. A well-anesthetized tooth (teeth) is essential. In rare instances, due to chronic inflammation, profound local anesthesia may be a problem. A few drops of local anesthesia so-

lution cautiously injected directly into the pulp can be of assistance in these instances. The bitewing radiograph in Fig 18-18 shows several primary molars where pulpotomy treatment is indicated.

2. Apply a rubber dam *(formocresol is a very caustic drug).* Note the formocresol burn in Fig 18-19. Do not allow the material to leak onto the adjacent tissue.

3. There are optimum locations for occlusal openings in the primary teeth. The openings are related to dental and pulpal morphology. *All coronal pulpal tissue should be removed.*

4. Place a No. 330 bur in the high-speed handpiece. Gain occlusal access to the pulp chamber by preparing a Class 1 cavity preparation. It is better to make too large an opening than one that is too small. Remove all overhanging enamel (Figs 18-20 and 18-21).

5. Use a sterile No. 4 or 8 round bur (slow speed) to remove all carious dentin (Fig 18-22). If possible, remove all carious dentin before exposing the pulp horns.

6. Visualize where the pulp horns should be beneath the pulpal wall (or floor). With a slow- or high-speed bur, connect the pulp horns. Harris (1969)

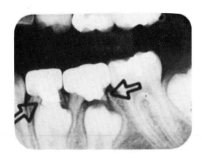

Fig 18-23 An overzealous removal of pulp tissue can result in *(arrows)* perforation of the pulp chamber.

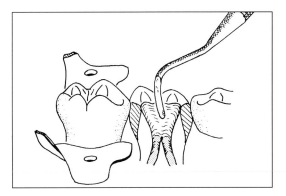

Fig 18-24 Remove the pulp tissue with a large spoon excavator.

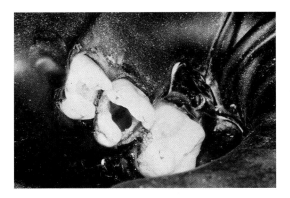

Fig 18-25 Hemorrhage should be minimal.

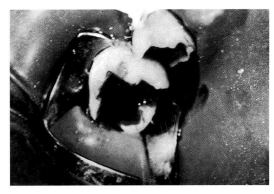

Fig 18-26 If hemorrhage is difficult to control, other methods should be considered.

found little histologic difference when pulps were amputated with a spoon excavator, low-speed bur, or high-speed bur (Harris, 1969). However, a novice should approach this part of the technique with caution because perforation of the pulp chamber can occur even with slow-speed burs (18-23).

7. Excise the pulpal tissue to the orifices of the root canal. Use a large spoon excavator to remove any remaining pulpal tissue (Fig 18-24). The pulpal tissue should be amputated to the entrance of the root canals. Gently wash out the debris with the water syringe.

8. After completing the amputation, evaluate the hemorrhage. If the pulpal tissue has been removed completely, hemorrhage should be minimal (Fig 18-25). A vital pulp with minimal chronic inflammation should achieve hemostasis in 3 to 5 minutes. If there is chronic hemorrhage, check for remaining pulpal tissue in the pulp chamber.

9. If there is purulent exudate, a fibrotic pulp, or uncontrollable hemorrhage, consider alternative pulp procedures (Fig 18-26).

10. Over the exposed pulp stump, place a sterile cotton pellet moistened (but not saturated) with formocresol, 20% dilution (Fig 18-27). Place a dry pellet over the first pellet to maintain maximum contact of the formocresol with the pulpal tissue. As previously mentioned, formocresol is very caustic.

11. Leave the formocresol in place for 2 minutes, then remove the pellet. The pulp stump should appear blackish brown (18-28). If there is bleeding, check for residual pulpal tissue. Reapply formocresol for 2 minutes.

12. Fill the pulp chamber to about half its volume with a thick mixture of zinc oxide–eugenol (Fig 18-29). Some clinicians advocate adding equal drops of formocresol to the eugenol, then mixing with zinc oxide powder. Beaver et al (1966) found this an unnecessary step.

13. Prepare the tooth for a stainless steel crown (Fig 18-30). Teeth where pulp therapy has been done seem to be brittle. This brittleness may be caused by removal of tooth structure or a change in the physical properties of the enamel or dentin after

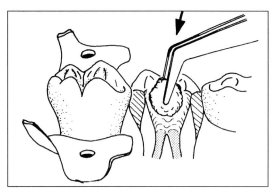

Fig 18-27 Place a moist cotton pellet of formocresol on the exposed pulpal tissue.

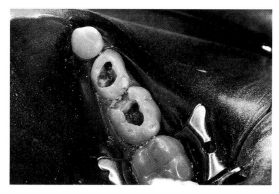

Fig 18-28 The tissue should appear blackish brown.

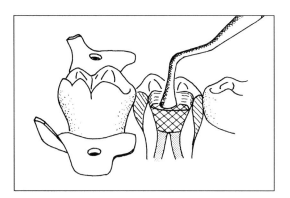

Fig 18-29 Obturate the pulp chamber with ZOE.

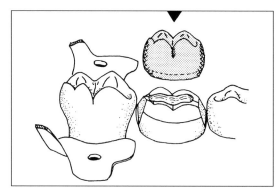

Fig 18-30 Prepare the tooth for a stainless steel crown.

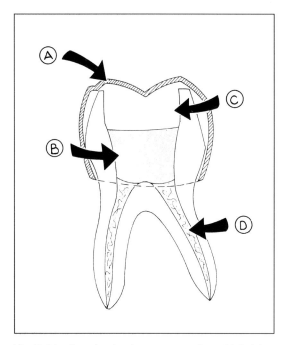

Fig 18-31 Completed pulpotomy procedure: *(A)* Stainless steel crown; *(B)* sub-base of ZOE; *(C)* cementing medium (Zinc phosphate cement); *(D)* remaining pulpal tissue.

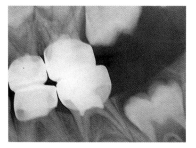

Fig 18-32 Postoperative radiograph of completed procedure.

removal of the coronal portion of the pulp. A stainless steel crown is the restoration of choice.

14. The completed pulpotomy (Fig 18-31) consists of the stainless steel crown, the sub-base of zinc oxide–eugenol, the cementing medium (zinc phosphate cement), and the remaining pulpal tissue.

15. The postoperative radiograph in Fig 18-32 shows pulpotomies, as indicated on all four primary molars, that were restored with stainless steel crowns.

Pulpectomy

Pulpectomy involves complete removal of necrotic pulpal tissue from the root canals and coronal portion of devital primary teeth to maintain a tooth in the dental arch.

The principal roadblock to pulpectomy success is the multiple tortuous root canals in primary teeth (Hibbard and Ireland, 1957). Because of the various morphologic configurations in the primary dentition, mechanical debridement and subsequent filling are difficult.

Another difficulty is the apparent connection between the coronal pulpal floor with the intraradicular area (Moss et al, 1965). These foramina allow necrotic products to pass into the bifurcation or trifurcation area, which is the apparent explanation for the usual occurrence of pathologic conditions in the intraradicular area of primary molars. Using dyes and a vacuum system, Ringelstein and Seow (1989) confirmed the findings of Moss et al. Forty-two percent of 75 extracted primary molars had foramina within the furcation area. There were no differences between primary first and second molars. But many of the foramina on the primary second molars were located on the root surfaces.

Marsh and Largent (1967) indicated pulpectomy procedures should be aimed at reduction of the bacteria in the contaminated pulp. Delay of treatment was condemned. An added problem is the range of different bacteria present in infected primary molars. They cultured 22 primary molars and found 15 different organisms. Streptococci of various types were found in 82% of the cultured teeth. Their opinion was that mechanical cleansing and irrigation are an effective means of reducing the number of bacteria. These data agree with those of a previous study reported by Cohen et al (1960).

In a laboratory setting, Seow (1991) suggested the use of an ultrasound method to biomechanically clean primary teeth prior to filling. A combination of mechanical cleaning and use of ultrasound removed 95% of the test bacteria. If ultrasound is used, caution should be exercised to avoiding overinstrumentation and prevent damage to the developing tooth bud.

Gould (1972) reported on 35 primary molars followed for 7 to 22 months after pulpectomy therapy. Clinically and radiographically, 29 were judged successful. The author did raise several as yet unanswered questions related to the best technique, sequelae to the succedaneous tooth, and long-term effect on the primary tooth itself.

There are few (if any) long-term clinical studies of pulpectomy methods and results in primary teeth. Spedding (1973, 1977), long an advocate, stated, "Once again, empiricism precedes scientific knowledge." Pulpectomies should be limited to primary incisors and primary second molars. Use in the primary incisors should be restricted to children under 4 years of age and use in primary second molars should be ex-

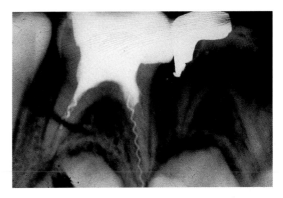

Fig 18-33 Two lentulo spirals broken during a pulpectomy procedure on a primary molar.

cluded after the eruption of the permanent first molar. The primary second molar is needed for the permanent first molar to erupt into its normal relationship. When one is faced with the alternatives of a distal shoe space maintainer, a removable acrylic resin space maintainer, or neglect, pulpectomy for a primary second molar is a positive alternative.

Zinc oxide–eugenol paste has been found to be more effectively bacteriostatic than formocresol, N-2-paste, and other commonly used pulpectomy materials (Cox et al, 1978). The recommendation is to mechanically debride the necrotic pulp. Use formocresol on a pellet for 5 minutes, then fill the canals with noncytotoxic resorbable zinc oxide–eugenol paste.

Placement of formocresol into the pulp canals should be discouraged, nor should ZOE reinforced with formocresol or straight ZOE be used (Coll et al, 1988; Ranly and Garcia-Godoy, 1991). Several studies have endorsed iodoform paste as a biocompatible substitute for the ZOE-formocresol combination (Rifkin, 1980; Garcia-Godoy, 1987). The idoform paste has several advantages:

1. It can be easily forced into the pulp canals and any accessory canals.
2. If any paste is accidentally expressed beyond the apices or foramina, the paste is readily resorbed.
3. Iodoform paste is an ideal pulpectomy agent: It disinfects, is managed well clinically, and resorbs simultaneously with the primary root (Ranly and Garcia-Godoy, 1991).

Condensing the material to fill the torturous canals has been a clinical problem. Aylard and Johnson (1987) evaluated five routinely used methods. Using a standard ZOE mixture, they placed the paste in straight and curved root canal models. The endodontic pressure syringe and the lentulo spiral were best filling the straight models, but the lentulo spiral was superior for the curved canals. A word of caution: because of the extremely curved canals of primary teeth, the lentulo spirals can be broken (Fig 18-33).

For a pulpectomy to be considered a success, any

radiolucent area at the apices of the tooth should be resolved with no accompanying root resorption (O'Riordan and Coll, 1979). If root resorption does occur, the tooth should be removed. Rifkin (1980) treated 45 nonvital primary teeth with a paste material containing p-chlorophenol, camphor, menthol, and iodoform. Using this material, he reported only three failures. A review of pulpectomy methods was reported by Goerig and Camp (1983). Current techniques produce success rates in excess of 90%. Teeth should be periodically recalled for evidence of swelling, ankylosis, or accelerated root resorption. As strong advocates of pulpectomies in primary teeth, Goerig and Camp concluded that there exists little evidence that coronal defects are created by these pulpal procedures in permanent teeth. Tagger and Sarnat (1984) described a two-step pulpectomy procedure, emphasizing debridement of the canals rather than instrumentation. Coll et al (1985) evaluated a one-appointment formocresol pulpectomy procedure. Forty-one pulpectomies were evaluated after an average recall period of 21 months, with 80.5% clinically and radiographically successful. Twenty-nine of the pulpectomies were available for a second evaluation (a mean of 70 months) with a success rate of 86%. Nearly one half of the treated teeth left zinc oxide–eugenol in the sulcus of the succedaneous tooth.

Coll et al (1988) in a retrospective study, reviewed primary incisors, comparing the results of pulpotomies, indirect pulp therapy, and pulpectomies. The teeth, over an 11-year period, were evaluated clinically and radiographically. When success rates of the primary incisors and primary molars were compared, there was not statistically significant difference. After an average follow-up of nearly 4 years, the success rates for the incisors were 86% for pulpotomies, 92% for indirect pulp therapy, and 78% for pulpectomies. Among those incisors treated with pulpectomy, on exfoliation, 73% retained the ZOE material. Again, the suggestion was made to examine iodoform as a legitimate substitute for a restorative material.

In two retrospective studies from the private practice sector, primary anterior and posterior teeth were evaluated for the success of pulpectomies (Flaitz et al, 1989; Barr et al, 1991). Both the primary incisors and the primary molars were filled with a ZOE paste plus formocresol. Pulpectomies in 84% of the primary incisors were judged successful after 37 months. However, 9% of the primary incisors demonstrated incomplete resorption of the restorative paste. After 40 months, treatment was considered successful in 82% of the primary molars.

Indications

1. Traumatized primary incisors with resultant pathologic conditions (in children younger than 4 to 4.5 years)

2. Primary second molars, before eruption of 6-year molars
3. Permanent immature teeth with immature roots
4. No evidence of pathologic conditions, with root resorption not more than two thirds or three fourths completed.

Justification

1. Removal of diseased pulp tissue
2. Space management

Contraindications

1. A tooth that is not restorable
2. Pathologic condition extending to the developing permanent tooth bud
3. Less than two thirds of the primary root structure remaining plus internal or external resorption
4. Internal resorption of the pulp chamber and root canals
5. Chronic illness with leukemia, rheumatic and congenital heart disease, chronic kidney disease, etc.

Disadvantages

1. Microbiology of infected teeth
2. Root canal morphology of primary teeth

Drugs or medicaments

1. Formocresol (20% dilution)
2. Camphorated monochlorophenol (CMCP)
3. Zinc oxide–eugenol, which is resorbable but is irritating to periapical tissue
4. Iodoform paste

Procedure for primary molars

1. A candidate for a pulpectomy procedure is seen in Fig 18-34. There is bifurcation involvement and minimal root resorption, and the permanent first molar has not erupted. Use local anesthesia and isolate with a rubber dam.
2. Prepare a cavity preparation as dictated by carious lesions.
3. Use a large round bur to remove the remaining carious lesions and the debris in the pulp chamber. Be extremely careful not to perforate the floor of the pulp chamber. Check that all coronal pulpal tissue has been removed.
4. After opening the pulp chamber, evaluate the hemorrhage or purulent exudate. If the hemor-

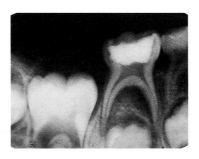

Fig 18-34 A candidate for a pulpectomy.

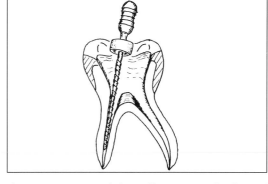

Fig 18-35 Use an endodontic file to remove the diseased pulpal tissue.

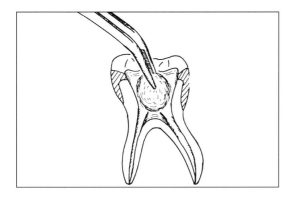

Fig 18-36 Dry the canals with cotton pellets and, if possible, paper points.

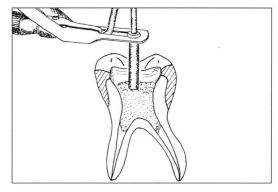

Fig 18-37 Obturate the canals with a ZOE mixture.

rhage is bluish or there is difficulty controlling the bleeding after 5 minutes, the pulp is chronically inflamed. If there is evidence of necrotic tissue breakdown, with accompanying suppuration, a pulpectomy is indicated.

5. With an endodontic file, remove the diseased pulpal tissue from all the canals (Fig 18-35). As the file is being withdrawn, it carries the pulpal material with it. Start with file No. 15 and finish with No. 35. In primary teeth, in contrast to permanent teeth, the filing is done only to remove pulpal tissue, not to enlarge the pulp canals. If a point of resistance is encountered, do not attempt to go beyond this point. Because of the tortuous root canals in the primary dentition, it may be impossible to remove all the remaining tissue. Note: it is not necessary to take a radiograph to determine file length as is done in endodontic procedures for permanent teeth.

6. Irrigate the canals. Dry the canals with cotton pellets and paper points (Fig 18-36). *Never put air directly into a pulp canal.* Repeatedly irrigate the canals. Gently rinse the canals with water, drying with cotton pellets and paper points.

At this point some clinicians recommend application of either formocresol or camphorated monochlorophenol for a period of 5 minutes to 7 days. We prefer to do the treatment procedures in one appointment.

7. If the hemorrhage is controlled and the canals are dry, fill the canals with a zinc oxide–eugenol cement. Mix it on a pad, lift it with an amalgam carrier, and insert it into the pulp chamber (Fig 18-37). The zinc oxide–eugenol cement should not have an accelerator. Zinc oxide is a resorbable material that will allow the tooth to exfoliate. Note: It is recommended not to incorporate formocresol in the zinc oxide–eugenol paste. Iodoform paste is a biocompatible substitute.

8. Use an amalgam plugger and constantly apply pressure to pack the zinc oxide–eugenol cement into the canals. Condensing pressure applied to the mass of zinc oxide–eugenol forces it into the root canals (Fig 18-38).

9. An alternative method is to use a thin mix of zinc oxide–eugenol cement on a file or paper point and place it in the pulp canals. Shape a thick mix of zinc oxide–eugenol in a cone and pack it in the canals (Fig 18-39) using a moist cotton pellet as the condenser.

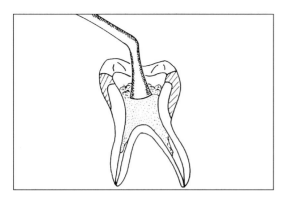

Fig 18-38   Apply constant pressure to the ZOE mixture.

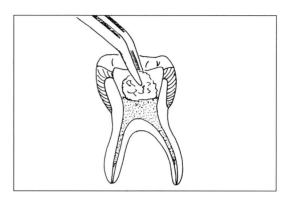

Fig 18-39   An alternative method is to use a moist cotton pellet to condense the mixture.

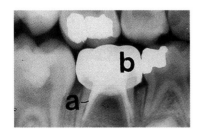

Fig 18-40   *(a)* Completed pulpectomy with *(b)* a stainless steel crown.

10. Obtain a periapical radiograph to be certain that the canals are filled with zinc oxide–eugenol. Because of calcification of the pulp canals, the zinc oxide–eugenol may not reach the apex of the teeth. But these teeth often remain in function until the permanent first molar erupts.
11. A completed pulpectomy procedure includes a zinc oxide–eugenol filled pulp chamber and root canals and a stainless steel crown (Fig 18-40).
12. Place the patient on a periodic recall program to evaluate the success of the procedure. Teeth that are symptom free clinically and radiographically with exfoliation within normal time limits are considered successful.

Procedure for anterior primary teeth

The need for pulpectomies on anterior primary teeth is seen in Fig 18-41. The 3-year-old child's primary central incisors have minimal root resorption. The process is similar to that for primary posterior teeth.

1. Isolate with a rubber dam and open into the pulp chamber with a No. 330 high-speed bur (Fig 18-42).
2. With a No. 15 endodontic file, remove the diseased pulpal tissue. Use as large a file as dictated by the size of the canal. A rubber stopper is used as a marker (Fig 18-43).
3. Irrigate the canal gently with a solution of sodium hypochlorite (Fig 18-44).
4. Dry the canal with paper points and cotton pellets (Fig 18-45).
5. Use a thick mix of zinc oxide–eugenol cement in the canal (Fig 18-46). A large endodontic condensor or amalgam plugger is applied to pack the cement up the canal. Again, the zinc oxide–eugenol cement does not have an accelerator. To check the success of the procedure, obtain a periapical radiograph. Again, iodoform is a recommended substitute.
6. Restore with a restoration such as a stainless steel crown or composite resin crown. The completed procedure is seen in Fig 18-47. The zinc oxide–eugenol paste has been condensed to the apices of the central incisors. The teeth should be evaluated periodically for normal exfoliation.
7. Spedding (1973) has recommended use of a pressure syringe to inject the zinc oxide material into the canals. A tin mix of the material is injected into the canals, followed by condensation of a thicker mix with a suitable instrument.

Table 18-8 summarizes the concepts of pulp therapy for children.

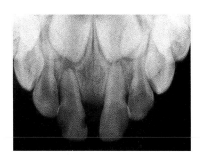

Fig 18-41 Anterior primary teeth that are candidates for pulpectomy procedure.

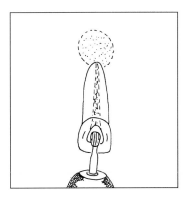

Fig 18-42 Open the tooth with a No. 330 bur.

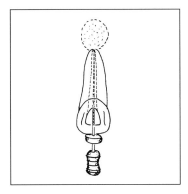

Fig 18-43 Use an endodontic file to remove the pulp tissue.

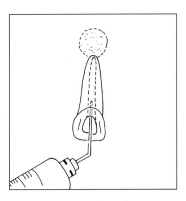

Fig 18-44 Irrigate the tooth.

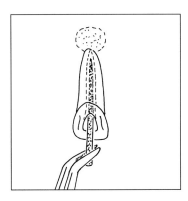

Fig 18-45 Dry the canal with paper points.

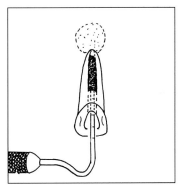

Fig 18-46 Condense a thick mix of paste in the

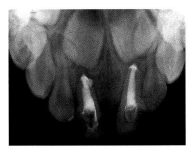

Fig 18-47 Completed pulpectomy procedure.

Table 18-8   Summary of pulp treatment

Procedure	Indications	Materials	Restoration
	Primary incisors		

Pulpotomy	Vital pulp
	Carious, mechanical or traumatic
	  exposure
	Tooth lacks mobility
	Has normal root length
	No periapical or soft tissue lesions
	Hemorrhage controllable
		Zinc oxide–eugenol
		Formocresol
			Composite resin
			Complete crown: Stainless
			  steel, open-faced

Pulpectomy	Nonvital pulp with discomfort History of trauma Evidence of apical root resorption Periapical lesion Hemorrhage lacking or uncontrollable Purulent exudate Patient younger than 4.5 y	Sodium hypochlorite Formocresol Zinc oxide–eugenol Iodoform paste	Composite resin Complete crown: Stainless steel, open-faced

Extraction	Nonvital tooth
	Extensive root resorption internal or
	  external
	Large periapical and soft tissue lesions
	Patient older than 4.5 y
			No space maintainer
			  needed

	Primary molars		
Pulpotomy	Vital pulp Carious or mechanical pulp exposure Tooth lacks mobility Normal root length Controllable hemorrhage No periapical or soft tissue lesions Lack of calcific degeneration	Formocresol Zinc oxide–eugenol	Stainless steel crown

Pulpectomy	Primary first molar before the second
	  primary molar erupts
	Primary second molar
	  (patient 6 y or younger)
	History of pain
	Evidence of root resorption (two thirds
	  of root left)
	Hemorrhage lacking or uncontrollable
	Purulent and putrescent exudate
	Tooth mobile
	Periapical lesion
		Sodium hypochlorite
		Zinc oxide–eugenol
		Iodoform paste
			Stainless steel crown

Extraction	Primary first molar if primary second molar is present Extensive resorption Nonrestorable tooth		Space maintainer
	Permanent molars		

Indirect pulp cap	Radiographic evidence of a probable
	  carious exposure
	Pain when eating sweets
	Nonmobile
	No gingival or periapical pathosis
		Calcium hydroxide
		Zinc oxide–eugenol
			Silver amalgam or
			  stainless steel crown

Direct pulp cap	Mechanical exposure (less than 1 mm) Hemorrhage controllable	Calcium hydroxide	Silver amalgam
Pulpotomy	Vital tooth Carious exposure Normal root development Economic factors Normal periapical tissue	Formocresol	Silver amalgam or stainless steel crown
Extraction	Nonrestorable tooth		Space maintainer

References

Aponte, A. J., Hartsook, J. T., and Crowley, M. C. Indirect pulp capping success verified. J. Dent. Child. 33:164, 1966.

Armstrong, R. L., et al. Comparison of Dycal and formocresol pulpotomies in young permanent teeth in monkeys. Oral Surg. 48:160, 1979.

Aylard, S. R., and Johnson, R. Assessment of filling techniques for primary teeth. Pediatr. Dent. 9:195, 1987.

Barr, E. S., Flaitz, C. M., and Hicks, M. J. A retrospective radiographic evaluation of primary molar pulpectomies. Pediatr. Dent. 13:4, 1991.

Beaver H. A., Kopel, H. M., and Sabes, W. R. The effect of zinc oxide–eugenol cement on a formocresolized pulp. J. Dent. Child. 33:381, 1966.

Berger, J. E. An evaluation of the effects of formocresol on the pulps of human primary molars following pulpotomies. Thesis. Ann Arbor: University of Michigan School of Dentistry, 1963.

Besic, F. C. Fate of bacteria sealed in dental cavities. J. Dent. Res. 22:349, 1943.

Block, R. M. et al. Cell-mediated immune response to dog pulp tissue altered by formocresol within the root canal. J. Endod. 3:424, 1977.

Block, R. M., et al. Systemic distribution of [14 C]-labeled paraformaldehyde incorporated within formocresol following pulpotomies in dogs. J. Endod. 9:176, 1983.

Chiniwalla, N. P., and Rapp, R. The effect of pulpotomy using formocresol on blood vessels architecture in primary anterior teeth of macaca rhesus monkeys. J. Endod. 8:205, 1982.

Cohen, M. M., Jaress, S. M., and Calisti, L. P. Bacteriologic study of infected deciduous molars. Oral Surg. 13:1382, 1960.

Coll, J. A., et al. An evaluation of pulpal therapy in primary incisors. Pediatr. Dent. 10:178, 1988.

Coll, J. A., Josell, S., and Casper, J. S. Evaluation of one-appointment formocresol pulpectomy technique for primary molars. Pediatr. Dent. 7:123, 1985.

Cox, S. T., Hembree, J. H., and McKnight, J. P. The bactericidal potential of various endodontic materials for primary teeth. Oral Surg. 45:947, 1978.

Davis, M. J., Myers, R., and Switkes, M. D. Glutaraldehyde: An alternative to formocresol for vital pulpotomy. J. Dent. Child. 49:176, 1982.

Dilley, G. J., and Courts, D. J. Immunological response to four pulpal medicaments. Pediatr. Dent. 3:179, 1981.

Dimaggio, J. J., and Hawes, R. R. Continued evaluation of direct and indirect pulp capping IADR abstract No. 4138, 1963.

Doyle, W. A., MacDonald, R. E., and Mitchell, D. F. Formocresol versus calcium hydroxide in pulpotomy. J. Dent. Child. 29:86, 1962.

Eidelman, E., Ulmansky, M., and Michaeli, Y. Histopathology of the pulp in primary incisors with deep dentinal caries. Pediatr. Dent. 14:372, 1992.

Fei, A., Udin, R. D., and Johnson, R. A clinical study of ferric sulfate as a pulpotomy agent in primary teeth. Pediatr. Dent. 13:327, 1991.

Fiskio, H. M. Pulpotomies in vital and non-vital permanent teeth J. Acad. Gen. Dent. 22:27, 1974.

Flaitz, C. M., Barr, E. S., and Hicks, M. J. Radiographic evaluation of pulpal therapy for primary anterior teeth. J. Dent. Child. 56:182, 1989.

Frank, A. L., Abou-Rass, M., and Glick, D. H. Changing trends in endodontics. J. Am. Dent. Assoc. 96:202, 1978.

Fuks, A. B., and Bimstein, E. Clinical evaluation of diluted formocresol pulpotomies in primary teeth of school children. Pediatr. Dent. 3:321, 1981.

Fuks, A. B., Bimstein, E., and Breechin, A. Radiological and histological evaluation of the effect of two concentrations of formocresol on pulpotomized primary and young permanent teeth in monkeys. Pediatr. Dent. 5:9, 1983.

Fuks, A. B., Bimstein, E., and Klein, H. Assessment of a 2% buffered glutaraldehyde solution in pulpotomized primary teeth of school children: A preliminary report. J. Pedod. 10:323, 1986a.

Fuks, A. B., Bimstein, E., and Michaeli, Y. Glutaraldehyde as a pulp dressing after pulpotomy in primary teeth of baboon monkeys. Pediatr. Dent. 8:32, 1986b.

Fuks, A. B., et al. Pulp response to collagen and glutaraldehyde in pulpotomized primary teeth of baboons. Pediatr. Dent. 13:142, 1991.

Fulton, R., and Ranly, D. M. An autoradiographic study of formocresol pulpotomies in rat molars using 3-H formaldehyde. J. Endod. 5:71, 1979.

Garcia-Godoy, F. Penetration and pulpal response by two concentrations of formocresol using two methods of application. J. Pedod. 6:102, 1981.

Garcia-Godoy, F. A comparison between zinc oxide–eugenol and polycarboxylate cements on formocresol pulpotomies. J. Pedod. 7:203, 1982.

Garcia-Godoy, F. Clinical evaluation of glutaraldehyde pulpotomies in primary teeth. Acta Odontol. Pediatr. 4:41, 1983.

Garcia-Godoy, F. Direct pulp capping and partial pulpotomy with diluted formocresol in primary molars. Acta Ordontol. Pediatr. 5:57, 1984.

Garcia-Godoy, F. Evaluation of an iodoform paste in root canal therapy for infected teeth. J. Dent. Child. 54:30, 1987.

Garcia-Godoy, F. Novakonic, D. P., and Carvajal, I.P. Pulpal response to different application times of formocresol. J. Pedod. 7:176, 1982.

Goerig, A. C., and Camp, J. H. Root canal treatment in primary teeth: A review. Pediatr. Dent 5:33, 1983.

Gould, J. M. Root canal therapy for infected primary molar teeth—Preliminary report. J. Dent. Child. 39:269, 1972.

Hargraves, J. A. A histopathological study following mortal amputation in seven deciduous teeth. Odontol. Rev. 10:351, 1959.

Harris, S. A preliminary histologic investigation of three amputation techniques with formocresol pulpotomies on normal primary teeth. Thesis. Los Angeles: University of Southern California, 1969.

Hawes, R. P., DiMaggio, J., and Soyegh, F. Evaluation of direct and indirect pulp capping. J. Dent. Res. 43:808, 1963.

Heilig, J., et al. Calcium hydroxide pulpotomy for primary teeth. J. Am. Dent. Assoc. 108:775, 1984.

Hernandez Pereyra J. R., deTello, H., Colafell, C. R. Clinical and radiographic evaluation of formocresol and glutaraldehyde pulpotomies in permanent teeth. Acta. Odontol. Pediatr. 8:59, 1987.

Hibbard, E. D., and Ireland, R. L. Morphology of root canals of the primary teeth. J. Dent. Child. 24:250, 1957.

Hicks, M. J., Barr, E. S., and Flaitz, C. M. Formocresol pulpotomies in primary molars: A radiographic study in a pediatric dentistry practice. J. Pedod. 10:331, 1986.

Hutchins, D. W., and Parker, W. A. Indirect pulp capping: Clinical evaluation using polymethyl methacrylate. J. Dent. Child. 39:55, 1972.

Jeng, H. W., Feigal, R. J., and Messer, H. H. Comparison of the cytotoxicity of formocresol, formaldehyde, and cresol, and glutaraldehyde using human pulp fibroblast cultures. Pediatr. Dent. 9:295, 1987.

Jepperson, K. Direct pulp capping on primary teeth—A long term investigation. J. Int. Assoc. Dent. Child. 2:10, 1971.

Jerrell, R. G., Courts, F. J., and Stanley, H. R. A comparison of two calcium hydroxide agents in direct pulp capping of primary teeth. J. Dent. Child. 51:34, 1984.

Johnson, D. C., Harshberger, J., and Nash, D. A. Vitalometer testing of primary and permanent canine teeth. Pediatr. Dent. 1:27, 1979.

Karp, W. B. Korb. P., Pashley, D. H. The oxidation of glutaraldelyde by rat tissues, Ped. Dent. 9:301, 1987.

Kerhove, B. C., et al. A clinical and television densitometric evaluation of the indirect pulp capping technique. J. Dent. Child. 34:992, 1967.

King, J. B., Jr. Crawford, J. J., and Lindahl, R. L. Indirect pulp capping: A bacteriological study of deep carious dentine in human teeth. Oral Surg. 20:663, 1965.

Kopel, H. M., et al. The effects of glutaraldehyde on primary pulp tissue following coronal amputation: An in vivo histological study. J. Dent. Child. 47:425, 1980.

Lazzari, E. P., and Ranly, D. M., and Walker, W. A. Biochemical effects of formocresol on bovine pulp tissue. Oral Surg. 45:796, 1978.

Lekka, M., Hume, W. R., and Wolensky, L. E. Comparison between formaldehyde and glutaraldehyde diffusion through the root tissues of pulpotomy-treated teeth. J. Pedod. 8:185, 1984.

Lewis, B. B., and Chester, S. B. Formaldehyde in dentistry: A review of mutagenic and carcinogenic potential. J. Am. Dent. Assoc. 103:429, 1981.

Loos, P. J., Straffon, L. H., and Han, S. S. Biological effects of formocresol. J. Dent. Child. 40:193, 1973.

Magnusson, B. Attempts to predict prognosis of pulpotomy in primary molars. Scand. J. Dent. Res. 78:232, 1970.

Magnusson, B. Therapeutic pulpotomies in primary molars with formocresol technique. Acta Odontol. Scand. 36:113, 1978.

Marsh, S. J., and Largent, M. D. A bacteriological study of the pulp canals of infected primary molars. J. Dent. Child. 34:460, 1967.

Mejare, I. Pulpotomy of primary molars with coronal or total pulpitis using formocresol technique. Scand. J. Dent. Res. 87:208, 1979.

Majare, I. Hasselgren, G., and Hammarstrom, L. E. Effect of formaldehyde-containing drugs on human dental pulp evaluated by enzyme histochemical technique. Scand. J. Dent. Res. 84:29, 1976.

Messer, L. B., Cline, J. J., and Korf, N. W. Long term effects of primary molar pulpotomies on succedaneous bicuspids. J. Dent. Res. 59:116, 1980.

Morawa, A., Straffon, H., and Corpron, R. Clinical evaluation of pulpotomies using dilute formocresol. J. Dent. Child. 42:360, 1975.

Moss, S. J., Addelston, R., and Goldsmith, E. D. Histologic study of pulpal floors of deciduous molars. J. Am. Dent. Assoc. 70:372, 1965.

Myers, D. R. et al. Tissue changes induced by the absorption of formocresol from pulpotomy sites in dogs. Pediatr. Dent. 5:6, 1983.

Myers, D. R., et al. Systemic absorption of 14 c-glutaraldehyde from glutaraldehyde treated pulpotomy sites. Pediatr. Dent. 8:134, 1986.

Myers, D. R., et al Histopathology of furcation lesions associated with pulp degeneration in primary molars. Pediatr. Dent. 9:279, 1987.

Mulder, G. R., van Amerogen, W. E., and Vingerling, P. A. Consequences of endodontic treatment of primary teeth. Part II. A clinical investigation into the influences of formocresol pulpotomy of the permanent successor. J. Dent. Child. 54:35, 1987.

Nirschi, R. F., and Avery, D. B. Evaluation of a new pulp capping agent in indirect pulp therapy. J. Dent. Child. 50:25, 1983.

Nordstrom, D. O., Wei, S. H. and Johnson, R. Use of stannous fluoride for indirect pulp capping. J. Am. Dent. Assoc. 88:997, 1974.

O'Riordan, M. W., and Coll, J. Pulpectomy procedure for deciduous teeth with severe pulpal necrosis. J. Am. Dent. Assoc. 99:480, 1979.

Pashley, L. L., et al. Systemic distribution of 14 C-formaldehyde from formocresol-treated pulpotomy sites. J. Dent. Res. 59:603, 1980.

Pruhs, R. J., Olen, G. A., and Sharma, P. S. Relationship between formocresol pulpotomies on primary teeth and enamel defects on their permanent successors. J. Am. Dent. Assoc. 94:698, 1977.

Ramos, D. L., et al. The effects of formocresol and glutaraldehyde on rat pulp respiration. J. Dent. Child. 38:114, 1980.

Ranly, D. M., A comparative study of the effects of formaldehyde, glutaraldehyde, and dimethylsuberimimidate on enzyme activity in the bovine dental pulp. Acta Odontol. Rev. 5:5, 1984.

Ranly, D. M., and Fulton, R. Reaction of rat molar pulp tissue to formocresol, formaldehyde, and cresol. J. Endod. 2:176, 1976.

Ranly, D. M., and Fulton, R. An autoradiographic study of the response of rat molar pulp to formocresol using 3H-thymidine. Pediatr. Dent. 5:20, 1983.

Ranly, D. M., and Garcia-Godoy, F. Reviewing pulp treatment for primary teeth. J. Am. Dent. Assoc. 122:83, 1991.

Ranly, D. M., and Lazzari, E. P. A biochemical study of bifunctional reagents as alternative to formocresol. J. Dent. Res. 52:1054, 1983.

Ranly, D. M., Garcia-Godoy, F., and Horn, D. Time, concentration, and PH parameters for the use of glutaraldehyde as a pulpotomy agent: An in vitro study. Pediatr. Dent. 9:199, 1987.

Ranly, D. M., Horn, D., and Hubbard, G. B. Assessment of the systemic distribution and toxicity of glutaraldehyde as a pulpotomy agent. Pediatr. Dent. 11:8, 1989.

Rayner, J. A., and Southerns, R. Pulp changes in deciduous teeth associated with deep carious dentine. Int. J. Dent. 7:39, 1979.

Redig, D. F. A comparison and evaluation of two formocresol pulpotomy techniques utilizing Buckley's formocresol. J. Dent. Child. 35:22, 1968.

Rifkin, A. A simple, effective, safe technique for the root canal treatment of abscessed primary teeth. J. Dent. Child. 47:435, 1980.

Ringelstein, D., and Seow, W. K. The prevalence of furcation foramina in primary molars. Pediatr. Dent. 11:198, 1989.

Rolling, I., and Lamjerg-Hansen, H. Pulp condition of successfully formocresol-treated primary molars. Scand. J. Dent. Res. 86:267, 1978.

Rolling I., and Paulsen, S. Formocresol pulpotomy of primary teeth and occurrence of enamel defects on the permanent successors. Acta Odontol. Scand. 36:243, 1978.

Rolling, I., and Thystrup, A. A 3-year clinical follow-up study of pulpotomized primary molars treated with the formocresol technique. Scand. J. Dent. Res. 83:47, 1975.

Rothman, M. S. Formocresol pulpotomy: A practical procedure for permanent teeth. Gen. Dent. 25:39, 1977.

Ruemping, D. R., Morton, T. H., Jr., and Anderson, M. W. Electrosurgical pulpotomy in primates—A comparison with formocresol pulpotomy. Pediatr. Dent. 5:14, 1983.

Rusmah, M., and Rahim, Z. H. A. Diffusion of buffered glutaraldehyde and formocresol from pulpotomized primary teeth. J. Dent. Child. 59:108, 1992.

Schroder, U. A 2 year follow-up of primary molar pulpotomies with a gentle technique and capped with calcium hydroxide. Scand. J. Dent. Res. 86:273, 1978.

Schwartz, E. A. Formocresol vital pulpotomy on permanent dentition. J. Can. Dent. Assoc. 46:570, 1980.

Seow, W. K. Comparison of ultrasonic and mechanical cleaning of primary root canals using a novel radiometric method. Pediatr. Dent. 13:136, 1991.

Seow, W. K., and Thong, Y. H. Modulation of polymorphonuclear leukocyte adherence by pulpotomy medicaments: effects of fromocresol, glutaraldehyde, eugenol, and calcium hydroxide. Pediatr. Dent. 8:16, 1986.

Shulman, E. R., McIver, F. T., and Burkes, E. J., Jr. Comparison of electrosurgery and formocresol as pulpotomy techniques in monkey primary teeth. Pediatr. Dent. 9:189, 1987.

Spedding, R. H., Root canal treatments for primary teeth. Dent Clin. North Am. 17:105, 1973.

Spedding, R. H. Endodontic treatment of primary molars. In Goldman, H. M., et al. Current Therapy in Dentistry. vol. 6 St. Louis: The C. V. Mosby Co., 1977.

Stark, M. M., et al. The localization of radioactive calcium hydroxide Ca45 over exposed pulps in rhesus monkey teeth: A preliminary report. J. Oral Ther. 1:290, 1964.

Sweet, C. A. Procedure for treatment of exposed and pulpless deciduous teeth. J. Am. Dent. Assoc. 16:1150, 1930.

Tagger, E., and Sarnat, H. Root canal therapy in infected primary teeth. Acta Odontol. Pediatr. 5:64, 1984.

Teplitsky, P. E. Formocresol pulpotomies on posterior permanent teeth. J. Can. Dent Assoc. 50:623, 1984.

Trask, P. A. Formocresol pulpotomy on (young) permanent teeth. J. Am. Dent. Assoc. 85:1316, 1972.

van Amerongen, W. E., Mulder, G. R., and Vingerling, P. A. Consequences of endodontic treatment in primary teeth. Part I. A clinical and radiographic study of the influence of formocresol pulpotomy on the life-span of primary molars. J. Dent. Child. 53:364, 1986.

Via, W. F., Jr. Evaluation of deciduous molars treated by pulpotomy and calcium hydroxide. J. Am. Dent. Assoc. 50:34, 1955.

Willard, R. M. Radiographic changes following formocresol pulpotomy in primary molars. J. Dent. Child. 43:414, 1976.

Wright, F. A. and Widmer, R. P. Pulpal therapy in primary molar teeth: A retrospective study. J. Pedod. 1195, 1979.

Additional readings

Feigal, R. J., and Messer, H. H. A critical look at glutaraldehyde. Pediatr. Dent. 12:69, 1980.

Flaitz, C. M., Barr, E. S., and Hicks, M. J. Radiographic evaluation of pulpal treatment for anterior primary teeth in a pediatric dentistry practice. Pediatr. Dent. 9:171, 1987.

Lazzari, E. P., and Ranly, D. M. The effects of formocresol on rat sponge implant tissue: A biochemical study. J. Dent. Res. 56:1027, 1977.

Magnusson, B. Pulpotomy in primary molars: A long-term clinical and histological evaluation. Int. Endod. J. 13:143, 1980.

Majare, I. Pulpotomy of primary molars with coronal or total pulpitis using formocresol technique. Scand. J. Dent. Res. 87:208, 1979.

Myers, D. R., et al. Distribution of 14C-formaldehyde after pulpotomy with formocresol. J. Am. Dent. Assoc. 96:805, 1978.

Ranly, D. M. Glutaraldehyde purity and stability: Implications for preparation, storage, and use as a pulpotomy agent. Pediatr. Dent. 6:83, 1984.

Ranly, D. M., and Garcia-Godoy, F. The diffusion of glutaraldehyde from zinc oxide–eugenol cement. Pediatr. Dent. 7:215, 1985.

Ranly, E. M., and Lazzari, E. P. The formocresol pulpotomy—The past, present, and the future. J. Pedod. 2:115, 1978.

Ranly, D. M., Montgomery, E. H., and Pope, H. O. The loss of 3H-formaldehyde from zinc oxide–eugenol cement—An in vitro study. J. Dent. Child. 42:128, 1975.

Straffon, L. H., and Han, S. S. The effect of formocresol on hamster connective tissue cells, a histologic and quantitative radioautographic study with proline-H. Arch. Oral Biol. 13:271, 1968.

Sun, H. W., Feigal, R. J., and Messer, H. H. Cytotoxicity of glutaraldehyde and formaldehyde in relation to time of exposure and concentration. Pediatr. Dent. 12:303, 1990.

Tagger, E., and Tagger, M. Pulpal and periapical reactions to glutaraldehyde and paraformaldehyde pulpotomy dressing in monkeys. J. Endod. 10:364, 1984.

Verco, P. J. W. Microbiological effectiveness of a reduced concentration of Buckley's formocresol. Pediatr. Dent. 7:130, 1985.

Wemes, J. C., Voldkamp, D. F., and Lewis, P. D. Glutaraldehyde of endodontic therapy: Philosophy and practice. J. Dent 11:63, 1983.

Questions

1. Despite excellent operative skills, you mechanically expose the mesiobuccal pulp horn (we told you so!) on the primary maxillary first molar. The carious lesion on the mesial and distal surfaces is moderate, the treatment now should be:

   a. Pulp capping with Dycal; restore with silver amalgam

   b. Pulpotomy; restore with a stainless steel crown

   c. Pulpectomy; restore the a stainless steel crown

   d. Pulp capping with Dycal; restore with a stainless steel crown

   e. Extraction and a space maintainer

2. A 5 year old, new to your office, has recurrent carious lesions under an occlusal amalgam restoration on the primary mandibular left second molar. There is a slight mobility but no history of pain. The radiograph shows a probable pulpal exposure. The primary first molar has been extracted previously. The treatment plan should be:

   a. Probable pulpotomy and stainless steel crown

   b. Indirect pulp therapy and silver amalgam restoration

   c. Pulpotomy and stainless steel crown with a fixed space maintainer

   d. Pulpectomy and stainless steel crown

   e. Extraction and removable space maintainer

3. The parent of a 7-year-old boy calls for an emergency appointment. The chief complaint is that a permanent mandibular first molar hurts when "I eat a Twinkie." Clinically, there is a large carious lesion, but surrounding tissues are normal. The radiograph reveals the carious lesion almost into the pulp, with the periapical areas normal. The pulp treatment for the tooth should be:

   a. Calcium hydroxide pulpotomy

   b. Formocresol pulpotomy

   c. Pulpectomy

   d. Direct pulp cap with Dycal

   e. Indirect pulp therapy with Dycal and a zinc oxide–eugenol cement

4. A 4-year-old girl is seen in your office with a history of trauma to the maxillary central incisors. One is discolored and black. The radiographs shows a small periapical area but no internal or external resorption. Clinically, the tooth is slightly mobile, but the soft tissue around the tooth is normal. The tooth ideally should be treatment planned for:

   a. Pulpectomy with zinc oxide–eugenol and a composite restoration

   b. Pulpotomy with formocresol and a composite restoration

   c. Pulp cap and a composite resin restoration

   d. Extraction only

   e. Extraction with space maintainer

5. The radiographs of a 4-year-old boy reveal a primary mandibular second molar with a bifurcation radiolucency. The roots appear to be normal. There is an obvious carious exposure. Opening the tooth reveals a purulent exudate in the pulp chamber with minimal hemorrhage. The treatment of choice is:

   a. Pulpectomy, root canal therapy, and stainless steel crown

   b. Removal of the tooth

   c. Opening the tooth, draining it, and using the tooth as an untreated space maintainer

   d. Pulpotomy with calcium hydroxide

   e. Pulpotomy with formocresol

Chapter 19

Trauma to Anterior Teeth

Objectives

After studying this chapter, the student should be able to:
1. Recognize the treatment indicated for various dental injuries to anterior teeth.
2. Examine means of preventing dental injury.
3. Appraise a fractured incisor using the patient's history, clinical examination, and radiographs.
4. Choose and employ appropriate treatment for dental injuries.
5. Recognize the typical factors associated with fractures of incisors.
6. Fabricate a splinting device for avulsed teeth.
7. Explain the importance of mouth guards for preventing dental injuries associated with traumas of the face and jaw.
8. Fabricate a mouth guard from an impression of the dental arch.
9. Evaluate stained permanent incisors, and where indicated, recommend appropriate methods for esthetic improvement.

Diagnosis and Assessment

The dentist should determine:
1. Time of injury and subsequent arrival for care; The results of treatment are highly dependent on the time elapsed.
2. The cause of the injury.
3. Where the injury occurred to determine need for a booster tetanus injection.
4. Whether the trauma was severe enough to cause other medical problems, such as headaches, vomiting, or other symptoms of head trauma.
5. What stimuli cause response in the injured area—thermal, percussion, or chemical.

Clinical examination

1. Visually observe the extent of the fracture to determine whether the pulp is exposed, whether there is soft tissue laceration, and whether teeth have been avulsed or displaced.
2. Take indicated radiographs of the fractured tooth, the adjacent teeth, and the opposing arch.
3. *Gently* palpate the surrounding tissue and teeth to check mobility, firmness, or loose alveolar bone.
4. Do not perform vitality tests at the initial appointment; they may be considered at subsequent visits.

Radiographic examination

Radiographs of excellent quality are a requirement for traumatized anterior teeth. They should be taken longitudinally to evaluate either the progress or the deterioration of the healing process. The radiographs should be evaluated for:

1. Root fracture.
2. Any fracture of supporting alveolar bone.
3. Proximity of the pulp tissue to the fracture.
4. Root maturity.

Direct trauma to primary anterior teeth

1. The most common age for fractures to primary anterior teeth is 1.5 to 2.5 years of age, when the child is learning to walk.
2. Displacement, not fracture, is the most common injury in the primary dentition.
3. Traumatic injuries to primary teeth should be examined as soon as possible to assess the extent of the damage.
4. The primary teeth should be examined for fractured enamel, damage to the opposing teeth, and pulpal trauma.

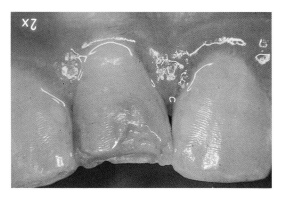

Fig 19-1 Localized enamel hypoplasia caused by trauma to the primary dentition.

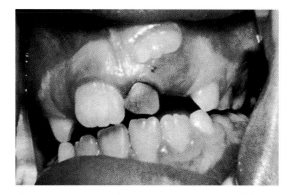

Fig 19-2 Overretained primary incisors can cause delays in eruption of permanent incisors.

5. Trauma to primary teeth often results in discoloration. The color indicates the response of the pulp to the trauma:

   a. A yellowish color indicates a calcific reaction that can result in complete calcification of the canal, known sometimes as an *endogenous root canal*. Treatment is observation for normal exfoliation.

   b. A blue-black color indicates degeneration of the pulp. Treatment should be either extraction or a pulpectomy to prevent damage to the developing permanent tooth bud.

6. Root fractures seldom occur in the primary dentition, but are possible. Extraction is the treatment of choice.

7. Displacement is treated:

   a. By repositioning and splinting, if the displacement is buccal or lingual with extreme mobility.

   b. By allowing the tooth (or teeth) to reerupt, if the tooth is intruded.

   c. By observation, if the involved tooth (teeth) is slightly mobile. In all of these situations, the tooth should be observed for subsequent color changes in the enamel.

8. If the tooth is completely avulsed, reimplantation is not a consideration. If the child is not in the complete primary dentition, a space maintainer may be indicated. Several types are available (see Chapter 17).

Sequelae to the developing permanent teeth

Injury to the primary dentition may cause obvious disturbances in the developing permanent dentition. The primary teeth, because of their close proximity to the permanent tooth buds, can transmit an injury to the permanent tooth buds (Fig 19-1).

Localized enamel hypoplasia caused during formation of a permanent tooth resulting from trauma to the preceding primary tooth is often referred to as *Turner's hypoplasia*, Turner being the first to describe the enamel defect. The defect shown in Fig 19-1 is a sequela of chronic inflammation or direct intrusion of the primary lateral incisor, whose apex was once labial to the developmental crypt of this permanent lateral incisor during formation. Thus, during critical periods of enamel deposition, the labial surface is particularly vulnerable to disturbances created by the overlying primary tooth. Treatment is restoration with a composite resin material.

Andreasen (1981) has classified these sequelae as follows:

1. *White or yellow-brown discoloration of enamel.* These discolorations are small to large opacities of hypocalcification in enamel. They are thought to be caused by periapical inflammation. The pH change evidently interferes with the maturation stage of enamel (also known as *Turner's tooth*).

2. *White or yellow-brown discoloration of enamel hypoplasia.* The findings with this type of hypoplasia show a horizontal indentation encircling the tooth. It is usually the result of intrusion of the primary incisor at age 2 years. It is a defect in enamel matrix formation.

3. *Crown dilaceration.* Malformed crowns occur in about 3% of injuries to the primary dentition. The trauma occurs at the time when the crown has been one half completed.

4. *Odontomalike malformations.* It is rarely seen, but seems to be a result of trauma. Radiographs will reveal a mass of hard tissue.

5. *Root dilaceration.* Root dilaceration appears as a marked curvature of the root portion. It usually involves permanent central incisors.

6. *Disturbances in eruption.* When primary incisors are lost prematurely, there is a delay in eruption of the permanent incisors, especially when the primary incisors are lost in younger children. Primary teeth that have calcified root canals may be overretained. These teeth can cause the permanent incisors to erupt lingually or labially (Fig 19-2). Treatment is extraction and orthodontic care.

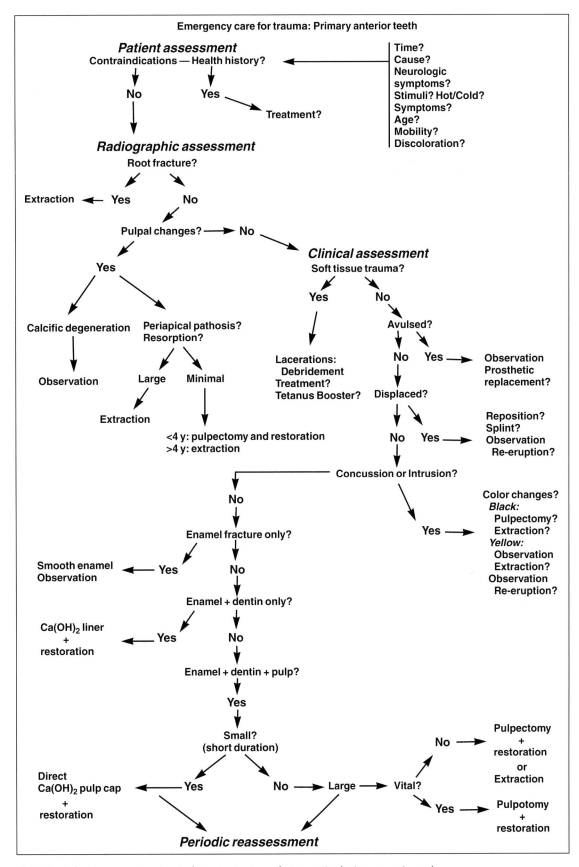

Fig 19-3   A decision-support system to determine treatment for traumatized primary anterior teeth.

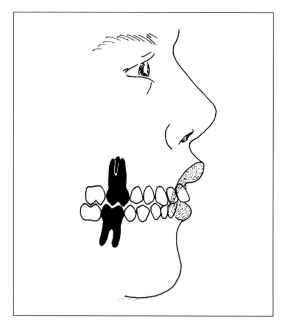

Fig 19-4 Children with Class II malocclusions are more prone to fractures.

Andreasen and Ravn (1971) evaluated 213 permanent teeth with a history of trauma to the primary incisors. They found 41% of the permanent teeth had a developmental disturbance. In the same study, they found a direct relationship with the severity of the injury, with intrusion resulting in a 69% disturbance to the underlying succedaneous teeth. Another factor is that the younger the child, the greater the chance of a developmental disturbance. Under age 2, there is a 63% chance of developmental disturbances.

Brin et al (1984) and Basset et al (1985) examined children who had experienced trauma to the primary teeth. They attempted to correlate the type of injury and the age of the patient when the injury occurred to defects observed on the permanent teeth. They found that patients with Class II malocclusions were prone to trauma. Trauma before age 5 was found to result in more defects of enamel mineralization, which were located in the incisal one third of the succedaneous permanent tooth. Intrusion with subsequent exfoliation was followed by discoloration and hypoplasia.

The effect of premature loss of primary teeth and the resultant effect on speech development was evaluated by Riekman and El Badrawry (1985) Fourteen children had primary maxillary incisors extracted because of rampant caries (nursing bottle caries). Using standard speech evaluation methods, they found four children to have some speech distortions, two severe. The other 10 children had normal speech patterns. They concluded that:

1. The premature loss of primary teeth does not have a long-term effect on speech development.
2. The younger the child is at the time of extraction, the greater the tendency for speech discrepancies.
3. Boys seem to be more prone to speech disharmonies.

Figure 19-3 is intended to assist the decision-making process for treatment of traumatized primary anterior teeth.

Treatment and restorations of permanent anterior teeth

Prevalence of dental injuries

1. In the primary dentition, it has been estimated that 54% of children aged 6 years or younger will have an injury to their anterior teeth.
2. In the permanent dentition, roughly 5% of children may have trauma to the anterior teeth.
3. The maxillary central incisors are most often involved.
4. Boys, aged 10 to 11, are the most susceptible group.
5. Figure 19-4 shows a fracture-prone profile (skeletal Class II malocclusion). Children with protruding anterior teeth have twice as many fractures as do children with other occlusions.
6. With the increased emphasis on recognition of the battered child, it has been noted that facial lacerations and trauma occur in roughly 50% of children who have been abused.

Meadows et al (1984) reviewed more than 300 cases of trauma to anterior teeth during a 1-year period. They concluded that the prime causes of trauma were falls of various types, and bicycles and sports were the major culprits. The greatest frequencies occurred in September, when school reopened.

Treatment of coronal fractures

Class I fracture (Fig 19-5)

Class I fractures involve enamel only.

1. Initial appointment should include:
   a. History of trauma
   b. Radiographs of affected, adjacent, and opposing teeth.
   c. Restoration: *(1)* smooth rough edges or *(2)* acid-etch composite resin restoration

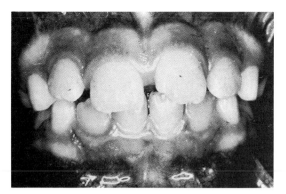

Fig 19-5 Class I fractures involve enamel only.

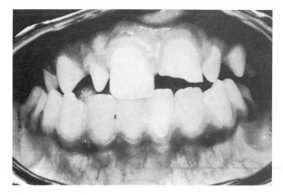

Fig 19-6 A Class II fracture involves both enamel and dentin.

d. Advice to parents that even though a fracture is minimal, there is always the chance that the tooth may become devital.
2. The patient should be recalled in 2 weeks for a brief check of any alterations in color or sensitivity of the tooth.
3. Any color change should be noted in the tooth. If there is a color change, the treatment needed must be reevaluated.

Class II fracture (Fig 19-6)

Class II fractures involve the enamel and dentin.

1. Initial appointment should include:
    a. History of trauma.
    b. Radiographs of affected, adjacent, and opposing teeth.
    c. Covering of the dentinal tubules with a calcium hydroxide preparation because of dentin exposure. It has been shown experimentally that the pulp has a dramatic increase in an inflammatory response if dentin is left exposed to bacteria (Brännström, 1960). The dentinal tubules serve as a direct route for bacteria and other noxious stimuli. Not to cover the exposed dentin should be considered a form of neglect.
    d. Provisional restoration: *(1)* an acid-etch composite resin restoration (primary choice), *(2)* open-faced stainless steel crown (unesthetic), or *(3)* an orthodontic band (unesthetic).
2. Recall appointment should include:
    a. Radiographs of the involved tooth.
    b. Notation of any color change, periapical change, or root resorption.
3. Final restoration should include one of the following:
    a. Use of an acid-etch composite resin restoration (with or without a pin).
    b. A heat-cured acrylic resin crown.
    c. A porcelain-fused-to-metal crown.

Class III fracture (Figs 19-7 to 19-9)

Class III fractures involve enamel, dentin, and pulp. The three variables considered during treatment of a Class III fracture are:

1. The size of the pulpal exposure.
2. The root development or level of root maturity.
3. The time lapse.

Pulp capping

1. Isolate the tooth with a rubber dam or cotton rolls.
2. Very gently dry the dentin and tooth structure with a cotton pledget.
3. Place a layer of calcium hydroxide over the exposed pulp and dentin.
4. Acid etch the enamel surface and place a layer of bonding material and composite resin over the calcium hydroxide and enamel.

The patient can be recalled to continue the completion of the restoration.

Several studies have reported success with capping minute pulpal exposures in permanent teeth (Kozlowska, 1961; Ravn, 1973, Andreasen, 1981). The success rates vary from 72% to 82%. Seventy-six fractured permanent incisors with pulpal exposures were treated either by pulp capping or pulpotomy (Fuks et al, 1982). Thirty-eight teeth with pinpoint exposures and complete root formations were treated by pulp capping with calcium hydroxide. Time lapse from the time of incidence to treatment did not seem to be a factor in the seven teeth that failed. Ravn (1982) pulp capped traumatized permanent incisors, finding a greater success rate with open apices than closed apices. Success or failure of treatment seems to depend on the presence of an associated periodontal ligament injury, the extent of the exposed dentin, and the duration of the pulpal exposure.

Pulpal healing is dependent on the extent of the luxation. With an open apex, the pulp survived more than

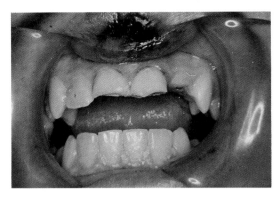

Fig 19-7   Class III fractures with pulpal exposures can be accompanied by lacerated lips.

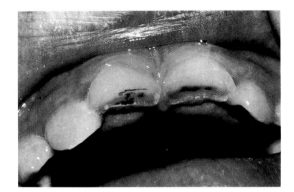

Fig 19-8   Severe Class III fractures that will require further pulp treatment.

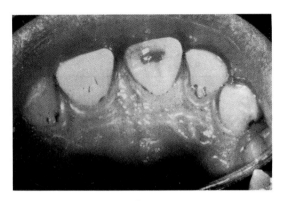

Fig 19-9   Extensive Class III fracture.

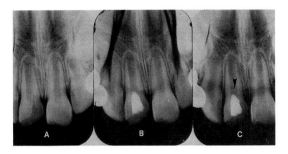

Fig 19-10   Calcium hydroxide was used to encourage apical closure.

50% of the time, with the exception of teeth that had been intruded; these failed nearly 100% of the time. With a closed apex, dependent on the type of luxation, success rates dropped dramatically; only those teeth with minimal luxation or concussion had a 50% or better survival rate (Andreasen and Andreasen, 1991).

Apexogensis (Pulpotomy)

Where there is an exposure on a vital permanent tooth with an open apex, the treatment of choice is a calcium hydroxide pulpotomy. The method is illustrated in Fig 19-10. An 8-year-old girl fractured her central incisor. The left central incisor (Fig 19-10,A) radiographically and clinically has a rather large pulpal exposure. To encourage continued root development, a calcium hydroxide pulpotomy is the treatment of choice. After local anesthesia is given, the tooth is isolated with a rubber dam. The procedure is as follows:

1. From a sterile endodontic kit, use a No. 6 bur to gain access to the pulp chamber.

2. Remove the pulpal tissue to the estimated level of the gingival crest of bone. Use a large sharp spoon excavator. It should be done without undue trauma to the remaining pulpal tissue.

3. Rinse out all residual and dentin debris.

4. Usually the hemorrhage is fairly well controlled. If not, place several moist cotton pledgets over the pulp to control hemorrhage.

5. Use a calcium hydroxide applicator and place a mixture of calcium hydroxide over the pulp stump Follow with a mixture of polycarboxylate cement (Fig 19-10,B).

6. You may place a composite resin restoration as a provisional restoration.

7. Follow up with periodic reviews, including radiographs. Figure 19-10, C shows a dentinal bridge and continued root formation.

When the root development is complete, a pulpectomy and a conventional root canal filling should be completed. If there is a long-standing large pulpal exposure and closed apex, a pulpectomy and root canal filling is the treatment of choice.

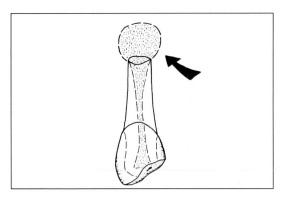

Fig 19-11 When a periapical lesion is present, apexification is needed.

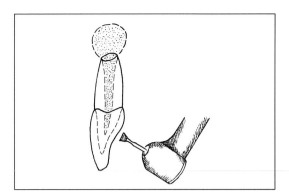

Fig 19-12 Gain access through the lingual surface.

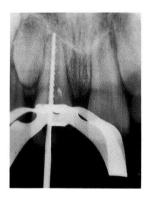

Fig 19-13 Establish file length.

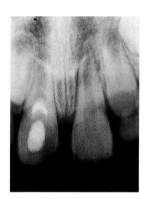

Fig 19-14 Seal in a pellet of CMCP for 1 week.

Apexification

Treatment of nonvital permanent teeth with incomplete apex formation is termed *apexification*, or *root-end closure*.

Permanent anterior teeth may become nonvital before apical closure. There is frequently evidence of a periapical lesion (Fig 19-11). In these instances where vital pulpotomy techniques are not successful for immature permanent teeth, apexification is indicated. The purpose is to stimulate root closure of the apex so that a conventional endodontic procedure with gutta-percha can be completed.

Frank (1966) was one of the first to describe the clinical methods using a calcium hydroxide paste and camphorated monochlorophenol (CMCP), as have Stiener et al (1968), to stimulate root closure.

The procedure for apexification is as follows:

1. After applying a rubber dam, gain access through the lingual portion of the crown of the tooth (Fig 19-12).
2. Using large reamers and files, remove the debris from the coronal half of the pulp. Establish the file length radiographically (Fig 19-13).
3. Clean the canal; irrigate it and then dry it with a paper point. Repeated gentle use of sodium hypochlorite assists debris removal.
4. Seal a pellet of CMCP in the pulp chamber with a provisional restorative material (Fig 19-14).
5. On recall, in 1 to 3 weeks, remove the provisional restoration and clean the canal.
6. Take care to avoid any instrumentation of the thin walls of the dentin near the apex.
7. Mix a paste of calcium hydroxide and CMCP on a glass slab. Carry the paste to the canal and force it into the apex with a large plugger or cone-shaped instrument (Fig 19-15). The initial objective is to fill the canal completely and obturate it with paste. Obtain a radiograph to check the accuracy of the root canal filling (Fig 19-16).
8. On 6-month recall, you should see radiographic evidence of apical closure. Weine (1976) noted five alternatives evident at this time (Fig 19-17):
   a. No apparent apical closure, but a resistance point when a file is inserted (Fig 19-17,*A*).
   b. Radiographic evidence of a calcified bridge at the apex (Fig 19-17,*B*).
   c. Apical closure without canal space changes (Fig 19-17,*C*).
   d. Normal continuance of apical closure (Fig 19-17,*D*).

e. Increased radiographic evidence of a pathologic apical change (Fig 19-17,*E*).

9. When you have accomplished apical closure, the root canal filling is completed (Fig 19-18).

10. If apexification has not been completed, repeat the cleaning and insertion of a Ca(OH)2 and CMCP paste.

The choices for treatment of fractured incisors are summarized in Table 19-1.

Treatment of root fractures

Root fractures occur less often in the cervical third, but they are the most difficult to treat. Root fractures occur the least, when types of trauma in the permanent dentition are compared. Clinically the tooth will be mobile and extruded. Often there is lingual displacement. Radiographs reveal a radiolucent line through the root of the tooth, disrupting the normal continuity of the root (Fig 19-19). The closer the fracture line is to the gingival

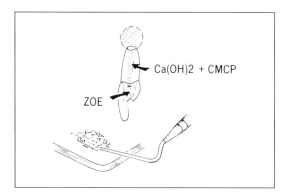

Fig 19-15 Mix a paste of calcium hydroxide and CMCP.

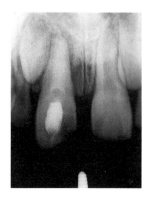

Fig 19-16 Fill the root canal with the mixture.

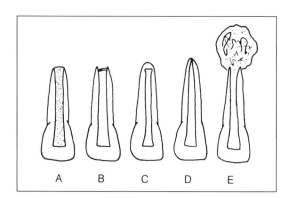

Fig 19-17 Five alternatives to root closure: *(A)* resistance point without apparent apical closure; *(B)* calcified bridge at the apex; *(C)* apical closure without canal space changes; *(D)* normal apical closure; *(E)* pathosis.

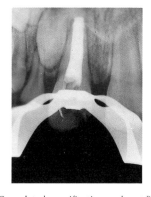

Fig 19-18 Completed apexification and root filled with gutta-percha.

Table 19-1 Choices of pulp treatment for Class III fractures

Procedure	Amount of pulpal exposure	Time lapse	Root maturity	Medicament
Pulp cap	Pinpoint–minute	Less than 2 hours	Closed apex	Calcium hydroxide
Pulpotomy	Small–large	NA	Open apex	Calcium hydroxide
Pulpectomy	Small–large	12 or more hours	Closed apex	Gutta -percha
Apexification	Nonvital pulp	NA	Open apex	Calcium hydroxide and CMCP*

*Camphorated monochlorophenol.

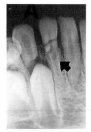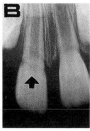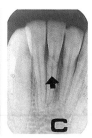

Fig 19-19 Root fractures *(arrows)*.

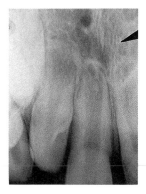

Fig 19-20 A concussion, as seen here, often includes thickening of the periodontal membrane *(arrow tip)*.

crest of bone, the less likelihood there is for successful treatment. The closer the fracture line is to the apex, the better the chance for success.

Bender and Freeland (1983) supported this statement. Following 14 patients with intra-alveolar root fracture, in some instances for 25 years, they found nearly 80% of the teeth remained intact. There was no need for endodontic therapy. Only teeth with pulpal pathosis should be considered for root canal treatment. Treatment includes:

1. Reduction of the displaced tooth.
2. Apposition of the fractured parts.
3. Splinting (as for avulsed teeth).
4. Observation for evidence of healing or pathologic changes.

The three accepted categories of root healing are healing of the fractured area with dentin, healing of the fractured area with a filling in of connective tissue, and healing of the fractured area with bone and connective tissue. The periodontal ligament is essential for root healing in all three types (Michanowicz et al, 1971). Failures are seen as a result of necrosis and root resorption.

Treatment of concussion

Symptoms include a painful tooth plus an elongated feeling of the involved tooth. Radiographically, there may be a thickening of the periodontal space due to injury to the periodontal membrane (Fig 19-20).

The effect of concussion on the blood supply is to sever the apical vessels, create edema or a hematoma at the apical tissues, and rupture the blood vessels within the tooth itself, which can lead to pulpitis, pulpal necrosis, and crown discoloration.

The younger the patient, the better the chances of the tooth's remaining vital. Treatment consists of a soft diet and analgesics.

Concussion can result in:

1. Asymptomatic pulpal necrosis.
2. Discoloration of the tooth.
3. Complete recovery.
4. Internal and external resorption.

Treatment of avulsion

Important: When a parent, teacher, or school nurse calls with a report of an avulsed tooth, instruct the person to place the tooth in *moist* gauze or a clean cloth if he or she cannot replant the tooth.

If possible, the avulsed tooth should be stored in milk until it can be replaced. In a laboratory study, milk was evaluated as the optimum medium to store avulsed teeth (Courts et al, 1983). Compared with saliva and water, milk is superior in maintaining vital tissues necessary to improve the chances for the success of reimplanatation.

The time the tooth is out of the host socket is the most important variable (Grossman and Ship, 1970). Success compared with time shows: *(1)* less than 30 minutes, 90% success; *(2)* 30 to 90 minutes, 43% success; *(3)* more than 90 minutes, 7% success. Thus, the question is one of whether endodontic treatment should be done at this time. Andreasen (1981) feels the following are the best choices:

1. Root canal treatment should be postponed for 1 to 2 weeks for teeth with a closed apex.
2. With an open apex, delayed endodontic treatment is justified. The hope is that there will be revascularization of the pulpal tissue. If root resorption begins, apexification can be attempted using calcium hydroxide as the filling material.
3. In the case of a closed foramen, endodontic treatment is indicated because pulpal necrosis is usually the outcome.
4. The prognosis for reimplanted teeth is guarded at best. External or internal root resorption or ankylosis may occur.
5. The tooth should be splinted for stabilization.

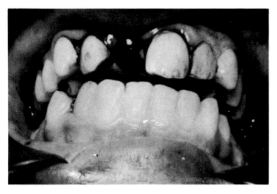

Fig 19-21 As a result of a sports accident, the central incisor was avulsed.

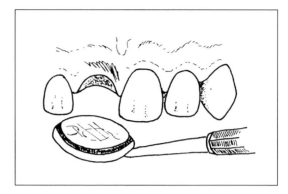

Fig 19-22 Examine the tooth socket for bony fractures.

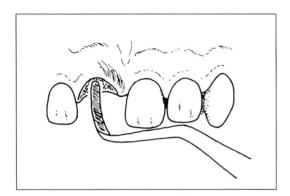

Fig 19-23 After administration of local anesthesia curette the area.

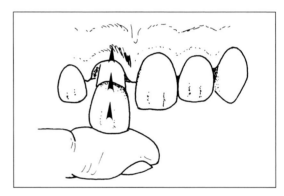

Fig 19-24 Reinsert the tooth with gentle pressure.

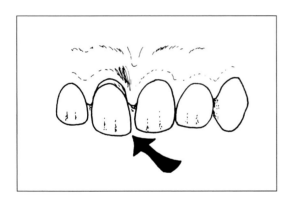

Fig 19-25 The inserted tooth may be somewhat longer.

When the patient arrives at the office, place the tooth in milk, if possible. Gently remove any debris from the tooth surface by rinsing. Radiograph the adjacent teeth as well as the tooth socket in question. Check for fractured alveolar bone, any remnants of a fractured root, and root fractures of adjacent teeth (Fig 19-21). Clinically examine the tooth socket and area for bony fractures (Fig 19-22). To stabilize the central incisor or incisors, plan a splint that includes the lateral incisors and canines. If the canines have not erupted, use the lateral incisors and remaining central incisor. A splint is used to provide stabilization until the tooth can reattach itself to the periodontal tissue.

The procedures for replanatation and splinting are as follows:

1. Administer local anesthesia. Use a soft tissue curette and remove any coagulated tissue from the socket (Fig 19-23). Carefully irrigate any tissue from the socket. *Do not scrape* the alveolar bone to remove any remains of periodontal membrane.
2. With gentle pressure, reinsert the tooth (Fig 19-24). A radiograph can be taken to verify the tooth's correct position.
3. In some instances, the incisor cannot be returned to its original position due to the accumulated clotted blood in the apex of the tooth socket (Fig 19-25). If so, equilibrate the incisal edge at a later date.
4. Use a piece of flexible stainless steel wire and adapt the wire to conform to the six teeth. The

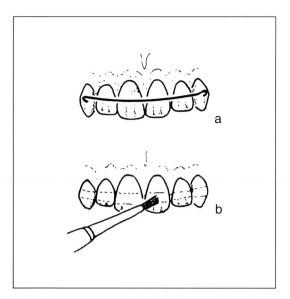

Fig 19-26 Stabilize the reinserted tooth with a wire-composite resin splint. Adapt the wire from canine to canine *(a)*. Use phosphoric acid to etch the anterior teeth *(b)*.

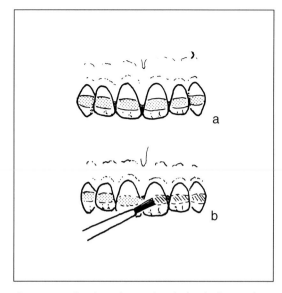

Fig 19-27 After the etching, a band of etched enamel appears *(a)*. Apply the bonding material *(b)*.

wire *must be passive* (Fig 19-26,*a*). First, bend the wire with your fingers. Second, use the No. 139 pliers to finish the adjustment to the teeth. About 3 mm from each end, bend small loops. These loops should go incisally to aid in retention and prevent lateral movement of the wire. Place cotton rolls in the buccal vestibule.

5. Etch the six teeth with 37% phosphoric acid. Confine the etched enamel to the middle third of the tooth (Fig 19-26,*b*).

6. After 1 minute, wash and dry the anterior teeth. A band of etched enamel with a chalky white appearance will be apparent (Fig 19-27,*a*).

7. Apply bonding agent to the etched surface (Fig 19-27,*b*)

8. Apply composite resin to the canines first to establish the position of the wire (Fig 19-28,*a*). Applying the composite resin to each canine first allows easy application to the remaining four teeth.

9. Apply the composite resin material to the remaining teeth (Fig 19-28,*b*). After polymerization is complete, check for adaptation and comfort to the patient's lip. Smooth off any rough edges with a diamond bur.

10. Allow the splint to remain in place for 10 to 14 days. Historically, splints such as these were left in place for 6 to 8 weeks. This period of time is not necessary. *As soon as possible, remove the splint to reduce the possibility of ankylosis or resorption.*

11. The patient should be instructed to maintain a soft diet while the splint is in place. An analgesic such as aspirin can be prescribed for any discomfort. A

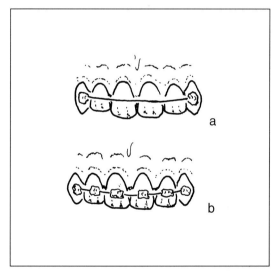

Fig 19-28 First attach the wire to the canines *(a)*. Apply the composite resin material to the remaining teeth *(b)*.

soft toothbrush should be used to keep the area clean of accumulated debris.

12. To remove the splint, cut the wires interproximally. Using a diamond bur, remove the composite resin and wire. Smooth the enamel surfaces, followed by fluoride paste polish. There may be need to equilibrate the incisal edge if it is too long. Evaluate periodically for success or failure. Figs 19-29a to c show a child with teeth that were reimplanted and splinted for 10 days.

Prognosis for avulsed teeth and successful healing is dependent on *(1)* minimal damage to the pulp and periodontal membrane; *(2)* the length of time the avulsed tooth was out of the mouth and how the tooth was stored; and *(3)* the level of root formation (Andreasen and Andraeasen, 1991).

Figs 19-29a to c An example of several avulsed teeth that were splinted for 10 days, after which the splint was removed.

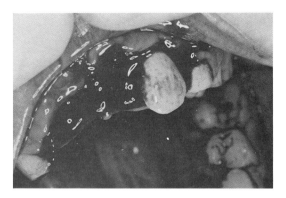

Fig 19-29a

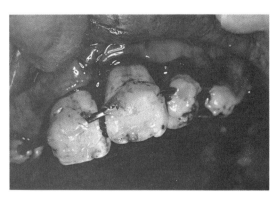

Fig 19-29b

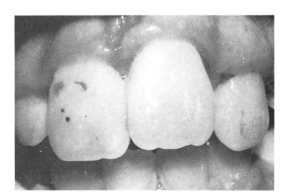

Fig 19-29c

Treatment of displacement

Displacement refers to bodily movement of the involved tooth to a labial, lingual, lateral, or intrusive position (Fig 19-30). Clinically the tooth will be mobile, have some gingival hemorrhage, and be displaced from the normal plane of occlusion or alignment. Radiographically, there will be a lack of periodontal space because the displaced tooth has obliterated the space.

Luxation is a severe loosening of the tooth, either minor (subluxation) or severe (luxation). The tooth is displaced labially or lingually.

If the displacement is minor and does not interfere with normal function, treatment is observation. The patient should be instructed to follow a soft diet for several days until the tooth tightens.

If the displacement is severe, local anesthesia is administered. As gently as possible, the tooth is repositioned and splinted. The splint should remain in place for 10 to 14 days. The patient should be instructed to eat soft foods, take analgesics for discomfort, and use warm saline rinses to cleanse the splint. The patient should be recalled periodically to note vitality, radiographic progress, and any color change. Depending on the severity of the displacement, pulpal necrosis is a constant concern. Unfortunately pulpal necrosis occurs with accompanying root resorption.

The sequelae to displacement are pulpal necrosis, root resorption, and root canal calcification. Andreasen (1970) found that 20% of subluxated teeth developed pulpal necrosis, and 64% of those with severe luxation developed pulpal necrosis. A subluxated tooth has minimal risk of pulpal necrosis; the tooth with an open apex has nearly a 100% survival rate. A luxated tooth displaced laterally or extruded is at high risk for pulpal necrosis; root resorption is a possibility (Andreasen and Andreasen, 1991).

The teeth should be checked periodically for any radiographic change and clinical color change.

Figure 19-31 is a decision-support system to assist in the selection of treatment for traumatized anterior permanent teeth.

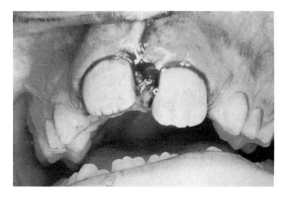

Fig 19-30 A tooth displaced to the labial surface. The tooth is also intruded.

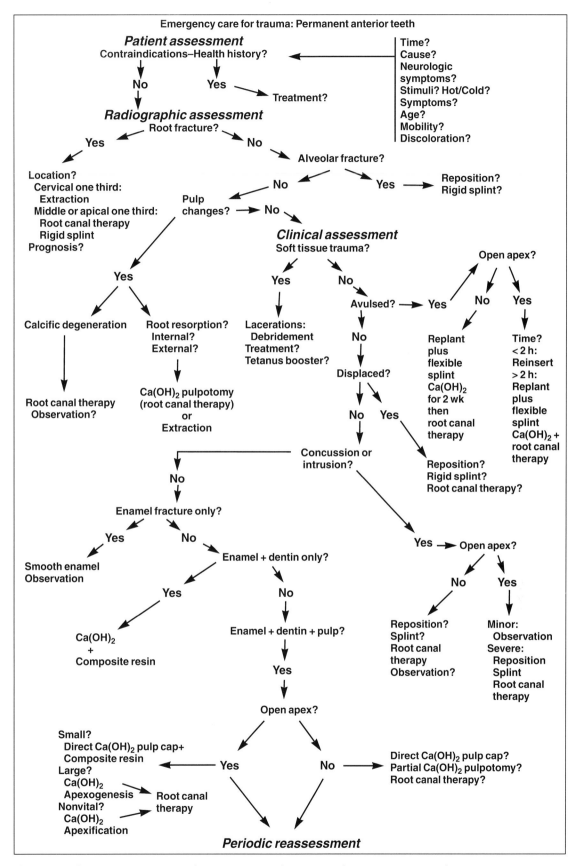

Fig 19-31 A decision-support system to determine treatment for traumatized permanent anterior teeth.

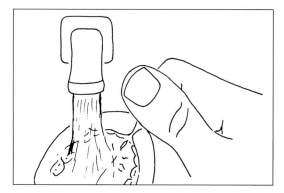

Fig 19-32 Rinse debris from the impression.

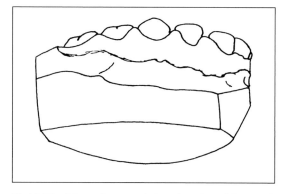

Fig 19-33 Trimmed cast ready for adaptation of the mouth guard material.

Mouth guards

For adolescents and young adults who participate in formal or intramural contact sports, wearing a mouth guard is an excellent method for preventing trauma to anterior teeth. Their use is mandated by law in a number of states. Three kinds of mouth protectors are available:

1. The ready-made mouth guard, sold at sporting goods stores, which is not specially fitted to the wearer.
2. The mouth-formed mouth guard, made from an arch-shaped shell of rubber or plastic that is softened and fitted to the mouth.
3. The custom mouth guard, which is made from an impression of the mouth.

The custom protector not only provides the greatest protection, comfort, and ease of speech and breathing, but also is better retained than the other kinds of protectors. Custom mouth guards can be made from various materials; the manufacturer's instructions should be followed exactly.

Custom mouth guard fabrication

Taking the impression

1. Select a tray that approximates the patient's maxillary arch. Try the tray in the mouth. If the tray does not fit, try others until a proper fit is obtained. Line the rim of the tray with periphery wax to aid retention of the tray. Measure out the alginate powder into a rubber mixing bowl. Add room-temperature water according to the manufacturer's directions. Stir with a broad spatula for 60 seconds.
2. With the spatula, lift alginate from the bowl and load the selected tray. Place the loaded tray over the dental arch. Rotate the tray into the mouth. Release

any air trapped in the buccal vestibule by lifting the lip and pushing out the cheek with a finger.
3. Hold the tray carefully in place for approximately 1 minute or until the alginate becomes semirigid.
4. While grasping the tray firmly with the fingers, snap it and the impression material off the teeth and remove from the mouth. Inspect the mouth for any remnants of alginate materials.
5. Wash any debris from the tray and impression in gently running water (Fig 19-32). Leftover debris will result in bubbles in the cast. A discrepancy in the cast results in a poorly fitting mouth guard. Check the impression to be sure that it includes all of the teeth, palate, and gingiva to the buccal vestibule. Look for any distortions or bubbles that would cause a faulty cast.

Preparing the cast

1. In a rubber bowl, mix the stone with water according to the manufacturer's directions. Stir with a spatula until the mixture is thick and creamy (approximately 60 seconds).
2. Place the stone mixture, a little at a time, in the impression. Vibrate the impression as it is being filled.
3. Allow the cast to set for several hours. Separate the tray and impression from the stone cast. Inspect for any defects or broken teeth.
4. Trim the base of the cast at the labial and buccal regions so that the vestibular area is readily accessible. Trim the distal palatal surface of the base to within 0.25 in. (0.63 cm) of the molar teeth. Trim the bottom of the base so that the palatal portion is not more than 0.25 in (0.63 cm) thick (Fig 19-33).
5. Using a pencil, draw a line along the labial and buccal surfaces of the cast to show the intended periphery of the mouth guard. The line should be 0.125 inch (0.31 cm) inside all gingival borders and frenula. Draw a line on the palate approximately 0.50 in. (1.25 cm) from the gingival margins of the teeth. Join the buccal and palatal lines approximately 0.125 in. (0.31 cm) distal to the most distal

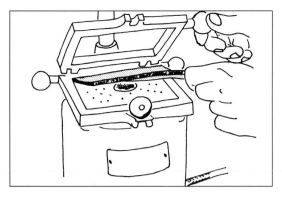

Fig 19-34　Place the mouth guard material and cast on the machine.

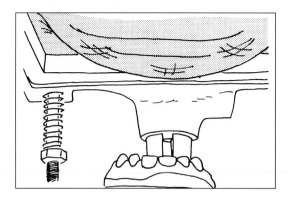

Fig 19-35　The mouth guard material, when heated, will sag on the cast.

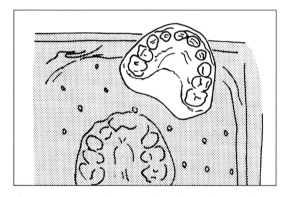

Fig 19-36　Separate the cast and mouth guard material.

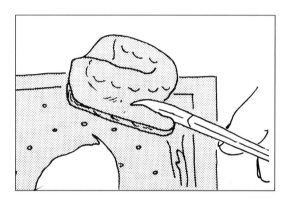

Fig 19-37　Remove the excess material with scissors.

teeth in the dental arch. Drill a hole in the palate portion of the cast. Use a vulcanite bur.

6. Completely immerse the cast in a pan of water for 5 minutes. A moist cast will not stick readily to hot (or overheated) vinyl.

Adapting the mouth guard

1. The Omnivac machine (Dental Manufacturing Co) has three main parts. On the top is a heating element that softens the vinyl sheet and can be held near the heating element or placed over the cast. At the bottom of the machine is a perforated platform that lies over a vacuum motor. When activated, the vacuum sucks air through the holes in the platform.

2. Place a vinyl-resin sheet in the middle plate; adjust the plate until it is as near the heating element as possible. Air dry the cast and place it in the center of the platform (Fig 19-34).

3. Turn on the heating element to begin softening the vinyl. As the vinyl softens, it will sag toward the cast (several centimeters below the vinyl sheet) (Fig 19-35). After about 3 minutes, the vinyl should have sagged to within 1.25 cm (0.50 in.) of the model. Readjust the middle plate to fit down tightly over the

platform on which the cast rests. Start the vacuum motor. Raise and lower the middle plate three to five times to release trapped air. Turn off the heating element and 30 seconds later stop the vacuum motor.

4. Keep the cast and vinyl-resin sheet together as you remove them from the machine. Allow them to cool; do not separate the vinyl from the cast at any time before both have cooled. If the vinyl is hot when it is removed from the cast, the mouth guard will be distorted.

5. Separate the vinyl mouth guard from the stone cast. Inspect the vinyl to make sure it has adapted well to the teeth, rugae, and outline (Fig 19-36).

6. Cut away excess material along the pencil outline scribed on the cast. Use curved or surgical scissors to cut the vinyl. Trimming is essential to prevent overextensions in the mouth (Fig 19-37).

7. Using a fine-grit carborundum arbor band in a slow-speed lathe, smooth the cut edge of the mouth guard (Fig 19-38). Polish the edge with wet pumice or a wet rag wheel. Light flaming of the peripheral edge with an alcohol torch will complete the polishing (Fig 19-39).

8. Place the mouth guard in the patient's mouth. Press to seat completely (Fig 19-40).

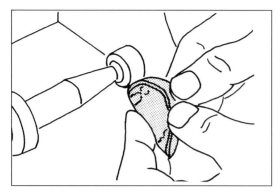

Fig 19-38 Smooth the edges of the mouth guard.

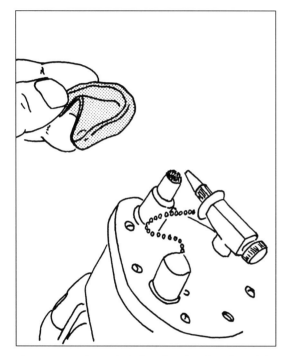

Fig 19-39 With an alcohol torch, refine the edges of the mouth guard.

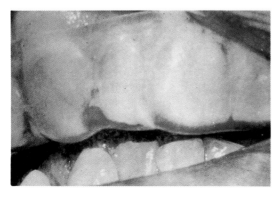

Fig 19-40 The mouth guard is seated in the patient's mouth for review of adaptation.

Observe the borders of the mouth guard to ensure that the tissues are not being blanched or restricted. Ask the patient whether there are areas of discomfort. If there is any tendency to gag or any impaired speech, trim the palatal border. Observe whether the mouth guard is retained tightly to the teeth. If the mouth guard falls off easily, if may need to be remade with greater palatal coverage. Light finger pressure should be required to dislodge it. If considerable pressure is required, trim the borders where there are heavy undercuts.

When the fabrication of a custom protector is completed, the patient should insert it so that it can be checked and adjusted if necessary. At the same time, the patient should be told how to keep the protector clean and fresh. After each wearing, it should be cleaned with soap and water or dentifrice and a soft nail brush or toothbrush; the wearer's teeth should also be brushed, if possible. The patient should be made aware that if cleaning is neglected, the appliance will become most unpleasant and possibly a source of irritation.

It is helpful if a storage container (denture holder or covered soap dish) for the protector can be kept in the locker. The container can be partially filled with a mixture of water and mouthwash to help keep the appliance fresh. Of greatest importance, however, if the cleaning after each wearing.

The wearer's name should be imprinted on the protector for identification. If the wearer attends school away from home, a duplicate protector should be made in case of damage to the original. For the same reason, the cast should be retained in the dental office.

Although the emphasis is usually on football, the owner of the mouth protector should be encouraged to wear it while engaged in any contact sport.

Summary

The following are the requirements in treating traumatized anterior teeth (Table 19-2):

1. Comprehensive history of the accident
2. Complete extraoral and intraoral examinations
3. Radiographs of involved teeth, adjacent teeth, and opposing teeth
4. Appropriate pulp treatment and provisional restoration
5. Relieving parent and patient discomfort and apprehension
6. For child abuse patients, ascertaining the frequency of trauma to the anterior teeth
7. Recall

Table 19-2 Summary for treatment of traumatized anterior teeth

Trauma present	Pulp treatment	Restoration
Primary incisor		
Enamel only (Class I)	Observation Note any color change	Smooth or rough edges
Enamel and dentin (Class II)	Calcium hydroxide liner Note any color change	Acid etch composite resin or open-faced stainless steel crown
Enamel, dentin, and pulp (Class III)	Formocresol pulpotomy Pulpectomy (if devital)	Open-faced stainless steel crown
Root fracture	Extraction	Space maintainer (?)
Avulsion	None	Space maintainer (?)
Displacement	Reposition	Splint
Concussion/intrusion	Observe for color change or reeruption: Black–nonvital pulp; pulpectomy Yellow–calcific pulp; observation	
Permanent incisor		
Enamel (Class I)	Observation	Smooth rough edges or acid-etch composite resin
Enamel and dentin (Class II)	Calcium hydroxide liner	Acid-etch composite resin
Enamel, dentin, and pulp (Class III)	Open apex: Calcium hydroxide pulpotomy (vital) Direct pulp cap (rare) Apexification (devital) Closed apex: Direct pulp cap (rare) Pulpectomy	Acid-etch composite resin Porcelain-fused-to-metal crown
Intrusion	Observe for color change, pulp vitality, and reeruption	
Concussion with mobility	Mild—observe Severe—splint	
Displacement	Mild—observe Severe—reposition splint	
Avulsion	Reimplant, splint for 10–14 days Observation	
Root fracture	Cervical one third: Root canal Extraction Middle one third: Splint Apical one third: Splint	Gold core with porcelain-fused-to- metal crown Space maintenance Fixed prosthetic appliance

Restoration of fractured incisors with an acid-etch composite resin system

In the past, restoration of fractured incisors was a haphazard procedure in dentistry for children. The restorations, when functional, were unesthetic. Orthodontic bands, stainless steel crowns with plastic windows, or fabricated acrylic resin crowns were used. If an esthetic crown, such as a celluloid crown form, was used, it was not functional. With the advent of the acid-etch method, a functional as well as esthetic restoration was created. Only minimal preparation (if any) if needed, thus restoring the fractured tooth's normal appearance. Both child and parent are pleased, the time the tooth is exposed to oral fluids is reduced, the pulp's chances of recovery are increased, and the cost to the patient is reduced.

In permanent teeth, improved retention of the composite resin can be accomplished by etching the enamel with 50% phosphoric acid for 30 seconds. (It is important to clean the permanent tooth enamel with a nonfluoridated prophylaxis paste *before* acid etching if surface preparation is not to be done.) The etching demineralizes the enamel surface, creating spaces in the surface layer of enamel (Gwinnet, 1973). The fluid composite resin flows in and around the enamel tags, thus increasing the retention of the restoration.

In a laboratory study, concentrations of phosphoric acid, type of fracture preparation, and restorative materials were compared (Nelson et al, 1974). It was found that a less-than-50% phosphoric acid, a scalloped preparation, and specific composite system (Nuva-Seal/Nuva-Fil) was optimum. Aker et al (1979) compared three methods of preparing enamel surfaces with five composite resin systems. Of the five systems, four were not influenced by the enamel surface preparation. For all the composite resin systems, roughing the enamel with a coarse diamond bur resulted in higher retentive values. In another laboratory study, the retention of a composite resin to enamel was thought to be related to the system's ability to wet and adapt to the etched enamel surface, not the physical strength properties (Mitchem and Turner, 1974). Ripa and Sheykholam (1978) have an excellent summary of clinical evaluations of acid-etch composite resin restorations for fractured incisors, with success rates from 80% to 100% after 11 to 36 months.

Marginal leakage around composite resin restorations is reduced by acid etching, as shown in several laboratory studies (Baharloo and Moore, 1974; Eliasson and Hill, 1977). In an attempt to reduce the roughness of a composite resin restoration, a glaze (unfilled resin) can be placed over the surface of a composite resin restoration after polishing. In a pilot clinical study of glazes, Calatrova et al (1976) found that after several months the glazes were gone from the restorations, which increased the roughness of the restorations and caused some marginal discoloration.

Donly and Browning (1992) placed bevels and chamfers on permanent teeth with Class IV cavity preparations, similar to fractures. In this laboratory study, half were restored with a microfilled composite resin, the other half with a macrofilled resin. Irrespective of the resin used, the chamfered preparation provided greater resistance to fracture. Andreasen and Andreasen (1991) also suggested use of a chamfer to increase ease of finishing and allow a greater bulk of material.

Tolley et al (1978) compared six finishing methods on five commercial composite resins. A silicon carbide disk provided the best finished surface, with a diamond bur resulting in the roughest surface finish. Composite resins should be inserted with as little excess as possible. The best finished surface was the result of the Mylar strip.

Mitchem (1983) evaluated concepts of cavity design and the influence of manipulation variables on clinical performance of anterior composite resin restorations. He found that:

1. The retention of a composite resin used to repair a fractured incisor is dependent extensively on the resin penetration of the etched enamel surface. It can be improved by beveling the preparation or adding a lingual dovetail. Use of pins is not recommended.
2. Exposed dentin must be protected with a calcium hydroxide liner because the etching material is a pulpal irritant and the acidic material opens the dentinal tubules, permitting access of the resin material to the pulp.
3. Use of intermediate bonding resins increases adaptation of the resin to the enamel because they are more fluid.
4. The visible light-curing resin systems have advantages compared with autopolymerizing resin systems. They remove the need for mixing, reducing the restoration's porosity, are more time efficient, increase the depth of cure, especially when applied in increments, can polymerize into undercuts, and require less working time than layered restorations.
5. Finishing should be kept to a minimum; 12-bladed finishing burs in combination with disks are the optimum method.
6. Occlusion should be carefully checked.
7. Glazing with an unfilled resin may be beneficial; however, bonding agents should not be used.

Ripa and Sheykholam (1978) described the advantages of the acid-etch composite technique as follows:

1. The dentin and pulp are protected while an immediate restoration of esthetic quality is placed.
2. The repair serves as both an immediate and long-term restoration.
3. Preparation of tooth structure is not required, nor is gross preparation of the tooth for mechanical retention necessary.
4. Anesthesia is not needed to place the restoration.
5. Treatment can usually be accomplished in 30 minutes or less.
6. The gingival area is usually not involved in the restoration so that later gingival recession will not affect the esthetic repair.
7. The restoration is economical.

The following describes one of the several techniques available to restore fractured incisors with an acid-etch composite resin restoration (Fig 19-41).

Armamentarium

Burs
    Flame-shaped diamonds
    Sandpaper disks/finishing strips

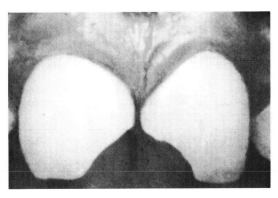

Fig 19-41 A Class II fracture on a permanent tooth: ideal for repair with a composite resin material.

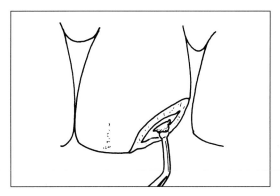

Fig 19-42 Place Dycal on the exposed dentin.

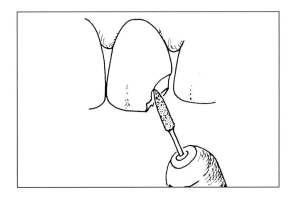

Fig 19-43 Place a 1.5-mm chamfer on the enamel margin.

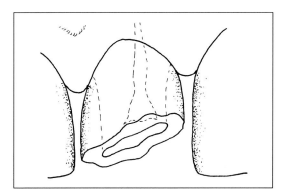

Fig 19-44 Place a bevel on a larger Class II fracture.

Materials
  Pin Kit (optional; Whaledent International)
  Composite resin material/kits;
  light-activated
  Celluloid crown form
  Plastic instruments
Calcium hydroxide liner (Dycal)
  Composite resin finishing kit
  37% phosphoric acid
  Prophylaxis paste

Procedure

1. Isolate the injured tooth and adjacent teeth with a rubber dam. With a moist cotton pledget, *gently* remove any saliva and other foreign material from the fracture site. *Do not* use compressed air to desiccate the dentin or enamel.

2. To protect the dentin from the acid penetration, cover the exposed dentin with a calcium hydroxide liner (Dycal, Fig 19-42). The calcium hydroxide should *not* extend onto enamel.

3. Clean the adjacent enamel of the tooth with a fine pumice paste. Remove the slurry with a gentle stream of warm water. The calcium hydroxide liner should remain in place. Gently dry the tooth.

4. To protect the medicament during the following procedures, place the bonding agent, which is an unfilled resin, over the dentin portion of the fracture. If a light-polymerizing material is used, the material should be exposed for 20 seconds.

5. Several options are available to prepare the tooth for the subsequent restoration with a composite resin material:
   a. If there is a minimal Class II fracture with just a small portion of dentin fracture, the only cavity preparation necessary is to remove only any overhanging or unsupported enamel. This type of preparation does not precipitate trauma by further instrumentation or require local anesthesia.
   b. A 1.5-mm chamfer can be placed on the enamel margin (Fig 19-43).
   c. A bevel is placed along the exposed enamel to prepare a butt-type joint (Fig 19-44). The bevel is placed in enamel at a 45° angle.

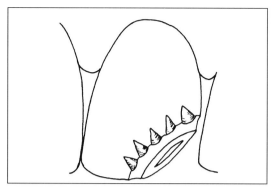

Fig 19-45 In addition to a bevel, a scalloped margin can be used to increase retention.

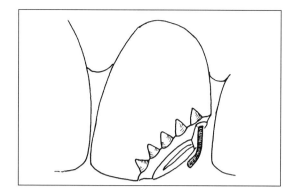

Fig 19-46 Place a pin in large fractures.

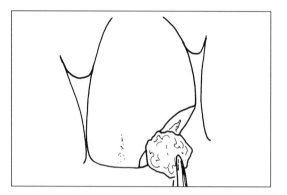

Fig 19-47 Etch the enamel with phosphoric acid.

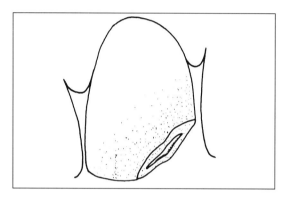

Fig 19-48 After etching, a chalky surface should appear.

    d. A bevel may be combined with a scalloped enamel effect. The rationale is to expose more surface area of enamel (Fig 19-45). Thus, when the enamel is etched, there is more retentive surface area for the composite resin to adhere to.

    e. If there is extensive tooth structure loss, a minipin (Whaledent) can be used to aid in retention. Anesthesia should be used for this technique. The pin should be masked with a masking material (Fig 19-46).

6. The optimal tooth preparation is to do little, if any, preparation to the fractured tooth. (This technique will follow that method.) Saturate a cotton pledget or a small brush with 37% phosphoric acid conditioner. Apply to the enamel surface, thoroughly wetting the adjacent enamel. Keep moist for 60 seconds (Fig 19-47).

7. Remove the conditioner by rinsing with warm water. Aspirate all fluids from the area. Gently dry the area with warm air. The acid-etched surfaces should appear chalky. If not, add the conditioning material for another 60 seconds (Fig 19-48).

8. Place a Mylar strip between the teeth to prevent excess flow of material. Place the bonding agent over the exposed dentin. If the composite resin material activated by a light is used, add small increments with the a plastic instrument. Polymerize each portion. Use a brush or the same plastic instrument to extend the composite resin onto the etched surface. The composite material can be placed directly over the bonding agent. When the desired anatomic form is completed, the last increment of composite resin is polymerized with the light.

9. To finish the composite resin, use the sandpaper disk supplied by the manufacturer or burs. Using the incremental buildup method should result in a restoration that needs minimal finishing. Remove any flash at the enamel margin. Overextension of the composite material will result in staining at margins because of marginal leakage.

10. If an autopolymerizing composite resin is used, a matrix is required and a celluloid crown form is used. Select a crown size that is slightly larger mesiodistally than the fractured tooth (Fig 19-49). Make a hole in the incisal edge to allow excess material and trapped air to escape. Load the crown form with mixed composite material and place over the tooth. Allow the material to polymerize. Use a scalpel to remove the celluloid crown. Finish as in step 9.

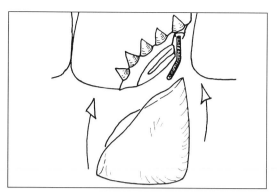

Fig 19-49 Use a crown with a self-curing composite resin material.

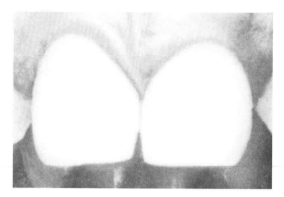

Fig 19-50 Completed composite resin restoration.

11. Remove the rubber dam. Check for any premature contacts in occlusion, during protrusion, and also in an end-to-end incisal relationship. If the tooth is left in hyperocculsion, early failure of the restoration can occur.
12. Rinse and dry the new restoration. Most manufacturers supply a glaze of unfilled resin to apply over the surface of the restoration (19-50). The sealant gives an initial shiny-looking tooth surface, which, unfortunately, may abrade in a short time.
13. Place the patient on recall for periodic review. The tooth should be reappraised for success of the restoration and continued pulpal vitality.

Restoration of discolored teeth

Causes

Trauma

Trauma to the primary teeth can result in displacement of primary teeth, causing localized enamel hypoplasia of the permanent tooth bud (see Fig 19-1), often referred to as *Turner's hypoplasia*. Andreasen (1970), looking at this risk after trauma to the primary dentition, found that intruded primary teeth produced malformed permanent teeth more than 75% of the time and that the younger the child when trauma occurred to the primary dentition, the greater the chance of damage to the permanent dentition.

Fluoride ion

When the fluoride content in the water exceeds 1.5 ppm, mild fluorosis can occur. When the fluoride content increases, the severity of the fluorosis increases. One theory is that the fluoride ion causes a disturbance in calcification of the tooth matrix.

Tetracycline

Even a casual glance at a representative list of articles in the dental literature reveals that clinicians are concerned about the use of the tetracycline antibiotics during the tooth formation period of a child's life. This concern arises from increasing evidence that the administration of these drugs during the developmental period often results in marked staining of either or both of the dentitions. Such stains are permanent.

The extent and color of the staining seem to depend on the type of drug, the dosage, the duration of administration, and the age of the patient at the time of administration. The following stain colors have been attributed to the drugs listed:

Yellow—tetracycline hydrochloride
Yellow to bright yellow—oxytetracycline
Orange to gray-brown—chlorotetracycline
Gray to blue-brown—dimethylchlortetracycline

Normal dosages or even less (250 to 500 mg/d or 20 to 75 mg/kg) are reported to produce vivid staining. Short-duration administration—once daily for 3 days—can result in a stained band across the middle one third of the anterior teeth.

There are also reports that these drugs cross placental barriers to produce characteristic tetracycline staining in primary teeth. Calcification of the teeth begins about the third month in utero, and the crowns of all permanent teeth, except the third molars, are usually completely calcified by the age of 9. If possible, other drugs should be used in the treatment of infections during pregnancy and the first 9 years of a child's life.

The patient's age at the time of administration apparently has a very important bearing on the clinical appearance of the staining. Many youngsters who receive tetracycline do not exhibit the characteristic stains; some authors suggest possible relationships between the disease being treated, the specific growth disturbances, and the drugs being used. Generally, the older the child is at the time of administration, the darker the stains are. Primary teeth are likely to stain pale to bright yellow; permanent teeth generally stain darker yellow to a gray-brown. Some investigators think that the pale yellow stains in the teeth of younger children tend to turn brown on exposure to sunlight. This darkening would help to explain why many permanent teeth erupt a normal color and gradually darken to gray-brown as the child grows older.

Treatment options

The following options are for improving the esthetic appearance in permanent teeth affected by tetracycline staining or fluorosis, or in hypoplastic, hypocalcific or otherwise unesthetic permanent anterior teeth:

1. Bleaching with a 30% hydrogen peroxide solution (Superoxol, Scientific Products, Inc). In some instances of lighter staining, this solution has dramatic results. The treatments consist of four or five visits. At each visit, the teeth are isolated with a rubber dam, and the Superoxol is applied for approximately 30 to 60 minutes and heated. The coloring in the teeth may decrease, especially the incisal one third. The parents and the patient should be advised that the color may return, and a touch-up is needed periodically. Discoloration caused by tetracycline staining and fluorosis are well managed by this method.
2. Bleaching with hydrochloric acid–pumice mixture. This mixture applied without heat, seems to result in permanent lightening of the enamel, according to recent research. The procedure can usually be completed in one office visit. It is not effective on stains caused by tetracycline, but on surface stains only.
3. Use of porcelain laminate veneers. Porcelain laminate veneers have increased in popularity (Faunce, 1975; Horn, 1983; Boksman et al, 1985; Hobo and Iwata, 1985). Produced in the laboratory to the described size, contour, thickness, and color, the veneer is attached to the enamel surface by a combination of mechanical and chemical bonding. The porcelain is etched with hydrofluoric acid on the inner surface; the enamel with the usual agents. A silane bonding agent is used to attach the resin chemically to the etched porcelain surface. A visible light-curing resin is used to complete the process.
4. Veneering with a composite resin system. This method entails removing a thin layer of enamel, acid etching the enamel surface, using an opaque material, and adding an appropriately shaded composite resin.

External bleaching methods (vital bleaching) include all types of bleaching on the external surfaces of teeth. Internal bleaching (nonvital bleaching) refers to bleaching from within the tooth.

Bleaching of vital teeth

Although clinical studies on humans have demonstrated that bleaching can be effective (Corcoran and Zillich, 1974, 1979; Boksman and Jordan, 1983), research on bleaching has been done primarily with animals. Myers et al (1980) found that rats' teeth stained with tetracycline returned to their original shade 4 days after treatment. Two studies in dogs (Wilson and Seale, 1985; Seale and Wilson, 1985) found that applying 35% hydrogen peroxide to tetracycline-stained teeth at 142° F for 15, 30, and 45 minutes produced the following results:

1. The teeth treated for 15 and 30 minutes became progressively lighter during the four bleaching appointments. The color of those teeth bleached for 45 minutes did not improve after the second appointment.
2. The color change was stable for all treated teeth at the end of day 92 after the bleaching cycle.
3. Severity of pulpal change, related mainly to odontoblastic cell change, was correlated to the length of application of the heat source and the bleaching agent.
4. After 92 days, evidence of cell repair was observed.

Armamentarium

Heat source (Union Broach)
Hydrogen peroxide, 30% (Superoxol)
Petroleum jelly
Extra-heavy rubber dam and floss
Phosphoric acid, 37%
Cavity varnish (Copalite, Harry J. Bosworth Co)

Procedure

The vital bleaching procedure may be used for tetracycline staining and fluorosis as follows:

1. *Tell the patient and parent that there may be little or no improvement in the color of the teeth.* Within 6 months the discoloration may begin returning. Do a prophylaxis with a rubber cup and unfluoridated pumice paste.
2. Lubricate the gingival tissues with petroleum jelly or topical anesthetic to prevent any tissue burning with the Superoxol.
3. Isolate the teeth with an extra-heavy rubber dam. Ligate the teeth with dental floss (Fig 19-51). Coat the ligatures with Copalite varnish to seal the dam.
4. Saturate the cotton pellet with Superoxol. Place the large cotton pellet on the tooth to be bleached (Fig 19-52). Keep the pellet moist but not supersaturated during the procedure.

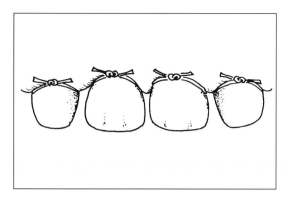

Fig 19-51 Isolate the teeth with rubber dam.

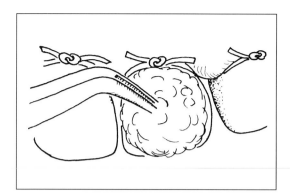

Fig 19-52 Saturate the teeth with Superoxol.

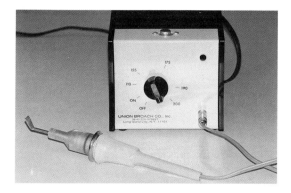

Fig 19-53 Heat source.

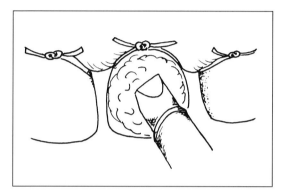

Fig 19-54 Apply the heat source to the Superoxol on the tooth.

5. Set the rheostat of the heat source at 135 F (Fig 19-53). Apply heat to the moist pellet (Fig 19-54). Ask the patient to raise a hand when the tooth begins to feel warm.
6. Repeat the procedure for each tooth. Treat each tooth on a rotating basis for 5 minutes at a time. Four or five 30-minute appointments are usually required to complete the bleaching procedure.
7. An option is to pretreat and postreat the enamel with 37% phosphoric acid for 1 to 2 minutes.
8. In Fig 19-55, note the difference in the young woman's teeth before and after treatment with 30% hydrogen peroxide.
9. Remove the dam and check to determine whether any of the bleaching material has leaked through. A whitish-appearing gingival tissue is an indication that leakage has occurred. This white appearance will disappear but can cause some tissue sloughing.

Bleaching for surface discolorations only

McCloskey (1984) described an effective method for removing surface discoloration from enamel. Although not thoroughly tested yet, the technique seems to be suitable for stains caused by fluorosis, idiopathic

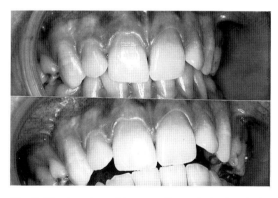

Fig 19-55 A patient with tetracycline stain *(top)* and after bleaching *(bottom).*

white and yellow enamel stains, and etching of enamel by orthodontic bands.

Armamentarium

Rubber dam and rubber dam material
Copalite varnish (L. D. Caulk Co.)
Hydrochloric acid, 18%
PREMA kit (Premier Dental Products)

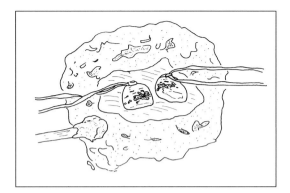

Fig 19-56   Sodium bicarbonate placed around the area.

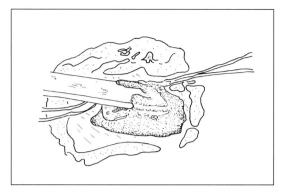

Fig 19-57   Burnishing the hydrochloric acid–pumice mixture.

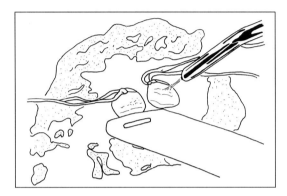

Fig 19-58   The teeth are rinsed. Note any color change.

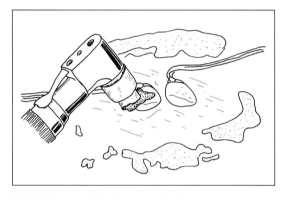

Fig 19-59   Smoothing the enamel surfaces.

PREMA compound
Contra-angle with rotary applicators
Hand applicators
Sodium bicarbonate
Dental floss
Tongue blade
Acidulated phosphate prophylaxis paste
Topical acidulated phosphate fluoride
Superfine aluminum oxide composite disk
Disposable eye protectors
Protective patient drape
Rubber gloves

Procedure

The following procedures are adapted from two excellent articles by Croll and Cavenaugh (1986a and b).

1. The dentist and assistant should both use rubber gloves. Protect the patient's, assistant's, and your own eyes with suitable eye protectors; drape the patient with a protective wrap.
2. Isolate the teeth to be modified with a rubber dam. Ligate the rubber dam with dental floss. Apply Copalite varnish to the margins of the rubber dam and teeth to seal the rubber dam (see Fig 19-42).

3. Mix the sodium bicarbonate to a thick paste in a disposable plastic mixing cup This paste is placed on the teeth around the rubber dam to protect the patient from any accidental spill of the hydrochloric acid (Fig 19-56).
4. Mix fine pumice and the 18% hydrochloric acid in a disposable plastic mixing cup to form a thick paste. An applicator is made by cutting a 0.5-in. wooden wedge from the tongue blade. With this wedge, burnish the hydrochloric acid mixture firmly into the stained labial enamel surface. Place a cotton swab on the lingual surfaces of the teeth to absorb the excess hydrochloric acid–pumice mixture (Fig 19-57).
5. Leave the hydrochloric acid–pumice mixture on for 5 seconds. Then rinse the teeth with adequate amounts of water and remove with high-velocity evacuation. Evaluate the teeth for any color improvement. This process of 5-second application and 10-second water rinse is repeated until the desired color improvement is noted (Fig 19-58).
6. The teeth are given a final water rinse for 30 seconds. Apply topical fluoride for 3 minutes.
7. Remove the rubber dam carefully.
8. Use an acidulated phosphate prophylaxis paste to smooth any remaining rough enamel surfaces (Fig 19-59).

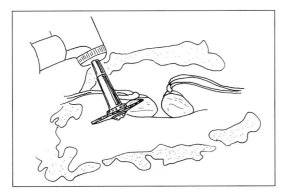

Fig 19-60   An aluminum oxide disk is used for final polish.

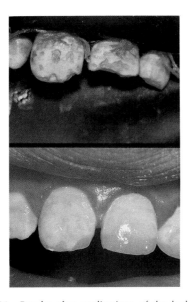

Fig 19-61   Results after applications of the hydrochloric acid–pumice mixture.

9. To restore normal luster to the enamel, a superfine aluminum oxide composite resin polishing disk can be used (Fig 19-60).
10. Dispose of the hydrochloric acid–pumice mixture by mixing it with the sodium bicarbonate. This should be done with extreme caution!

Because of poor oral hygiene, white, opaque decalcified areas become apparent when orthodontic appliances are removed. The hydrochloric acid–pumice mixture can be used with success to remove these opaque lesions (Kapila, 1988).

A young man who lived on a farm with excessive fluoride in the water source had fluorosis (Fig 19-61). The teeth were bleached with the hydrochloric acid–pumice mixture, and then restored with a composite resin.

Advantages

1. Unlike combination hydrogen peroxide and heating methods, there is no heat applied to the tooth. This eliminates pulpal changes caused by heating.
2. The method does not require multiple office visits or limit appointment time to 30 minutes.
3. There is no significant loss of tooth structure.
4. The patient tolerates the procedure well.
5. Using the described precautions, the method is easily accomplished by the dentist.
6. The color change in the enamel surface seems to be permanent.

Disadvantages

The method is limited to enamel stain removal only; intrinsic staining of dentin caused by tetracycline is not altered by this method.

"Home" bleaching

Referred to a "home" bleaching method, this is a conservative method for stained permanent anterior teeth. This bleaching method uses a customized night guard and either carbamide peroxide or hydrogen peroxide as the bleaching agent. This technique was introduced by Haywood and Heymann (1989).

Armamentarium

Two bleaching materials are available:

1. Ten percent carbamide peroxide. An unstable solution, it dissolves into 3% to 5% hydrogen peroxide which acts as the bleaching agent. Carbopol, a polymer, is added to several products to thicken the carbamide peroxide solution, slowing the release of the hydrogen peroxide. The solutions of 10% carbamide peroxide plus Carbopol are marketed as Proxigel (Reed & Carnrick) and Rembrandt (DentMat Corp). Solutions without Carbopol are Gly-Oxide (Marion-Merril-Dow) and White and Brite (Omni). A product with 15% carbamide peroxide plus Carbopol is Nu Smile (M&M Innovations).
2. Hydrogen peroxide. These are available in gel form with 1% to 10% hydrogen peroxide, depending on the manufacturer. Available as gels are Peroxygel, 1.5% hydrogen peroxide (Colgate Hoyt), Brite Smile, 2%, 5%, or 10% hydrogen peroxide (Brite Smile, and Natural White, 6% hydrogen peroxide (Aesthete).

Procedure (Haywood and Heymann; 1989; Haywood, 1992)

1. After a prophylaxis, use a standard shade guide to determine the pretreatment shade of the patient's anterior teeth.

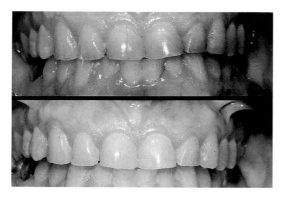

Fig 19-62 Results after bleaching with carbamide peroxide solution.

2. For documentation purposes, take intraoral photographs as references for change. Place the selected shade button adjacent to the teeth to be bleached.
3. After taking an impression of the arch to be bleached, make a cast. From the cast, fabricate a custom night guard (see "mouth guards" in this chapter).
4. After the night guard is adjusted, the bleaching agent of choice is prescribed or given to the patient with the following printed instructions:
   a. At bedtime, brush and floss as usual, rinsing the teeth well.
   b. Place 2 to 3 drops of the solution in the night guard.
   c. Insert the night guard, removing any excess solution.
   d. Repeat the process until the desired result is achieved.
   e. Wash and clean the night guard each morning; brush and floss as usual.
   f. Discontinue the treatment if the process becomes uncomfortable.
5. The shade changes should be evaluated every 2 to 5 weeks. Intraoral photographs are taken at each visit and at the end of treatment. Another option for the patient is to use the same process but wear the night guard for 4 to 6 hours during the day.
6. The patient should be advised that there are no guarantees that the teeth will be lightened. Fig 19-62 shows a patient who used a carbamide peroxide with Carbopol to bleach stained teeth.

Advantages

1. Cost effective
2. Can improve esthetics
3. Easily performed procedure

Disadvantages

1. Question as to permanent change
2. Irritation of gingiva?
3. Depends on patient compliance
4. In older patients, may cause some thermal sensitivity

Bleaching of nonvital teeth

Teeth that have been traumatized with a follow-up endodontic procedure often discolor. Discoloration may be due to the disintegration of the blood by-products from the pulp, hemosiderin and hematoidin. A relatively simple method is to seal a mixture of sodium perforate and 30% hydrogen peroxide (Superoxol) in the stained tooth. The secret of success is to remove all stained enamel and dentin.

The root canal filling material is sealed over with a polycarboxylate cement. The mixture of the sodium perborate–hydrogen peroxide is placed in the discolored pulp chamber. A provisional restoration of improved zinc oxide–eugenol is placed over the mixture (Fig 19-63).

After 7 days, the tooth is examined for color change. A second or third bleaching procedure may be needed. It is advisable to overbleach by one or two shades because there is a tendency for the color to regress. When the bleaching process is completed, a light-shade composite resin is used to restore the tooth (Fig 19-64).

Laminate veneers

Indications

Patients with tetracycline stain, fluorosis, hypoplastic or hypocalcific teeth, or other unesthetic anterior teeth may benefit from laminate veneers.

Contraindications

1. Teeth in severe labial version
2. Mouth breathers
3. Exposed dentin
4. Poor oral hygiene (low dental IQ)

Preformed laminate veneers

Because of the weakness of the preformed laminate veneers, use of this type of restoration is no longer recommended. Disadvantages were:

1. Laminated teeth were bulky in appearance.
2. The process was time consuming.
3. Poor gingival adaptation could result in inflammation.
4. Replacement was difficult.

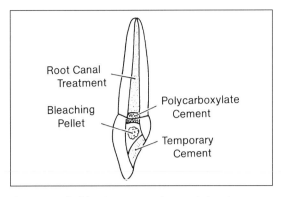

Fig 19-63 The bleaching process for nonvital teeth.

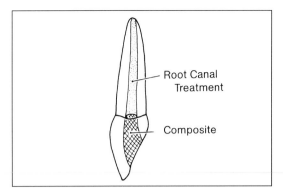

Fig 19-64 The final step in the nonvital bleaching process.

Porcelain laminate veneers

An alternative treatment for extremely hypoplastic or discolored teeth is the use of porcelain veneers. Due to limitations of acrylic resin laminate veneers, porcelain veneers are an excellent alternative for badly discolored permanent incisors.

Advantages (Christensen, 1985)

1. The patient's enamel color and surface texture are re-created.
2. Preparation is conservative.
3. The underlying defects in enamel are easily corrected.
4. Periodontal tolerance is excellent.
5. If the procedure is done properly, little finishing is needed.

Disadvantages

1. Unlike a composite resin veneer, porcelain laminate veneers require a two-appointment procedure.
2. The technique requires meticulous attention to detail.
3. They are more expensive, because of laboratory fees.

Problems (Sheets and Taniguchi, 1990)
1. If done improperly, marginal integrity is poor.
2. The veneers can have an unesthetic monochromatic color.
3. Cementing techniques are poor.
4. Surface textures are unnatural.

Procedure (Calamia, 1985; Quinn et al, 1986; Sheets and Taniguchi, 1990)

1. Tooth preparation. Cut a conservative preparation in the enamel surface to a depth of about 0.5 to 1.0 mm. Mesiodistal extension is 0.5 mm into enamel, but stays facial to the patient's own contacts. A 0.5-mm incisal reduction is recommended to form a slight incisal overlap. Place a chamfer finish 0.5 to 2.0 mm supragingivally.
2. Instrumentation. Select the shade prior to tooth preparation. Remove the enamel surface with a depth-cutting stone. Polish only the margins with a 12-fluted finishing bur. Leave the enamel surfaces roughened for maximum bond strength.
3. Impression. Use an elastomeric impression is used to create master dies. A silicone impression material is an excellent choice. For one or two veneers, Sheets and Taniguchi (1990) suggested taking two impressions, for three to six veneers, three impressions, and for seven to ten veneers, four impressions.
4. Provisional restoration. If a provisional laminate is indicated, place a layer of microfilled resin on the unetched enamel.
5. Casts. Construct epoxy casts of the impression; these seem to produce a smoother surface.
6. Try-in and cementation. Pre-etch the completed veneer. Clean the teeth receiving the veneers with pumice, and rinse them prior to try-in. Place the veneers on the teeth and check them for marginal integrity. Ask the patient to review the veneers, then clean the veneers. Coat the etched veneer with the silane coupling agent, used in accordance with the manufacturer's instructions. Etch the enamel surfaces of the teeth with 37% orthophosphoric acid. If dentin is exposed, a dentin bonding agent may be used as well. Place composite resin on the lingual surface of the veneer. Place each veneer individually.
7. Finishing. Only light finishing is needed. Gently remove excess composite resin. Finishing strips can be used interproximally.

An adolescent with tetracycline staining now has a pleasing smile, improved by the use of porcelain veneers (Fig 19-65).

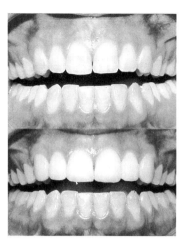

Fig 19-65 An adolescent with tetracycline staining *(top).* The preparations were 0.5 mm into enamel. Results after placement of porcelain veneers *(bottom).*

Acid-etch composite resin veneer

Another alternative for treatment of tetracycline stain or any other severe stain is to use a veneer of composite resin etched to the enamel surface.

Advantages are:

1. It is a one-appointment procedure.
2. The microfilled composite resins are well adapted to such a procedure.
3. The composite resins are excellent esthetically.
4. It is economical and easily repaired.

Disadvantages are:

1. A rough surface may appear after several months.
2. Some surface stain may appear.
3. The method requires a precise technique.

Use of composite resin restorative materials (Collard et al 1991)

The ideal composite resin restorative material would be one that demonstrates excellent esthetics, complete fracture and wear resistance, marginal seal and bond-ability to enamel and to dentin, easy handling, and usage in both anterior and posterior situations. Such a composite material does not exist.

Dental composite restorative systems consist of a bonding resin and a composite material. Bonding resin is applied to the clean, dry cavity preparation and allowed to polymerize before the composite resin is placed. This process may be either chemically initiated (self cured) or photoinitiated (light cured). Bonding resin and composite resin in self-curing systems are formulated in two parts, usually paste-paste. Clinically, polymerization begins when equal amounts of the two pastes are brought together and mixed to a uniform consistency according to the manufacturer's instruc-

tions. The bonding resin and composite resin in light-curing systems generally are single components, although some products require mixing of the bonding resin. These composite resins offer numerous advantages over self-curing materials, including (1) reduced curing time, (2) greater color stability, and (3) curing on command.

A problem common to all resin materials is contraction during polymerization. The material tends to pull away from the tooth margins when it cures, resulting in the formation of a gap between the tooth and the restorative material. Conventional composite resins have been used extensively in the past. They are still available and have been refined and improved for the last several years., The most noticeable improvement is in the surface roughness of the finished composite resin. The new smooth-surface composite resins appear specifically to solve the problem of surface polishability.

Composite restorative materials are categorized into four types: (1) large-particle macrofilled, which includes conventional composite resins; (2) microfilled; (3) small-particle macrofilled; and (4) hybrids. The materials in these categories differ in the size and amount of the inorganic filler particles used. In general, the finer the particle size, the better will be the surface polishability. Also, the lower the percentage of inorganic filler particles, the lower will be the resistance of the composite resin to stress. Conversely, the heavier the fill, the stronger the composite resin will be. Composite systems within these groups may be either self curing or photocuring.

Manufacturers have tried to control the physical properties of their resin materials by adjusting the percentage and size of the filler particle content, resulting in an enormous number of individual products that are available to the dental practitioner. This is the reason that it is so important to understand the basic types of composite resins and their advantages, disadvantages, indications, and limitations. A material that works well in one situation may not work well in another. The following is a summary of the physical properties of composite resins by category.

Large-Particle Macrofilled. In general, composite resins that have 75% or greater filler content are considered to be macrofilled. The larger-particle macrofills are heavy filled composite resins with particle sizes that range from about 8 to 50 um. These materials exhibit excellent fracture resistance because of their highly loaded nature, but they are virtually unpolished because of the large particle sizes. The large-particle macrofills are indicated in demanding stress-bearing areas.

Microfilled. Microfilled dental composite resins are essentially the opposite of the large-particle macrofills. Composite materials that are loaded with less than 66% inorganic filler are lightly filled, or microfilled. In addition, true microfills contain extremely small particles of colloidal or fumed silica, 0.04 um in size. This small size enables the material to be polished to a very high luster. However, the low filler level results in a material that is less resistant to fracture and should not be used in stress-bearing areas.

Microfilled composite resins may be indicated for the following:

1. Protected Class III and Class V cavity preparations
2. Hypoplastic and white-spot lesions on facial surfaces
3. Small, protected, Class IV cavity preparations.
4. Closing small diastemas
5. Direct labial veneers

Small-Particle Macrofilled. The small-particle macrofilled composite resins are heavily loaded composite resins with a particle size of about 1 to 5 um. These materials offer strength and can be used in areas where fracture resistance is a consideration. They can be finished to a very smooth surface, although the surface will be somewhat duller than the surface of a microfill.

Small particle macrofills may be indicated for the following:

1. Large Class IV cavity preparations
2. Incisal edge of mandibular incisors
3. Closing wide diastemas
4. Posterior restorations

Hybrid. The hybrid composite resins were developed in an attempt to combine the best features of both the macrofilled and microfilled materials, strength and polishability. The filler particles in a true hybrid composite resin are two types: microparticles (0.04 um) and macroparticles (5 um or less). They have a high degree of fracture resistance in stress-bearing situations. The combination of filler particle sizes gives a material that is more polishable than the small-particle macrofills but less polishable than the microfills. The indications for the use of hybrid composite resins are the same as for the small-particle macrofills; however, a smoother, higher-luster surface can be obtained.

Another way to achieve high fracture resistance and polishability is the *piggy back*, or *light on heavy*, technique. The main part of the restoration is built up in macrofilled material; the surface is then veneered with a microfilled composite resin for a very smooth, gloss finish.

Most of the new composite materials developed today are of the hybrid variety, utilizing a blend of particle sizes to achieve the desired physical properties. This is especially true of the posterior composite resins. At this time, it appears that the hybrids are the composite material of the future. Depending on the particle size and percentage of fill, they can be used in both anterior and posterior situations.

Procedure

1. Local anesthesia is optional but may be indicated to allow placement of the shoulder beneath the gingival tissue. Use a rubber dam to keep salivary contamination to a minimum and protect the gingival tissues from the etching material.
2. Use a rubber dam clamp usually reserved for gold foil restoration or any rubber dam clamp that will aid in tissue reflection (Fig 19-66). It is best to restore one tooth at a time. Normal contours of the adjacent teeth can be used to contour the replacement.
3. Use a long, tapered diamond stone to prepare a veneer window (Fig 19-67). The facing should be about 1 mm *only in enamel*. Leave a collar of enamel completely around the labial aspect of the tooth. It is not necessary to carry the preparation interproximally.
4. Apply 37% phosphoric acid to the enamel surfaces (Fig 19-68). The etching material should be in contact with the enamel for 60 seconds. Rinse gently with water and evacuate the area. Again, gently dry the area. The area of etched enamel should have a chalky white appearance.
5. Place a Mylar strip between the teeth (Fig 19-69). This step is important, especially after the first composite resin veneer is completed to prevent an unintended welding of the composite resin facings.
6. The composite system that uses a visible light source as the means of polymerization is the composite system of choice. The composite material should be microfilled or one of the hybrids. Place the bonding agent over the etched surface. Gently dry with an air syringe.
7. The resin material should be dispensed from the syringe. Using a plastic instrument, adapt the resin to the etched surface of the tooth. Each increment should be polymerized with the light source. The final step includes polishing with abrasive disks and a fine polishing material in a rubber cup.
8. After the composite material is polymerized, regardless of the kind of composite resin used, complete the finishing and contouring of the labial facings of the composite resin veneer using recommended polishing procedures. Normal ridges and developmental grooves can be added to enhance the esthetic appearance.
9. Add a glaze for the final finish. The teeth will be thicker buccolingually. These surfaces will feel a little fuller to the patient and may appear so. Time will adjust this feeling.

A patient with anterior hypoplastic defects is pictured in Fig 19-70. The composite resin veneers were completed with the use of a microfilled composite resin, giving excellent esthetic results.

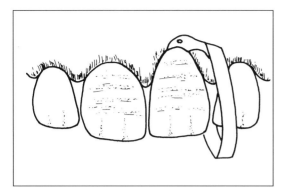

Fig 19-66 Isolate the tooth with a rubber dam clamp and rubber dam.

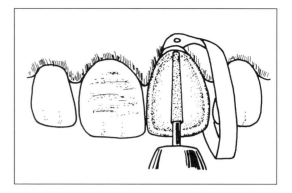

Fig 19-67 Remove a minimal amount of enamel.

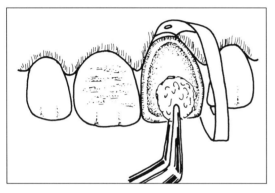

Fig 19-68 Apply phosphoric acid to the enamel surface.

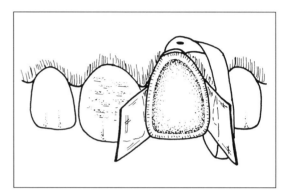

Fig 19-69 Place a Mylar strip between the teeth.

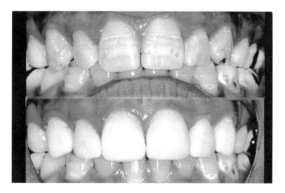

Fig 19-70 Hypoplastic defects *(top)* restored with composite resin veneers *(bottom).*

References

Aker, D. A., Aker, J. R., and Sorensen, S. E. Effect of methods of tooth enamel preparation on the retentive strength of acid-etch composite resins. J. Am. Dent. Assoc. 99:185, 1979.

Andreasen, J. O. Luxation of permanent teeth due to trauma. Scand. J. Dent. Res. 78:273, 1970.

Andreasen, J. O. Traumatic injuries of the teeth. 2nd ed. Philadelphia: W. B. Saunders Co., 1981.

Andreasen, J. O., and Andreasen, F. M. Essential of Traumatic Injuries to the Teeth. Copenhagen: Munksgaard, 1991.

Andreasen, J. O., and Ravn, J. J. The effect of traumatic injuries to primary teeth on their permanent successors II. A clinical and radiographic follow-up study of 213 teeth. Scand. J. Dent. Res. 79:284, 1970.

Baharloo, D., and Moore, D. L. Effect of acid-etching on marginal penetration of composite resin restorations. J. Prosthet. Dent. 32:152, 1974.

Basset, Y. B., et al. Effect of trauma to the primary incisors on permanent successors in different development stages. Pediatr. Dent. 7:37, 1985.

Bender I. B., and Freeland, J. D. Clinical conditions in the diagnosis and treatment of intra-alveolar root fractures. J. Am. Dent. Assoc. 107:595, 1983.

Boksman, L., et al. Etched porcelain labial veneers. Ont. Dent. 62:1, 1985.

Boksman, L., and Jordan, R. E. Conservative treatment of the stained dentition: Vital bleaching. Aust. Dent. J. 28:67, 1983.

Brannstrom, M. Dental and pulpal response. Acta Odontol. Scand. 18:234, 1960.

Brin, I., et al. Trauma to primary incisors and its effect on the permanent successors. Pediatr. Dent. 6:78, 1984.

Calamia, J. R., Etched porcelain veneers: The current state of the art. Quintessence Int. 16:5, 1985.

Calatrova, J., Dennison, J. D., and Charbeneau, G. T. Clinical evaluation of two glazing agents for composite resin: A preliminary report. Oper. Dent. 1:82, 1976.

Christensen, G. J. Veneering of teeth: State of the art. Dent. Clin. North Am. 29:373, 1985.

Collard, E. W., et al. Fundamentals of Operative Dentistry. Oklahoma City: Oklahoma University Press, 1991.

Cororan, J. F., and Zillich, R. M. Bleaching of vital tetracycline stained teeth. J. Mich. Dent. Assoc. 56:340, 1974.

Cororan, J. F., and Zillich, R. M. Update on vital bleaching. J. Mich. Dent. Assoc. 61:583, 1979.

Courts, F. J., Mueller, W. A., and Tabeling, H. J. Milk as an interim storage medium for avulsed teeth. Pediatr. Dent. 5:183, 1983.

Croll, T. P., and Cavanaugh, R. R. Enamel color modification by controlled hydrochloric acid–pumice abrasion. I Technique and examples. Quintessence Int. 17:81, 1986a.

Croll, T. P., and Cavanaugh, R. R. Enamel color modification by controlled hydrochloric acid–pumice abrasion. II. Further examples Quintessence Int. 17:157, 1986b.

Donly, K. J., and Browning, R. Class IV preparation design for microfilled and macrofilled composite resin. Pediatr. Dent. 14:34, 1992.

Eliasson, S. T., and Hill, G. L. Cavosurface design and marginal leakage of composite resin restorations. Oper. Dent. 2:55, 1977.

Faunce, F. The use of laminate veneers for restoration of fractured and discolored teeth. Tex. Dent. J. 93:6, 1975.

Frank, A. L. Therapy for the divergent pulpless tooth by continued apical formation. J. Am. Dent. Assoc. 72:87, 1966.

Fuks, A. B., Bielak, S., and Chosak, A. Clinical and radiographic assessment of direct pulp capping and pulpotomy in permanent teeth. Pediatr. Dent. 4:240, 1982.

Grossman, L. I., and Ship, I. I. Survival rate of replanted teeth. Oral Surg. 29:899, 1970.

Gwinnett, A. J. Structural changes in enamel and dentin of fractured anterior teeth after acid conditioning in vitro. J. Am. Dent. Assoc. 86:117, 1973.

Haywood, V. B. History, safety and effectiveness of "current" bleaching techniques and applications of the nightguard vital bleaching techniques. Quintessence, Inc. 23:471, 1992.

Haywood, V. B. and Heymann, H. O. Nightguard vital bleaching. Quintessence Int. 20:174, 1989.

Hobo, S., and Iwata, T. A new laminate veneer technique using a castable apatite ceramic material. I. Theoretical considerations. Quintessence Int. 7:451, 1985.

Horn, H. R. Porcelain laminate veneers bonded to etched enamel. Dent. Clin. North Am. 27:671, 1983.

Kapila, S., and Currier, G. F. Hydrochloric acid–pumice treatment for post-orthodontic localized decalcification. Am J. Dent. 1:15, 1988.

Kozlowska, I. Direct pulp capping. Dent. Abstr. 6:214, 1961.

McCloskey, R. J. A technique for removal of fluorosis stains. J. Am. Dent. Assoc. 109:63, 1984.

Meadow, D., Needleham, H., and Linder, G. Oral trauma in children. Pediatr. Dent. 6:248, 1984.

Michanowicz, A. E., et al. Cementogenic repair of root fractures. J. Am. Dent. Assoc. 82:567, 1971.

Mitchem, J. C. Resin restoration: Factors affecting clinical performance. Dent. Clin. North Am. 27:713, 1983.

Mitchem, J. C., and Turner, L. R. The retentive strengths of acid-etched retained resins. J. Am. Dent. Assoc. 89:1107, 1974.

Myers, D. R., et al. The effectiveness of bleaching for the removal of tetracycline from rat incisors. J. Pedod. 4:227, 1980.

Nelson, S. R., Till, M. J., and Hinding, J. H. Comparison of materials and methods used in acid-etch restorative procedures. J. Am. Dent. Assoc. 89:1123, 1974.

Quinn, F., McConnell, R. J., and Byrne, D. Porcelain laminates: A review. Br. Dent. J. 161:61, 1986.

Ravn, J. J. Follow-up study of permanent incisors with complicated crown fractures after acute trauma. Scand. J. Dent. Res. 90:363, 1982.

Riekman, G. A., and El Badrawry, H. E. Effect of premature loss of primary incisors on speech. Pediatr Dent. 7:119, 1985.

Ripa, L. W., and Sheykholam, Z. Acid etch technique of fracture repair: Description and current status. J. Pedod. 2:128, 1978.

Seale, N. S., and Wilson, C. F. G. Pulpal response to bleaching of teeth in dogs. Pediatr. Dent. 7:209, 1985.

Sheets, C. G., and Taniguchi, T. Advantages and limitations in the use of porcelain veneer restorations. J. Prosthet. Dent. 64:406, 1990.

Steiner, J. C., Dow, P. R., and Cathey, G. M. Inducing root-end closure of nonvital permanent teeth. J. Dent. Child. 35:47, 1968.

Tolley, L. G., O'Brien, W. J., and Dennison, J. B. Surface finish of dental composite restorative materials. J. Biomed. Mater. Res. 12:223, 1978.

Weine, F. S. Endodontic Therapy. 2nd ed. St. Louis: The C. V. Mosby Co., 1976.

Wilson, C. F. G., and Seale, N. S. Color change following vital bleaching of tetracycline-stained teeth. Pediatr. Dent. 7:205, 1985.

Additional readings

American Dental Association Council on Dental Materials, Instruments, and Equipment. Status report on enamel bonding of composite, preformed laminate, and laboratory fabricated resin veneers. J. Am. Dent. Assoc. 109:762, 1984.

Berman, L. H. Intrinsic staining and hypoplastic enamel. Etiology and treatment alternatives. Gen. Dent. 30:484, 1982.

Calatrova, L., Dennison, J. D., and Charbeneau, G. T. Clinical evaluation of two glazing agents for composite resin: A preliminary report. Oper. Dent. 1:82, 1976.

Cohen, S. C. Human pulpal response to bleaching procedures of vital teeth. J. Endod. 5:134, 1979.

Croll, T. P. Enamel Microabrasion. Chicago: Quintessence, 1991.

Croll, T. P. Enamel microabrasion for removal of superficial dysmineralization and decalcification defects. J. Am. Dent. Assoc. 120:411, 1990.

Fountain, S. B., and Comp, J. H. Traumatic injuries. In Pathways of the Pulp. 4th ed. St. Louis: The C. V. Mosby Co., 1987.

Harley, K. E., and Ibbetson, R. J. Anterior veneers for the adolescent patient. 1. General indications and composite veneers. Dent. Update 18:55, 1991.

Harley, K. E., and Ibbetson, R. J. Anterior veneers for the adolescent patient. 2. Porcelain veneers and conclusions. Dent. Update 18:112, 1990.

Haywood, V. B., and Heymann, H. O. Nightguard bleaching: How safe is it? Quintessence Inc. 22:515, 1991.

Helpin, M. L. The open-faced stainless steel crown restoration in children. J. Dent. Child. 50:34, 1983.

Johnson, W. W. Use of laminate veneers in pediatric dentistry: Present status and future development. Pediatr. Dent. 4:32, 1982.

Khanna, S. L., and Chow, J. Comparison of four composite materials and effect on tooth preparation. J. Dent. Child. 46:379, 1979.

Krakow, A. A., Berk, H., And Gron, P. Therapeutic induction of root formation in the exposed incompletely formed tooth with vital pulp. Oral Surg. 43:755, 1977.

Larson, T. D., and Phair, C. B. The use of direct bonded microfilled composite resin veneer. J. Am. Dent. Assoc. 115:449, 1987.

Mathewson, R. J. Morrison, J. T., and Carpenter, R. Modification of stained enamel surfaces: Use of hydrochloric acid and pumice mixture. Okla. Dent. Assoc. J. Spring: 22, 1987.

McCloskey, R. J. A technique for removal of fluorosis stain. J. Am. Dent. Assoc. 109:63, 1984.

Mitra, S. S. Decision Support System: Tools and Techniques. New York: Wiley, 1986.

Powell, V. L., and Boles, D. J. Tooth bleaching: Its effect on oral tissues. J. Am. Dent. Assoc. 122:50, 1991.

Thorton, J. B., Wright J. T., and Fritcher, B. P. Microfilled composite restorative resins in pediatric dentistry. Compend. Cont. Educ. Dent. 5:665, 1984.

Watson, S. R. Decision Synthesis: The Principle and Practice. New York: Cambridge University Press, 1987.

Zadik, D., et al. Traumatized teeth: Two-year results. J. Pedod. 4:16, 1980.

Questions

1. The maxillary central incisors of a 2-year-old child were traumatically intruded 2 mm apically. Immediate treatment would require:

    a. Carefully removing both incisors
    b. Repositioning the intruded teeth
    c. Making the patient as comfortable as possible without disturbing the teeth
    d. Repositioning and splinting the intruded teeth with preformed bands on the central and lateral incisors and a soldered contoured labial arch wire attached to the bands

2. A 4.5-year-old child has fallen within the past 2 hours and traumatized both maxillary central incisors to the point that they are extremely mobile. The treatment of choice would be to:

    a. Extract them because they would be lost soon anyway
    b. Do nothing and observe periodically
    c. Immobilize them with a splint and do nothing more
    d. Check radiographically for root fractures, and if none, proceed with a splint and periodic examination

3. A 3-year-old child has a central incisor that has turned bluish black. There is a small radiolucent area at the apex of the tooth. The ideal treatment is:

    a. Extraction
    b. Pulpotomy with formocresol
    c. Pulpectomy; fill with zinc oxide-eugenol
    d. Pulpotomy with calcium hydroxide

4. A 6-year-old girl fractures her left central incisor. There is a large pulpal exposure of 6 hours' duration. Radiographs show no root fracture but verify the pulpal exposure. The tooth is not excessively mobile. The soft tissue and lip and bruised but not lacerated. The pulp treatment should be:

    a. Pulp cap with calcium hydroxide
    b. Pulpotomy with formocresol
    c. Pulpotomy with calcium hydroxide
    d. Pulpectomy and apexification
    e. Extraction

5. A 7-year-old boy is seen in your office. The right central incisor is darkly discolored, and the mother relates a history of trauma "about 1 year ago." The radiograph shows a small area of periapical involvement. The pulp treatment at this time should be:

    a. Formocresol pulpotomy
    b. Calcium hydroxide pulpotomy
    c. Extraction
    d. Root canal treatment
    e. Pulpectomy and apexification technique

6. A 17-year-old comes to your office with a history of long-term use of a tetracycline; the anterior teeth are a mild yellowish brown. What method would you use to remove the tetracycline stain?

    a. Hydrochloric acid–pumice microabrasion
    b. At-home bleaching method
    c. Superoxol with or without heat
    d. Composite resin veneers

7. A 18-year-old has just completed orthodontic therapy. To the amazement of the orthodontist, removal of the orthodontic bands revealed a number of white decalcifications around the anterior teeth. The orthodontist calls you. "Can you do something?" he asks. What method would you use to remove the decalcified spots?

    a. Hydrochloric acid–pumice microabrasion
    b. At-home bleaching
    c. Superoxol with or without heat
    d. Composite resin veneers

8. A 17-year-old with hypoplastic defects on the maxillary incisors sought consultation for a means to improve the appearance of these teeth. A contraindication for use of a laminate veneer method is:

    a. High cost
    b. Mouth breathing
    c. The need to remove a minimal amount of enamel
    d. Acid etching of the enamel
    e. None of the above

317

Chapter 20

Extraction Techniques

Objectives

After studying this chapter, the student should be able to:
1. Identify and describe offending oral problems through objective symptomatology.
2. Discuss factors to be considered regarding an impacted supernumerary tooth.
3. Discuss the role of antibiotic therapy in the course of acute, subacute, and chronic dental infections.
4. Describe postoperative care following the surgical removal of a tooth.
5. Describe the contraindications to removal of a primary tooth.
6. Demonstrate the technique for removing a primary incisor, canine, or molar.
7. Describe the surgical sectioning of a primary molar to facilitate its atraumatic removal.
8. Demonstrate effective removal of a fractured primary tooth root.

Considerations for and the technical procedures involved in the extraction of primary and permanent teeth in both simple and moderately complex situations are discussed in this chapter.

What might ordinarily be a simple extraction of a primary tooth may become a rather difficult problem should the clinical crown be destroyed or weakened by caries or trauma or should the tooth be severely ankylosed. The woefully impaired clinical crown of a permanent first molar can also produce complexity.

Overall considerations

Until recent years, the study and development of established minor oral surgical procedures for the child patient have been minimal. Authorities in oral surgery compared removals of primary teeth with those of the permanent dentition. Some considered the technique for removal of a primary tooth no different than that for a permanent tooth. Others made the point that the extraction of the primary tooth was easier to perform if the root system exhibited appreciable resorption.

With the advent of pediatric dentistry, more viable principles of diagnosis began to surface. The dentist now realizes that when a good understanding of oral surgery principles is coupled with a sound management technique, the procedures, as related to the child

can be accomplished with adequate skill and confidence (Archer, 1975).

The indications for tooth removal for the child are related to extensive caries, root pathosis, fractured roots or crowns, ankylosed teeth, and supernumerary and overretained primary teeth.

As previously stated, management of the child is a concern linked with the oral surgical measure. Law et al (1969) consider fear the leading obstacle and possible impasse to required dental treatment. If a child who is fearful or who has been managed poorly in the dental office realizes he or she is to have a tooth extraction, the child's "anxiety titer" can be quite high. Law et al (1969) contend in this instance that the child should be informed 1 week or so in advance of the pending oral surgery procedure. In this way, the psychologic stress will be lessened.

We have observed when dealing with the fear within some children that the circumstances presented at the moment and the degree to which the child may control his or her own emotions casts a deciding influence on the treatment procedure. The patient's internal and external responses to the stress will be the guide to the practitioner's decision of approach and time of treatment. With adequate patient management and sensible measures of pain control, the patient's fear of a tooth extraction may be kept to a low level of concern.

Care and planning must go into any minor oral surgery procedure for the child. The dentist must identify the problem, plan the best course of treatment, and skillfully execute the procedure according to plan. Clinical identification of the offending tooth is the prime requisite. It may be readily identified through the objective symptoms of acute or subacute discomfort, such as the pain of pulpal deterioration, or periodontal ligament inflammation, as indicated by tenderness to pressure or marked tooth mobility.

On the other hand, the symptoms may be subjective. The patient is usually comfortable, and clinical signs are more subdued. Close observation, however, may indicate some sign of gingival inflammation along with a suggestion of pathologic tooth mobility. Cervical lymphadenopathy may be apparent. The patient's condition may be accompanied by a draining fistula associated with chronic inflammation.

Whether the symptoms are subjective or objective, clinical signs are an important means of identifying or substantiating the problem.

Antibiotic therapy

The need for and the type of antibiotic therapy selected should be carefully determined in cases of severe chronic or acute oral infection of odontogenic origin. The choice of the agent will depend on the site of infection, the kind of microorganisms present, and the severity of the infective process (Megran et al, 1984).

Pyogenic infections are best treated with penicillin or amoxicillin in conjunction with removal of necrotic pulpal tissue or the tooth itself. If the pediatric patient is subject to unfavorable response to the agent, the substitution of clindamycin as the antimicrobial vehicle is acceptable. The cephalosporins are another group that is highly active with the anaerobes prevalent in the infective process. Neither erythromycin nor tetracycline is considered an effective antimicrobial vehicle in the presence of mixed oral infections because their in vitro action is subpar against some forms of anaerobes.

Fever alone should not be an indication for the use of antibiotics. It is essential that the microbiology of the oral flora in the infective state be determined, and the information should be procured through a blood culture, if necessary. The antimicrobial agent with the narrowest antimicrobial spectrum should be considered when the vehicle is chosen.

Armamentarium

The surgical instruments designed for adult procedures can be used effectively for the child patient. Some forceps are specifically designed for the small mouth. Thoma (1958) states that the small forceps are easily concealed and less fear inspiring. The Nos. 150-S and 151-S forceps are excellent instruments for the removal of primary teeth.

Forceps and elevators that by virtue of their design and function threaten the underlying developing permanent teeth should be avoided. Such a forceps is the cowhorn. Its beaks descend into the furcal areas of, for example, a primary mandibular molar as pressure is applied and proves destructive. Large root elevators are also contraindicated. Narrow root picks and mosquito-beaked forceps are the instruments of choice for root removals.

Postoperative considerations

Postoperative concerns are the same for the most part. Occasionally there may be some postsurgical hemorrhage associated with tooth removal, but not of much significance in the well child. Localized osteitis (dry socket) is even more infrequent.

Postsurgical discomfort following the majority of procedures is negligible. Should there be discomfort, the use of a mild analgesic, such as acetaminophen (Tylenol), in recommended dosage should provide the needed relief.

The patient should allow the clean gauze pack that was placed on the wound before dismissal to remain in place for at least 10 minutes. The precaution will usually suffice during the postoperative bleeding period, thus permitting a firm blood clot to form. A soft diet the first day postoperatively will be kinder to the surgical wound and be less likely to disturb the newly established clot.

The parent should exercise caution and observe the child during the effective period of the local anesthetic. The young patient may unknowingly or through curiosity chew on and traumatize the anesthetized area of the lip, tongue, or cheek.

Warm saline mouth rinses should be used at least four or five times daily beginning on the day following the operation. The rinse should consist of a glass of warm water, as warm as can be held comfortably in the mouth, with 40 mg (¼ teaspoon) of salt added to it. The rinsing action should be gentle and should be continued for 2 or 3 days following surgery.

Rationale for tooth removal

A number of conditions predispose the need for removal of primary teeth. They are as follows (Archer, 1975):

1. Acute pathologic involvement. This involvement represents an acute periapical infection of a carious primary tooth. The microorganisms may be virulent enough to produce an infection that is diffused and distended, such as cellulitis. The operator will need to carefully consider a pulpectomy for such a tooth. However, extraction is more often the measure of choice.

2. Chronic pathologic involvement. The primary molar is usually carious with apical or furcal pathosis, whereas the primary anterior tooth may have apical involvement, the culmination of caries or trauma. Either of these conditions will likely demonstrate a parulis. The position of the developing permanent tooth in the infective environment threatens the maturing tooth's normalcy. Tooth removal, therefore, is the accepted procedure.

3. The overretained primary tooth. The resorptive mechanism is contingent on the eruption process of the developing permanent tooth. If the erupting succedaneous tooth is malposed, the resorptive process on the primary tooth may be irregular. Should the erupting tooth be completely displaced and the eruptive forces directed elsewhere, root resorption on the primary tooth may not take place. The resorptive process may also be affected by endocrine disturbances or vitamin deficiencies. Atypical resorption of a primary tooth root may cause it to be overretained. The offending tooth should be eliminated before it complicates normal eruption.

4. The ankylosed primary tooth. When the cessation of vertical alveolar bone growth is observed, as evidenced by primary tooth submergence, close supervision is necessary. The ankylosed tooth should be removed at a propitious time and space maintenance should be considered.

5. The cariously involved, nonrestorable primary tooth. When caries has seriously involved the clinical crown of a tooth in the primary dentition, the tooth should be removed. Use of an appliance to retain the space should be studied.

6. The natal or neonatal primary tooth. The natal tooth, which has erupted before birth, or the neonatal tooth, usually erupting 1 month following birth, must be considered for extraction if *(1)* the tooth is mobile and there is a chance of aspiration; *(2)* the tooth is a source of mechanical irritation, causing ulceration on the ventral surface of the tongue; or *(3)* there is interference with breastfeeding. The natal or neonatal tooth may be a supernumerary tooth.

7. The supernumerary tooth. The supernumerary tooth, erupted or impacted, is capable of diverting eruption of a permanent tooth from its normal path, impacting it, or delaying its eruption. It should be removed. If it does not interfere directly with eruption of the permanent tooth, its extraction may be delayed. Critical observation during this interim period is necessary to guard against possible cystic formation.

8. The fractured or traumatized tooth. Toddlers and preschoolers often injure their anterior teeth, fracturing crowns, exposing vital pulpal tissue, fracturing roots, and intruding or luxating teeth. Trauma and injury to teeth often create concern about what should be done. With toddlers there is scant opportunity to treat and retain severely damaged teeth, the problem being immaturity in both dentitional and mental development. The decision will usually be tooth removal. The preschool-

er has an increased mental maturity, along with a significant change in dental development. With the preschooler there is more opportunity for pulpal and restorative treatment for the injured tooth.

9. The impacted tooth. The impacted tooth may be a supernumerary tooth, a malformed tooth, or an unerupted, ectopically placed tooth. For the young child, its removal is complicated and requires the decision and performance skill of a well-trained professional.

Contraindications to tooth removal

The removal of a tooth is contraindicated where acute symptoms of oral or systemic disease are manifested in the child patient. Acute infection requires consultation with the child's physician, and subsequent tooth elimination will be dependent on a more improved general health (Hertz et al, 1979).

1. Acute systemic infections. After the acute stages of systemic infections, such as glomerulonephritis, congenital heart disease, rheumatic fever, rheumatic heart disease, are reduced to chronicity, regimens of chemoprophylaxis will be required before extractions.

2. Blood diseases. The hemophilic or leukemic child will require a well-trained general dentist, a pediatric dentist, or an oral surgeon along with a hematologist to perform satisfactorily the measures required during tooth removal.

3. Uncontrolled diabetes mellitus. Tooth removals should be avoided. Surgical wounds heal poorly, and postoperative pain can be extreme. Recurrent hemorrhages may result.

4. Irradiated bone. Tooth removal should be avoided. If an extraction is necessary, it should be accomplished before radiation therapy. Osteomyelitis usually develops following an extraction in an irradiated patient because of osseous avascularity.

5. Acute oral infection. In the presence of oral infections, such as acute necrotizing ulcerative gingivitis, acute herpetic stomatitis, acute dentoalveolar abscessing, and other acute forms of oral disease, tooth removals are definitely contraindicated until the infections are eliminated.

Technique for tooth removal

Precautions

Immediately following the local anesthetic procedure, the dentist should explain to the child the sensations and experiences to be encountered. To the uninformed child the sensation of pressure from the forceps during the extraction procedure can be interpreted as pain, and extraneous noise and osseous sound conduction associated with luxation seem to aggravate the anxieties of the moment. Explain and demonstrate to the child that pressures and noises associated with tooth extractions are not to be feared.

Undue pressure should never be placed on a tooth when it is being luxated. The forces from the forceps should be firmly but gently applied. The forceps and hand must be allowed to feel the alveolar bone distend as pressure is exerted. The delivery should not be hurried. Precautions such as this minimize root fracture while effectively loosening the tooth from its periodontal attachments.

When a mandibular tooth is removed, it is prudent to stabilize the mandible during the manipulative action. Stabilization may be provided by support under the mandible or by the use of a rubber bite block or mouth gag.

The precautions necessary to avoid the unintentional removal of a permanent tooth bud during the extraction of a primary molar tooth should be understood. The dentist must know what the root system is like. Is the permanent tooth bud closely involved with the root system? Radiographic confirmation is essential before tooth extraction.

Another measure of precaution is the use of a safety screen of gauze over the oropharynx to guard against swallowing or aspiration of an extracted tooth. A gauze sponge, either 5 x 5 cm (2 x 2 in.) or 10 x 10 cm (4 x 4 in.) is unfolded and placed along the tongue adjacent to the extraction site to gently cover the oropharynx.

Primary incisors and canines

Armamentarium

Straight elevator, No. 301
Forceps
    No. 151 or 151-S
    No. 150 or 150-S
Gauze sponges, 5 or 10 cm (2 or 4 in.)
Rubber bite block

Procedure

1. Use a No. 301 straight elevator to free the attached gingiva from the cervix of the tooth labially and lingually. Luxate the tooth slightly.
2. For mandibular teeth, apply and maintain firm apical pressure with the No. 151 or 151-S forceps. Support the mandible with your free hand. Gently direct the initial luxative force lingually and carefully apply the next toward the labial side. Apply a rotative force along the tooth's long axis, delivering it through its path of least resistance.
3. For maxillary teeth, apply firm apical pressure with the No. 150 or 150-S forceps as the beaks engage

the tooth. Direct the initial luxative movement toward the palate and then, carefully, labially. Rotate the tooth on its long axis in one continuous direction, delivering it with the rotation.
4. Mold the labial and lingual or palatal plates of the alveolar bone into normal conformity with digital pressure.
5. Fold and place a sterile gauze sponge over the wound to help establish hemostasis. Immediately before patient dismissal, place a fresh sterile sponge over the wound with instructions to remove it after 10 minutes.

Primary molars

Armamentarium

Elevators
    Straight, Nos. 301 and 34-S
    Periosteal, No. 9
Forceps
    No. 151 or 151-S
    No. 150 or 150-S
Rubber bite block
Gauze sponges, 5 or 10 cm (2 or 4 in.)

Procedure

1. Use a straight or periosteal elevator to free the attached gingiva. Luxate the tooth slightly.
2. For mandibular teeth, apply the beaks of a No. 151 or 151-S forceps to the clinical crown and establish firm apical pressure while supporting the mandible with the free hand. Initial luxation is toward the buccal side. Hold pressure momentarily, permitting buccal alveolar plate expansion. Return the luxating force lingually. Hold pressure to permit lingual alveolar plate expansion. Alternate the buccal and lingual movements to further expand the cortical plate. When there is adequate freedom of movement, deliver the tooth to the buccal or lingual side, exercising slow, firm, continuous pressure.
3. For maxillary teeth, apply the beaks of a No. 150 or 150-S forceps to the clinical crown and secure a positive apical pressure. Initial luxative movement is toward the buccal side while maintaining a strong apical pressure. Hold buccal pressure for a moment to permit slight cortical plate expansion. Return luxative force toward the palate. Momentarily hold compression to afford cortical plate expansion. Continue alternate buccal and lingual movements, pausing briefly with each one. With a freedom in buccal and lingual movement, you can deliver the tooth palatally or buccally.
4. Mold the labial and palatal cortical plates into normal conformity with finger pressure.
5. Place a folded sterile gauze sponge over the wound during the hemostatic process.

Aberrant primary molar roots

Not infrequently, the primary mandibular second molar tooth will have diverging mesial and distal roots. In more rare instances, the roots are so developed as to interfere with a developing tooth bud. In either situation, the primary second molar should be sectioned and removed one half at a time, preventing possible oral damage from excessive force (Fig 20-1).

Armamentarium

Elevators
  Straight, No. 301
  Periosteal, No. 9
Bur, No. 169L, 330 or narrow, tapered diamond stone
Gauze sponges, 5 x 5 cm (2 x 2 in.) or 10 x 10 cm (4 x 4 in.)
Rubber bite block
Forceps No. 151 or 151-S

Procedure

1. Place the bur or tapered diamond stone at the buccal groove of the tooth to be removed and section the crown buccolingually, carrying the slice to the floor of the pulp chamber and beneath the free margin of the gingiva (Fig 20-2).
2. Place the No. 301 straight elevator into the slice and rotate it on its long axis, splitting the tooth through its bifurcation (Fig 20-3).
3. Remove one half of the tooth and then the remaining half, with an extraction forceps. Use a buccal-to-lingual movement to luxate and deliver each half.
4. Place a sterile 5 x 5-cm (2 x 2-in.) sponge over the wound to aid hemostasis.

Fractured or residual root tips

Similar to a primary tooth extraction, root removal can be simple or time consuming and complex. The degree of difficulty depends on the circumstances of its existence in the oral cavity. The root may be the remains of a primary tooth involved in a destructive carious process, or a root may fracture during tooth removal. There may be a root remnant from a previous extraction. Trauma, such as a avulsion of luxation, may be the predecessor of a fractured root tip.

A root or multiple root particles may be observed clinically when a child's mouth is examined, the remnants of a severe, destructive caries process (Fig 20-4). These roots will vary in size and condition depending on the amount of time they have been in the oral cavity and the manner of resorption. The root particles are usually mobile in that their support is largely that of inflammatory tissue. They are easily removed.

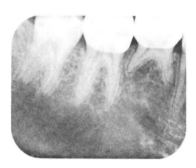

Fig 20-1 The primary mandibular right second molar has diverged roots. It is to be removed for orthodontic purposes, but for removal without a possible tooth or patient mishap, the choice extraction procedure should be sectioning. Note that the mandibular right second premolar is congenitally absent.

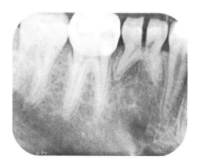

Fig 20-2 The cleft extends from the buccal groove through the lingual groove, dividing the crown in half buccolingually. Its depth is to the floor of the pulp chamber, extending buccally and lingually into the free gingival space.

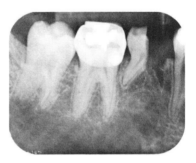

Fig 20-3 A No. 301 straight elevator is inserted into the cleft and rotated slightly, splitting the tooth in half. One half is removed with No. 151 forceps.

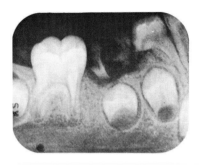

Fig 20-4 Root remnants of a severe, destructive carious process. The radiograph indicates that the roots are supported in inflammatory tissue.

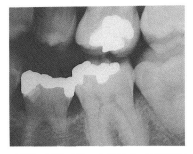

Fig 20-5 The primary mandibular second molar is ankylosed, leading to mesial tipping of the permanent mandibular first molar, thus causing a loss of arch length.

Armamentarium

Straight elevator, No. 301
Right and left narrow root picks
Mosquito-beak forceps
Rubber bite block
Gauze sponges, 5 x 5 cm (2 x 2 in.) or 10 x 10 cm (4 x 4 in.)
Rosenthal and duckbill Rongeurs

Procedures

1. Place an unfolded gauze sponge over the tongue, lightly covering the oropharynx.
2. Use an elevator to probe about the root, separating it from the tissue, thus removing the root. Or wedge the elevator between an adjacent tooth and the root. Gently rotate the elevator blade, lifting the root from the tissue.
3. You can use mosquito-beak forceps to grasp a small root, thereby lifting it out.
4. The Blumenthal rongeur is shaped somewhat like a No. 150 forceps and is useful in grasping and removing roots, particularly in the maxilla. The duckbill rongeur resembles a No. 151 forceps and is well suited for removal of roots in the mandible.

Inaccessible root tips

There will be occasions when a primary tooth root is inaccessible for removal unless a surgical bone-removal procedure is exercised. If the root is hopelessly unattainable through normal means but will not interfere with normal growth and eruption, sound judgment supports leaving the root to resorb or eventually exfoliate on its own. Should obvious difficulties be created with the presence of the fractured root, the choice procedure would be surgical intervention. Law et al (1969) stated, "the better part of valor is to leave the embedded root tip and let it be exfoliated or resorbed."

Ankylosed teeth

Protection of the underlying permanent dentition must also be thought of in cases of ankylosis. The ankylosed primary tooth may be completely submerged and adjacent to the developmental tooth bud. The task of removing the tooth can be difficult in itself, but special surgical care and skill must be exercised to prevent injury to the developing dentition during the procedure.

The phenomenon of the so-called submerging-type tooth anomaly is not completely understood. It is evident that the gradual sinking of a tooth is somehow associated with failure of vertical bone growth, caused by fusion of the cementum of the root with bone and the accompanying loss of periodontal ligament attachment. The results are loss of arch length, extrusion of teeth of the opposite arch, and interference with eruption of the succedaneous teeth.

If observed ankylosed teeth are left until submergence is almost complete, a tipping of the tooth distal to the space will occur, thus causing a loss of arch length (Fig 20-5). The space may be protected by placing a crown on the ankylosed tooth to preserve the mesiodistal dimension. A better procedure may be to remove the tooth and place a space maintainer.

Supereruption of a tooth in the opposite arch must be guarded against. Again, the placement of a stainless steel crown may keep the ankylosed tooth in occlusal function and prevent extrusion of a tooth in the opposite arch. A space maintainer that will not only protect mesiodistal dimension but also supply an occlusal function, preventing supereruption, may be placed.

An ankylosed primary tooth may also prevent timely eruption of the succeeding permanent tooth. The condition can establish an impaction of the permanent tooth or divert its direction of eruption—either one causing an affection of total arch length. An ankylosed primary tooth should be observed closely and be removed at the normal exfoliation time, providing the tooth is not jeopardizing normal development.

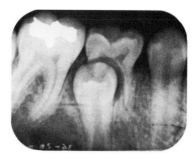

Fig 20-6 The primary mandibular second molar is overretained because of failure of the mesial root to resorb. The condition is caused by the ectopic positioning of the developing second premolar. The second premolar will very likely erupt in lingual version. Arch length development can be affected.

Overretained teeth

Ordinarily the primary tooth moves through an orderly, timed system of root resorption with eventual exfoliation along with its antimere. It is not rare to observe that a particular tooth is overretained. A radiograph will reveal a root that has failed to resorb or a resorption process that is incomplete. There may be a history of repeated injury to anterior primary teeth. In the case of the primary mandibular second molar, one root may resorb completely while the other is unaffected. Occasionally this failure to resorb is due to an ectopically positioned developing tooth (Fig 20-6).

When a primary tooth is obviously overretained, it should be removed.

Supernumerary teeth

The supernumerary tooth may erupt into normal alignment and divert the position of the regular successor in its eruption. A dentist may examine a child 4 years of age exhibiting a well-aligned maxillary dentition, only to take a second look and observe two primary lateral incisors on one side of the arch. A supernumerary tooth may erupt in the midline, occupying the interproximal space between the permanent maxillary central incisors. This type of tooth is referred to as a *mesiodens*. A supernumerary tooth may be impacted or lay in almost any posture, diverting or preventing eruption of a permanent tooth.

The removal of a supernumerary tooth may at times require careful consideration (Primosch, 1981). In some instances a determination must be made as to which tooth is the supernumerary and which, therefore, should be sacrificed. The tooth removal will vary from the simple elimination of a well-positioned tooth to the complicated extraction of a malposed or impacted tooth.

References

Archer, W. H. Oral and Maxillofacial Surgery, Vol. 1. 5th ed. Philadelphia: W. B. Saunders Co., 1975, pp. 110-128.

Hertz, R. S., Saunders, B., and Wolk, R. S. Dentoalveolar surgery. In Saunders, B. Pediatric Oral and Maxillofacial Surgery. St. Louis: The C. V. Mosby Co., 1979.

Law, D. B., Thompson, M. L., and Davis, J. M. An Atlas of Pedodontics. Philadelphia: W. B. Saunders Co., 1969.

Megran, D. W., Scheifele, D. W., Chow, A. W. Odontogenic infections. Pediatr. Infect. Dis. 3:3, 257, 1984.

Primosch, R. E. Anterior supernumerary teeth assessment and surgical intervention. Pediatr. Dent. 3:204, 1981.

Thoma, K. H. Oral Surgery, 3rd ed. St. Louis: The C. V. Mosby Co., 1958, pp. 202-203.

Questions

1. A 3-week-old infant has been appointed for dental examination. A prematurely erupted primary mandibular left incisor is noted. Which of the following factors will help determine the correct treatment?

    a. The tooth has only soft tissue attachment with marked mobility
    b. The tooth is natal in development
    c. Ventral surface of infants's tongue is traumatized
    d. Mother's breasts are traumatized and tender due to infant's nursing
    e. Clinical crown is well calcified
    f. a,c,d
    g. b,e
    h. c,d

2. The correct treatment for the infant referred to in question 1 should be to leave the tooth in the arch and permit the root to develop.

    a. True
    b. False

3. Jimmy aged 6 years, exhibits a parulis apical to the primary maxillary right lateral incisor. He has a history of prior, unpleasant dental experiences. He is fearful of the tooth's removal. The logical procedure in this instance will be to:

    a. Remove the tooth at this time
    b. Prescribe a conscious sedation procedure, with tooth removal at a subsequent appointment
    c. Explain to Jimmy the reasons for removal of the tooth, how it will be performed, and reappoint in 1 week
    d. Refer him to an oral surgeon for the tooth removal

4. A 9-year-old is appointed on the emergency schedule. The primary mandibular left second molar is infected. Radiographically, there is evidence of a furcal lesion. He has a fever of 39°C (102.2°F), malaise, and chills. A moderate, generalized swelling is palpable extending mesially and distally along the buccal surface of the soft tissue adjacent to the affected tooth. The appropriate decision before tooth removal will be:

    a. To prescribe an antibiotic
    b. To prescribe a broad-spectrum antibiotic
    c. Not to prescribe an antibiotic
    d. To establish drainage into the pulp chamber
    e. To prescribe warm saline irrigation hourly or after meals
    f. To prescribe a narrow-spectrum antibiotic
    g. c,d,e
    h. a,d,e,f

5. Jane, aged 7, has a carious primary maxillary left first molar that is causing discomfort. The buccal soft tissue is inflamed and spongy to palpation. A furcal bone lesion is evident radiographically. The appropriate treatment will be:

    a. Pulpectomy
    b. Tooth removal and placement of a space maintainer appliance
    c. Tooth removal
    d. Pulpotomy
    e. To establish drainage into the pulp chamber and permit the tooth to remain until exfoliated

Chapter 21

Space Maintenance

Objectives

After studying this chapter, the student should be able to:
1. Discuss the scope of arch length and occlusal discrepancies.
2. Recognize the problems of arch length discrepancy.
3. Identify the factors contributing to abnormal arch form development.
4. Effectively manage a condition of premature primary tooth loss.

Purpose of a space maintainer

The function of a space maintainer is to preserve arch length following the premature loss of a primary tooth (or teeth). The space maintainer allows the permanent tooth to erupt unhindered into proper alignment and occlusion. A space maintainer is recommended after the extraction of a primary molar. Just "watching" often results in the creation of a more difficult arch length problem (Fig 21-1).

Types of space maintainers

Fixed or removable appliances can be used to maintain space to prevent arch length loss. If restorable abutment teeth are available, a fixed appliance is the appliance of choice. A fixed appliance reduces the incidence of broken and lost appliances; a fixed appliance is somewhat less reliant on patient cooperation.

There are four basic types of space maintainers (Pedodontic Appliances, 1977):

1. The band (crown) and loop is used to maintain the loss of a single primary first or second molar (Fig 21-2).
2. The Nance holding arch maintains the maxillary arch length after the premature loss of more than one primary maxillary molar in the same quadrant or after a bilateral loss of primary molars (Fig 21-3).
3. The fixed lingual arch is used to maintain mandibu-

lar arch length and prevent mesial tipping and/or rotation of the permanent first molars (Fig 21-4). The fixed lingual arch prevents lingual tipping of the permanent incisors.
4. The intra-alveolar ("distal shoe") appliance is used to prevent mesial migration of the unerupted permanent first molar after premature loss of the primary second molar (Fig 21-5).

Band and loop appliances

Band and loops are not active appliances.

Indications (Currier and Austerman, 1992; Moyers, 1988; Nanda, 1993; Profitt and Fields, 1993)

1. Premature loss of any primary first molar in the primary dentition or the primary maxillary first molar in the transitional dentition. In these cases the unerupted premolar usually is more than 2 years from clinical eruption and its root length is less than one third mature.
2. Premature loss of a primary second molar as the permanent first molar is erupting clinically. These cases must be followed up with other types of appliance therapy as the entire occlusal portion of the permanent first molar erupts.

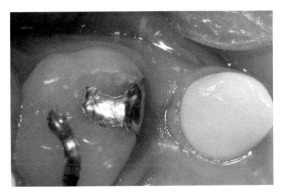

Fig 21-1   Loss of space from the failure to maintain the space of the primary maxillary second molar.

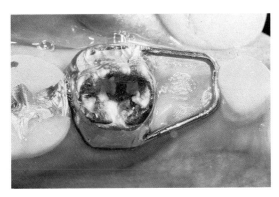

Fig 21-2   Crown and loop space maintainer.

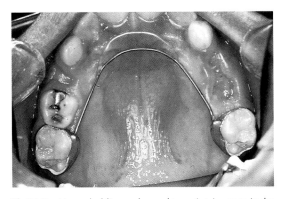

Fig 21-3   Nance holding arch, used to maintain space in the maxillary arch. Note the small acrylic resin button in the palatal area.

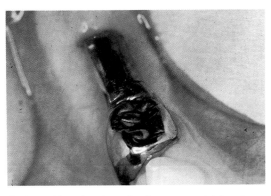

Fig 21-4   Fixed lingual arch used to maintain the space for the loss of mandibular primary teeth.

Contraindications

1. An occlusion that is extremely crowded or already exhibits marked space loss
2. High dental caries activity
3. Replacement of primary anterior teeth
4. Replacement of primary second molars in the primary dentition without partial clinical eruption of the permanent first molar
5. Replacement of primary second molars in the transitional dentition with the permanent molar banded (rare exception)
6. Cases that need guidance of eruption (sequential extraction of primary teeth without removal of permanent teeth); eg, ectopic loss of a primary canine, which indicates arch perimeter shortage on one side of the arch and necessitates removal of the contralateral primary canine in the mandibular arch for correction of the midline discrepancy

The important point is that these appliances are not direct substitutes for an amalgam or stainless steel crown restoration (Figs 21-6a and b).

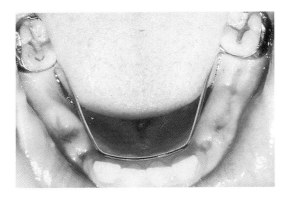

Fig 21-5   Use of an intra-alveolar space maintainer to replace a lost primary second molar

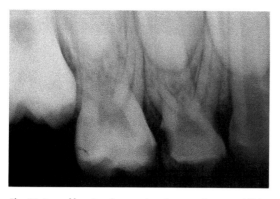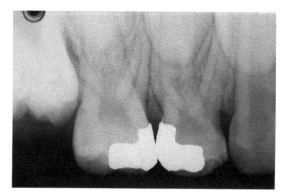

Figs 21-6a and b   Amalgam restorations used to reestablish normal contour and space.

Construction

1. Select an appropriate band or stainless steel crown. Use a tongue blade or a band seater to seat the band. Use a band pusher to adapt and burnish the band. A well-adapted band or crown is essential to prevent decalcification or recurrent dental caries.

2. Construction of the appliance by the indirect method requires an impression of the fully seated band or crown. Make sure the quadrant impression tray extends 5 to 6 mm beyond the distal abutment tooth. Use either an alginate material or a low-fusing compound material. Stabilize the crown or the band in the impression before pouring a stone cast. Use a piece of wire to stabilize the band in the alginate material. A compound impression requires the band to be "luted" with a hot instrument to the compound (Fig 21-7). If a stainless steel crown is the abutment, adapt a provisional crown; cement with a mixture of petroleum jelly and zinc-oxide eugenol cement.

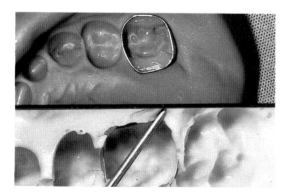

Fig 21-7   Stabilize the bands with wax in the compound impression *(top)*; with a piece of wire in the alginate impression *(bottom)*.

3. Pour the impression in stone. Carefully remove the cast from the impression. Trim a flat base on the cast, and trim the stone distal to the abutment tooth, so the cast does not interfere with wire bending (Fig 21-8). If the tooth in question has not been extracted, cut the tooth from the cast.

4. Using a three-pronged plier or a No. 139 pliers, bend a 3-in. length of 0.036 wire into a loop (Fig 21-9). The wire is held at right angles to the beaks of the pliers. A word of caution: Do not repeatedly bend the wire. Excessive bending increases the hardness and brittleness of the wire, and this increases the tendency for failure of the wire. The loop is bent so that it is slightly off the soft tissue. The loop should dip toward the ridge and is parallel to the soft tissue. The finished loop should be in about the middle third of the band or crown, but above the soft tissue (Fig 21-10). Leave about 0.25 in. of wire distal to the band as an aid to soldering (Fig 21-11).

5. Use an orthodontic blow pipe or electrosolder the wire to the band.

6. Immerse the cast in water; remove the stone from the appliance. Cut off the excess wire. Smooth and polish the appliance.

7. Try-in the appliance. Check the occlusion to make sure the wire or solder does not impinge on the soft tissue. Remove the appliance and clean and dry it.

8. Mix a creamy mix of cement. Seat the appliance first with finger pressure and then use the band seater and band adaptor to complete the cementation process. Remove the excess cement (Fig 21-12).

9. Place the child on a periodic-recall program. The appliance should be checked periodically to see if *(1)* The succedaneous tooth has erupted (Fig 21-13); *(2)* the appliance is impinging on the soft tissue (Fig 21-14); or *(3)* the appliance is not functioning as intended (Fig 21-15).

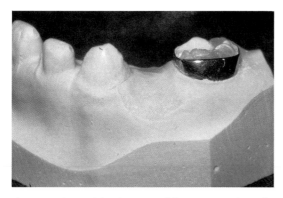

Fig 21-8 The tooth has been cut off the cast. Note the sticky wax around the band.

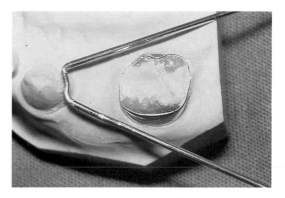

Fig 21-9 Bend the wire into a loop adjacent to the primary canine.

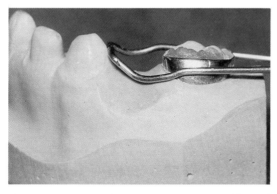

Fig 21-10 The finished loops should end in the middle third of the band.

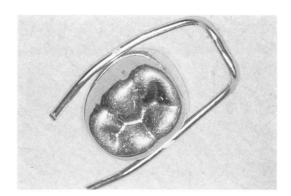

Fig 21-11 Completed wire, bent before soldering.

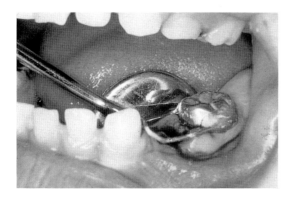

Fig 21-12 The primary first molar has been extracted and the crown and loop have been cemented.

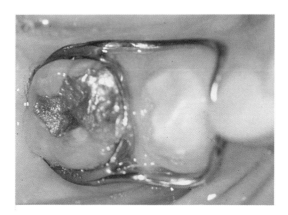

Fig 21-13 The space maintainer has served its purpose; now the maintainer should be removed.

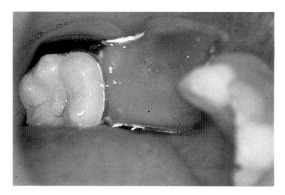

Fig 21-14 The mandibular space maintainer has slipped beneath contour of the primary canine, irritating the tissue along the buccal surface.

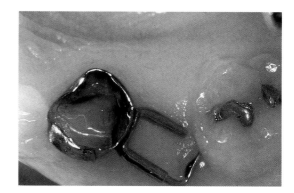

Fig 21-15 Note the recurrent caries around the band on the primary first molar. In addition, the wire has imbedded in the tissue, allowing mesial drift of the permanent first molar.

Bilateral fixed space maintainers

Maxillary appliances that do not interfere with the occlusion are the Nance holding arch and the transpalatal bar. The Nance appliance has its wire bent from the molar and into the anterior palate at the junction of the horizontal and anterior vertical, or premaxilla-maxilla junction. The wire is free except for the solder joints on the bands and a small piece of acrylic resin as a button over the anterior extension. The transpalatal bar has its wire bent directly from one molar band to the other, but the wire is contoured to the outline of the hard palate, just off the tissues (Fig 21-16).

The fixed lingual arch is most often used in the mandibular arch. It is a passive wire, soldered from a band on one side of the arch to a band on the other side. Its problems in the maxillary arch are related to overbite: The mandibular incisors occlude into the wire at the cingula or the maxillary incisors. This is not a problem in the mandibular arch.

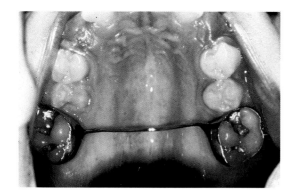

Fig 21-16 Transpalatal bar from one permanent first molar across the palate to the opposite permanent first molar.

Fixed lingual arch

Indications

1. Maintenance of arch perimeter, not just quadrant perimeter, because of premature loss of primary teeth. It is used almost exclusively in the mandibular arch. Maxillary arch perimeter is usually maintained with a bilaterally designed appliance, ie, Nance holding arch or transpalatal bar.
2. Maintenance or prevention of mandibular changes in arch length, overjet, and overbite from incisor repositioning in the traditional dentition.
3. Retention or stabilization of the positions of the mandibular anterior teeth after tooth movement to prevent relapse in mandibular anterior crowding and changes in bite depth.

Contraindications

1. Anything that would require frequent adjustments, eg, tooth movement or space regaining
2. Rampant dental caries, high plaque scores, and/or poor patient cooperation
3. Anterior or posterior crossbite, if the mandibular teeth are contributing factors and need to be corrected prior to lingual arch placement
4. Extreme mandibular anterior crowding or lingually erupting succedaneous teeth

Construction

In the transitional dentition, the lingual arch is most often placed on permanent first molars. The primary second molars can be used in the primary dentition (Fig 21-17).

One large advantage of banding the primary second molars is that the permanent first molars are left free from the adverse decalcification or demineralization that may develop around the bands over a long period

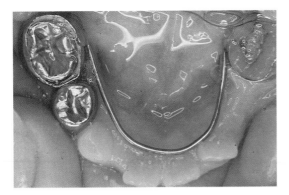

Fig 21-17 Fixed lingual wire using the primary second molars as abutments.

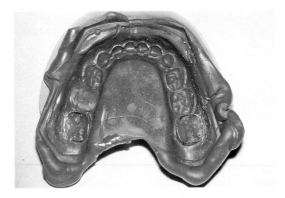

Fig 21-18 Complete arch compound impression with the bands waxed in place.

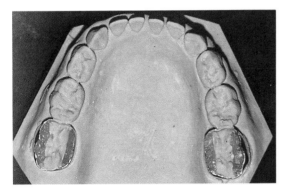

Fig 21-19 Cast of the mandibular arch with bands in place.

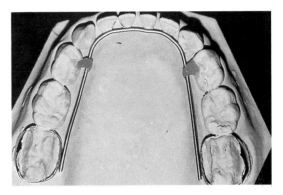

Fig 21-20 Completed arch wire on the cast. Note the form and position of the wire.

of time. It is not advisable to band one permanent first molar on one side and a primary second molar on the other in the transitional dentition; such placement is probably related to poor treatment planning.

The lingual arch is fabricated indirectly, ie, on the cast rather than in the mouth.

1. Select the appropriate band sizes for the permanent first molars. Similar to adapting the band for the band and loop space maintainer, use a tongue blade or a band seater to seat the bands.

2. Use a complete-arch impression (Fig 21-18). An alginate impression or low-fusing compound impression can be used. The impression should indicate the outline of the molar bands. If the margins cannot be seen, retake the impression.

3. Use a posterior band remover and remove the bands. The best procedure is to remove one band and set it in the impression; then remove the other band and place it in the impression. This reduces the possibility of confusing the two bands.

4. Use hot sticky wax and "lute" the bands to the impression. The sticky wax holds the bands in place and provides a space to facilitate soldering.

5. Pour up the impression in stone. Carefully remove the impression material. Make a flat base for the cast (Fig 21-19).

6. On the cast, draw the position of the intended lingual arch wire. The wire runs from the middle third of the molar bands along the gingival one third of the primary molars. The wire continues across the cingula of the incisors slightly above the gingival papillae. The wire should not interfere with the occlusion, tongue, or erupting permanent teeth. In general, the wire should be close to the tissue, but not tissue borne.

7. Use 0.036 stainless steel wire or Elgiloy wire. Use No. 139 pliers or a three-pronged plier to bend a U-shaped wire. Bend the wire so it contacts the cingula of the incisors slightly above the gingiva, contacts the gingival third of the primary molars (if present), and then runs parallel to the middle third of the molar bands (Fig 21-20). *The wire should be passive.* If the wire is not passive, when seated, tooth movement might occur.

8. Secure the wire to the cast with stone or some other material (Fig 21-21). Remove the sticky wax from the bands. The bands should be clean, free of wax and stone. Use an orthodontic blow pipe or electrosolder the wire to the bands. The solder joint should be free of pits and cover the wire completely.

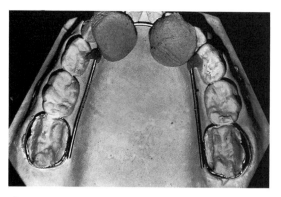

Fig 21-21   Secure the lingual arch wire in place prior to soldering.

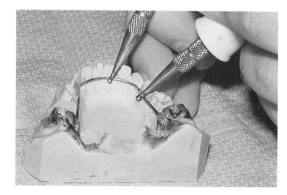

Fig 21-22   After soldering, heat treat the wire to reduce stresses induced in the wire during bending.

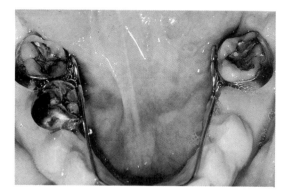

Fig 21-23   The lingual arch wire is impeding the eruption of the second premolar. It is time for removal of the lingual arch wire.

9. Use a spot welder to heat treat the wire (Fig 21-22). This step is necessary to reduce any stresses in the wire caused by bending. If Elgiloy is used, heat treating increases the effectiveness of the wire.
10. Remove the appliance from the cast. Clean and polish the appliance.
11. Try-in the appliance. Seat the appliance in the mouth. Ensure that the wire is passive, the bands fit well, the wire does not impinge on soft tissue, and there are no occlusal interferences.

There are numerous reasons that the wire might not fit as exactly as bent on the cast: bands improperly fitted on the teeth; distorted impression; bands not seated properly in the impression; bands mobile during pour up; inaccurately bent wire; distortion during removal of the appliance from the stone; tight contacts during appliance placement; unwanted biting forces or pushing forces during appliance fitting; and a poor cementing process, allowing incomplete seating of the appliance, open margins or occlusal interferences to remain or allowing a bath of saliva during cementation.

12. Similar to the procedure for the band and loop appliance, clean the fixed lingual arch wire. Dry the abutment teeth. Mix a creamy mix of cement. Seat the appliance with a tongue blade and a band seater. Remove excess cement.
13. Place the child on a periodic-recall program to check for loose bands. Make sure that the lingual wire is not preventing tooth eruption (Fig 21-23) or impinging on the soft tissue.

Premature loss of a primary second molar

The premature loss of a primary second molar and the potential problems that arise are a reminder that rationale and approach to treatment may vary from time to time. Careful thought must be exercised to select the treatment that is best at that particular period in time. The objective in the event of early loss of a primary second molar is the prevention of mesial drift of the permanent first molar.

If the permanent first molar has erupted into the oral cavity before the loss of the primary second molar, usually a band or crown and loop retainer that uses the primary first molar as the abutment and extends the loop to the mesial surface of the permanent first molar is the acceptable procedure (Fig 21-24). Should the primary first molar also be absent, a band and loop appliance that initiates on the permanent first molar and extends to the distal surface of the primary canine is the appliance of choice (Fig 21-25).

In the event there are bilateral losses of teeth in the arch, a lingual or palatal holding arch appliance is perhaps the best treatment.

In all likelihood, a child patient 3 to 5 years old will not have an erupted permanent first molar. Should the primary second molar become abscessed and require early removal, the use of an intra-alveolar (distal shoe) appliance to retain the permanent first molar in position and provide it with eruptive guidance is a prime consideration.

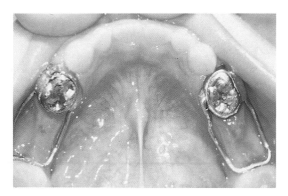

Fig 21-24 Bilateral use of band and loops.

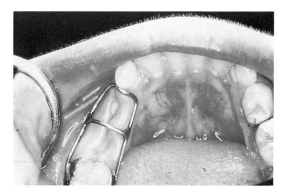

Fig 21-25 A modified band and loop space maintainer replacing the loss of the primary first and second molars.

Intra-alveolar (distal shoe) appliance

The main objective is to retain and guide the permanent first molar into normal eruptive position.

The intra-alveolar appliance consists of a stainless steel crown placed on a primary first molar. A stainless steel L-shaped bar, manufactured specifically for this procedure, is spot welded and soldered to the distal surface of the crown. The bar extends posteriorly to a position even with the mesial surface of the permanent first molar or the distal root socket of the primary second molar. The horizontal extension is off the gingival tissue, occluding somewhat with the maxillary dentition. A right-angle bend is established in the bar, directing it along the mesial surface of the permanent molar or into the distal root socket (Fig 21-26).

The indication for this appliance is as a replacement for a primary second molar, irretrievably impaired by caries or infection, which is abutted to an unerupted permanent first molar. Contraindication for the appliance would be a hopelessly damaged abutment, which in this case would be the primary first molar.

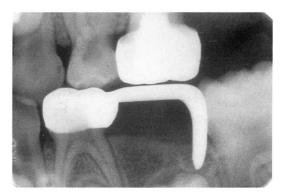

Fig 21-26 An intra-alveolar appliance replacing the primary mandibular left second molar prevents the mesial drift of the permanent first molar.

Advantages

1. It is a proved and efficient appliance for the purpose.
2. It prevents elongation of opposing dentition.
3. It may be fabricated by indirect or direct means.
4. The cost is moderate.

Disadvantages

1. The patient must be under close scrutiny while the appliance is in place.
2. There is no allowance for inaccuracy in measurement or fabrication.

Armamentarium

Stainless steel crowns
Occlusal bar material

Pliers
   No. 104 (UBECO)
   No. 139
   No. 110
Orthodontic blowpipe
Spot welder with solder electrodes
Silver solder
Flux
Zinc phosphate cement
Rag wheels, pumice, and gold rouge

Direct method

1. Prepare the primary first molar for a stainless steel crown, and then adapt a suitable stainless steel crown as previously described.
2. Take a unit of the bar material and fit it to the distal surface of the stainless steel crown. If the bar material extends beyond the gingival margin of the crown, trim off the excess and spot weld the bar to the crown (Fig 21-27). Electrosolder the crown and

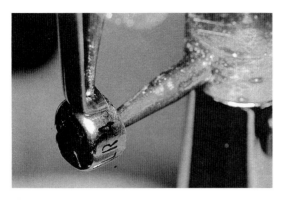

Fig 21-27　Fit a maintainer bar to the distal surface of stainless steel crown. Usually the abutment portion of the bar extends below the cervical margin of the crown, making it necessary to shorten it before spot welding.

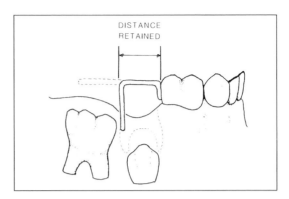

Fig 21-28　Accurate radiographic and clinical measurement of the distance from the distal surface of the primary first molar posteriorly to the distal root socket of the primary second molar is required.

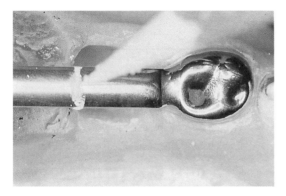

Fig 21-29　From the measurements established, mark the location for the bend on the bar.

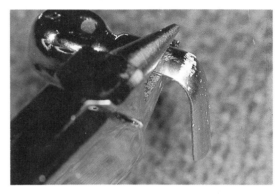

Fig 21-30　Use a No. 139 pliers to hold the appliance and place a No. 104 pliers on the mark to produce a right angle bend.

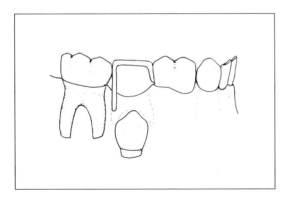

Fig 21-31　The bar should extend distally to approximately the mesial surface of the permanent first molar. The depth of the bar should not interfere with the developing second premolar.

bar and smooth and polish with the rag wheel and pumice, then rag wheel with gold rouge.

3. From clinical or radiographic measurement, record the distance from the distal surface of the primary first molar to the distal wall of the distal root socket of the primary second molar or the mesial surface of the permanent first molar (Fig 21-28). Mark this measurement on the bar material (Fig 21-29). Use two pliers. Hold the bar with the No. 139 pliers at the mark and bend the material at that point with the No. 104 pliers (Fig 21-30).

4. Unless previously removed, extract the primary second molar. Allow time for hemostasis. Put the appliance into place and adjust where required. Take a radiograph to check the position of the distal shoe projection. The bar should extend distally to approximate alignment with the mesial surface of the permanent first molar and extend alveolarly into the distal root socket or adjacent to the mesial surface of the molar to retain and guide it into place (Fig 21-31). If the bar is too short, the permanent

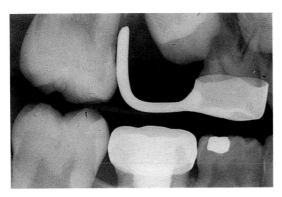 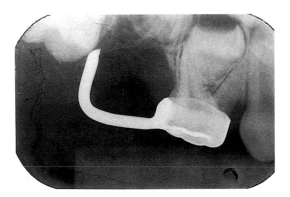

Figs 21-32a and b Note the overextended bar on this distal shoe and the deflection of the second premolar.

first molar will erupt beneath it. If it is too long, it may in time interfere with the developing second premolar (Figs 21-32a and b).

5. After eruption of the permanent first molar, the appliance should be removed. A conventional crown and loop space maintainer should be fabricated and cemented into place.

Indirect method

The indirect method requires two appointments, coupled with a laboratory procedure. From one aspect it is an optional procedure, but from another it is the only method. The indirect procedure is necessary when the primary second molar has been absent for some time.

First appointment

1. Prepare the primary first molar for a stainless steel crown. Fabricate a suitable crown. If the primary second molar has not been extracted, follow the procedure in step 2.
2. With the fitted crown in place on the abutment tooth (primary first molar), take an impression. In

addition, take an impression of the opposing dentition, and place a provisional crown on the abutment tooth.

Laboratory

1. With the crown in place in the impression, add sticky wax to the inside of the crown at its distal surface (the wax is added to create a void as an aid to soldering). Pour a stone cast. Additionally, pour the opposing impression (Fig 21-33).
2. From the radiograph, measure the distance from the distal surface of the primary first molar to the mesial surface of the permanent first molar. This measurement should be close to the mesiodistal width of the missing primary second molar. Transfer this measurement to the cast with the Boley gauge (Fig 21-34).
3. Cut the primary second molar from the cast and fabricate the bar, trimming and abutting it to the distal surface of the crown. Using the opposing model, adjust the bar height so that its occlusal plane does not interfere with the opposing occlusion. Do not establish the alveolar bend at this time. (Figs 21-35 and 21-36).

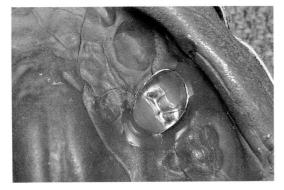 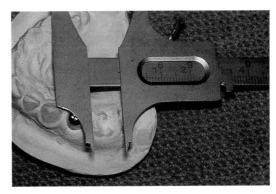

Fig 21-33 Place the crown in the compound impression, with sticky wax on the buccal and lingual surfaces.

Fig 21-34 From the radiograph, use a Boley gauge to measure the length of the bar.

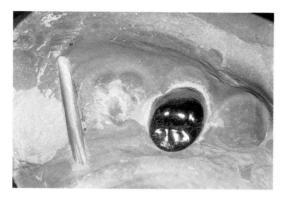

Fig 21-35   Cut the cast to accommodate the bending of the bar.

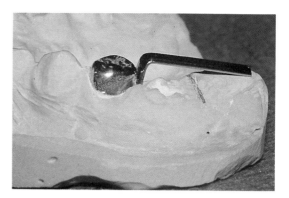

Fig 21-36   Bar material in place ready to bend.

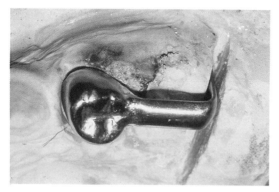

Fig 21-37   Completed distal shoe after the bar material has been soldered to the stainless steel crown.

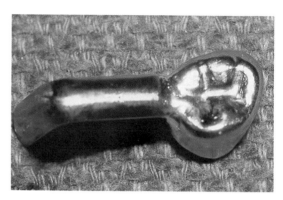

Fig 21-38   Polished appliance.

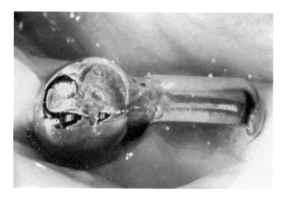

Fig 21-39   Intra-alveolar appliance in place.

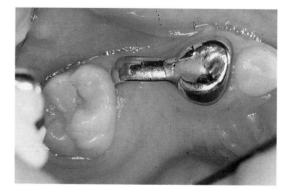

Fig 21-40   An example of the need for periodic recall. This appliance needs to be removed and replaced with a crown and loop space maintainer.

4. Anchor the bar in place with stone or an investment material and flame solder the crown and bar. Smooth and polish the appliance. Anchor the bar to the crown and solder. Then smooth and polish the appliance (Figs 21-37 and 21-38).

5. An appropriate local anesthetic procedure is achieved. Quite often it is unnecessary to incise the alveolar tissue, particularly if the distal shoe extension has a relatively sharp edge. After placement, the insertion should be checked radiographically to determine accuracy of the bend. Adjust if necessary (Fig 21-39).

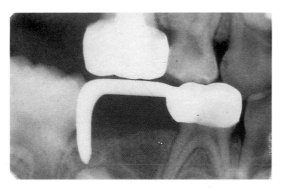
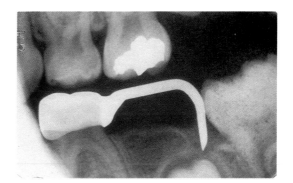

Fig 21-41a Distal shoes were placed when the patient was 4 years old.

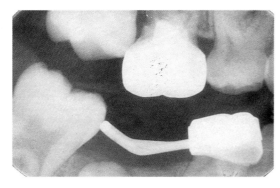
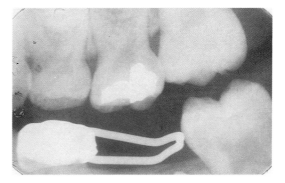

Fig 21-41b After 1 year, the distal shoes were replaced with crown and loops.

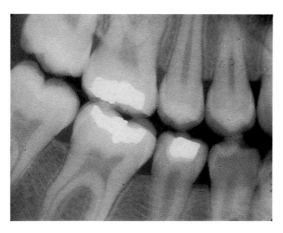
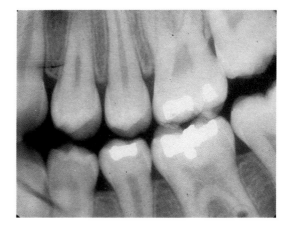

Fig 21-41c Final permanent dentition.

Periodic recall

It is very important to impress on the child's parent the need for periodic recall. Observing the patient at 3-month intervals is most appropriate. Fig 21-40 illustrates the need for periodic recalls. Note how the bar portion has "slipped" to the buccal segment. It is time for removal of the appliance and replacement with another space maintainer.

The distal shoe space maintainer, when used in the appropriate situation and with parents who are cooperative, prevents a potential orthodontic problem. A 4-year-old girl had bilateral distal shoes replacing both mandibular primary second molars (Fig 21-41a). One year later, these appliances were replaced with crown and loop space maintainers (Fig 21-41b). Seen in a recall program every 6 months, she was in the early permanent dentition 6 years later (Fig 21-41c).

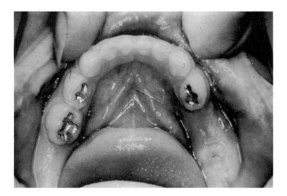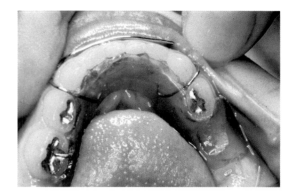

Figs 21-42a and b Use of a removable space maintainer to replace a primary mandibular second molar.

Removable appliances

Removable appliances such as the acrylic resin space maintainer or the modified Hawley appliance are occasionally useful in replacing prematurely lost primary second molars (Figs 21-41a to c). These appliances are suited for multiple tooth replacement unilaterally or bilaterally. They have three disadvantages: *(1)* the patient may not tolerate wearing the appliance, *(2)* the appliance is not as effective in preventing mesial drift of the permanent molar, and *(3)* the appliance can offer problems of poor oral hygiene. The principal advantage of these types of appliances is that they are functional and will prevent supereruption of the teeth of the opposing arch (Figs 21-42a and b).

Acknowledgements

Drs Theresa M. White and Daniel P. Dalzell, Department of Pediatric Dentistry, University of Oklahoma, College of Dentistry, for photographs used in this chapter. Drs Ram S. Nanda, C. Frans Currier, and Pramod Sinha, Department of Orthodontics, University of Oklahoma, College of Dentistry, for manuscript advice during this chapter's development, plus the use of photographs.

References

Currier, G. F., and Austerman, J. A., Fabrication of Appliances for Preventive, Interceptive, and Adjunctive Orthodontics. 4th ed. Oklahoma City: Oklahoma University Health Science Center Press, 1992.

Moyers, R. E., Handbook of Orthodontics. 4th ed. Chicago: Year Book Medical Publishers, Inc., 1988.

Nanda, R. S., Basics of Undergraduate Orthodontics. 4th ed. Oklahoma City: Oklahoma University Health Science Center Press, 1993.

Pedodontic Appliances. Hayward, Colo.: Quercus Corp., 1977.

Profitt, W. R., and Fields, H. W., Jr. Contemporary Orthodontics. 2nd ed. New York: The C. V. Mosby Co., 1993.

Questions

1. Jennifer, aged 4, must have a primary second molar extracted because of pulpal degeneration. What type of space maintainer is indicated?

   a. A band and loop, from the primary first molar to the approximate area of the permanent first molar

   b. A removable appliance, replacing the space of the primary second molar

   c. A distal shoe intra-alveolar space maintainer

   d. None is indicated at this time; wait until the permanent first molar erupts

2. Mark, aged 9, has had both the primary maxillary first and second molars on the left and right sides removed. What is the optimum type of space maintainer?

   a. A removable space maintainer with a Hawley-type wire

   b. A Nance holding arch

   c. A transpalatal bar

   d. None—the succedaneous teeth will erupt soon

3. Sue, aged 5, has lost both the primary mandibular first molars to dental caries. What is the best type of space maintainer to use?

   a. None; the space loss is not a problem at this age

   b. Two band and loop space maintainers, with the primary second molars serving as abutments

   c. A removable appliance

   d. A fixed lingual wire with the primary second molars as abutments.

4. Jimmy, aged 7, has lost the primary maxillary second molar. What is the optimum type of space maintainer to use?

   a. None is needed at this time; the permanent first molar is erupted at this age

   b. A band and loop with the permanent first molar as the abutment tooth

   c. A band and loop with the primary first molar as the abutment tooth

   d. Either a transpalatal bar or a Nance holding arch

5. Arthur, aged 8, has lost the primary mandibular first molar on the left side and primary canine, first, and second molars on the right side. The mandibular left canine is to be extracted. What type of space maintainer is indicated?

   a. A removable appliance with a Hawley-type wire

   b. A fixed lingual wire from the permanent first molars on the right and left sides

   c. None at this time; he will need orthodontic treatment in the future

Prosthodontics

There are instances where a removable prosthodontic appliance is needed instead of a single-tooth replacement that is accomplished with a band and loop space maintainer or a fixed lingual wire. This chapter deals with replacement of multiple tooth loss with either a removable or fixed appliance. The advantages and disadvantages of the various types of replacement are listed in Table 22-1.

Indications

Some of the typical causes are:

1. Caries resulting in multiple extractions of primary teeth. A usual instance is a child with nursing bottle caries.
2. Trauma from tooth avulsion or displacement.
3. Teeth absent because of a congenital of genetic defect. An example is ectodermal dysplasia.
4. Dentinogenesis imperfecta or amelogenesis imperfecta and cleft palate.

Table 22-1 Advantages and disadvantages of types of replacements for primary and permanent anterior teeth

Type	Advantages	Disadvantages
Fixed lingual wire	Fixed Esthetic	Age of child?
Removable partial denture	Cost	Easily lost
Fixed bridge	Fixed Esthetic	Cost Time to fabricate Rationale for use

Considerations

Nanda (1976) suggested that the following questions be asked before a removable prosthodontic appliance is fabricated for a child:

1. Will the child adapt to the change in the oral environment caused by the insertion of the removable appliance?
2. Will the appliance be capable of preventing tooth migration, extrusion, and adverse oral habits?
3. What is the anticipated eruption time of the succedaneous teeth?
4. If needed, what type of appliance is indicated?
5. Is there any evidence of psychologic trauma because of the early loss of anterior primary teeth? Is the child embarrassed because of the lack of teeth?
6. Will the absence of anterior teeth have any detrimental effect on speech development? (The effect on speech development may vary from child to child).
7. What influence will the absence or insertion of a removable appliance have on the growth and development of the child?

Requirements

If the answers to the previous questions indicate the need for a removable appliance, the following should be considered for an acceptable prosthodontic device. It should:

1. Be stable and strong enough to function in the process of chewing.
2. Restore esthetics.
3. Prevent overeruption of opposing teeth or drift of the adjacent teeth.
4. Be easily cleaned.
5. Be noncariogenic and nonirritating to the supporting tissues.
6. Be easily and economically fabricated with minimal tooth preparation.

Removable Partial Dentures

As a rule, the younger the child, the easier will be the adaptation to the appliance or appliances. There are some distinct advantages and disadvantages when a removable appliance is selected.

Advantages

1. Facial profile as well as function and esthetics are improved.
2. It facilitates cleaning of the adjacent teeth.
3. Material costs are minimal.

Disadvantages

1. There is complete dependence on patient and parent cooperation.
2. Failure to maintain good oral hygiene produces pathologic changes and gingival inflammation. Increased caries can be expected.
3. If the appliance is removed the rationale for the construction of the appliance—esthetics, function, space maintenance, or prevention—is lost.

Impression methods

For younger children, trays are selected from the various sizes commercially available. The procedure is introduced to the younger child by using simple terms to describe what is going to be done, how it is to be done, and indicate that the child can be a "helper" to accomplish the impression procedure. Periphery wax is added to the rim of the impression tray. For young children (less than 6 years), a fast-setting alginate impression material in a stock tray is recommended for the final impression and working cast. For older children, a custom tray fabricated from a working cast can be used. The final impression can be made with a silicone or rubber base impression material.

While making the impression, the operator should have a mirror or tongue blade handy to remove excess impression material from the posterior palatal area. Gagging by the child often can be prevented by using tactics to distract. For example, asking the child to raise one leg and count to five (or the assistant can count to five), and then to raise the other leg, and so on. Usually by the count of 30, a fast-set alginate will have gelatinized. Another method that works well is to have the child lean forward and breath through his or her mouth, and "pant like a puppy dog." Often a small dab of alginate placed over the child's thumb will distract him or her. When the material sets, the child can raise the hand. The thumb impression can be sent home as one of the "prizes" for the day. The mandibular impression is accomplished in a similar manner.

The interarch relationship is best accomplished by the use of a soft wax to record a centric relation. Lindahl (1961) suggests having the child practice several times before using a wax bite so that the child will have the feel of where to close. The impressions are poured in an improved stone material using recommended water-powder ratios. The impressions should be poured as soon as possible to reduce distortion of the working cast. There is no known method for storing an alginate impression. Stone must be poured within 15 minutes of the impression's gelatinizing or distortion will occur.

Using the centric wax bite, the operator mounts the trimmed casts on a suitable articulator. A word of caution: articulators are manufactured for use in fixed and removable prosthodontics. The movements, condylar settings, and function of the articulator are calibrated with adults in mind. To transpose these manufactured adult averages into use for children is a mistake. The articulator should only be used as an aid approximating the maxillomandibular relationship to the arrangement of the teeth.

Clasp design

Several types of clasps are available to aid in retention of removable appliances. The clasp is placed in an undercut area to aid in resisting removal.

Birnbaum et al (1978) described a method that uses a light-cured composite resin to increase clasp retention. Recontouring primary or partially erupted permanent teeth with composite resin improves retention by creating recesses for clasps. They did not observe any increase in food impaction or gingival response. These authors believed the use of composite resin lugs is biologically more efficient than use of orthodontic bands.

Several types of clasps are available (Fig 22-1). The circumferential clasp is best used as an auxiliary clasp. It can be used on primary canines or molars. Its retentive potential can be increased by use of the composite resin retentive lug. The Adam's clasp is an excellent all-around clasp. It is easily adjusted, seldom interferes

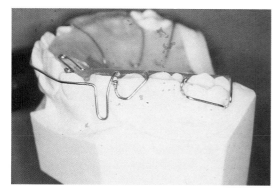

Fig 22-1　The several types of clasps used are seen on this cast.

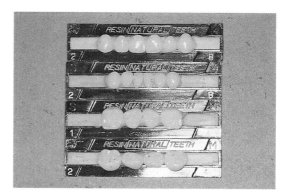

Fig 22-2　Commercially available denture teeth manufactured for the primary dentition.

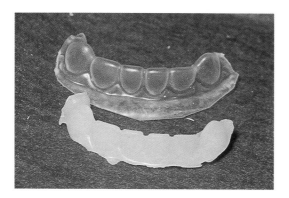

Fig 22-3　Teeth fabricated from a typodont in tooth-colored resin.

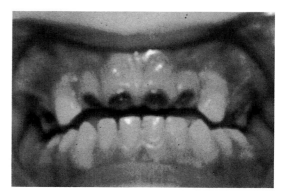

Fig 22-4　A child needing prosthetic replacement.

with occlusion, and, above all, is retentive. Ball clasps are purchased as a commercial item and are adapted to the cast. The ball clasps fit interproximally between the teeth. It is a good idea to remove a small portion of the cast before adaptation of the ball clasps. An added aid to retention is the use of labial bow or Hawley wire. This wire increases anterior retention and is best used on the mandibular arch. All of the clasps and arch wires are fabricated from 0.028 to 0.030 stainless steel orthodontic wire. With the exception of the circumferential wire, all of the clasps and Hawley wires can be purchased prefabricated in several sizes.

Replacement teeth

There are teeth commercially available similar to those used for adult dentures (Fig 22-2). The teeth are available in one size and shades 59 or 61. The light primary teeth are well matched with this shade unless stained with an intrinsic agent (tetracycline).

Teeth can be fabricated from a typodont model by taking an impression of the teeth and duplicating the teeth with a tooth-colored resin (Fig 22-3). The teeth are cut and used as individual teeth.

Procedure

A girl, aged 4.5 years was found to have four carious primary incisors (Fig 22-4). The teeth were extracted, and, after 10 days, impressions and casts were completed to fabricate a removable appliance to replace the anterior primary teeth because the mother was concerned about the appearance and "crooked permanent teeth." The casts were mounted on a simple articulator because only the anterior primary teeth were going to be replaced.

1. Using preformed primary denture teeth, make an esthetic arrangement of the teeth. Set the primary teeth according to the usual dentition of the child or what it should be for his or her age (Fig 22-5). The teeth are set with spaces and in a more vertical axis than in adult dentures. Wax the teeth together and to the buccal surface of the cast.
2. Adapt clasps to the primary first and second molars.
3. Apply separating medium to the cast before the clasps are attached to the cast. Separating media on the clasps will cause the orthodontic resin to lack adherence. Wax the clasps to the buccal surface of the cast.

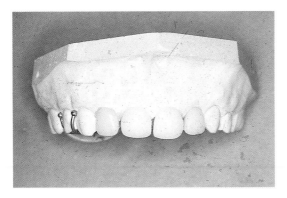

Fig 22-5 Denture teeth adapted to the cast.

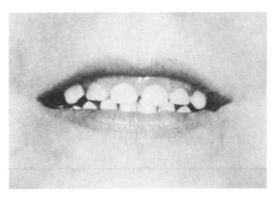

Fig 22-6 The fabricated appliance in the child's mouth.

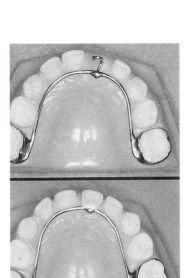

Fig 22-7 Stainless steel bands adapted *(top)*. Teeth cured to the wire *(bottom)*.

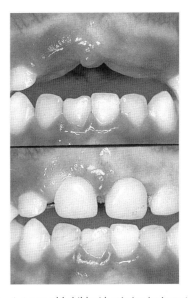

Fig 22-8 A 4-year-old child with missing incisors *(top)*. The appliance in place *(bottom)*.

4. Apply orthodontic acrylic resin by adding powder and liquid according to the manufacturer's instruction. To reduce porosity, place the cast in a pressure cooker until the resin is cured.

5. Finish and polish the anterior appliance on the cast. Trim the appliance on the cast so that the acrylic resin will extend into the embrasures of the teeth, thus increasing retention of the appliance. The appliance should be finished and polished to reduce all porosity, rough edges, and potential food traps.

6. Fig 22-6 shows the appliance in the child's mouth. The teeth may be butted to the alveolar ridge and the labial flange omitted. As the child grows, it may be necessary to remove portions of the appliance to allow for eruption of the permanent successors.

Fixed anterior appliances

Steffen et al (1971) described a method of fabricating an anterior fixed appliance. The advantage of this appliance is that there is less dependency on patient and parent cooperation. Removing the teeth as the successors erupt allows the appliance to remain in function. For example, a fixed appliance was fabricated for a 4-year-old child who lost the primary incisors to caries (Fig 22-8, *top*).

Procedure

1. Adapt stainless steel bands to the primary second molars (Fig 22-7, *top*). Make an impression in alginate or compound with the band in place. Remove the bands and place them in the impression; pour the stone.

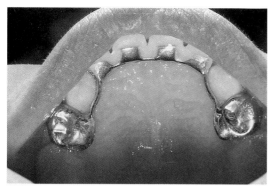

Fig 22-9 Palatal view with the replacement teeth attached to the mesh. Note the omega loops.

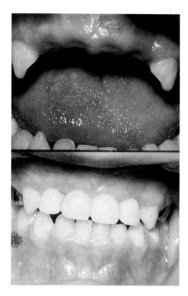

Fig 22-10 Before *(top)* and after *(bottom)* views of the fixed anterior appliance.

2. Bend a lingual arch from 0.036 stainless steel wire. Adapt the wire to the lingual surface of the primary molars. Solder the lingual wire to the bands.
3. Prepare a lug for each tooth to be replaced by soldering the lug of 0.028 wire to the lingual wire. Place the lug to approximate the center of the replacement tooth. The lug can be adjusted after soldering to its best position. Repeat this process for each tooth to be replaced. Note: Adjacent teeth on the cast should be protected with moist asbestos during the soldering process.
4. If plastic teeth are used, drill a hole in the center of the tooth to accept the lug. Usually the preformed acrylic resin primary teeth used in the previous example are the teeth of choice.
5. Coat the cast with separating medium. Attach the tooth or teeth by filling the hole in the acrylic resin tooth with self-curing acrylic resin. The wire is posi-

tioned on the model, the teeth are aligned, and the resin is allowed to cure (Fig 22-7, *bottom*).
6. Trim the teeth to the cast and polish them. Figure 22-8, *bottom* shows the incisors replaced with a fixed appliance. Function, appearance, and facial contour have been restored.

Groper (1992) describes a more durable fixed space maintainer for missing primary incisors. A solid direct bond pad is soldered with a mesh base and eyelet to the lingual wire (Fig 22-9). Breakage is reduced because the stainless steel, rather than acrylic resin, is used to retain the acrylic resin teeth. The omega loops allow for needed adjustments. Figure 22-10 illustrates the missing teeth and cementation of the appliance.

Complete dentures

Children with genetic diseases in which missing teeth are part of the syndrome often need complete dentures to restore the primary and permanent dentitions (Figs 22-11 and 22-12).

Figure 22-13 shows a 7-year-old boy with ectodermal dysplasia. The child has three primary canines and two cone-shaped primary central incisors. Johnson and Stratton (1980) have described a method for construction of these prosthetic appliances.

Procedure

1. Complete the preliminary impressions using stock trays and alginate impression material. After the impressions are poured, construct custom trays.
2. Take the final impressions with a polysulfide impression material.
3. Pour the final casts in an improved stone. In this patient, because there were no primary teeth in the area, alveolar bone growth to date has been minimal.
4. The next step is to fabricate wax occlusion rims to attempt to make a centric relation record. This step is difficult because children do not have the same musculature, temporal mandibular joint function, or growth maturity as adults. Unfortunately, articulators and prosthetic principles are directed toward adults. The use of wax occlusion rims, however, does reduce the error.
5. On one side, remove a portion of the occlusion rim and replace it with soft wax (Aluwax Dental Products). This wax is used to have the patient close and to register the maxillomandibular relationship.
6. Mount the casts on an articulator. Arrange zero-degree plastic denture teeth to a flat occlusal plane.
7. After the denture setup is completed, a try-in with the teeth in wax is very advantageous. It was de-

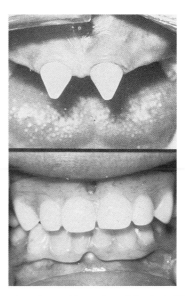

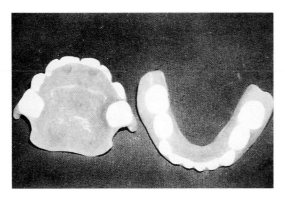

Figs 22-11 and 12 Total or partial lack of teeth (anodontia or oligodontia) is seen in patients with ectodermal dysplasia. The patient will have dysfunction of sweat glands, sparse hair, low bridge of the nose, protruding lips, and other ectodermally related defects. The most striking oral feature is total or partial lack of teeth and the conical shape of any teeth present. The more common ectodermal dysplasia is an inherited, sex-linked, recessive gene; males are more severely affected. The care for these children is periodic prosthetic replacement of the missing teeth. These children continue to exhibit normal facial growth except for alveolar bone disposition (Sarnat et al, 1953). There is need to periodically remake the appliance and esthetically customize the dentures to the child's current stage of dental development. Note the use of the existing maxillary teeth for retention of the denture.

cided to overlap the maxillary teeth with the denture. This same procedure is often used in children with dentinogenesis imperfecta to prevent further abrasion of the teeth.

8. During the wax try-in, complete all necessary adjustments to improve esthetics and ensure accurate vertical and horizontal relationships. When all discrepancies are corrected, the dentures are ready for waxing, processing and finishing. When growth of the jaws is anticipated, the wax-up should be enlarged so that future relines are possible.

9. At delivery, check the completed dentures internally for any small bubbles that would cause irritation. Insert the dentures and check for gross errors. Use indicator paste to remove pressure areas in the denture bases. Refine the occlusion by remounting the dentures and equilibrating them on the articulator.

10. The completed dentures are seen in Fig 22-13. The patient and parent should be instructed in home care of the prosthodontic appliances. They need to be informed of the need for periodic recall and refabrication of the dentures as growth occurs.

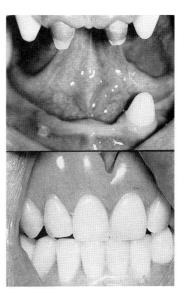

Fig 22-13 A patient with ectodermal dysplasia, an indication for a prosthetic appliance *(top).* An overlay denture is used to improve appearance and function *(bottom).*

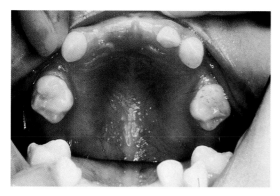

Fig 22-14 A patient with missing teeth caused by arrested infantile rickets.

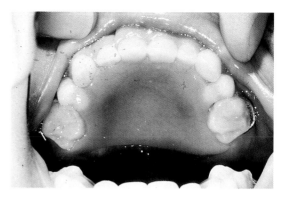

Fig 22-15 The completed partial denture in the child's mouth.

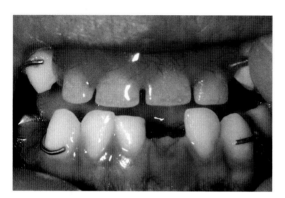

Fig 22-16 The use of circumferential clasps for retentive purposes.

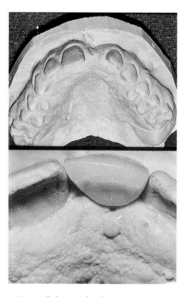

Fig 22-17 Cast of the avulsed permanent central incisor *(top)*; replacement tooth adapted to the cast *(bottom)*. (Courtesy of Dr Theresa White.)

Patient instructions

Ettinger and Pinkham (1976) suggested the following instructions for parents and patients:

1. The child should not sleep with the appliance. When removed, the appliance should be kept moist.
2. The appliance should be removed for sports activities.
3. When the dentures are first inserted, the child should be given food that is enjoyed, but that requires chewing.
4. The child should be encouraged to wear the dentures.
5. The parents should check the child's mouth for supporting tissue irritation and erupting teeth.
6. The parents and patient should be instructed in home care of the appliance and the remaining teeth.
7. The child should be evaluated every 3 months for changes. Children constantly grow and the dentures need to be evaluated periodically for accommodation to this growth change.

Clinical examples

The following demonstrate alternative forms of appliance construction.

Figures 22-14 and 22-15 are of a girl with arrested infantile rickets. A partial denture replaced the missing three anterior teeth and two posterior teeth. Circumferential clasps were used on the primary second molars for retention.

Figure 22-16 shows prosthodontic replacement of teeth removed because of dental caries. Circumferential clasps were used for retention. Primary posterior teeth were used on one side to assist in maintaining occlusion.

A patient, aged 13, avulsed a central incisor, which could not be reimplanted. An acrylic resin tooth, of the appropriate shade, is adapted to the cast (Fig 22-17). A "channel" is cut in the lingual surface of the replacement tooth; a wire with retentive loops is adapted and attached to the acrylic resin tooth with a composite resin material (Fig 22-18). The lingual surfaces of the

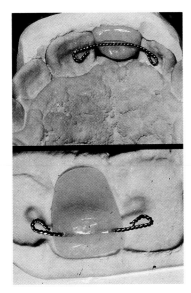

Fig 22-18 Wire, with retentive loops, adapted to the cast *(top)*; wire attached to the replacement tooth *(bottom)*. (Courtesy of Dr Theresa White.)

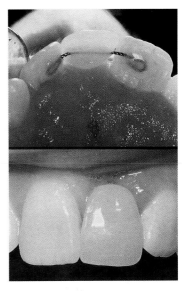

Fig 22-19 Palatal *(top)* and labial *(bottom)* views of the replacement tooth, attached with a composite resin material. (Courtesy of Dr Theresa White.)

permanent teeth are etched with phosphoric acid; composite resin is used to attach the wire and replacement tooth to the adjacent permanent teeth (Fig 22-19).

Acid-etch resin-retained metal prostheses

Rochette (1973) was the first to advocate the use of a perforated metal-resin bonded appliance for use as a periodontal splint. Howe and Denehy (1977) advocated a method for the replacement of missing teeth with a cast perforated framework and a porcelain-fused-to-metal pontic. For bonding, a filled and unfilled composite resin system was used. Livaditis and Thompson (1982) introduced the next phase, a nonperforated casting that has been electrolytically etched. These retainers are then bonded to an etched enamel surface. These innovative authors, as well as Wood (1983), are from the Baltimore College of Dental Surgery, University of Maryland, Baltimore, Maryland. Because they are recognized as proponents and advocates of this type of restoration, popularizing its use, this type of restoration is often referred to as the *Maryland bridge.*

Two studies have evaluated the longevity of the cast-metal, resin-bonded fixed restorations. Eshleman et al (1984) evaluated 39 anterior appliances that had a perforated metal retainer. The length of service in the patient's mouth varied from 3.5 years to less than 1 year, with the majority in the 1- to 2-year range. Of the 39 in service, all were still functioning, although eight required rebonding. They felt the most common clinical failure is the bond to enamel, suggesting that the metal

should cover the largest enamel surface possible. Williams (1984) reviewed 63 acid-etch–retained bridges. The appliances had been in the patients' mouths for an average of 2.7 years, with a range of less than 1 year to 7 years. He reported a small loss of attachment (15.8%), with greatest loss in the first year. Periodontal problems were not evident, but some color change in the pontics was noted. Only two appliances had fracture of the porcelain.

Olin et al (1991) evaluated 103 resin-bonded bridges. After an average service of 3 years, approximately 12% failed (or debonded). Crispin (1991), who evaluated 71 bonded appliances after 5 years, suggested that the fixed appliances are very technique sensitive. Success is dependent on meticulous attention to detail of the complete process.

Indications

1. Congenitally missing teeth such as lateral incisors and premolars
2. Teeth lost to trauma
3. Anterior teeth missing because of congenital defects such as cleft palate
4. Carious teeth that have been extracted, if there is strong evidence of behavior alteration in philosophy of prevention by parent or patient

Contraindications

1. Poor oral hygiene
2. Large carious lesions in abutment teeth
3. Malpositioned teeth that do not allow for improved esthetics by bonding

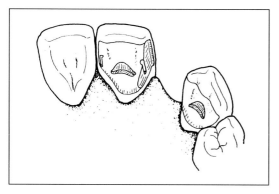

Fig 22-20 The anterior preparations for an acid-etch cast bridge.

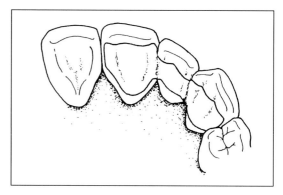

Fig 22-21 The framework covers as much of the lingual surface as possible.

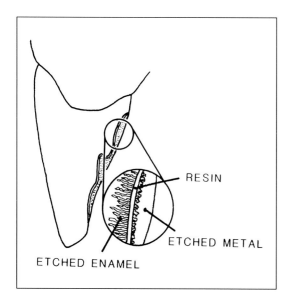

Fig 22-22 A cross section of a completed acid-etch cast bridge.

Advantages (Barrack, 1985)

1. Cost effective; less than comprehensive porcelain-fused-to-metal restorations
2. Conservative in enamel reduction, reducing trauma to pulp and periodontal tissue
3. Can be done without local anesthesia
4. Excellent esthetics
5. Time efficient
6. Failure easily repaired

Disadvantages

1. Contraindicated where large, restored, carious lesions exists
2. Relatively new technique; few long-term studies available
3. May be some grayness of etched abutment teeth

4. Difficult to determine efficacy of etched metal before acid-etch bonding

Procedure

For a more in-depth description, see Simonsen et al (1982).

Anterior teeth replacement

1. With the use of a flame-shaped diamond on the lingual surface, break the contacts interproximally (Fig 22-20) to provide a wraparound effect. Reduce the lingual surface to enhance the occlusion. If the occlusal forces may be excessive, shallow grooves can be used. Each abutment must have its own retention. A small chamfer placed about 1 mm from the gingival crest assists in a smooth transition from the cast metal and tooth structure. Cingulum notches or rests also can be used.
2. Make an impression of the final preparation and pour it in die stone. Construct the framework, covering as much of the lingual surface as possible, yet minimizing the incisal show of material (Fig 22-21). The framework should be fabricated so the connectors for the pontic can be easily cleaned.
3. On the second appointment, try-in the framework and check occlusion and esthetics.
4. Wood (1983) suggested mixing the composite resin with a material such as eugenol to check the color of the final cemented appliance. It may be necessary to use an opaque material to mask the metal.
5. Polish the oral side of the casting. Etch the enamel side of the metal but block the nonetched surfaces blocked out with wax. Attach the metal casting to an electrode, and etch the bridge on the surface to be bonded to the tooth structure. Rinse off the acid after the etching is completed.
6. Care must now be exercised in handling the etched metal surface. If it is contaminated, it must be

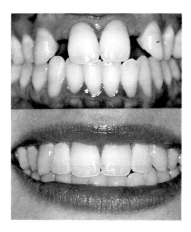

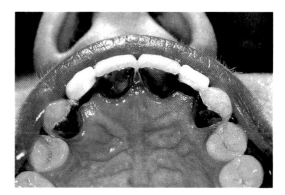

Fig 22-23 An adolescent with congenitally missing lateral incisors *(top)*. The teeth have been replaced with an acid-etch cast bridge *(bottom)*.

Fig 22-24 Occlusal view of the completed prosthesis.

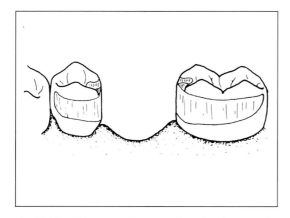

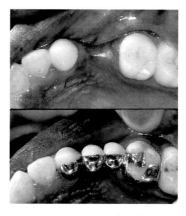

Fig 22-25 "Wraparound" preparations for the posterior teeth.

Fig 22-26 Missing premolars *(top)* have been replaced with an acid-etch cast bridge *(bottom)*.

cleaned with a solvent. Bonding must be done in a dry environment. Apply a bonding agent (unfilled resin) to the etched enamel and metal surfaces. Mix the composite resin pastes and apply the mix to the metal only. Seat the bridge before complete polymerization, carefully remove any excess composite resin (Fig 22-22). After polymerization, use finishing burs to remove excess material.

A patient with congenitally missing lateral incisors is an ideal candidate for this type of restorative procedure (Fig 22-23). Figure 22-24 is an occlusal view of the completed prosthesis. Both the central incisors and canines were used as abutments for the prosthodontic appliance.

Posterior teeth replacement

1. The wraparound design as advocated by Thompson and Livaditis (1982) should cover each tooth by 180°. The height of contour should be lowered to within 1 mm of the gingival crest (Fig 22-25). The preparation should be as thick as possible yet remain in the enamel to avoid overcontouring.
2. Shallow occlusal rests can also be used, remaining in enamel only. The walls of these occlusal rests must be nearly parallel.

The steps of try-in, casting, etching, and resin polymerization are similar to the steps for the anterior restoration.

An example of the replacement of missing premolars is seen in Figure 22-26.

The acid-etch–retained cast prothesis has filled a void in the treatment of adolescents with missing teeth, whether the cause of tooth loss is trauma or congenital defect. In the past, these teeth were replaced by removable appliances that were easily broken or by extensive and expensive fixed prosthodontic appliances. The acid-etch–retained cast appliance is an excellent substitute that requires minimal tooth reduction and provides excellent resultant appearances.

References

Barrack, G. Etched cast restorations. Quintessence Int. 1:27, 1985.

Birnbaum, R., Carrel, R., and Binns, W. H. Recontouring teeth with adhesive resin for added retention of cleft palate appliances. J. Pedod. 2:237, 1978.

Crispin, B. J. A longitudinal clinical study of bonded fixed partial dentures: The first five years. J. Prosthet. Dent. 66:336, 1991.

Eshleman, J. R., Mann, P. C., and Barnes, R. F. Clinical evaluation of cast metal resin-bonded anterior fixed partial dentures. J. Prosthet. Dent. 6:761, 1984.

Ettinger, R. L., and Pinkham, J. R. Modifications in restorative dentistry for the handicapped patient. In Nowak, A. J. Dentistry for the Handicapped. St. Louis: The C. V. Mosby Co., 1976.

Groper, J. N. An adjustable, nonbreakable, fixed anterior space maintainer. Pediatr. Dent. 14:60, 1992.

Howe, D. F., and Denehy, G. E. Anterior fixed partial dentures utilizing the acid etch technique and cast metal. J. Prosthet. Dent. 37:28, 1977.

Johnson, D. L. and Stratton, R. J. Fundamentals of Removable Prosthodontics. Chicago: Quintessence Publ. Co., 1980.

Lindahl, R. L. Denture techniques suitable for growing arches. Dent. Clin. North Am. Nov.: 659, 1961.

Livaditis, G. J. Etched metal resin-bonded restorations: Principles in retainer design. Int. J. Periodont. Rest. Dent. 3(4):35, 1983.

Livaditis, G. J. and Thompson, V. P. Etched castings: An improved retentive mechanism for resin bonded retainers. J. Prosthet. Dent. 47:52, 1982.

Nanda, R. S. Basic of Undergraduate Orthodontics. Oklahoma City: University of Oklahoma Press, 1976.

Olin, P. S., Hill, M. E. E., and Donahue, J. L. Clinical evaluation of resin-bonded bridges: A retrospective study. Quintessence Int. 22:873, 1991.

Rochette, A. L. Attachment of a splint to enamel of lower anterior teeth. J. Prosthet. Dent. 30:418, 1973.

Sarnat, B. G., et al. Year report of facial growth of complete anodontia with ectodermal dysplasia. Am. J. Dis. Child. 64:106, 1953.

Simonsen, R. Thomson, V., and Barrack, G. General considerations in framework design and anterior tooth modification. Quintessence Dent. Technol. 7:21, 1982.

Steffen, J. M., Miller, J. B., and Johnson, R. An esthetic method of anterior space maintenance. J. Dent. Child. 38:154, 1971.

Thompson, V., Barrack, G., and Simonsen, R. Posterior design principles in etched cast restorations. Quintessence Int. 3:311, 1983.

Williams, V. D. Acid-etched retained cast metal prosthesis: A seven year retrospective study. J. Am. Dent. Assoc. 108:629, 1984.

Wood, M. Anterior etched cast-resin bonded bridges: An alternative for adolescent patients. Pediatr. Dent. 5:172, 1983.

Additional readings

Denehy, G. E. Cast anterior bridges utilizing composite resin. Pediatr. Dent. 4:44, 1982.

Denehy, G. E., and Howe, D. F. A conservative approach to missing anterior teeth. Quintessence Int. 7:23, 1979.

Klopper, B. J., and Strizak-Sherman, R. Esthetic anterior space maintenance. Pediatr. Dent. 5:12, 1983.

Laird, W. R. E. Immediate dentures for children. J. Prosthet. Dent. 24:358, 1970.

Law, D. B., Lewis, T. M. and David, J. M. An Atlas of Pedodontics. Philadelphia: W. B. Saunders Co., 1981.

Livaditis, G. J. Cast metal resin-bonded retainers for posterior teeth. J. Am. Dent. Assoc. 101:926, 1980.

Roa, S. R. Removable partial dentures for children. In Finn, S. B. Clinical Pedodontics. 4th ed. Philadelphia: W. B. Saunders Co., 1973.

Simonsen, R., Thompson, V., and Barrack, G. Etched Cast Restorations: Clinical and Laboratory Techniques. Chicago: Quintessence Publ. Co., Inc. 1983.

Thompson, V., and Livaditis, G. J. Etched castings acid-etched composite bonded posterior bridges. Pediatr. Dent. 4:38, 1982.

Wood, M. Etched castings: An alternative approach to treatment. Dent Clin. North Am. 29:393, 1985.

Yanover, L., Craft, W., and Pulver, F. The acid-etched fixed prothesis. J. Am. Dent. Assoc. 104:325, 1982.

Questions

1. A 3-year-old girl has a central incisor removed because of trauma. What is the best appliance to use to replace this missing tooth?

   a. A removable appliance
   b. A fixed lingual wire with a tooth attached
   c. A fixed lingual wire only
   d. A Hawley appliance with replacement tooth

2. A 3-year-old child has a removable appliance fabricated. What is the biggest disadvantage of this appliance?

   a. It is caries inducing
   b. It is irritating to the supporting tissues
   c. Wearing of the appliance is completely dependent on the child and parents
   d. It is difficult to clean

3. When an overdenture is fabricated for a child with dentinogenesis imperfecta, which of the following steps are used?

   a. Preliminary maxillary and mandibular alginate impressions are taken for fabrication of custom trays
   b. Final impressions are completed with polysulfide impression material
   c. Wax occlusion rims are fabricated, and an intraocclusal record is taken
   d. The casts are mounted on an articulator
   e. The teeth are set using plastic teeth, they are tried in wax, and processing is completed
   f. a,c,d
   g. b,e
   h. c,d,e
   i. b,d,e
   j. All of the above

4. Separating medium is applied to a working cast:

   a. After the clasps and teeth are waxed to the cast
   b. Before the clasps and teeth are adapted to the cast
   c. Before the clasps are adapted and after the teeth are adapted

5. In which of the following patients is a prosthodontic appliance not indicated?

   a. A 5.5-year-old child who has two central incisors avulsed
   b. An 8-year-old child with ectodermal dysplasia
   c. An 11-year-old child with dentinogenesis imperfecta
   d. A 3-year old child who has four primary maxillary incisors extracted as a result of nursing bottle caries
   e. A 2.5-year-old child who avulsed a primary central incisor

Chapter 23

Guidance of the Developing Occlusion

> **Objectives**
>
> After studying this chapter, the student should be able to:
> 1. Discuss the aims and scope of arch length and occlusal discrepancies.
> 2. Identify the causative factors contributing to abnormal arch form development.
> 3. Identify the causative factors associated with crossbites.
> 4. Discuss the differences between eruptive guidance procedures and serial exaction procedures.

Prevention, as the family dentist and pediatric dentist see dentistry for the child, focuses on three essential aspects of child dental health: *(1)* caries control, *(2)* maintenance of periodontal integrity, and *(3)* preclusion of developing malocclusions.

The dentist recognizes that *complete* control of these three antagonists to sound dental health is impossible for reasons beyond human endeavor. He or she does realize, however, that with knowledge and understanding of the problems, the dentist can exercise measures that will attenuate or resolve them in most instances.

Preventive orthodontics "requires a continuing long-range approach." During the primary dentition period, the child should be observed and closely supervised for evidence of incipient problems of abnormal symmetry or occlusion.

Many unpredictable factors can affect the management of the developing dental arches and minimize the overall success of any treatment (AAPD, 1993). The variables that can affect the outcome of treatment may include:

1. The chronologic or emotional age of the patient.
2. The intensity, frequency and duration of oral habits.
3. Parental interest, support, and compliance.
4. Variations in facial growth.
5. Accuracy of the clinician's diagnosis and the appropriateness of care.

Oral habits

Oral habits are learned patterns of muscular contraction. Abnormal habits can interfere with regular patterns of facial growth. Oral habits may include the following:

1. Finger habit
2. Lip wetting or sucking
3. Abnormal swallowing or tongue thrusting
4. Abnormal muscle habits, eg, the mentalis muscle

The prevention of deleterious oral habits starts with proper nursing. Translated, this means that if the infant is breast-fed, time, love, and patience on the part of the mother are essential to allow the fulfillment of feeding and the gratifications that are concomitant with the activity. Should the baby be placed on bottle feeding, again, the importance of love, time, and patience on the parents' part is essential. This means holding the infant during the feeding and using a physiologically designed nursing nipple and exerciser (pacifier) to augment normal functional and deglutitional maturation (Fig 23-1). The correct exhibition of kinesthetic and neuromuscular activity on the infant's part may significantly reduce any tendencies toward anomalous tongue, lip, and finger habits.

The effects of the different types of feeding and non-nutritive sucking in infants from birth to 18 months of age were studied (Bishara et al, 1987). The authors found no differences in arch dimensions among groups in the study. Adair et al (1992) compared the occlusions of 24- to 59-month-old children who used either orthodontic pacifiers or conventional pacifiers. The children were examined for malocclusions involving overbite, overjet, canine and molar relationships, and posterior crossbites. The orthodontic pacifier users had a significantly higher incidence of overjet and the

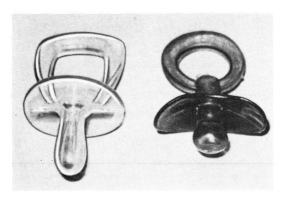

Fig 23-1 Nursing nipples and exercisers should be designed to meet the physiologic needs of the infant and provoke correct kinesthetic and neuromuscular activity. The exerciser on the right is the Nuk's Sauger, which is widely accepted by pediatricians and pediatric dentists.

conventional pacifier users had a significantly higher incidence of open bites. There were only minor differences in the occlusions of the two pacifier groups.

Sucking mechanism

In infancy, sucking is the most well-developed avenue of sensation. The infant not only receives sustenance but also derives sensory pleasures that are transmitted from the mouth to the brain. This gratification is a feeling of security, warmth, and euphoria. With further development, other neural pathways establish themselves, and the sucking mechanism is less important.

The infant who is impatiently nursed or who is given a bottle with a poorly designed nipple loses the warmth and feeling of well being and therefore is deprived of the suckling pleasures. This deprivation may motivate the infant to suck on the thumb or finger for additional gratification.

If the child persists with the finger habit but desists from it within the first 3 years of life, the damage incurred, such as an open bite, is temporary, provided the child's occlusion is normal.

The type of malocclusion produced by digit sucking is dependent on a number of variables (Sorokolit and Nanda, 1989):

1. Position of the digit
2. Associated orofacial muscle contractions
3. Mandibular position during sucking
4. Facial skeletal pattern
5. Amount, frequency, and duration of force applied

During the first 3 years, the damage is largely confined to the anterior segment, producing an anterior open bite. With a normal occlusion, damage is usually temporary. However, damage can be detrimental to the occlusion if the habit continues beyond the age of 3.5 years.

After 4 years of age, a finger habit becomes strongly established. Psychogenic effects take form, frequently motivated by persistent parental nagging. The oral structures take on further deformation because of the length of time the child has had the habit, its increased consistency, and the vigor involved in the activity (Figs 23-2a and b). With a marked change in the occlusion, compensatory muscular forces appear and create a fully developed malocclusion, such as the posterior crossbites associated with finger habits. Moreover, the finger or thumb involved will show evidence of the habit.

To answer the question of a parent, physician, psychologist, or other person as to the permanency of damage to the oral structures, the dentist must consider three factors, according to Graber and Swain (1985): duration, frequency, and intensity of habit. Likewise, many of these children can be treated by simple means.

Finger-sucking habits

A finger- or thumb-sucking habit in the infant or young child may be disconcerting for one parent and disregarded by another. It is frustrating to one professional and accepted by another. The habit is believed to be destructive by the dentist and a transient deformity by the physician. It is a highly controversial issue.

Tongue and lip habits

Tongue and lip habits are often associated with a finger habit and in large part are the added compensatory forces that produce full-blown malocclusions.

With an increase in overjet produced by a finger habit, it is increasingly hard to purse the lips over the teeth during the swallowing act. The mentalis muscle constricts the lower lip firmly against the mandibular incisor teeth and tightly against the lingual surface of the maxillary incisors. The tongue thrusts forward in concert with the lower lip to close off the mouth during the process of swallowing. The upper lip is functionless (Fig 23-3).

After the lower lip's abnormal intrusion into the swallowing act, the finger habit becomes secondary, and lip sucking becomes the supplier of the gratification process. In addition, a tongue that is larger than normal can produce marked malocclusions.

Oral habit therapy

When the need for active intervention, particularly appliance therapy is considered, a number of factors are involved:

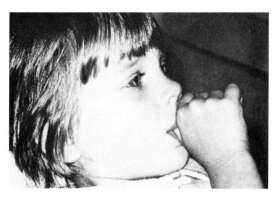

Fig 23-2a A child patient, aged 4 years, exhibits a pernicious finger-sucking habit.

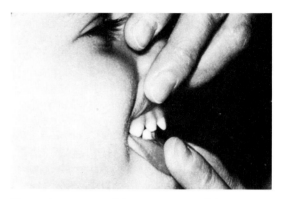

Fig 23-2b Because of the vigorousness of the activity, a marked overjet has resulted.

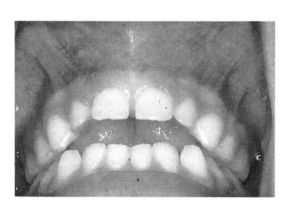

Fig 23-3 The patient has developed a severe anterior open bite because of a tongue thrust associated with swallowing.

1. *Age of the patient.* The patient should be at least 7 years old. It is important that the child be old enough to reason and understand.
2. *Maturity of the patient.* It is important that the patient understand the problem and have a desire to help correct it. Any evidence of immaturity on the patient's part may contradict any desire of the dentist's to treat the problem.
3. *Parent cooperation.* A child who elects to accept appliance therapy should have all the support and encouragement necessary from parents to help through the treatment period.
4. *Timely deliberation.* The dentist should have observed and thoroughly acquainted himself or herself with the patient over a period of several months or longer, noting the patient's general attitude and, more specifically, ability to cope with or break the habit on his or her own. The dentist should be alert to suggestive psychologic problems.
5. *Assessment of the deformity.* The dentist must assess the extent of deformity. Should there be other complexities associated with the habit deformity, it would be sound procedure to refer the patient to the specialist for evaluation and guidance. If the de-

formity is negligible, the dentist should give serious thought to avoidance of therapy. If, however, the deformity is apparent and there is an absence of other contributory factors, serious consideration should be given to appliance therapy.

Habit-correcting appliances

Thumb- and finger-sucking appliance

The use of a palatal appliance is referred to as a *tongue screen.* It is a crib-type appliance that is also effective for tongue-thrusting habits. The crib is constructed of chrome alloy wire. It fits palatally to the maxillary incisors, and its raised rigid design keeps the thumb or finger from laying snugly against the palate. It is secured to stainless steel crowns or stainless steel bands cemented to the primary maxillary molars or permanent first molars (Figs 23-4a to c). In essence, it is a lingual arch appliance with short spurs so placed on the crib as to remind the neuromuscular system that the thumb should not be there.

Tongue retrainer

The same appliance used for thumb and finger habits can be used to retrain the tongue (Fig 23-5). Moyers (1988) reported the use of myotherapy in early phases of the treatment, following by the application of a lingual arch wire carefully adapted to the teeth with "strategically placed spurs" about 2 mm in length to afford the tongue a neuromuscular reminder. The stages of Moyers' total treatment comprise three phases:

1. The learning of a new reflex (swallowing) at the conscious level.

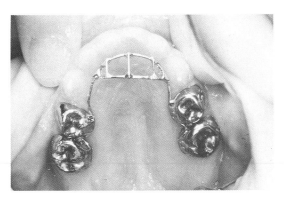

Fig 23-4a The crib is anchored to stainless steel crowns on both left and right primary first and second molars. The crib can be designed with spurs as a greater reminder for the thumb.

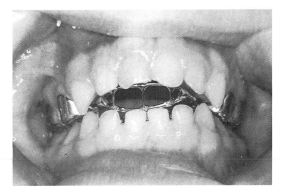

Fig 23-4b The appliance does not interfere with normal closure.

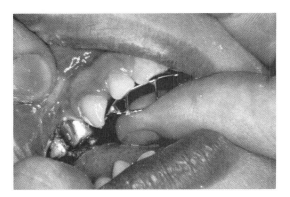

Fig 23-4c The reminder.

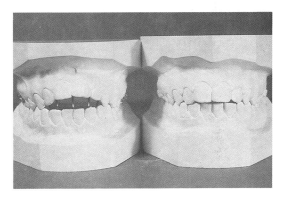

Fig 23-5 Before and after casts of a patient. The crib was effective in controlling the tongue thrust for this patient.

2. The transition of the conscious level to a subconscious swallowing reflex using the following, often repeated, exercise. A sugarless, citric acid–flavored, biconcave fruit drop is placed on the dorsum of the tongue and held between the tongue and palate until it dissolves.
3. Reinforcement using a lingual arch wire.

For detailed information on the technique of tongue retraining, see the *Handbook of Orthodontics* (Moyers, 1988).

Crossbites

The *crossbite* exists when there is an abnormal labial or lingual relationship of a tooth or teeth when the teeth of the maxilla and mandible are in occlusion (Nanda, 1993). The crossbite may include one or more teeth and can be unilateral or bilateral. There are three types of crossbites (AAPD, 1993):

Indications

1. Dental crossbites. These involve tipping of a tooth or teeth. This type is localized and does not involve basal bone.
2. Skeletal crossbites. These involve abnormal growth, size, and shape of the craniofacial skeleton. The possible causes are *(1)* Overgrowth of the mandible and/or arrested growth of the maxilla, or *(2)* Lack of equal growth in the length or width of the maxilla or mandible.
3. Functional (muscular) crossbites. These crossbites are produced by shifting of the mandible to achieve occlusion. Muscular contractions may also result in distorted growth of facial bones or abnormal positions of teeth.

Primary dentition

Anterior crossbites sometimes need treatment. However, check the eruption time of the permanent incisors. The crossbite may correct itself when the permanent teeth erupt.

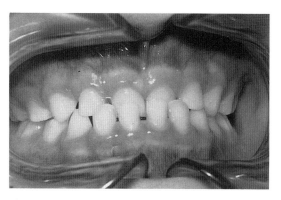

Fig 23-6 An anterior crossbite in the primary dentition involving the maxillary central and lateral incisors.

Posterior crossbites may be treated with selective grinding or appliance therapy. However, patients with a Class III skeletal relationship, and a posterior crossbite should receive comprehensive therapy.

Mixed dentition

Anterior crossbite in the mixed dentition usually needs correction.

In a patient with a Class I malocclusion a posterior crossbite should be corrected. Skeletal crossbites and Class III skeletal relationships would receive comprehensive care.

Permanent dentition

As in the primary and mixed dentitions, anterior crossbites usually should be corrected.

Appliances should be used to correct posterior crossbites. Again, children with Class III skeletal relationships should receive comprehensive care.

Appliances

Correction of a crossbite should result in improved occlusion and acceptable interarch relationships. The prognosis is improved when the crossbite is caused by dental factors.

Procedure

1. Measure the space available. This is the most important step. The space must be available before the crossbite can be corrected.
2. Design the appliance for the crossbite present. Appliances can be designed for single- or multiple-tooth crossbites.
3. Check and classify the interarch and molar relationships.

Anterior crossbites

The simple anterior crossbite is a dental-type arch length discrepancy caused principally by axial inclinations of maxillary incisors that have deviated from normal (Fig 23-6). This crossbite is simple as long as it is found in a Class I molar relationship. If, however, the malocclusion registered is a Class II or III, it is not classified as simple.

The dentist must ask certain questions before an accurate diagnosis and treatment plan can be devised. The dentist will require acceptable complete-mouth radiographs or a panoramic radiograph, study casts, and front-on and profile photographs, along with the patient for assessment.

Passive appliances

Inclined plane

The inclined plane of acrylic resin is an effective appliance in selected instances. It is fitted and cemented to the mandibular incisors, the incisal portion supporting an inclined plane. The maxillary incisor in lingual crossbite abuts the incline plane and is the only tooth in the oral cavity in functional contact. Repeated occlusal pressure of the tooth against the inclined plane gradually carries the tooth down the incline, leveraging it labially. In a few days the device should be removed. Very likely the tooth position will be corrected. If not, the appliance should be readjusted and recemented for another few days. Once posterior occlusion is back in contact, the tooth is usually forward and the appliance may be removed. Graber and Swain (1985) stated that under no circumstance should the appliance be in the mouth for longer than 6 weeks (Figs 23-7a and b).

The inclined plane appliance has its advantages and disadvantages and for some operators is not a treatment of choice.

Advantages
1. There is ease of construction.
2. Correction is of short duration, depending on function and muscle force.
3. During movement there is no soreness or looseness of the tooth.
4. Relapse is rare.

Disadvantages
1. Diet is limited.
2. There is a temporary speech defect.
3. An open bite may be created if the appliance is left in place too long.
4. The appliance may become loose and may require recementation.
5. Alignment of the malposed tooth may be imperfect when the appliance is removed.

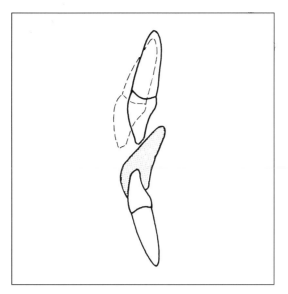

Fig 23-7a Mechanics of the incline plane when placed on the mandibular incisors.

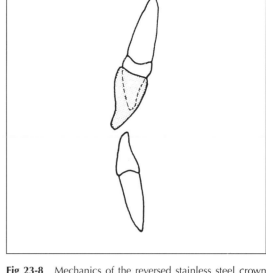

Fig 23-8 Mechanics of the reversed stainless steel crown functioning as an incline to move the maxillary incisor out of crossbite.

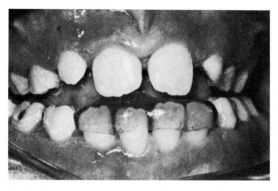

Fig 23-7b The acry lic resin inclined plane fitted to the mandibular incisors. The inclined plane engages the permanent maxillary right central incisor.

The appliance can be constructed directly or indirectly in quick-curing acrylic resin. Bulk is added to the splint only in the areas that are to be the inclined plane. Adjustments will need to be made on the appliance before cementation to afford the desired plane angle and functional contact area.

Reversed stainless steel crown

Another appliance that can be readily adapted for use as an inclined plane to correct the lingual crossbite of the maxillary incisor tooth is the reversed stainless steel crown. When placed on the affected incisor in a reversed position, it will create its own inclined plane and produce a functional contact and a leverage force (Fig 23-8).

There are some disadvantages to this particular appliance or any of similar design.

1. It is difficult to check the degree of tooth movement accomplished during treatment because the appliance is not easily removed. Graber and Swain (1985) suggested that a postcementation wax or compound core be used to compare change.
2. The opposing mandibular incisors become mobile and uncomfortable from the constant incisal pressure exerted by functional contact.
3. The compensatory lingual movement of the opposing mandibular incisor or incisors is evident. Graber and Swain (1985) contended that this movement is quite often a beneficial response.
4. If the clinical crown is only partially erupted, little retention will be offered for a stainless steel crown adaptation.
5. Should the maxillary incisor erupt palatally to the line of occlusion, suitable leverage may be difficult to obtain.

Active appliances

Two types of active appliances may be effectively used to correct the maxillary incisor crossbite. One is a removable palatal appliance using S or helical springs, and the other is one of several designs of the fixed labial arch wire and maxillary molar band attachment.

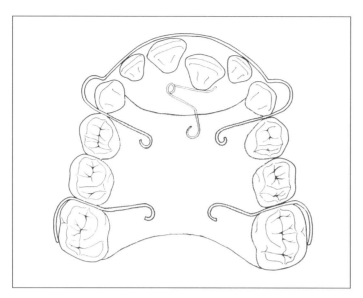

Fig 23-9 Permanent maxillary left central incisor in crossbite. A Hawley appliance with a helical spring that exerts a labially directed force against the lingual surface of the inlocked tooth is an effective tool.

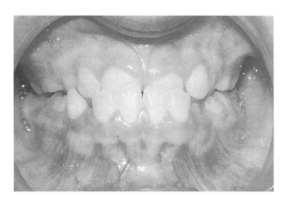

Fig 23-10a Patient with anterior crossbite in the permanent dentition, a candidate for treatment with a removable appliance.

Removable appliances

The removable palatal appliance consists of a modified Hawley apparatus with S or helical springs built into its palatal section lingual to the affected tooth or teeth. The springs exert a labially directed force on the lingual surface of the tooth or teeth in crossbite. The spring's force will require adjustment at frequent intervals until the desired labial tooth movement is accomplished (Fig 23-9).

The advantage of this particular appliance rests in its action. Unlike the inclined plane devices that depend on functional contact to produce the desired forces for tooth movement, a constant force is exerted when the appliance is satisfactorily activated (Figs 23-10a to c).

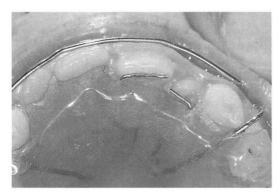

Fig 23-10b Hawley-type appliance with a helical spring exerting pressure on the permanent incisor in anterior crossbite.

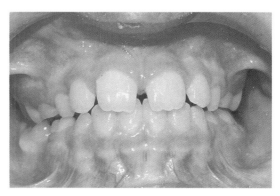

Fig 23-10c The patient in Fig 23-10a after treatment with a removable appliance.

There is one disadvantage to the use of this type appliance. The child patient must be well motivated to wear it. Poor cooperation by the patient in wearing it either delays the ultimate completion of the project or spells total failure for the treatment.

Fixed appliances

The fixed appliance consists of a labial or lingual arch wire with molar bands or crowns (Fig 23-11).

For the labial arch wire, the molar bands will have horizontal buccal tubes. The 0.040-in. buccal tubes and 0.040-in. round stainless steel wire are recommended. The arch wire should be well adapted to the buccal and labial surfaces of the teeth, with bilateral, adjustable vertical spring loops attached. The procedure consists of banding the four maxillary incisors, placing spot-welded edgewise brackets, and using 0.020-in light wire for tooth movement and control.

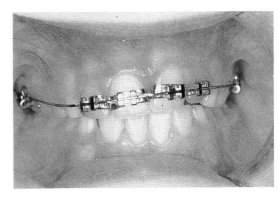

Fig 23-11 Use of a 2 x 4 appliance, where the two molars and the four incisors are banded. The arch wire is expanded to move the central incisors that are in crossbite into normal occlusion.

Posterior crossbites

Kutin and Hawes (1969) have figured that 1 in 13 children can be expected to exhibit some form of posterior crossbite (Fig 23-12).

Individual teeth

Use of cross elastics is effective for single molars and premolars in crossbite, as long as space is adequate (Fig 23-13).

Procedure (Nanda, 1993)

1. Select and fit the appropriate band to the maxillary and mandibular teeth. Burnish and adapt the bands.
2. Spot weld or solder hooks to the bands. The direction of forces is related to the direction in which you wish the teeth to move.
3. Cement the bands. Instruct the patient in the use of the rubber elastics (usually 0.25-in. heavy rubber elastics) (Fig 23-13).
4. The elastics should be changed periodically.

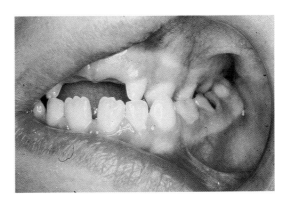

Fig 23-12 Posterior crossbite in the mixed dentition.

Multiple teeth (Fig 23-14)

Use the quadhelix (Currier and Austerman, 1993) to correct dental malocclusions that result in posterior crossbite of multiple teeth.

Indications

1. Bilateral crossbites in the primary and transitional dentitions
2. A unilateral crossbite in the primary or transitional dentition

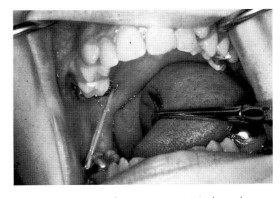

Fig 23-13 Use cross elastics to correct a single-tooth crossbite.

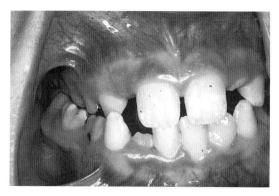

Fig 23-14 Patient with a unilateral posterior crossbite, a candidate for a quadhelix fixed appliance.

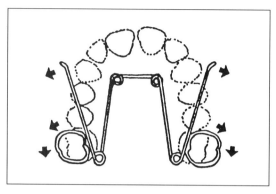

Fig 23-15 Activate the quadhelix by moving the posterior helical loops buccally.

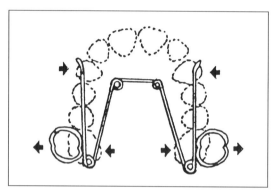

Fig 23-16 Continue the activation of the quadhelix by activating the anterior helical loops.

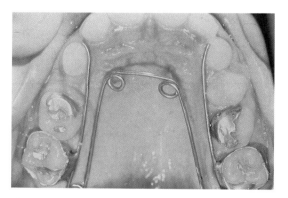

Fig 23-17 Quadhelix cemented in position.

Contraindications

1. Skeletal crossbites
2. Single-tooth crossbites

Procedure

1. Fit bands to either the primary second molars or the permanent first molars.
2. Take a complete-arch impression with low-fusing compound or an alginate material.
3. Remove the bands from the teeth and seat them in their proper position. Seal in place. Make a working cast of stone.
4. Use 0.032 stainless steel wire. The wire should contact all the posterior teeth and the canines (if present). The contact is close to, but not touching, the soft tissue at the cervical margin. The loops or helixes and the palatal portion should be 2 to 3 mm distal to the banded teeth. The anterior aspect of the wire is just distal to the primary canines. The helical loop should be 2 to 3 mm in diameter.
5. Secure the wire to the working cast. Solder the wire to the molar bands. Clean and polish the appliance.

6. Activate the appliance prior to cementation: Step 1—Activate the posterior helical loops, moving the free wires buccally (Fig 23-15). Step 2—Activate the anterior helical loops moving the molar bands buccally (Fig 23-16).

When the wire has been activated, the lingual surface of the molar bands will be above the central fossa of the molars (Fig 23-17). The anterior portion of the wires will be above the canine cusp tips. Both anterior and posterior crossbites should be overcorrected using the appliance for a period of retention (Figs 23-18a and b).

Note: Not only do crossbites cause orthodontic problems, but they also can cause periodontal problems (Fig 23-19).

Ectopic eruption

Ectopic eruption reflects the abnormal eruption of a permanent tooth wherein the tooth is out of normal alignment and causes abnormal resorptive processes on a primary tooth. This phenomenon affects primarily

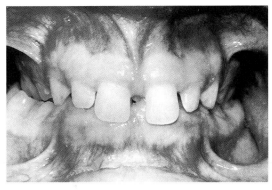

Fig 23-18a Posterior crossbite before treatment with a quadhelix.

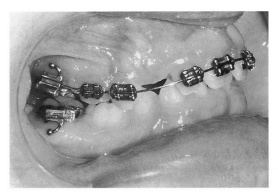

Fig 23-18b The same patient as in Fig 23-18a, comprehensive treatment, after treatment with a quadhelix.

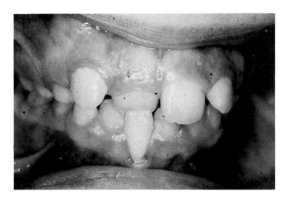

Fig 23-19 Because of repeated trauma from the maxillary central incisor, which is in crossbite, the mandibular central incisor has experienced tissue loss.

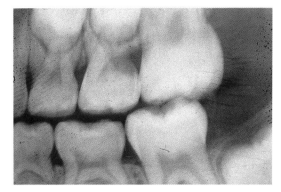

Fig 23-20 Young (1957) observed that 66% of the ectopically erupted teeth correct themselves without treatment intervention. This radiograph is an example of a jump-type ectopia wherein the maxillary first permanent molar, which was entrapped, freed itself. Note the resorptive destruction on the distobuccal root of the second primary molar.

the permanent maxillary first molar and the permanent mandibular lateral incisor. It is observed on occasion in other locations of the mouth, notably the permanent mandibular first molar area.

Etiology

The permanent maxillary first molars, the maxillary canines, the mandibular incisors and other teeth, including the permanent mandibular first molars, are the most frequently affected by ectopic eruption.

Permanent maxillary first molar

1. The tooth in question is frequently larger than normal.
2. The tooth erupts at an abnormal angle to the occlusal plane, indicative of ectopic positioning of the tooth germ.
3. Tuberosity growth lags, therefore producing abnormal arch length.

4. Morphology of the distal surface of the primary second molar crown and root lends perfectly to the entrapment of an abnormally tilted permanent first molar.
5. In certain instances, the size of the primary second molar may be a significant factor in causing arch length shortage and entrapment of the permanent maxillary first molar.
6. Pulver (1968) has pointed to an additional factor to consider, "delayed calcification of some affected first permanent molars."

Young (1957) reported that 66% of the observed ectopic entrapments finally erupted into an acceptable position without corrective intervention (Fig 23-20).

Maxillary canine

The maxillary canine in its early development becomes ectopic or may be forced into ectopic eruption because of a shortage of space.

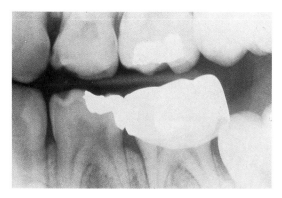

Fig 23-21 Ectopic eruption of a permanent maxillary first molar. An ill-fitted or oversized stainless steel crown can produce an ectopic eruption. The ledge created by a poorly contoured gingival margin on the crown can entrap the permanent molar. Often replacement with a smaller, carefully contoured crown will free the molar.

Other teeth

The permanent mandibular first molar is also seen in ectopic eruption with the resultant destruction of the primary second molar. There are other permanent teeth that erupt in an ectopic manner, only to become impacted.

Clinical evidence

Usually the evidence of an ectopic eruption will be seen initially during radiographic examination. In this instance (Fig 23-21), a clinical and radiographic examination have revealed a primary second molar with the distal portion of the root destroyed by resorptive processes. The permanent first molar is in ectopic eruption.

When the ectopic condition is evident, a determination needs to be made whether the eruptive states reflects early-on development or an irreversible entrapment. In the first instance, one may observe the ectopic development to determine its prospects. If it is evident that the abnormal angulation of the ensnared tooth is such that it will not erupt, treatment should be inaugurated.

An ectopic eruption can be produced artificially by an oversized or poorly finished stainless steel crown. The erupting permanent first molar may become entrapped against a marginal overhang. Quite often the condition is correctable by replacing the defective crown with one of more suitable size and gingival contour. There may or may not be distal root destruction on the primary second molar (Fig 23-21).

Treatment

A number of treatment procedures or appliances are effective in certain ectopic eruptions. The simplest of these is the use of brass separating wire. Other appliances, more elaborate in design, are better adapted to the more severe complications. In most instances, the primary objective is to distalize the permanent molar from entrapment and provide it with eruptive guidance. At other times, the primary second molar is sacrificed, the permanent molar is permitted to erupt, and then it is distalized to normal position.

Procedures

Brass ligature wire (0.026 in.)

To distalize the permanent molar, the operator may use brass ligature effectively where the degree of angulation of the permanent molar is not too severe and the entrapments are not too excessive.

Method
1. Local anesthesia is optional.
2. Use 5-cm lengths of ligature wire.
3. Establish a semicircular loop at one end of the wire, and then bend it at a 90° angle to the right or left side of the crown.
4. A forceps such as a mosquito-beak or hemostat will be most helpful in threading the ligature wire interproximally. Place the beak of the forceps near the bend of the loop positioned for interproximal passage.
5. Direct the curve of the loop subgingivally beneath the contact of the two teeth to the opposite side of the alveolar ridge, exiting by way of the interproximal space. Several attempts may be necessary, adjusting the curvature of the loop for better access and passage (Fig 23-22).
6. Twist the two ends of the ligature wire together to establish a separating force at the contact area (Figs 23-23a and b).
7. Tighten the wire every 3 or 4 days. At times it may be necessary to place new ligature wire.

Stainless steel crown

A stainless steel crown with an extended distal surface acting as an inclined plane has proved effective in freeing deeply angulated and entrapped permanent molars (Figs 23-24a to c).

The objective is to distalize the permanent molar and restore the primary second molar for maintenance of arch length.

Method (Figs 23-25a to d)
1. Complete the pulpotomy on the primary second molar.
2. Do the routine crown preparation on the primary second molar. The distal slice is a modified slice that converges from the occlusal surface subgingi-

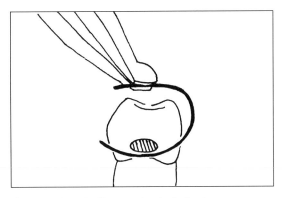

Fig 23-22   Pass the ligature wire gingival to the contact.

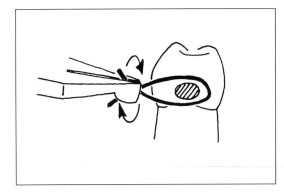

Fig 23-23a   Use a Howe pliers to twist the two ends of the separating wire together. The mosquito-beak forceps can also be used effectively for the procedure.

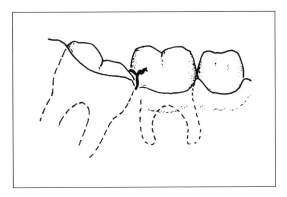

Fig 23-23b   How a separation force is produced to distalize the permanent molar.

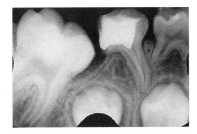

Fig 23-24a   The permanent mandibular right first molar is entrapped. A pulpotomy is performed on the primary second molar. Note complete resorptive destruction of the distal root.

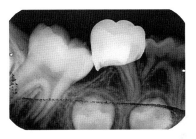

Fig 23-24b   The primary mandibular right second molar is prepared and fitted with a stainless steel crown. The distal surface of the crown remains untrimmed while the mesial, buccal, and lingual surfaces are trimmed. The distal surface is designed as an inclined plane to guide the eruption of the permanent first molar.

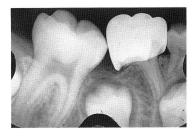

Fig 23-24c   Over a period of time, the ectopic eruption is nearly corrected, without space loss.

vally and mesial surface to the ectopically erupted permanent first molar. Keep as much mesiodistal dimension as possible occlusally.

3. Trim the crown conventionally on the mesial surface and the mesial two thirds of the buccal and lingual surfaces while curving and extending it subgingivally at the distal surface, resting mesially to the ectopic molar. The untrimmed distal surface of the crown lends itself well to this purpose.

4. The gingival margin of the distal surface of the crown may need inordinate crimping to move it mesially to and beyond the mesial marginal ridge of the ectopic molar. Thus an inclined plane is established.

Other devices

There are other devices that in certain instances work well in freeing ectopically erupted molars.

Humphrey appliance. The Humphrey appliance (Humphrey, 1962) consists of an orthodontic band

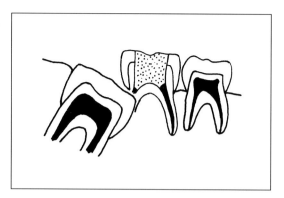

Fig 23-25a Permanent mandibular right first molar in ectopia. Perform a pulpotomy on the primary second molar.

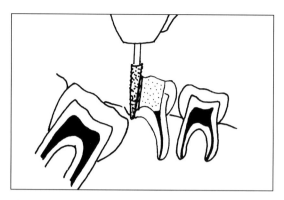

Fig 23-25b Produce the distal slice on the primary second molar with a narrow, tapered diamond stone. Direct the diamond stone subgingivally with care, avoiding the mesial surface of the permanent molar.

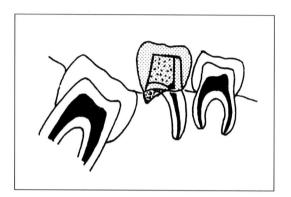

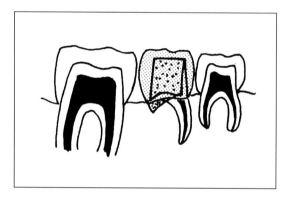

Figs 23-25c and d Eruption of the permanent molar along the distal surface of the primary second molar.

adapted and fitted to the second primary molar. An S loop of soft round Elgiloy wire is soldered to the buccal surface. The loop is then heat treated. A small occlusal opening is placed in the central pit of the ectopic molar. Before cementation, the appliance is activated to exert a distalizing force. The terminal end of the S loop is inserted into the occlusal opening. Reactivation of the spring loop may be necessary to complete distalization of the tooth. If so, the appliance will need to be removed and then recemented.

Helical springs. Helical springs have also been substituted for the S loop. The forces exerted by the helical spring are more continual and reactivation of the spring is less a problem and procedure. The appliance need not be removed for adjustment (Figs 23-26a to f).

These types of appliances when constructed unilaterally will cause the abutment tooth to respond to reciprocal forces. If the primary second molar has sustained marked damage and resorption from the ectopic eruption, it is better to use a more passive treatment, such as the stainless steel crown.

Serial extraction and eruptive guidance procedures

In certain instances, the specialist uses the method of the serial extraction procedure to selectively remove teeth in both the mixed and permanent dentition. The purpose is to minimize the early complications of certain malocclusions, thus reducing the length of treatment time and some of the complexities associated with appliance therapy (Hertz, 1979).

The specialist may use the procedure from an eruptive guidance standpoint whereby only the teeth of the primary dentition are eliminated and holding arch appliances are used to maintain the credibility of the space already established and prevent drifting or tipping of certain teeth.

Before serial extraction of eruptive guidance procedures, an arch length and cephalometric analysis must be accomplished to determine that either of these procedures is essential in treatment of the malocclusion. The orthodontist or pediatric dentist is qualified to carry out the procedures necessary for arch length assessments and cephalometric analysis.

Fig 23-26a A modification of the Humphrey appliance is the use of a helical spring rather than the S loop. Its forces are more continual and adjustment less a problem. The first step is banding the primary second molar.

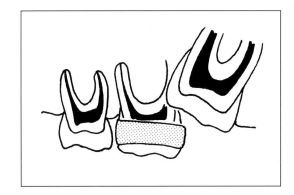

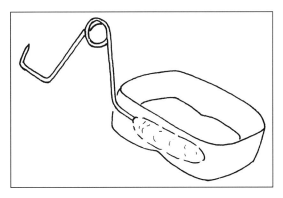

Fig 23-26b The second step is the development of the helical spring using 0.022-in round wire. With the helical loop formed, one free end is adapted and soldered to the buccal surface of the band.

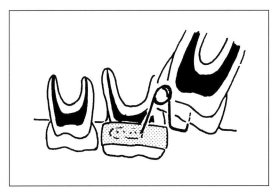

Fig 23-26c The coil of the helical is directed toward the mucobuccal fold but free of it. The free end of the helical spring can be anchored to the central pit area of the permanent molar with acid-etch composite resin.

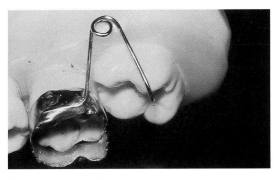

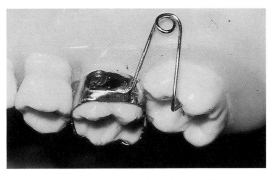

Figs 23-26d and e Following cementation of the appliance, the free end of the helical spring is anchored occlusally with acid-etch composite resin.

Fig 23-26f Cemented appliance to correct ectopic eruption, after the correction has been completed. In this patient, the appliance and primary second molar were removed, and a space maintainer was placed to hold the space.

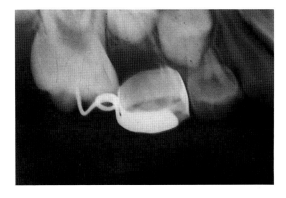

Figs 23-27a to d to 23-29a to d Eruptive guidance. Eruptive guidance case and casts are courtesy of R. S. Nanda.

Figs 23-27a to d The patient was 9 years old and in the mixed dentition period. The occlusion was a Class I molar relation. A mandibular lingual holding arch was placed.

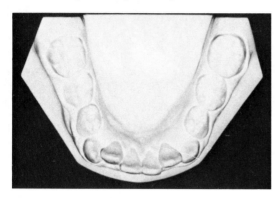

Fig 23-27a

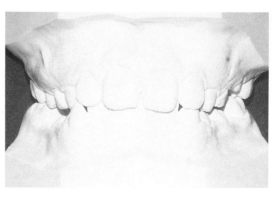

Fig 23-27b

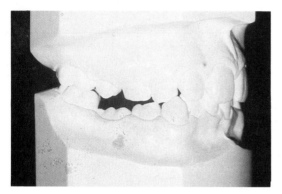

Fig 23-27c

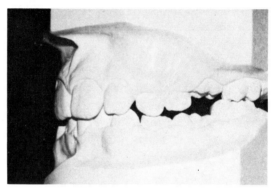

Fig 23-27d

Serial extraction procedures are most often launched by the orthodontist when diagnosis clearly indicates that corrective measures for the malocclusion will necessitate the removal of four premolars along with comprehensive therapy. In most instances, these cases for treatment are Class I malocclusions, whereas other malocclusions may demand a different kind of treatment.

Almost all cases of eruptive guidance procedure involve strategically selected primary teeth removals to allow the orderly and unencumbered eruption of the permanent teeth. All cases involving eruptive guidance procedure are instituted from Class I malocclusions wherein the arch length and cephalometric analyses indicate available or potentially available space.

In that eruptive guidance extends over a period of several years, it is necessary to reassess the growth patterns from time to time to determine whether alternatives in treatment are required. Retentive appliances are most likely needed. Appliance therapy involving minor tooth movement may be required in some situations (Figs 23-27a to d to 23-29a to d).

Indications

Nanda (1993) indicated that dentoalveolar discrepancies in the mixed dentition or eruptive guidance measures are dependent on a number of factors that may exist simply or in combination, and all are associated with a shortage of arch length. These factors are:

1. Anterior crowding.
2. Protrusion.
3. Distal terminal plane relationship of the primary second molars of a Class II molar relation.
4. Impinging deep overbite (usually not present in the primary or mixed dentition).

Arch length shortages of 7 to 12 mm will require the serial extraction procedure and comprehensive appliance therapy to close the spaces created by the removal of four premolars.

Arch length discrepancies of 3 to 7 mm are borderline as to management. It will require a more indepth look at the skeletal growth pattern of the child, careful

Figs 23-28a to d At this stage of active exfoliation of primary teeth, the patient, 11 years old, has developed a Class II molar relationship. Maxillary cervical headgear was placed to distalize the permanent maxillary first molars. A maxillary labial arch wire was placed and the maxillary first premolars were banded and rotated into normal position.

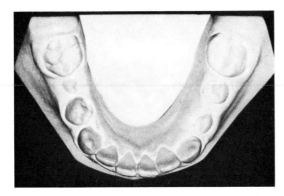

Fig 23-28a

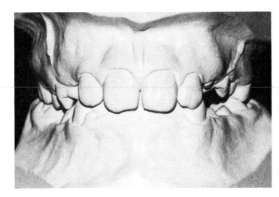

Fig 23-28b

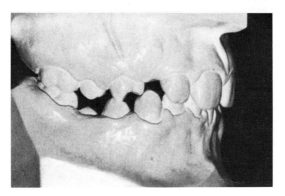

Fig 23-28c

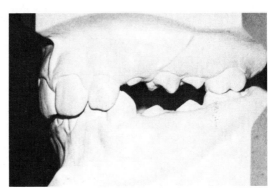

Fig 23-28d

supervision of the leeway spaces, and possibly a reclamation of lost space by a small degree of distalization of the molars. As such, reassessment may indicate the route of the serial extraction procedure or a small amount of minor tooth movement, or even some slight interproximal reduction of enamel in the contact areas, preceded by eruptive guidance procedure. Shortages of less than 3 mm are easily corrected with eruptive guidance measures (Nanda, 1993). A flow chart has been devised and should permit a more vivid picture of the points previously discussed (Nanda, 1993).

Note: the individual patient will be categorized in the flow chart according to age and stage of development.

Six years

Signs. Erupting mandibular incisors are rotated; space is inadequate.

Action. Remove primary lateral incisors.

Logic. The permanent lateral incisors will erupt within a short period of time. Further assessment will be necessary.
Note: at the time the incisors erupt, even in normal situations, slight crowding is a norm that is accommodated by growth in the anterior section of the arch.

Follow-up. Recall in 6 months to observe eruptive and developmental progress.

Figs 23-29a to d The mandibular arch was virtually untreated other than placement of the lingual holding arch appliance. The maxillary teeth, with minor tooth manipulation, moved into acceptable position.

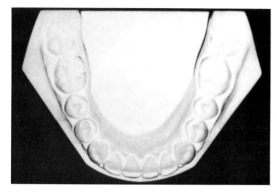

Fig 23-29a

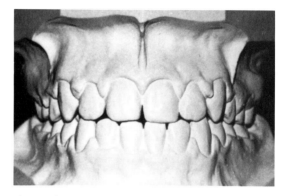

Fig 23-29b

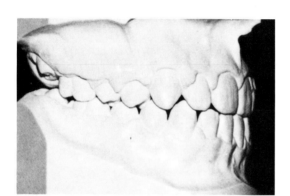

Fig 23-29c

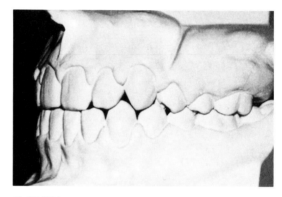

Fig 23-29d

Seven years

Signs. Erupting mandibular permanent lateral incisors are lingually placed and crowded.

Action
1. Slice mesial surface of primary canines (even into the dentin if necessary).
2. If this procedure appears to be an inadequate measure, wait until the lateral incisors are erupted and perform a space analysis.
3. In cases of excessive shortage, remove the primary canines. The mandibular incisors are usually in protrusion and will self-correct their alignment.

   Note: if the cephalometric analysis indicates that the mandibular incisors will require uprighting, no corrective action will be necessary because the uprighting will occur automatically. However, if the mandibular incisor inclination is correct, place a lingual holding arch to prevent the mandibular incisors from linguoversion.

4. In some instances, because of lack of space, an erupting lateral incisor may cause root resorption and premature loss of a primary canine. This unilateral loss of a canine will relieve crowding but will shift the midline of the arch.

Alternatives. Consider removing the mandibular canine on the opposite side of the arch and follow up with sequential removals of the maxillary canines.

If the mandibular canine or the opposite side should not be removed, place a lingual holding arch with a soldered stop against the distal surface of the lateral (if erupted) or central incisor on the side of the exfoliated canine to prevent a shift of the midline.

Follow-up. In the event a lingual arch appliance had been placed, recall the patient every 2 to 3 months to make certain the bands are well cemented. You must not run a chance of decalcification of the molars. If an appliance is not placed, recall the patient in 6 months.

Eight to 9 years

Evaluate the dentinofacial complex and develop a diagnosis.

Premise
1. The growth of the dental arch is almost completed.
2. Arch length from the permanent first molar to the permanent first molar is fixed (it can only shorten, never increase).
3. Permanent incisors have erupted; use their size to estimate the size of the unerupted canines and premolars.
4. Unerupted canines and premolars have crown forms completed. Use periapical radiographs to determine their size.

Because tooth size and arch length are fixed, you can determine whether or not there is adequate arch length.

Result
1. If total arch length is adequate, the patient will require guided eruption through a supervised extraction procedure, but extraction is confined to the primary dentition.
2. If the patient has not had a lingual holding arch placed previously, it may be advisable to place one before the primary second molars exfoliate to preclude late mesial shift.
3. If the arch length is inadequate:
   a. By 0.0 to 3.0 mm. Guide eruption of the teeth by slicing the interproximal surfaces of the primary canines and molars.
   b. By 4.0 to 7.0 mm. Consult a specialist. The overall skeletal and facial profile and growth pattern may need study, with consideration toward extraction procedures for the primary teeth.
      In the upper limits of space shortage in this category, the need for the removal of the first premolars may begin to appear but not before another assessment at about 10 to 11 years of age is accomplished.
   c. By 7.0 to 12.0 mm. The case will require some form of managed extractions with full orthodontic consultation.

Follow-up. Recall in 6 months to observe developing dentition.

Ten to 12 years

Reevaluate the growth of the dentition and face and the previous diagnosis.

Option A: Eruptive guidance. Option A should be used of the patient is reaffirmed as requiring the eruption guidance procedure.

1. Continue the sequential process of strategic removal of primary teeth to provide a favorable eruption pattern of permanent teeth.
2. Use the leeway space and place a fixed lingual arch appliance in the mandibular arch to prevent late mesial shift.
3. To correct the cusp-to-cusp interarch relationship, use maxillary cervical headgear to distalize the maxillary first molar by 2.0 to 3.0 mm and establish correct intercuspation. A palatal arch may be used to hold the maxillary molars once they have been distalized and to permit unencumbered eruption of the premolars and canines.
4. Observe the patient every 3 months until the eruption process is completed.

Option B: Managed extractions. Option B should be used if the patient's need for a serial extraction procedure, requiring the removal of all first premolars, is reaffirmed.
   Consult with an orthodontist to:

1. Recheck the diagnosis.
2. Develop a strategy for the extraction procedure.
3. Determine the need to preserve the arch length and find out if lingual arch placement is necessary. In more serious cases of arch length shortage, the space needs to be fully guarded.
4. Schedule frequent consultations.
5. Take over treatment of the malocclusion at the most opportune time.

Acknowledgment

Drs. Ram S. Nanda and G. Frans Currier, Department of Orthodontics, University of Oklahoma College of Dentistry for the use of materials and drawings for this chapter.

References

Adair, S. M., Milano, M., and Dushku, J. C. Evaluation of the effects of orthodontic pacifiers on the primary dentitions of 24-to-59 month old children; preliminary study. Pediatr. Dent. 14:13, 1992.

American Academy of Pediatric Dentistry (AAPD). Reference Manual. Chicago: AAPD, 1993.

Bishara, S. E., et al. Influence of feeding and non-nutritive sucking methods on the development of the dental arches: Longitudinal study of the first 18 months of life. Pediatr. Dent. 9:13, 1987.

Currier, G. F., and Austerman, J. B. Fabrication of Appliances for Preventive, Interceptive, and Adjunctive Orthodontics. Oklahoma City: Oklahoma University Health Science Center Press, 1992.

Graber, T. M., and Swain, B. F. Orthodontics: Current Principles and Techniques. St. Louis: The C. V. Mosby Company, 1985.

Hertz, R. S. Serial Extractions. In Saunder, B. Pediatric Oral and Maxillofacial Surgery. St. Louis: The C. V. Mosby Co., 1979.

Humphrey, W. P. A simple technique for correcting an ectopically erupting first permanent molar. J. Dent. Child. 29:176, 1962.

Moyers, R. E. Handbook of Orthodontics. 4th ed. Chicago: Year Book Medical Publishers, Inc., 1988.

Nanda, R. S. Basics of Undergraduate Orthodontics. Oklahoma City: Oklahoma University Health and Science Center Press, 1993.

Pulver, F. The etiology and prevalence of ectopic eruption of the maxillary first permanent molar. J. Dent. Child. 35:138, 1968.

Sorokolit, C. A., and Nanda, R. S. The influence of function on the development and correction of malocculsions. J. Okla. Dent. Assoc. Fall:22, 1989.

Young, D. H. Ectopic eruption of the first permanent molar. J. Dent Child. 24:153, 1957.

Additional readings

Dewel, B. F. Serial extraction: Precautions, limitations and alternatives. Am. J. Orthod. 69:95, 1976.

Garcia-Godoy, F. Correction of ectopically erupting maxillary permanent first molars. J. Am. Dent. Assoc. 105:244, 1982.

Harrison, L. M., Jr., and Michal, B. C. Treatment of ectopically erupting permanent molars. Dent. Clin. North Am. 28:57, 1984.

Hirayama K., and Chow, M. H. Correcting ectopic first permanent molars with metal or elastic separators. Pediatr. Dent. 14:342, 1992.

Yuen, S., Chan, J., and Tay, F. Ectopic eruption of the maxillary permanent first molar: The effect of increased mesial angulation on arch length. J. Am. Dent. Assoc. 111:447, 1985.

Questions

1. Jane, aged 21 months, has been sucking her thumb since infancy. Her mother brings her to the dental clinic because the parents are quite concerned and have been trying to break Jane of the habit. Clinically, Jane has a slightly open bite. As near as you can determine, there is no evidence that a tongue thrust is developing. Jane's mother believes their child is using her thumb less except when she's upset or not feeling well. She appears to be a well-dispositioned child. You determine that:

   a. The thumb sucking is quite normal for this stage of the child's growth
   b. A thumb habit appliance should be considered when the primary second molars have erupted to correct the developing malocclusion
   c. Mittens may be taped to the hands before naps and at bedtime.
   d. The oral defect will correct itself at this age with diminishment of the thumb habit
   e. The parents should avoid the early forms of nagging that can affect the child's emotional make-up, intensifying the oral habit
   f. a,c
   g. a,d,e

2. Rebecca, aged 8 years, is in the dental office for examination. In addition to a minor carious condition, an anterior crossbite is noted. The patient has a Class I occlusal relationship. The permanent maxillary right lateral incisor is inlocked palatally. The permanent central incisors and permanent left lateral incisor are in alignment. Your determination to treat the crossbite is based on the clinical finding and the fact(s) that:

   a. The case is a Class I occlusal relationship, making it therefore a simple anterior crossbite
   b. The parents want the crossbite treated if at all possible
   c. There is no maxillary midline deviation to the right, and it appears that there is enough room for the lateral incisor in the space
   d. The path of closure of the well-formed jaws is uninhibited, and the permanent maxillary right lateral incisor, which is the only tooth malposed, will be easily accepted in the space allotted
   e. a,c
   f. a,c,d

3. Crossbites may arise from the following:

   a. Tipping of teeth
   b. Skeletal asymmetry
   c. Functional shifting of the mandibular muscles
   d. None of the above
   e. d
   f. a,b,c
   g. a
   h. b,c

4. Pauline, aged 7 years, has an ectopic permanent maxillary fight first molar. The radiograph reveals negligible resorptive damage to the subgingival portion of the distal surface of the primary second molar. The permanent molar is about 20° mesial to its normal eruptive attitude. The treatment of choice will be:

   a. The Humphrey unilateral appliance
   b. A stainless steel crown with distal surface incline
   c. A 0.026 brass ligature wire
   d. Periodic observation for possible self-correction

5. The term crossbite is applied when:

   a. There is an absence of occlusion
   b. There is an abnormal buccolingual relationship of the teeth
   c. There is excessive vertical overlap of the incisors
   d. There is excessive overjet of the incisors
   e. There is a tight cusp and fossa relation in centric occlusion

Chapter 24

Treatment Planning

Planning the approach to pediatric dental care is initiated only after a complete and comprehensive diagnosis is obtained. This diagnosis implies the gathering of all necessary medical records and clinical and radiographic dental findings. Once the correct diagnosis is achieved, the operator may proceed with the development of an organized and efficient sequence to providing care. The development of a treatment plan is the most critical step in the successful future management of the child and parent. Without advanced planning, treatment rendered will be disorganized and inefficient and can lead to dissatisfaction and confusion for both the dentist and the parent.

The formation of a treatment plan has many advantages. First, it commits the operator in advance to a certain sequence of care. Although this commitment is not absolutely rigid and may be modified during the treatment phase, it does provide a step-by-step guideline for the operator to follow. The written treatment plan eliminates the decision-making process as to what procedure should be completed next at each appointment period and helps the dental staff plan in advance the equipment and materials that will be required for the procedure. Second, it provides an estimate of the time required for each appointment and the number of appointments required to complete the treatment. This information is especially helpful to the parents, who will need to schedule appointments. Because dental appointments often constitute a major inconvenience to the parents as a result of the need to arrange for transportation and baby sitting, as well as the consideration of lost time from school and work, treatment sessions should be planned as efficiently and effectively as possible to minimize the number and length of visits. Third, fee payments can be arranged. Often this arrangement is best accomplished by dividing the total fee by the number of expected appointments so that a set, predetermined fee per appointment can be established, and there is no confusion as to what payment is required at each appointment on a pay-as-you-go basis.

In addition, when planning treatment where there is a questionable diagnosis, you should always assume the worst and plan for the more extensive treatment alternative. For example, a radiographically deep carious lesion that approaches but does not have obvious penetration into the pulp should be treatment planned for a pulpotomy and stainless steel crown. If during carious lesion removal there is no evidence of pulpal exposure, the more conservative treatment of calcium hydroxide placement and amalgam restoration can be completed. The parents will be delighted to learn that the treatment will cost less. This approach is psychologically better than if the reverse were to occur.

Every dentist should strive to restore the dentition to its normal form and function. Where individual teeth cannot be satisfactorily restored, their removal and subsequent placement of a space maintainer, when indicated, is the treatment of choice. Since effective use of time is essential in the dental management of the child, maximize the delivery of a local anesthetic by performing quadrant dentistry. Quadrant dentistry implies the completion of all required procedures in one fourth, or quadrant, of the mouth, for example, the maxillary right quadrant during one session. On occasion, restoration of maxillary anterior teeth may necessitate the use of a "fifth quadrant." In other words, consideration of time and local anesthesia may require division of the treatment sessions into four posterior quadrants and one anterior quadrant. Assuming that all quadrants are of equal priority, reserve treatment of the anterior quadrant until last because: (1) posterior quadrants serve greater importance in masticatory function and space maintenance and are retained for longer periods of time, and (2) anterior teeth are primarily of esthetic concern to the parents and may well be their chief complaint. Early restoration of anterior teeth may result in early departure of the patient from your practice once this concern is satisfied.

In cases where minimal procedures are required, consider complete-arch (horizontal division—left and right side of one arch) or half-mouth (vertical division—maxillary and mandibular of one side) dentistry.

The preference to avoid administering bilateral mandibular blocks in young children is a matter of individual judgment.

Diagnostic evaluation of oral disease conditions in children is often concrete and absolute. Generally, a lesion is present or it is not. There is usually little room for discussion or disagreement. However, in the determination of a plan for treatment, there is considerable flexibility and subjective assessment. For example, when is it appropriate to restore an incipient carious lesion? The factors that must be weighed are the patient's susceptibility to carious lesion formation (past dental caries experience), prognosis for cooperation in prevention-oriented practices, and the tooth's approximation to exfoliation. If the patient has a high carious lesion prevalence and poor orientation toward prevention, the incipient lesion on a primary tooth beyond 1 year from normal exfoliation should be restored. In addition, the necessity for closely evaluating adjacent and bilateral sites in primary teeth should be appreciated. Incipient lesions should always be restored in those caries-active children who require other operative procedures in that quadrant to facilitate the maximal use of the local anesthetic and access under the rubber dam. Realizing the infectious and transmissible nature of dental caries and the low potential for its arrest in primary teeth, you would be ill advised to dismiss incipient lesions in children. The philosophy of "wait and see" (observe on recall) is poorly supported because the probability is high that you are only going to watch the lesion expand. The concept of consciously leaving an active disease process untreated could be questioned on ethical and moral grounds.

Therefore, after thorough diagnosis of the problem and determination to treat it, a sequence of appointments must next be established. This area encompasses personal preferences and individual treatment philosophies. However, certain guidelines can be used to meet this challenge successfully. The following is a standard format that may be used in establishing treatment priorities.

Determination of treatment priorities

Step one

Emergency procedures must be dealt with immediately, which implies rendering only the minimal necessary treatment to relieve pain and infection. Conservative treatment approach at an emergency visit is advantageous because the child is often under stress and of low tolerance level. If possible, delay extraction or extensive pulpal therapy, provided that the pain can be relieved by some other means. This delay will allow time to gather complete diagnostic records and plan for treatment, thus not denying other potential dental problems. Usually the condition of the offending tooth has been present for a long time. An additional week without care until records can be obtained is probably of little consequence.

Step two

A plaque-control program should be introduced. This program includes plaque identification and removal, diet counseling, topical fluoride application, and child-parent education on home care oral hygiene practices. The advantage of this approach is the opportunity to place emphasis on prevention, development of patient rapport, evaluation of patient behavior, and introduction of an initial atraumatic experience for the child patient. The emphasis on prevention should be reinforced at every future appointment. However, some practitioners feel that for patients with extensive dental needs, prevention at initial appointments should not be overemphasized because it is often not a priority from the patient's viewpoint. Instead, emphasis should be placed on returning the patient to sound dental health first, then interest can be generated in its maintenance following the restorative therapy.

Step three

Restorative therapy is usually begun at the third dental visit. A procedure that is short and simple should be selected first during this initial appointment to allow the development of the patient's trust and confidence. If management of the child's behavior becomes overwhelming, arrangements have been made to terminate the procedure quickly. This step is especially important if the appointment is the child's first dental experience. In this case, there is sufficient introduction of new experiences, such as the injection of the local anesthetic and corresponding numbness, the rubber dam, and the sound and vibration of the handpiece, that the burden of a prolonged visit may be expecting more tolerance and ability to cope that the child is able to manifest. Although it is correct to set treatment priorities so that the most severe or compromised condition is treated first, it may be more prudent to postpone this consideration until the second restorative visit. For example, an isolated occlusal amalgam restoration in one quadrant may be the initial treatment procedure of choice over a pulpotomy and stainless steel crown in another quadrant, even though its prompt treatment is deemed more necessary. Similarly, the last restorative visit in the sequence should be of minimal effort on the assumption that it leaves the child with a favorable memory of the dental visits. In a clinical situation where all quadrants display a similar level of treatment needs, the selection of the initial treatment quadrant varies according to your personal preference and comfort. Generally, the side opposite the operator's handedness (left side for right-handed operator) is selected because of ease in patient stability during the injection procedure. However, whether the maxillary or the mandibular quadrant is selected first may reflect the level of the operator's experience. The student may have to select between the lesser of two evils: difficulty in using a mirror for the maxillary arch or lack of confidence in the administration of a successful mandibular block. Whatever decision is finally made, the determined sequence of treatment should remain absolute and be followed in a precise manner.

Finally, it should be mentioned that restorative dentistry can also be prevention oriented. If some predictive judgments regarding the patient's future caries prognosis are made, a considerable amount of unnecessary re-treatment may be avoided. For example, the consideration to place stainless steel crowns instead of multiple surface amalgam restorations in a 3-year-old with poor home care is valid. Stainless steel crowns seldom require additional treatment, in contrast to amalgam restorations, which have the potential to fail because of marginal deterioration, or which must be replaced because of cervical demineralization. Despite the initial additional expense of stainless steel crown placement, over the span of time it may, in fact, be the more economical restoration.

Step four

Following completion of the restorative phase of treatment, orthodontic and prosthodontic care may be rendered if needed. Although minor oral surgical procedures are accomplished during the restorative phase of treatment using the quadrant approach, complex surgical endeavors should be delayed until this phase.

Step five

No treatment plan is completed until provision is made to provide a recall appointment for evaluation and necessary follow-up care.

Summary

The formation of a treatment plan may make the difference between success and failure in management of the child dental patient. Arrange procedures in sequence according to priority when forming the treatment plan. The treatment plan can be likened to a navigational chart or road map in that it sets a direction and a goal. When establishing a treatment plan, consider the external factors that might influence parental acceptance. These factors include dental I.Q. and interest level, past experiences, finances, availability for appointments, and overriding medical or social problems. Also realize your own limitations; do not attempt to treat beyond your capabilities. Proper use of

referral should not be considered as an admission of incompetence but rather as a realization that the patient's needs might be best handled elsewhere and that you are concerned enough about the patient's welfare to make the necessary referral.

Presentation of treatment plan to the parents

Effective care presentation to the parents requires that the dentist be able to communicate so that the parent not only understands the dental problems of the child but also approves of the services you recommend for treatment. The importance of the environment during the presentation should not be disregarded. The atmosphere should be relaxed and informal. Visual aids demonstrating the recommended procedures may be helpful during your explanation. A view box for examination of radiographs should also be present. The panoramic radiograph is a very effective patient-parent educational aid. An organized, relaxed, and concerned presentation will help impress your patients and their parents with your sincerity and thoroughness, which will in turn help motivate them toward accepting your advice.

The successful presentation will accurately inform the parents of (1) the dental needs of their child, (2) the restorative procedures required, (3) the amount of time required to perform the projected procedures, (4) the total cost for rendering the services, and (5) the preventive measures necessary to maintain the completed treatment. However, merely to list the patient's problems and their solutions is ineffective. In general, each problem should be discussed in the following manner (1) point out the problem using casts, radiographs, or the patient's mouth; (2) state the probable cause of the problem, such as plaque or insufficient arch length; (3) state the outcome of the problem for the individual, such as its effect on function, health, or appearance; (4) show how the problem will be resolved; and finally, (5) stress the benefit the patient will receive from the treatment.

Unless the presentation is performed in an orderly, precise, and concise manner, valuable time will be lost. Explanations become repetitious. The presentation should reflect an air of pleasantness and self-assurance. A dentist who possesses genuine concern for the child's welfare will handle the presentation in a natural and understandable way. So—relax, allow sufficient time to talk, and relate in general terms some of the procedures that need to be done (eg, pulpotomy), the number of teeth involved, the number of visits required, and the costs involved.

Do not react dramatically to the conditions you have found, and do not criticize the parent for the existing conditions. Reasonable explanation of the causes, how they can be treated, and the preventive suggestions offered will provide for a better-educated parent and child. Although the ability to produce the services necessary creates self-confidence, you should not "guarantee" your treatment or the prevention of further recurrence of the condition. You should imply that the services to be rendered will "help" prevent further difficulties but that the real preventive measures will come from the awareness and care rendered by the patient and the parent. Everyone has a responsibility in good prevention—the dentist, the patient, and the parent.

A parent or an older patient will listen and learn. He or she should also be allowed to participate and to respond, particularly if there are any questions. Actually, the presentation may be given through a series of questions with answers applied to the particular patient's dental needs. For example:

1. What is the problem?
2. Can it be corrected?
3. How can it be corrected?
4. How long will it take?
5 Will it bother me?
6. How much will it cost?
7. How can it be paid?

Criteria and protocol for referral

In the general practice of dentistry, 80% of the children seen are excellent patients, usually better patients than their parents. However, some types of patients would receive better care if referred to a pediatric dentist:

1. The very young child, younger than 2 years with rampant caries requiring hospitalization
2. The child with a developmental disturbance affecting the oral cavity, such as a cleft palate or dentinogenesis imperfecta
3. The child with a concurrent medical problem, such as cystic fibrosis, chronic heart disease, or kidney disease
4. The child or adolescent with a congenitally or developmentally handicapping condition (mental, emotional, or physical) that influences quality dental care
5. The child who is a severe management problem

You should not be reluctant to refer a patient or consider it a reflection on your qualifications as a dentist. The patient's best interest should be served. The pediatric dentist has the advantage of being specially trained and equipped, both emotionally and physically, to manage the unusual child patient or difficult treatment requirements.

When a generalist refers a patient to a specialist, the generalist is, in fact, "lending" the patient to the specialist. The specialist is requested to perform independent judgement and care, for example, the referral to an oral surgeon for removal of third molars, an endodontist for a specific root canal procedure, or the orthodontist for care of malocclusion. In each instance, the specific procedure is performed and the patient returns to the referring generalist. However, the pediatric dentist is unique because the patients are usually referred for complete patient care and seldom for a specific procedure, unless specifically requested otherwise by the referring generalist.

The referral process

1. If it is decided that the child is best managed by referral to a pediatric dentist, discuss the rationale with the parent or parents. Most parents want to do what is best for their child and will accept your decision. The parents will respect the practitioner who recognizes that it would be best for all concerned if someone else tries to solve the problem for them.
2. Have the office receptionist contact the specialist's office and arrange the appointment. Better yet, the generalist can call the specialist and discuss the patient's immediate problem and how this problem might best be solved. Do not send the parent and patient unannounced to the specialist's office. It is difficult to decide what the patient needs when they appear in an office with only a wet, underexposed radiograph.
3. Inform the specialist of the specific problem. Does the patient need to be seen for an emergency? The emergency could be a fractured incisor, an infected tooth, or a tooth that is causing discomfort. Does the child have a medical problem or a developmental disability? How old is the child?
4. Forward any radiographs or records available to the specialist's office. Do not give the records to the parent to hand deliver to the office.
5. Conversely, the specialist in turn should send you a note thanking you for the referral, describing what the problem is and how it best can be solved. Part of any referral process should involve confirmation and affirmation of the treatment plan.

If these simple rules are followed, there is a harmonious relationship among the generalist, specialist, patient, and parents. The important factor is that there will be quality care for the special child patient.

Sample treatment plan cases

The following section presents the diagnosis and treatment plans for two pediatric dental patients who are representative of those you can expect to see in your practice. A third case is presented to test your skills and judgment in arranging a treatment plan based on your diagnostic ability.

Table 24-1 Existing restorations and carious lesions according to surface for patient in Case 1

| Quadrant | Tooth (No.) | Restoration | Carious surfaces | |
			Clinical	Radiographic
Maxillary right	Second molar (55)	Occlusal		Mesial
	First molar (54)			Distal
Maxillary left	First molar (64)			Distal
	Second molar (65)	Occlusal	Occlusal	Mesial
Mandibular left	Second molar (75)	Occlusal	Occlusal	Mesial
	First molar (74)	Occlusal		Distal
Mandibular right	First molar (84)		Disto-occlusal	Disto-occlusal
	Second molar (85)	Occlusal		Mesial

Please keep in mind when viewing both the radiographs and the maxillary and mandibular arch photographs that the left-hand side is the patient's right side and vice versa.

Case 1 (Figs 24-1a to f)

History and examination

Subject. Five-year-old black girl

Chief complaint. None; routine dental checkup.

Social history. Only child of concerned parents, both living at home and both employed. She appears friendly and cooperative, with some slight anxiety toward dental treatment. The family has just moved into town (which has an optimally fluoridated water supply), and she participates in a preschool program.

Medical history. Negative.

Dental history. Previous treatment rendered 1 year ago. Radiographs were not taken at that time. Behavior displayed during treatment was acceptable by parental assessment—no known negative outcome.

Physical examination

Head and neck. Within normal limits.

Intraoral soft tissue. Within normal limits with the exception of very mild gingivitis in the presence of minimal plaque accumulation. Plaque accumulation is present mostly on the proximal surfaces of the molars.

Occlusion. Early mixed dentition displaying mesial step molars, Class I canines, midline shift 2 mm to the right and acceptable overjet and overbite relationships. There is lingual ectopic eruption of the permanent mandibular left central incisor and overretained primary central incisor. Both arches have symmetric form with prominent primate spaces. Dental development is appropriate for chronologic age.

Dental tissue. Normal size, shape, color, and number. Maxillary occlusal radiograph reveals calcific pulpal metamorphosis of right central incisor, but positive history of trauma is not confirmed by the parents. A summary of existing restorations and carious lesions according to surface is found in Table 24-1.

Recommended treatment plan

Appointment 1. Diagnosis and patient-parent dental health education (prevention).

Appointment 2. Case presentation and reinforcement of dental health education (prevention).

Appointment 3. Tooth 84, formocresol pulpotomy and stainless steel crown; tooth 85, mesio-occlusal amalgam restoration.

Appointment 4. Tooth 75, mesio-occlusal amalgam restoration; tooth 74, disto-occlusal amalgam restoration; tooth 71, extraction; tooth 81, extraction.

Appointment 5. Tooth 55, mesio-occlusal amalgam restoration; tooth 54, disto-occlusal amalgam restoration.

Appointment 6. Tooth 64, amalgam restoration; tooth 65, mesio-occlusal amalgam restoration.

Appointment 7. Polish amalgam restorations; give oral hygiene instructions, apply topical fluoride.

Appointment 8. Recall in 6 months; observe pulpal status of teeth 51 and 61 and eruption of mandibular incisors.

Figs 24-1a to f   Case 1.

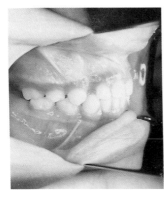 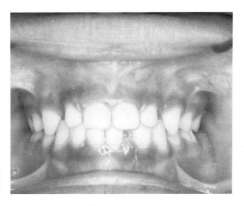 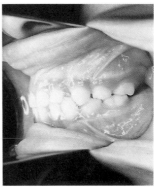

Fig 24-1a   Right lateral view.   **Fig 24-1b**   Frontal view.   **Fig 24-1c**   Left lateral view.

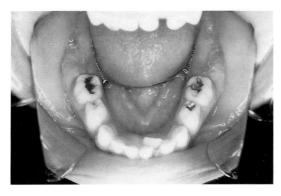 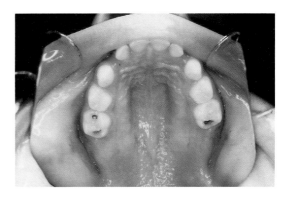

Fig 24-1d   Mandibular arch.   **Fig 24-1e**   Maxillary arch.

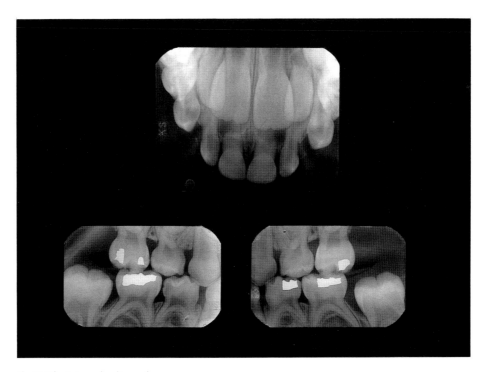

Fig 24-1f   Intraoral radiographs.

Comments

Appointment 1. This patient has routine diagnostic problems. There are no medical conditions to precaution or contraindicate dental treatment. Past dental history is noncontributory, and you should not expect any behavioral problems provided that sound management procedures are employed. Oral hygiene instruction should stress the use of dental floss to remove plaque between the molars. The bilateral and adjacent-surface pattern of carious attack should be noted. In addition, the waste created by the replacement of all amalgam restorations might have been avoided if radiographs were originally taken to detect the proximal lesions during the previous treatment phase.

Appointment 3. This quadrant is treated first because the deep carious lesion on tooth 84 holds priority over all others. Since this is not the patient's initial dental experience, a simpler quadrant need not be selected first. Besides, if problems occur in patient management, you may elect to complete the pulpotomy only and provisionally restore the tooth for later crown placement. If the entire quadrant is completed, the crown should be cemented before condensation of the amalgam in the adjacent tooth to prevent possible amalgam fracture during crown seating and to ensure tight proximal contact.

Appointment 4. A mandibular occlusal radiograph must be taken before tooth extraction. Both primary incisors are removed at this time to take advantage of the mandibular block. The right central incisor may be anesthetized by local infiltration which ensures adequate anesthesia if cross innervation exists. The right central incisor is removed because the permanent right incisor is likewise erupting lingually. This condition can be confirmed radiographically. Note the occlusal carious lesion on tooth 75 would have been prevented if the original outline of the preparation design had included all susceptible pits and fissures as recommended.

Appointment 5. This appointment is interchangeable with appointment 6 because they have similar priority.

Appointment 7. Topical fluoride application should be applied after the amalgam restorations are polished, to maximize its benefits. No treatment is indicated at this time for the maxillary central incisors because they are nonsymptomic. Future observation should be directed at providing treatment if abscess formation or delayed exfoliation should occur. The treatment of choice would then be extraction, with no need for space maintenance.

Case 2 (Figs 24-2a to g)

History and examination

Subject. Eight-year-old black boy.

Chief complaint. Carious lesions; thermal sensitivity in mandibular left quadrant of low intensity and short duration.

Social history. Youngest of five siblings of divorced parents; lives with his mother, who works at a factory having dental insurance for dependents of employees. His older brothers have prepared him for his first dental visit. Immediately on greeting him in the operatory, he begins crying and insisting that he does not want a "shot."

Medical history. There is history of one episode of convulsions, at 1.5 years of age, caused by high fever. No other episodes have occurred since that time. He is myoptic and allergic to dust and sulfonamides.

Dental History. None.

Physical examination

Head and neck. Within normal limits.

Intraoral soft tissues. There is evidence of marginal gingivitis, hypertrophic maxillary labial frenum and tonsillar tissue. Plaque index shows plaque accumulation on 87% of the dental surfaces. Oral hygiene practices are not stressed at home.

Occlusion. Early mixed dentition with Class I molars and canines and a developing overjet-overbite relationship. Both arches have symmetric form and adequate space for permanent tooth eruption. There is a diastema between the maxillary central incisors. His mother exhibits a similar diastema.

Dental tissue. All teeth present and developing are of normal size, shape, color, and number. The primary maxillary lateral incisors and mandibular right first molar are mobile. There is an anesthetic, hypoplastic enamel defect on the labial surface of the maxillary left central incisor. A summary of existing carious surfaces is found in Table 24-2.

Recommended treatment plan

Appointment 1. Diagnosis and patient-parent dental health education.

Appointment 2. Case presentation and reinforcement of dental health education; tooth 36 excavate carious lesion and provisionally restore with zinc oxide–eugenol.

Table 24-2 Existing carious lesions according to surface for patient in Case 2

Quadrant	Tooth (No.)	Carious surfaces	
		Clinical	Radiographic
Maxillary right	Second molar (16)	Occlusolingual	
	Second molar (55)	Occlusolingual	Occlusal
Maxillary left	Central incisor (21)	Labial	
	First molar (64)		Distal
	Second molar (65)		Mesial
	First molar (26)	Occlusolingual	Occlusal
Mandibular left	First molar (36)	Mesio-occlusobuccal	Occlusal
	Second molar (75)	Occlusobuccal	
	First molar (74)	Disto-occlusal	Distal
Mandibular right	First molar (84)	Disto-occlusobuccolingual	Disto-occlusal
	Second molar (85)	Mesiocclusobuccal	Occlusal
	First molar (46)	Occlusobuccal	

Figs 24-2a to g   Case 2.

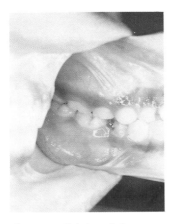

Fig 24-2a   Right lateral view.

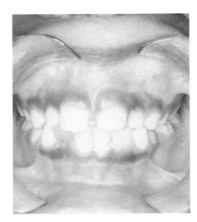

Fig 24-2b   Frontal view.

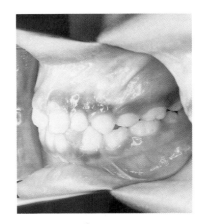

Fig 24-2c   Left lateral view.

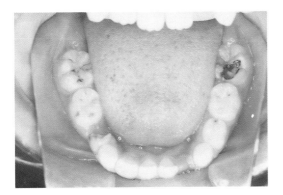

Fig 24-2d   Mandibular arch.

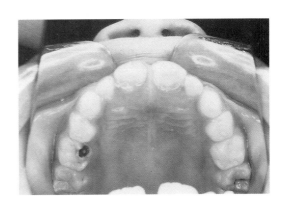

Fig 24-2e   Maxillary arch.

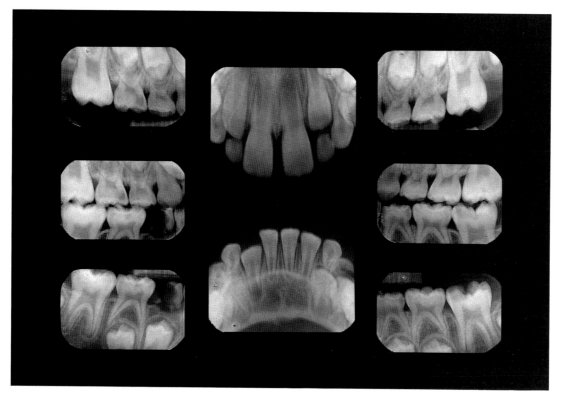

Fig 24-2f Intraoral radiographs.

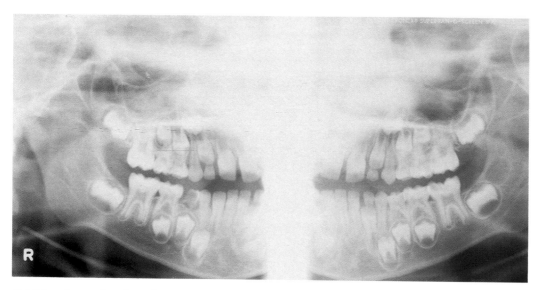

Fig 24-2g Panoramic radiograph.

Appointment 3. Tooth 46 occlusobuccal amalgam restoration; tooth 85, stainless steel crown; tooth 84, extract. Compound wax impression for fabrication of crown and loop space maintainer on tooth 85.

Appointment 4. Tooth 85, cement crown and loop space maintainer; tooth 36, stainless steel crown; tooth 75, occlusobuccal amalgam restoration; tooth 74, formocresol pulpotomy and stainless steel crown.

Appointment 5. Tooth 16, occlusolingual amalgam restoration; tooth 55, formocresol pulpotomy and stainless steel crown.

Appointment 6. Tooth 26, occlusolingual amalgam restoration; tooth 65, mesio-occlusal amalgam restoration; tooth 64, disto-occlusal amalgam restoration.

Appointment 7. Tooth 21, labial composite resin restoration; polish amalgam restorations; give oral hygiene instructions; apply topical fluoride.

Appointment 8. Recall in 6 months.

Comments

Appointment 1. This patient has multiple large carious lesions and some thermal sensitivity associated with the permanent mandibular left first molar. There are no medical conditions that contraindicate dental treatment on a routine basis. However, he does display subjective fear and anxiety related to the injection procedure.

Appointment 2. Oral hygiene practice at home must be stressed along with diet counseling. Since obvious fear has been displayed during the previous visit and there is history of some discomfort associated with tooth 36, it is prudent at this time to consider use of nitrous oxide-oxygen inhalation during the injection procedure and carious lesion excavation of tooth 36. Because the alleviation of pain is your only goal at this time, the placement of a provisional restoration is sufficient. Also, this short but necessary procedure will allow you to evaluate the patient's behavior during dental treatment. If the patient's response is not satisfactory, another pharmacotherapeutic modality can be selected for the next appointment.

Appointment 3. This quadrant was selected first because the badly resorbed primary first molar needs to be extracted. The decision to maintain this space and what appliance to use in doing so is a difficult one to make. The possibility of mesial migration and consequent loss of arch length in this area is slight mainly because it has not occurred before this time even though the right condition (loss of proximal contact) has been present. Nevertheless, it was decided to maintain the space just to be safe because the patient cannot afford to lose any space from an arch that is just barely of sufficient length. The crown and loop appliance was selected over the band and loop type because the tooth needed to be restored, and crown placement avoids the problem of cervical demineralization from dissolution of cement under an orthodontic band. Although a fixed lingual arch is normally the treatment of choice in this situation, it is not absolutely recommended because the first premolar will succeed eruption of the canine. When the premolar erupts, the appliance can be removed simply by cutting off the wire and smoothing the solder joint intraorally.

The procedure for fabrication of a crown and loop using the indirect technique is as follows: *(1)* prepare tooth for crown; *(2)* adapt crown; *(3)* take impression of area; *(4)* remove crown and place in impression to be poured up as a working cast; and *(5)* adapt and provisionally cement a second crown until next appointment.

Appointment 4. The provisional crown is removed and the crown and loop is cemented. Although a stainless steel crown has been selected to be placed on tooth 36, a pin amalgam restoration is a reasonable alternative choice for treatment.

Appointment 5. The operator should exercise care when excavating carious lesions on tooth 55 because the chances are good that a pulpotomy will not be needed. The radiographic appearance of the carious lesion can be misleading because the lesion occurs on the lingual surface, which is superimposed on the pulp in the two-dimensional view provided by the bitewing radiograph.

Questions

The following history, photographs, and radiographs of a 5-year-old white boy are provided for your examination.

The patient is cooperative but somewhat shy and apprehensive. He has a past history of a functional heart murmur and borderline diabetes. Past dental treatment was rendered when he was 3 years old. A plaque index of 70% is found on initial visit. There is no chief complaint.

On a separate sheet of paper, first list your diagnosis by tooth number, then propose a sequence of treatment by appointments as previously demonstrated. (See the answers in the appendix for your review).

Figs 24-3a to e   Case 3.

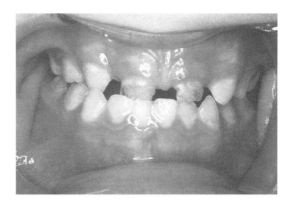

Fig 24-3a   Frontal view.

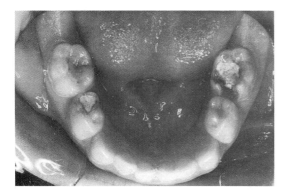

Fig 24-3b   Mandibular arch.

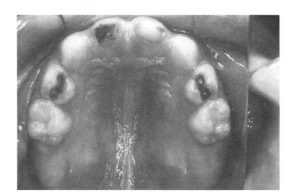

Fig 24-3c   Maxillary arch.

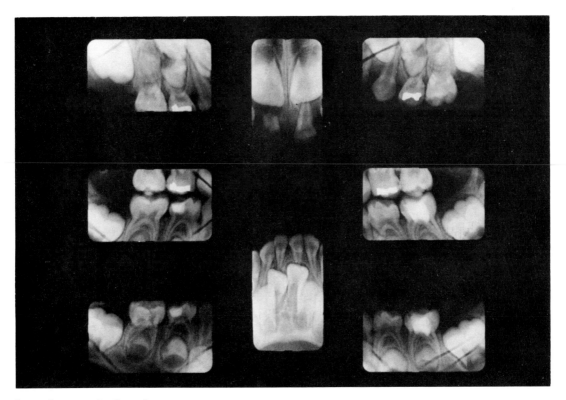

Fig 24-3d   Intraoral radiographs.

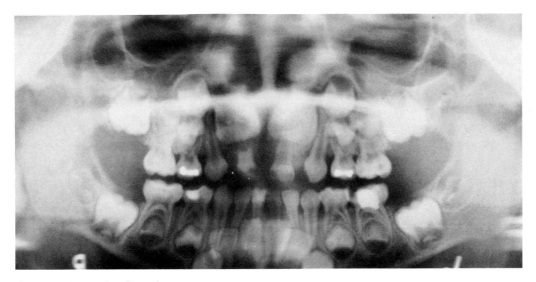

Fig 24-3e   Panoramic radiograph.

Review Answers

Chapter 1

1. **(e)** All of the above. The health history is intended to introduce the patient and parent to the dentist. Only by personal interview with the patient/parent can the dentist determine interrelated medical factors that should be explored in-depth, the need for consultation, and further influences on dental care.

2. **(d)** The normal sequence of calcification for primary teeth begins by the 14th week in utero and occurs as follows: central incisor, first molar, lateral incisor, canine, and second molar.

3. **(b)** The normal sequence of eruption for primary teeth is central incisor, lateral incisor, first molar, canine, and second molar. Note that the sequence of eruption differs from the calcification sequence because the first molar—lateral incisor positions are reversed.

4. **(h)** The teeth undergoing calcification at the time of birth include all the primary teeth and the permanent first molars (see Fig. 1-1) in varying stages of enamel completion. A traumatic systemic insult, such as the history of anoxia in this child, during the critical period of enamel deposition would be sufficient to disrupt ameloblastic function, thus resulting in hypoplastic enamel of the teeth undergoing calcification at that time.

5. **(b)** The factors which directly influence child behavior are growth and development, family and peer influences, past medical and dental experiences and dental office environment. The most potent factor influencing human behavior is that emanating from the family unit.

6a. **(b)** Carlos is 4 years of age and is classified, according to Stone and Church, as a preschooler.

6b. **(a)** The age range of the preschooler is 2 to 5 years. The child age 2 to 3 years still manifests immaturities that may affect his cooperative potential. The child age 3 to 5 years will usually exhibit cooperative behavior.

7. **(d)** As a rule the preschool child is one with whom verbalization is easy and who responds acceptably to modeling procedures. Dental personnel cannot be too certain of the child's behavioral response to the dental experience, however, although the reception area behavior supplies some strong leads.

Chapter 2

1. In the maxillary arch, the primate space is mesial to the maxillary canine. In the mandibular arch, the primate space is distal to the mandibular canine.

2. The leeway space in the maxillary arch is about 0.9 mm.; in the mandibular arch about 1.7 mm.

3. **(c)** In the primary dentition, this relationship is based on the distal surfaces of the second primary molar.

4. **(e)** All of the above are indications of the need for a mixed dentition analysis.

5. **(e)** A mesial step based on the relationships of the distal surfaces of the primary molars.

Chapter 3

1. **(b)** The maxillary anterior occlusal would be the choice, with a periapical a good substitute. The occlusal would give a somewhat better overall view.

2. **(h)** The best surveys at this time would be occlusal radiographs plus bite wings. A panoramic radiograph is also usable at this age. If for any reason there are questionable areas, periapicals can be obtained for further evaluation.

3. **(a)** Bitewing: (*j*) None of the above. The bite wing angulation is + 10 through the interproximal contacts perpendicular to the film packet.
(b) Maxillary molar: (f) + 40°
(c) Mandibular molar: (j) None of the above. The angulation is – 10°.
(d) Mandibular occlusal: (g) – 30°
(e) Maxillary occlusal: (h) + 60°

4. **(b)** The easiest to take would be the anterior occlusal radiographs, one maxillary occlusal to check the fracture sites and one mandibular occlusal for any fractures.

5. **(e)** Because the child is in the low risk category, radiographs can be postponed for six months. If the child should happen to develop caries, the frequency of radiographs could then be increased because of the higher risk of caries.

5. **(c)** The inclusion cysts contain squamous epithelial remnants from the time of palatal closure. No treatment is required because they will exfoliate spontaneously without complication within a few weeks. For additional information consult Table 3-1 and Fig. 3-38.

6. **(d)** This traumatic ulcer is the result of lip chewing following the administration of a left mandibular block. The unaccustomed loss of sensory sensation provoked the child into biting the anesthetized lip. Treatment is palliative with the exception of using topical antibiotics if the lesion should develop a secondary bacterial infection. Prevention through proper patient warning is mandatory in young children.

7. **(b)** This ulcer, commonly known as a canker sore, can be extremely sensitive in some patients and treatment is largely symptomatic. It is self-limiting, having a duration of 7 to 14 days. See Fig. 3-42.

Chapter 4

1. **(e)** All of the above answers are correct. The reported values for the prevalence of gingivitis in children varies greatly according to the study examined and the criteria used. However, regardless of the study examined, the prevalence of gingivitis increases as the child grows older. Marked increases occur during the period of permanent tooth eruption (mixed dentition) and prevalence reaches a peak at puberty, after which it slightly declines.

2. **(d)** Loe, et al. (1965), demonstrated that gingivitis is a reversible process which can be resolved in 7 days following institution of proper oral hygiene procedures. If oral hygiene is suspended, gingivitis will develop within 15 to 21 days with a marked increase in the number of cultured organisms. Filamentous forms and spirochetes were late, not early, colonizers of the gingival plaque.

3. **(e)** All of the above statements are correct. Due to the thinner, less keratinized epithelium with its greater vascularity, the attached gingiva in children appears less dense and is redder. Its texture is less stippled and its width is comparatively greater.

4. **(d)** The key to solving this diagnosis is the recognition of the systemic involvement, including elevated temperature and lymphadenopathy and the clinical presence of multiple, sore vesicles of short duration in a young patient (peak incidence occurs around 2 years of age).

Chapter 5

1. **(e)** *S. mutans* has been identified as the causative agent in the initiation of caries. *Lactobacillus acidophilus* has been isolated from deeper lesions and is probably more responsible for progression than initiation of caries. All of the other selections are contributory in nature but not the causative agent.

2. **(c)** If a positive answer is given to this question, then you can safely diagnose this condition as "nursing bottle syndrome." The remaining questions may contribute as genetic or environmental components in the formation of caries but the key is the selective involvement of the teeth noted indicating assault prior to 18 months of age.

3. **(e)** Mandibular molars are more susceptible to caries formation than maxillary molars. The remaining answers are all true.

4. **(c)** The occlusal surface represents 12.5% of the total susceptible surfaces but accounts for approximately 45% of the detectable lesions. However, the occlusal surface of the first molar is the correct answer because the second premolar is not present in a 9-year-old child.

5. **(d)** Occlusal caries are first to develop because of the rapid susceptibility of pit and fissures to caries. The mesial surface is next because it is in contact with the distal surface of the first molar from as early as 2 years of age, but has less rapid onset than occlusal lesions. On the other hand, the distal surface of the second molar does not have an adjacent contact until the first permanent molar erupts at age 6.

Chapter 6

1. **(e)** According to a review by Melcer and Feldman (1979) of various educational approaches, the best approach is closely supervised teaching on a multiple visit basis which allows for periodic reinforcement.

2. **(d)** With increased frequency of toothbrushing, there is a corresponding improvement in oral hygiene status and gingival health but little reduction in caries prevalence. It is probable that only a few highly motivated, well instructed individuals can reach and maintain the required level of oral hygiene efficiency necessary to prevent caries. Any minor reduction in caries experience is most likely related to the increased exposure of the fluoride in the dentifrice, rather than any direct improvement in the oral hygiene level. In addition, it is recommended that parents assume the primary role and responsibility for cleaning their children's teeth if they are younger than 9 years of age. Children younger than age 9 have not developed the conceptual ability or dexterity necessary to remove plaque effectively. Oral irrigation does not remove plaque and therefore is not an effective substitute for toothbrushing.

3. **(d)** Since no one toothbrushing technique is superior in its ability to remove plaque, the horizontal scrubbing method is recommended because it is the most comfortable and acceptable to both parents and children.

4. **(g)** The use of supervised toothbrushing is sufficient for plaque removal prior to topical fluoride application because removal of the acquired pellicle is not necessary. Aside from not removing the fluoride-rich surface layer, a toothbrush prophylaxis is more educational for the patient. However, a rubber cup prophylaxis must be used to remove extrinsic stain, if present, but this rarely occurs in children.

5. **(g)** The immunization of humans with bacterial antigen to produce an antibody reaction against plaque formation has not occurred because these problems need to be overcome.

Chapter 7

1. **(a)** Optimally fluoridated water produces caries reduction mainly on the smooth surfaces, but does render the occlusal surface less susceptible by enhancing the coalescence of the pits and fissures. However, this will only occur during the preeruptive stage of crown formation. Topical fluoride application has no effect during this process. The depth of pits and fissures is determined during formation before fluoride can be topically applied after eruption.

2. **(b)** The optimal level of fluoride concentration in the drinking water is adjusted according to the average annual maximum daily air temperature of the community. A community located in a cold climate would receive higher levels of fluoride (up to 1.2 ppm) because less water is consumed, whereas in warmer climates, where more water is consumed, the level would be lower (adjusted down to 0.7 ppm).

3. **(d)** The benefit derived from continuous exposure to optimally fluoridated water since birth, in terms of percent caries reduction, ranges between 50–70%, depending upon the study examined.

4. **(c)** Prior to prescribing supplemental fluoride therapy, the dentist must ascertain the natural fluoride content of the child's drinking water as well as chronologic age. The child' chronologic age roughly reflects his or her body mass and therefore his or her capacity to utilize fluoride.

5. **(b)** For a child aged 2 to 3 years, living in a fluoride deficient community, the recommended daily dose of fluoride is 0.5 mg. This dosage is one-half that required for children older than 3 years of age.

Chapter 8

1. **(e)** All of the above are correct. Occlusal caries in children have a rapid onset and high prevalence. The occlusal surface has enhanced susceptibility because its surface is least benefitted by fluoride and because of the bacterial harboring capacity of its anatomy.

2. **(d)** Occlusal sealants are mechanically retained by penetration of the sealant into the etched enamel, forming resin tags up to 40 microns in length.

3. **(e)** All of the above factors will inhibit retention of occlusal sealants. For these reasons, isolation is mandatory and additional enamel preparation by prolonged acid conditioning may be required.

4. **(b)** A 60-second application of acid etchant is required for permanent teeth. A successfully conditioned enamel surface has a dull and chalky appearance.

5. **(a)** Occlusal sealants should be placed prior to topical fluoride treatments, not after. An enamel surface that has just received topical fluoride will not etch as successfully as one that has not. In addition, a fluoride treatment following sealant placement will help remineralize those etched areas not covered by the sealant.

Chapter 12

Chapter 9

1. **(d)** On occasion, a dentist will encounter a child or adolescent, physically normal, but exhibiting problems which are sociologic in nature and negative in behavior. Such behavior may suggest some phase of intellectual impairment. The autistic child is a good example. Mental retardation may or may not be a factor.

2. **(a)** Retraining is the method of behavior change required. The modifying techniques developed by Eysenck and others and Wolpe's densensitization process, both of which relieve a child of his or her anxiety, have proven valuable contributions to retraining and behavior shaping. Addleston's Tell, Show, and Do sequence can be applied in a meaningful and unsurprising manner in retraining.

3. **(b)** A new patient may evince anxiety over a contemplated visit to the dentist. On the other hand, if anxiety is a factor, it may be covertly managed by the patient. Therefore, the introductory approach to the dental experience should be nonthreatening. Getting acquainted and presenting some form of modeling of cooperative behavior is the accepted process.

Chapter 10

1. **(b)** The child should be seen for your evaluation. Perhaps with your personality and child management techniques the child can be treated without any conscious medication.

2. **(e)** All of the factors are interrelated for acceptable desired results from the use of medication, irrespective of the drug used.

3. **(a)** For the shy, timid child hydroxyzine in either commercial form would be best to use. This drug is safe and best given in divided doses.

4. **(a)** The choice is naloxone (Narcan) since it does not further depress respiration. This drug should be used if depression is suspected. The best route is S.Q. or just beneath the tongue.

5. **(e)** For this child the co-medication of chloral hydrate and either hydroxyzine HCl (Atarax) or hydroxyzine pamoate (Vistaril) would be the choice. This can be given as a mixture prior to the operative procedure.

Chapter 11

1. **(j)** All of these are typical examples of the types of patients that should be treated in the hospital.

2. **(c)** If there are any carious lesions involving two or more surfaces, they should be restored with stainless steel crowns. Back-to-back amalgams are contraindicated.

3. **(c)** The first step is to place a throat pack before any other oral procedures are done. Then the radiographs, oral prophylaxis, and diagnosis can be completed.

4. **(a)** The 5.5-year old child should have permanent incisors erupting in the near future. Since the child is having the restorative care done in the hospital it can be assumed that behavior is a problem. Thus, the best procedure would be extractions.

5. **(d)** Remove the throat pack. It is somewhat embarrassing to suddenly realize the throat pack is in place and the child is beginning to wake up from the general anesthesia procedure.

Chapter 12

1. **(d)** When a surgical procedure is involved, the inferior alveolar, the lingual nerve, and the buccal nerve must be anesthetized. The lingual nerve supplies the soft tissues lingual to the tooth being removed while the buccal nerve innervates the buccal soft tissues from the most posterior tooth anteriorly to the first primary molar.

2. **(b)** When removing a maxillary first primary molar, it is essential that the posterior superior alveolar infiltration be performed in addition to the middle superior alveolar infiltration. Mink and Spedding (1966) report that the congenital absence of the middle superior alveolar nerve is not rare and its absence may alter anesthetic profundity if one depends solely on that innervation.

3. **(i)** A patient must be prepared prior to rendering any anesthetic procedure, and the technical procedure must be performed expertly.

4. **(f)** In addressing the child patient, the dentist's explanation should be uncomplicated and easily comprehended. Cooperation is most often established when communication is understandable and free of threat.

Chapter 13

1. **(b)** You may proceed with the administration of the local anesthetic at this time because the patient displays attainment of the diagnostic signs of sedation achieved by nitrous oxide at the 40% level. After the injection, the patient can be maintained at a 20% to 30% nitrous oxide level.

2. **(e)** All of the above choices should be completed prior to placing the nasal mask. In fact, all should be done before the patient is even seated, except for choice (a). It is beneficial to the anxious child that the operator be prepared and organized in advance.

3. **(b)** Total calculated flow rate is less for children than adults because their tidal volume is less. To achieve adequate sedation, the patient should be placed on 2 to 4 liters/minute nitrous oxide (40%) plus 3 to 5 liters/minute oxygen (60%). However, the flow rate should be adjusted according to the degree of inflation observed in the reservoir bag.

4. **(e)** The use of nitrous oxide is rarely contraindicated. None of the conditions listed are considered contraindications but rather precautions. In fact, nitrous oxide–oxygen may be helpful for patients with respiratory difficulties because it alleviates anxiety and promotes high levels of oxygenation.

5. **(d)** Nitrous oxide is carried by the serum and thus does not compete with oxygen or carbon dioxide for hemoglobin in the red blood cells.

Chapter 14

1. **(c)** Indirect pulp capping is limited to the permanent dentition; direct pulp capping is contraindicated in the primary dentition; and extraction with a space maintainer is somewhat radical at this stage.

2. **(b)** The cervical bulge on the mesiobuccal surface is the most prominent anatomical feature on this tooth. This anatomical landmark repeatedly causes frustration in crown adaption.

3. **(a)** The mesiobuccal pulp horn is the most prominent. This is true in most primary teeth, but more so in the first primary molars.

4. **(b)** The child is within normal limits. The first primary teeth to erupt by 6 months of age are the mandibular central incisors. So, the mother is somewhat anxious and needs reassurance that all is well with her child.

5. **(h)** The primary pulp is proportionately larger than the permanent pulp, so the primary pulp is closer to the enamel surface. It does follow the surface contour and the mesial pulp horn is closer to the dentinoenamel function.

Chapter 15

1. **(e)** Any one of the mentioned factors could contribute to the defective restoration. It is most important to control these variables.

2. **(b)** Burlew or rubber disks produce heat which can be detrimental to the pulp.

3. **(c)** Burnishing is beneficial to all amalgam restorations. Once thought to be detrimental to amalgam restorations, recent studies have shown it to be of significant benefit.

4. **(a)** The main cause for the overhang is improper wedging. The goal of the wedge is to tightly adapt the band material to the cervical margin. The force of amalgam condensation will not extrude the amalgam beyond the matrix band if properly wedged. Deep caries is not an excuse since a matrix retainer can be adapted for this purpose.

5. **(b)** If possible, try to remove the overhang with a scaler or a curved scalpel blade. Do not turn the attempt to remove the excess material into a bloody surgical procedure. If it is small, it can be watched. A gross overhang is solved by redoing the amalgam restoration.

Chapter 16

1. **(c)** The crown is still too long. It needs to be marked at the gingival level and extended one or two millimeters beneath the scratch. Recrimping the crown (answer b) because it is not adapted is a good second choice because in some instances this may remedy the blanching of the gingival tissue. To do nothing is wrong because the child will have a very uncomfortable tissue reaction.

2. **(d)** Usually when the crown rotates freely on the crown preparation, it means that the crown selected is too large. Try the next smaller crown. If all else fails, yell, "Help."

3. **(b)** Due to the inherent weakness of amalgam plus the morphology of primary teeth, a stainless steel crown is indicated. With a few exceptions, multiple surfaces of caries indicate the need for a stainless steel crown.

4. **(e)** You may have answered (a) which in truth may be the answer, but academically it is wrong. The 800-417 plier is a crimping plier used to crimp the gingival margins. All is not lost. Simply crimp the open margin and recheck the crown on the tooth. Usually this does the trick. The 800-417 plier is used to crimp the gingival 1/3 of the crown.

5. **(h)** The likely causes are a poor mix of cement, usually too thick, and improper path of insertion. The crown should be seated on the lingual and "snapped" over to the buccal. If the crown is seated too far on the lingual, there is insufficient crown surface on the buccal.

Chapter 17

1. **(h)** All of the factors listed are valid. Acid etching is effective in increasing retention in permanent teeth, reducing marginal leakage, but it is of questionable value in primary teeth.

2. **(b)** The crown is selected before removal of carious lesions or tooth preparation. The incisal width is used to determine crown size.

3. **(d)** This is the first choice, because of the ease of access; **(e)** is the second choice, but it is a more difficult preparation.

4. **(b)** If the crown preparation, adaptation, and cementation follow suggested methods, there is no reason for the crown not to remain in the child's mouth until the primary tooth exfoliates.

Chapter 18

1. **(b)** Direct pulp capping is contraindicated in the primary dentition. Dycal or calcium hydroxide causes internal root resorption with failure. Since direct pulp capping is contraindicated in the primary dentition, pulpotomy is the pulp treatment of choice. The child's age is not important. A stainless steel crown is indicated for the reasons that *(1)* the tooth has multiple surfaces involved and *(2)* all primary teeth with pulpotomies should have stainless steel crowns.

2. **(c)** A 5-year-old child does not have a first permanent molar, thus it becomes important to maintain the space of the first primary molar. Why not combine the stainless steel crown with a space maintainer? The second primary molar will need a pulpotomy because of the pulp exposure.

3. **(e)** This case history represents a typical patient where the indication is an indirect pulp cap. The radiograph shows a near exposure with all other clinical and radiographic findings normal. Chances of success are in the 90% plus range.

4. **(a)** The ideal treatment for this patient would be pulpectomy and a composite restoration. The tooth may resorb a little faster than its antimere, but at least it will last until the permanent incisors erupt. Extraction with a space maintainer is a second choice. However, the space maintainer would be mainly for esthetics. Pulpotomy is a poor choice because the tooth is devital.

5. **(a)** A pulpectomy is the treatment of choice. Because the child is under 5, the first permanent molar has not erupted, thus a pulpectomy is the optimum choice.

Chapter 19

1. **(c)** More than likely the teeth will reerupt. The best thing at this time is to do nothing. You should advise the mother that the teeth may become devital in the future. The teeth may turn black or even yellow. The most important matter is to reassure the parent and the child.

2. **(d)** In this instance, a simple splint using a wire and an acid etch method is the treatment of choice. The splint should be left on for 10 to 14 days. A soft diet is also indicated.

3. **(c)** With the small area of pathology, the treatment of choice is pulpectomy with a zinc oxide–eugenol paste. The paste should be a material without an accelerator. The color is the tipoff that the pulp has degenerated.

4. **(c)** The goal of the treatment is to allow the apex of the tooth to reach maturity. The $Ca(OH)_2$ pulpotomy, it is hoped, will do this. Pulp capping is contraindicated due to the size of the exposure. Pulpectomy and apexification are only indicated if the tooth becomes nonvital. The point to remember is that at age 6 the root of the central incisor has not completely formed.

5. **(e)** As in question 4, the goal is to allow the root to complete development. Formocresol pulpotomy will not accomplish this goal. Extraction is not the treatment of choice. Pulpectomy and apexification (Frank's Technique) is the choice. Since the tooth is devital with the area of pathology at the apex and the dark discoloration, there is no doubt the tooth is devital.

6. **(b)** Home bleaching might be the first option with superoxal with or without heat the second option.

7. **(a)** With mild decalcification, a mixture of hydrochloric acid-pumice mixture can remove the areas of decalcification.

8. **(b)** This is a contraindication because mouth breathers have a tendency to dessicate the veneers, resulting in discoloration.

Chapter 20

1. **(f)** If a natal or neonatal tooth is present in the oral cavity and is extremely mobile with little more than soft tissue attachment, there is a danger that the tooth may become detached and aspirated by the infant. On the other hand, it the tooth is firm enough to resist the nursing action of the tongue, the thrusting tongue may become traumatized on its ventral surface producing ulceration. Furthermore, it is very likely the mother cannot nurse the infant in comfort. Factors such as these will strongly determine the fate of any precociously erupted tooth.

2. **(b)** The threat of undesirable results from any of the circumstances presented should preclude the continued existence of the natal or neonatal tooth in the infant's mouth.

3. **(c)** For a child who is 6 years old and capable of reasoning, communication on his or her level is most helpful. Explain to the child the need for and method of removing the tooth, and reappoint in one week. Law, et al, contend that the psychological stress will be diluted by this technique.

4. **(h)** Whenever acute dental infection is accompanied by fever, malaise, and chills, it is strongly recommended that the patient be placed on antibiotic therapy to reduce the infection. Congruous dental treatments, such as establishing both drainage for the infective process and saline irrigations, are essential.

5. **(b)** A primary molar, having furcative damage, will seldom be a good candidate for a pulp procedure. In the instance of a first primary molar, the appropriate treatment procedure is its removal and replacement with a fixed space maintainer appliance. The appliance is usually a band/loop or crown/loop maintainer anchored to the second primary molar.

Chapter 21

1. **(c)** If the first permanent molar has not erupted, a distal shoe (or intraalveolar space maintainer) is the choice.

2. **(a)** or **(c)** Either appliance will maintain the space. A poor second choice is a removable type appliance.

3. **(b)** or **(d)** The two band and loop space maintainers or the lingual arch will maintain the space.

4. **(b)** or **(d)** The decision might rest on the caries rate of the child: one might hesitate on banding both first permanent molars waiting for the premolars to erupt.

5. **(b)** At age 8 it is important to maintain the spaces.

Chapter 22

1. **(b)** A fixed appliance is the appliance of choice. At this age a removable appliance is the second choice.

2. **(c)** The success of a removable appliance is dependent upon the child and parental supervision.

3. **(j)** This briefly follows the steps used to construct an overdenture.

4. **(b)** The separating media should be applied before the clasps and teeth are waxed to the model. If applied after, the orthodontic resin will not adhere to the clasps or teeth.

5. **(a)** This child does not need a replacement since the permanent incisors will be erupting in the near future. The other examples are valid indications for prosthodontic appliances.

Chapter 23

1. **(g)** Gesell and Ilg (1943) observe that finger sucking is normal in the early periods of the child's growth and damage to the primary dentition is temporary and will correct itself providing the occlusion is normal (Graber, 1972). Persistent parental nagging can encourage psychogenic effects in the child.

2. **(c)** Graber (1972) points out that the dentist must answer several questions in order to ascertain whether or not the case at hand is a simple anterior crossbite: *(1)* how many teeth are involved in the crossbite?; *(2)* do the upper or lower teeth appear to be malposed?; *(3)* is the crossbite purely dental or are there skeletal involvements?; *(4)* is the path of closure uninhibited or is there a midline shift?; and *(5)* is there ample room to labialize the inlocked tooth?

3. **(f)** All three can contribute to the crossbite relationships.

4. **(c)** At age 7 years it is better not to delay treatment. Where distal damage to the second primary molar is minimal and the entrapment angulation of the first permanent molar is not great, the treatment of choice is brass ligature wire.

5. **(b)** When there is abnormal labial or lingual relationship of the tooth and or teeth.

Chapter 24

The following is one approach to the treatment of this case.

Appointment 1
Diagnosis and oral hygiene education.

Appointment 2
Case presentation and oral hygiene education with concentration on diet counseling.

Appointment 3
No. 51–extract
No. 54–DO amalgam
No. 55–OL amalgam

Appointment 4
No. 75–SSC
No. 74–DO amalgam

Appointment 5
No. 85–MO amalgam
No. 84–formocresol pulpotomy and SSC
No. 71–M composite resin
No. 81–M composite resin

Appointment 6
No. 61–openface SSC
No. 64–DO amalgam
No. 65–MOL amalgam

Appointment 7
Polish amalgams, give oral hygiene instructions and apply topical fluoride.

Appointment 8
Recall in six months. Note the photographs taken at this time. The right bitewing radiograph reveals a mesial lesion on No. 55

Future appointments will be needed to evaluate and manage the esthetic problem created by the congenitally missing maxillary lateral incisors.

Index

Entries in italics refer to pages with illustrations.